Advances in the Diagnosis and Treatment of Thyroid Carcinoma

Advances in the Diagnosis and Treatment of Thyroid Carcinoma

Editors

Fabio Medas

Pier Francesco Alesina

MDPI • Basel • Beijing • Wuhan • Barcelona • Belgrade • Manchester • Tokyo • Cluj • Tianjin

Editors

Fabio Medas
Department of Surgical Sciences
University of Cagliari
Cagliari
Italy

Pier Francesco Alesina
Clinic for Endocrine Surgery
Helios Universitätsklinikum Wuppertal
Wuppertal
Germany

Editorial Office
MDPI
St. Alban-Anlage 66
4052 Basel, Switzerland

This is a reprint of articles from the Special Issue published online in the open access journal *Cancers* (ISSN 2072-6694) (available at: www.mdpi.com/journal/cancers/special_issues/Diagnosis_Thyroid_Carcinoma).

For citation purposes, cite each article independently as indicated on the article page online and as indicated below:

LastName, A.A.; LastName, B.B.; LastName, C.C. Article Title. *Journal Name* **Year**, *Volume Number*, Page Range.

ISBN 978-3-0365-5334-4 (Hbk)
ISBN 978-3-0365-5333-7 (PDF)

Contents

Preface to "Advances in the Diagnosis and Treatment of Thyroid Carcinoma"

Dear Colleagues,

In the last 40 years, the incidence of thyroid carcinoma has considerably increased, making it the most common endocrine malignancy. Even though, in most cases, the initial treatment is curative, a certain number of patients experience a poor course of disease, with local or distant recurrence, and require further medical or surgical treatment, which considerably worsens their quality of life.

Indeed, thyroid cancer represents a heterogeneous disease, comprising different molecular and histological subtypes with distinct clinical behavior and prognosis.

In the last two decades, great efforts have been made to improve its diagnosis and surgical outcomes. Molecular biomarkers have been studied and introduced in clinical practice, and new pathological and clinical classifications have been proposed to consider tumor behavior and the risk of disease recurrence. At the same time, new devices and surgical approaches have been developed to improve radicality and reduce surgical trauma, including mini-invasive and remote access surgery, the intraoperative monitoring of recurrent laryngeal nerves, and the use of indocyanine green fluorescence to identify parathyroid glands.

Nevertheless, many issues remain a matter of debate, regarding, for example, the indication and extent of lymphectomy of the central compartment, the treatment of microcarcinoma, the therapeutic options for poorly differentiated and anaplastic carcinomas, and the indications and strategies in cases of recurrent disease.

In this Special Issue of *Cancers*, we report the latest research on the diagnosis and therapy of thyroid cancer.

Fabio Medas and Pier Francesco Alesina
Editors

cancers

MDPI

Article

Prophylactic Central Lymph Node Dissection Improves Disease-Free Survival in Patients with Intermediate and High Risk Differentiated Thyroid Carcinoma: A Retrospective Analysis on 399 Patients

Fabio Medas [1,*], Gian Luigi Canu [1], Federico Cappellacci [1], Giacomo Anedda [1], Giovanni Conzo [2], Enrico Erdas [1] and Pietro Giorgio Calò [1]

1 Department of Surgical Sciences, University of Cagliari, 09124 Cagliari, Italy
2 Division of General and Oncologic Surgery, Department of Cardiothoracic Sciences, University of Campania "Luigi Vanvitelli", 80131 Naples, Italy
* Correspondence: fabiomedas@gmail.com or fabiomedas@unica.it

Received: 19 May 2020; Accepted: 20 June 2020; Published: 23 June 2020

Abstract: The role of prophylactic central lymph node dissection (pCLND) in the treatment of differentiated thyroid cancer (DTC) is controversial and still a matter of debate. The primary outcome of our study was to assess whether pCLND is effective in reducing the incidence of recurrent disease, and the secondary goal was to estimate the incidence of postoperative complications in patients who underwent pCLND and to evaluate the prognostic value of occult node metastases. In this retrospective study, we included patients with preoperative diagnosis of DTC and clinically uninvolved lymph nodes (cN0). The patients were divided into two groups, depending on the surgical approach: total thyroidectomy alone (TT group) or total thyroidectomy and pCLND (pCLND group). Three hundred and ninety-nine patients were included in this study, 320 (80.2%) in the TT group and 79 (19.8%) in the pCLND group. There were no significant differences in morbidity among the two groups. Histopathological evaluation demonstrated a similar distribution of aggressive features, especially regarding multicentricity, extrathyroidal extension, and angioinvasivity between the two groups. Occult lymph node metastases were found in 20 (25.3%) patients in the pCLND group. Prophylactic CLND was effective in improving disease-free survival in patients with intermediate and high risk of disease recurrence ($p = 0.0392$); occult lymph node metastases resulted as a significant negative prognostic factor ($p < 0.001$).

Keywords: thyroid carcinoma; prophylactic central lymph node dissection; lymph node metastases

1. Introduction

Differentiated thyroid carcinoma (DTC) is traditionally considered as a tumor with good prognosis, with an overall survival nearly comparable to the general population. Nevertheless, a certain number of patients experience a poor clinical outcome, with local recurrence requiring further medical or surgical treatment, with a considerable worsening of the quality of life.

The incidence of local recurrence is widely variable; the American Thyroid Association (ATA) guidelines for patients with differentiated thyroid cancers, published in 2015, report an incidence of local recurrence in 3–13% of patients with low-risk tumors, 21–36% in cases of intermediate-risk tumors, and in 68% of high risk tumors [1]; similar findings have been extensively reported in literature [2–7].

The most important risk factors for local recurrence have been reported in the literature and are the presence of lymph node metastases, the extrathyroidal extension of the tumor with invasion of perithyroidal tissues, the presence of BRAF V600E mutation, and the incomplete resection of the tumor [1,2,8,9].

In fact, one of the outstanding issues is the role of lymphectomy of the central compartment in cases of clinically uninvolved lymph nodes. In fact, the incidence of occult node metastases is high, with a reported incidence up to 90% [2,10–14]. Furthermore, the real prognostic value of lymph node metastases in DTC is still uncertain, with some authors suggesting that lymph node metastases do not decrease the survival rate [3,15–18], while others have reported a worsening in both overall and in disease-free survival [8,19–23].

For these reasons, a prophylactic central lymph node dissection (pCLND) has been proposed for tumors with clinically uninvolved lymph nodes, but suspected of having aggressive behavior at preoperative and intraoperative evaluation. Nevertheless, this suggestion is met with considerable resistance due to the higher incidence of postoperative complications including hypoparathyroidism and recurrent laryngeal nerve (RLN) injury, and to the doubtful role of lymph node metastases on prognosis [24–26]. Consequently, the most important guidelines on DTC are discordant on this topic, with the ATA guidelines and National Comprehensive Cancer Network (NCCN) guidelines suggesting a prudent approach [1,27], while the Japanese Association of Endocrine Surgeon and the Japanese Society of Thyroid Surgeons recommend routine pCLND [28].

The aim of this study was to assess whether prophylactic CLND is effective in reducing the incidence of recurrent disease, to evaluate the incidence of postoperative complications in patients who underwent pCLND, and the influence of occult node metastases on the prognosis.

2. Methods

In this retrospective observational study, we included patients who underwent thyroidectomy for DTC at our department from January 2011 to December 2016. Ethical approval was obtained from our local ethics committee. Patients were identified from a prospectively maintained institutional database including all patients who underwent thyroidectomy. Inclusion criteria were preoperative diagnosis of DTC and the absence of clinically involved lymph nodes both on Ultrasound (US) and on intraoperative examination (cN0). Exclusion criteria were distant metastases, incidental diagnosis of DTC at pathological evaluation, and surgery performed for recurrent disease.

Patients were divided into two groups: in the first group, we included patients who underwent total thyroidectomy alone (TT group), while in the second group, patients who had undergone thyroidectomy and prophylactic CLND (pCLND group). The design of the study is reported in Figure 1.

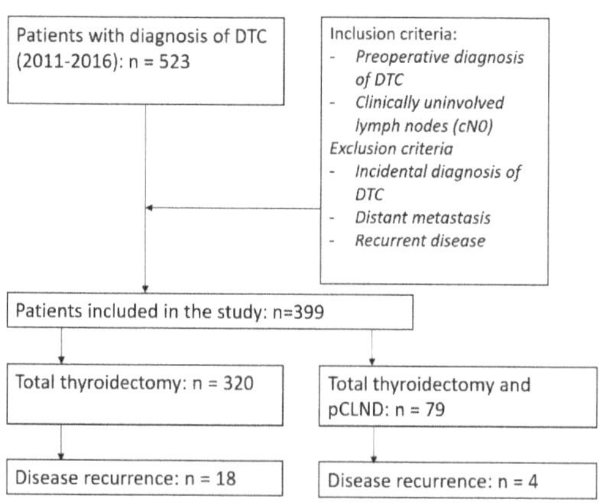

Figure 1. Design of the study. DTC: differentiated thyroid carcinoma; pCLND: prophylactic central lymph node dissection.

2.1. Outcome of the Study

The primary outcome of the study was to evaluate whether prophylactic CLND improves disease-free survival in patients with DTC. The secondary outcomes were to assess whether prophylactic CLND is burdened by a higher incidence of postoperative complications, specifically RLN injury and hypoparathyroidism, and to evaluate the prognostic significance of occult lymph node metastases.

2.2. Preoperative Evaluation

Preoperative evaluation included clinical history, physical examination, and blood tests to assess thyroid function and autoimmune thyroiditis. Fine-needle aspiration cytology (FNAC) was performed in all patients, and the results were classified according to the Consensus Statement of AIT (Italian Thyroid Association), AME (Medical Endicronologist Associaction), SIE (Italian Endocrinology Association), and SIAPEC-IAP (Italian Society of Pathological Anatomy) for the Classification and Reporting of Thyroid Cytology [25]. Hyperthyroidism status was defined in the case of low serum Thyroid-Stimulating Hormone (TSH) (<0.4 mIU/L), use of thyrostatic drugs or positivity for Anti-TSH receptor antibodies (TRAb). Autoimmune thyroiditis was defined in the case of positivity for anti-thyroglobulin antibodies (Tg-Ab) or anti-thyroid peroxidase antibodies (TPO-Ab) and on the basis of histopathological examination.

High-resolution US of the neck was always performed before surgery by an experienced surgeon, with careful evaluation of the central and the lateral compartment. Preoperative laryngoscopy was routinely performed to assess vocal fold mobility.

Indication for surgery was preoperative cytologic diagnosis or suspicion of DTC or, in the case of negative cytology, the presence of a highly suspicious nodule based on family history, physical examination, and US features of the nodule.

2.3. Surgical Treatment

All procedures were performed by three endocrine surgeons with high experience in thyroid surgery, each performing at least 100 thyroidectomies per year. The surgical procedures were extracapsular total thyroidectomies. The RLNs were routinely exposed until their insertion into the larynx to avoid injury. Intraoperative neuromonitoring (IONM) of RLNs was routinely used in order to facilitate nerve identification and confirm its functional integrity. Parathyroid glands were searched at the usual sites and any attempt to preserve them was made.

Prophylactic CLND (pCLND) was performed in cases of clinically uninvolved lymph nodes (cN0) in tumors considered at high risk for recurrence based on family history, US features of the nodule, results of FNAC, and intraoperative examination of the thyroid gland, especially in cases of suspected extracapsular extension of the tumor. The choice to perform a pCNLD was planned and concerted among surgeons and endocrinologist preoperatively, and then discussed with the patient. CLND consisted of excision of all lymphatic structures included in level VI and level VII, on the basis of the recognized anatomic continuity between the superior mediastinum and neck. The anatomical limits of the dissection were represented anteriorly by the superficial layer of the deep cervical fascia, superiorly by the hyoid bone, laterally by the carotid arteries, inferiorly by the innominate artery, and posteriorly by the pre-vertebral layer of the deep cervical fascia. The central compartment included the pretracheal, prelaryngeal (Delphian), paratracheal, and paralaryngeal lymph nodes. Level VII was comprised of the superior anterior mediastinal lymph nodes, located above the innominate artery and below the level of the upper border of the sternal manubrium.

Patients in which only some perithyroidal lymph nodes were excised, without the clear intention to perform a pCLND, were included in the TT group.

2.4. Pathologic Examination

The surgical specimen was fixed with formaldehyde; sections were stained with hematoxylin-eosin (H&E) and analyzed by a dedicated pathologist. Immunohistochemical analysis was performed with the streptavidin-biotin technique on paraffin sections using anti-pan-cytokeratin antibody.

In cases of multifocal carcinoma, the tumor size was defined as the largest diameter among the malignant nodules. A microcarcinoma was defined as a tumor with larger diameter equal or inferior to 10 mm. Extrathyroidal extension was defined as the presence of gross infiltration of perithyroidal tissues found in pathological examination. Vascular invasion was defined as invasion of vessels in the tumor capsule or beyond it, with intravascular tumor cells attached to the vessel wall.

The lymph node yield was defined as the number of lymph nodes harvested after lymphectomy, and lymph node ratio was defined as the ratio between metastatic lymph nodes and total lymph nodes retrieved, calculated only in patients with metastatic lymph nodes.

Lymph node micrometastasis was defined as a metastasis with maximum dimension ≤0.5 cm.

2.5. Postoperative Management and Follow-Up

Serum calcium and (Parathyroid Hormone) PTH levels were assayed pre- and postoperatively. Postsurgical hypoparathyroidism was defined as PTH < 10 pg/mL following the operation (normal range = 10–65 pg/mL).

Postoperative fibrolaryngoscopy was performed in the case of loss of signal at IONM or in patients experiencing dysphonia after surgery, even in the case of normal signal at IONM.

Hypoparathyroidism and RLN injury were considered permanent if lasting for more than 12 months after surgery.

All patients were referred to an endocrinologist for postoperative management and were stratified in ATA groups for risk of disease recurrence, following the 2009 and then 2015 ATA Guidelines. Radioactive iodine was routinely administrated after total thyroidectomy in case of ATA intermediate and high risk tumors.

Serum thyroglobulin (Tg) and anti-Tg antibodies measurements and neck ultrasound (US) were used for postoperative evaluation. During initial follow-up, serum Tg and anti-Tg antibodies were measured every 6–12 months. More frequent Tg and anti-Tg antibody measurements were performed in ATA high risk patients. In ATA low and intermediate-risk patients that achieved an excellent response to treatment, Tg measurements were repeated every 12–24 months. ATA high risk patients (regardless of response to therapy) and all patients with biochemical incomplete, structural incomplete, or indeterminate response to treatment continued to execute Tg and anti-Tg antibodies measurements at least every 6–12 months for several years.

In patients with DTC of any risk level with significant comorbidity that precluded thyroid hormone withdrawal prior to RAI therapy, recombinant human TSH (rhTSH) preparation was done; these situations included medical or psychiatric conditions that could be acutely exacerbated in the case of hypothyroidism (leading to a serious adverse event) or inability to mount an adequate endogenous TSH response with thyroid hormone withdrawal.

Disease-free status was defined as a no evidence of disease (NED) and included the following features: no clinical evidence of tumor, no imaging evidence of disease by RAI imaging and/or neck US, and low serum Tg levels during TSH suppression (Tg < 0.2 ng/mL) or after stimulation (Tg < 1 ng/mL) in the absence of interfering antibodies.

Disease-free survival was defined as the time elapsed from surgery to the detection of recurrent disease.

For the purpose of this work, risk stratification for disease recurrence was reviewed for every patient that underwent surgery until 2015 and was eventually adapted to the latest ATA guidelines.

2.6. Statistical Analysis

Statistical analysis was performed with MedCalc® vers. 19.2.1. The Chi-squared test and Student's t-test were used for categorical and continuous variables, respectively. Log-rank test was used to estimate the differences in Kaplan–Meier curves for independent risk factors. Results were considered statistically significant in the case of a p-value <0.05. Continuous variables are expressed as mean ± standard deviation of the mean.

3. Results

We included in this study 399 patients with clinically uninvolved lymph nodes (cN0) and pathological diagnosis of DTC (Table 1). There were 101 (25.3%) males and 298 (74.7%) females with a mean age of 50.5 years. Autoimmune thyroiditis was present in 146 (36.6%) cases, and hyperthyroidism in 28 (7%). A familiar history of thyroid carcinoma was present in seven (1.8%) patients, none of these were in the context of Multiple Endocrine Neoplasia Syndrome. In 148 (37.1%) patients, FNAC demonstrated atypia of undetermined significance (including Tir3, Tir3a, and Tir3b), and in 178 (44.6%) FNAC indicated a suspicious malignancy (Tir4) or a malignant nodule (Tir5). In the remaining 73 (18.3%) patients, despite the fact that FNAC was not suspicious or indicative for malignancy, a thyroidectomy was planned based on family history of the patient, physical examination, or US features of the nodule.

Table 1. Univariate analysis of demographic, preoperative, operative data, and outcomes of patients with differentiated thyroid carcinoma and clinically uninvolved lymph nodes.

	Patients (n = 399)	TT Group (n = 320)	pCLND Group (n = 79)	p
Sex				0.1493
Male	101 (25.3%)	86 (26.9%)	15 (19.0%)	
Female	298 (74.7%)	234 (73.1%)	64 (81.0%)	
Age, years	50.5 ± 14.4 (15–83)	52.4 + 14.0	42.6 ± 13.5	p < 0.001
Hyperthyroidism	28 (7%)	25 (7.8%)	3 (3.8%)	0.314
Autoimmune thyroiditis	146 (36.6%)	97 (30.3%)	49 (62.0%)	p < 0.001
US findings				
Multinodular disease	250 (62.7%)	204 (63.8%)	46 (58.2%)	0.436
Peri- and intra-vascularization of the nodule	243 (60.9%)	195 (60.9%)	48 (60.8%)	0.920
Hypoechoic nodule	70 (17.6%)	48 (15%)	22 (27.8%)	0.011
Microcalcification	34 (8.5%)	29 (9.1%)	5 (6.3%)	0.579
FNAC				<0.001
Tir1-2	73 (18.3%)	66 (20.6%)	7 (8.9%)	
Tir3	148 (37.1%)	131 (40.9%)	17 (21.5%)	
Tir4-5	178 (44.6%)	123 (38.4%)	55 (69.6%)	
Operative time, minutes	94.4 ± 22.2	92.5 ± 22.6	102.3 ± 18.9	p < 0.001
Postoperative stay, days	2.8 ± 1.1	2.8 ± 1.0	3.0 ± 1.3	0.068
Transient hypoparathyroidism	136 (34.1%)	102 (31.9%)	34 (43.0%)	0.081
Permanent hypoparathyroidism	39 (9.8%)	27 (8.4%)	12 (15.2%)	0.109
Transient RLN injury	10 (2.5%)	7 (2.2%)	3 (3.8%)	0.675
Permanent RLN injury	3 (0.8%)	2 (0.6%)	1 (1.3%)	0.891
Postoperative bleeding	5 (1.3%)	4 (1.3%)	1 (1.3%)	0.580
RAI therapy	331 (82.9%)	258 (80.6%)	73 (92.4%)	0.019
Follow-up, months	55.4 ± 15.9	56.1 ± 16.1	52.6 ± 15.2	0.087
Recurrent disease	22 (5.5%)	18 (5.6%)	4 (5.1%)	0.936

TT: total thyroidectomy; pCLND: prophylactic central compartment lymph node dissection; US: ultrasound; FNAC: fine-needle aspiration cytology; RLN: recurrent laryngeal nerve; RAI: radioactive iodine. Continuous variables are reported as the mean ± standard deviation of the mean.

The surgical procedure consisted of total thyroidectomy alone in 320 (80.2%) patients, and total thyroidectomy and prophylactic CLND in 79 (19.8%).

Patients were divided into two groups based on the surgical approach. Those who underwent prophylactic CLND were significantly younger (42.6 y.o. vs. 52.4 y.o.; p < 0.001) and more frequently affected with autoimmune thyroiditis (62% vs. 30.3%; $p < 0.001$). Furthermore, FNAC was significantly more frequently diagnostic for DTC in the pCLND group (69.6% vs. 38.4%; $p < 0.001$).

The mean operative time was significantly longer in the pCLND group (102.3 min vs. 92.5 min; $p < 0.001$) as well as postoperative stay (3.0 days vs. 2.8 days). The incidence of transient hypoparathyroidism (43% vs. 31.9%), permanent hypoparathyroidism (15.2% vs. 8.4%), transient RLN injury (3.8% vs. 2.2%), and permanent RLN injury (1.3% vs. 0.6%) was higher in the pCLND group, but these differences were not statistically significant. The mean follow-up time was 55.4 months.

Full histopathologic findings are reported in Table 2. Nodule size and thyroid weight were similar between the two groups. Conversely, the histotype was significantly different between the two groups ($p < 0.001$). In the pCLND group, the incidence of the tall cell variant of PTC (TCV-PTC) was nearly quadruple that in the other group (25.3% vs. 6.3%), whereas the incidence of follicular variant of PTC (FV-PTC) was less than half (16.5% vs. 37.5%) when compared to the TT group. The presence of aggressive features of the tumor including multicentricity, angioinvasivity, and extrathyroidal extension was similar between the two groups.

Table 2. Univariate analysis of pathological data of patients with differentiated thyroid carcinoma and clinically uninvolved lymph nodes.

	Patients (n = 399)	TT Group (n = 320)	pCLND Group (n = 79)	p
Nodule size (mm)	16.8 ± 10.9	16.9 ± 11.1	16.3 ± 9.8	0.681
Thyroid weight (gr)	26.7 ± 22.5	27.4 ± 24.2	24.1 ± 13.3	0.252
Histotype				<0.0001
PTC	151	115 (35.9%)	36 (45.6%)	
FV-PTC	133	120 (37.5%)	13 (16.5%)	
TCV-PTC	40	20 (6.3%)	20 (25.3%)	
FTC	53	47 (14.7%)	6 (7.6%)	
HCC	21	18 (5.6%)	3 (3.8%)	
Low differentiated carcinoma	1	0	1 (1.3%)	
Microcarcinoma	109 (27.3%)	87 (27.2%)	22 (27.8%)	0.981
Multicentricity	151 (37.8%)	117 (36.6%)	34 (43%)	0.350
Angioinvasivity	15 (3.8%)	13 (4.1%)	2 (2.5%)	0.756
Extrathyroidal extension	27 (6.8%)	23 (7.2%)	4 (5.1%)	0.672
LN yield	5.1 ± 5.3	2.1 ± 1.1	8.9 ± 6.0	$p < 0.001$
LN metastasis	35 (8.8%)	15 (4.7%)	20 (25.3%)	$p < 0.001$
Number of positive LN	0.5 ± 1.3	0.2 ± 0.7	0.8 ± 1.7	0.006
LN ratio	0.5 ± 0.3	0.6 ± 0.2	0.3 ± 0.3	0.004
ATA risk class of disease recurrence				$p < 0.001$
Low	310 (77.7%)	268 (83.8%)	42 (53.2%)	
Medium	64 (16%)	30 (9.4%)	34 (43.0%)	
High	25 (6.3%)	22 (6.9%)	3 (3.8%)	

TT: total thyroidectomy; pCLND: prophylactic central compartment lymph node dissection; PTC: papillary thyroid carcinoma; FV-PTC: follicular variant of PTC; TCV-PTC: tall cell variant of PTC; FTC: follicular carcinoma; HCC: hurtle cell carcinoma; LN: lymph node; ATA: American Thyroid Association. Continuous variables are reported as the mean ± standard deviation of the mean.

As defined in the Methods section, all patients in the pCLND group underwent lymphectomy of the level VI and level VII lymph nodes, whereas in the other group, an excision of some perithyroidal lymph nodes was performed in 99 (30.9%) patients.

Lymph node yield (8.9 vs. 2.1; $p < 0.001$) and lymph node metastases (25.3% vs. 4.7%; $p < 0.001$) were significantly higher in the pCLND group. In contrast, the lymph node ratio was lower in the pCLND group (0.3 vs. 0.6; $p < 0.001$).

Patients were classified according to the ATA stratification for risk of structural disease recurrence. Patients in the pCLND group were ranked more frequently in the intermediate class of risk (43% vs. 9.4%; $p < 0.001$) than those in the other group, whereas low and high risk classes were similar between the two groups.

Radioactive iodine (RAI) therapy was administrated significantly more often in the pCLND group (92.4% vs. 80.6%; $p = 0.019$).

Overall, 22 (5.5%) patients experienced recurrent disease; 16 of these were localized in the central compartment, whereas the others were in the lateral neck compartment. The crude incidence of disease recurrence was similar between the two groups: 5.6% in The TT group and 5.1% in the pCLND group ($p = 0.936$). Log-rank test on Kaplan–Meier curves, reported in Figure 2a, did not show any significant difference between the two groups ($p = 0.0883$; HR 0.9267, 95% CI 0.3203–2.6814).

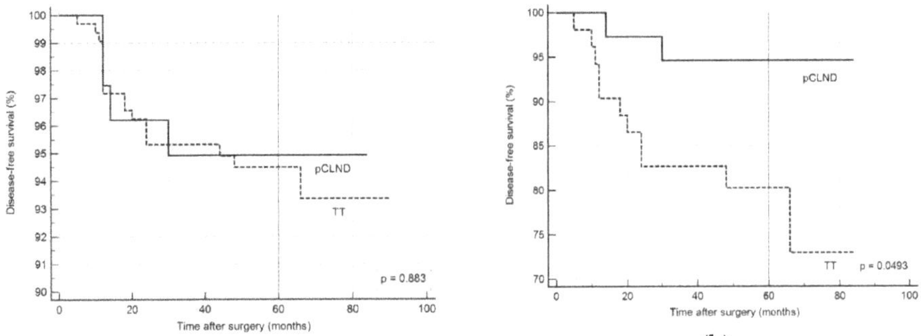

(a) (b)

Figure 2. Kaplan–Meier curves estimating disease-free survival according to surgical procedure, (**a**) including all the patients regardless of ATA class risk of recurrence: $p = 0.883$, HR 0.9267 (95% CI 0.3203–2.6814); (**b**) including only patients with moderate and high risk for disease recurrence according to ATA guidelines: $p = 0.0493$, HR 0.3299 (95% CI 0.1092–0.9967). pCLND: prophylactic central lymph node dissection; TT: total thyroidectomy; HR: hazard risk.

A subset analysis was performed considering the ATA stratification for risk of disease recurrence, as reported in Table 3. Considering the patients in the intermediate and high class of risk, the incidence of recurrent disease was significantly lower in the pCLND group (5.4% vs. 21.2%; $p = 0.0392$) than in the TT group. On the other hand, no significant differences were observed in the low class of risk. Log-rank test on Kaplan–Meier curves for patients in intermediate and high class of risk, reported in Figure 2b, demonstrated a significant difference between the two curves ($p = 0.0439$; HR 0.3299, 95% CI 0.1092–0.9967).

Table 3. Univariate analysis of recurrent disease in patients stratified for risk of structural recurrence according to the American Thyroid Association guidelines.

ATA Risk	Low			Medium–High		
	TT	pCLND	Total	TT	pCLND	Total
Patients	268	42	310	52	37	89
Recurrent disease	7 (2.6%)	2 (4.8%)	9 (2.9%)	11 (21.2%)	2 (5.4%)	13 (14.6%)
p (TT vs. CLND)		0.441			0.0392	

ATA: American Thyroid Association guidelines; TT: total thyroidectomy; pCLND: prophylactic central compartment lymph node dissection.

Overall, occult lymph node metastases in our series were found in 35 (8.8%) patients. As reported in Table 4, the incidence of disease recurrence was 20% in patients with lymph node metastases (pN+), 2.8% in patients with uninvolved lymph nodes in which an evaluation of N status was possible because at least one lymph node was excised (pN0), and 5% in patients in which N status was not assessed (pNx) ($p < 0.001$). The log-rank test on Kaplan–Meier curves representing patients with and without lymph node metastases (Figure 3) demonstrated a significant difference between the two groups ($p < 0.001$; HR 15.160, 95% CI 3.444–566.7289).

Table 4. Univariate analysis of recurrent disease in patients stratified according to N status.

	pNx	pN0	pN+
Patients	221	143	35
Disease recurrence	11 (5%)	4 (2.8%)	7 (20%)

pNx: pathological nodal status not assessed; pN0: lymph nodes uninvolved at pathological examination; pN+: lymph node metastases at pathological examination. Statistical significance: overall $p < 0.001$; pNx vs. pN0: $p = 0.1132$; pNx vs. pN+: $p < 0.001$; pN0 vs. pN+ $p < 0.001$.

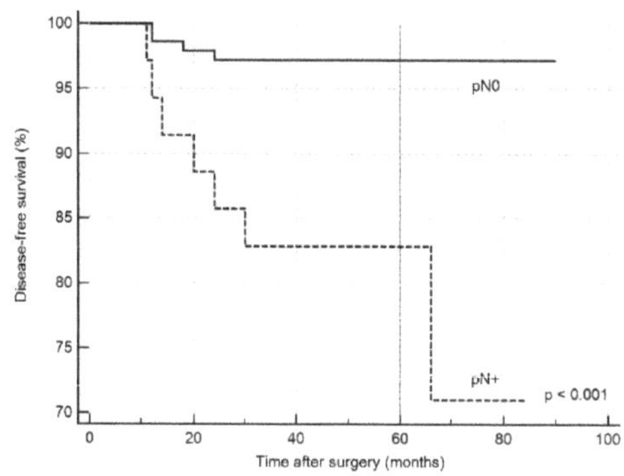

Figure 3. Kaplan-Meier curves estimating overall disease-free survival according to N status: $p < 0.001$ (HR 15.160, 95% CI 3.4445–66.7289). pN0: No evidence of lymph node metastases at pathological examination. pN+: Lymph node metastases at pathological examination.

4. Discussion

In this work, we focused our attention on prophylactic CLND and the influence of occult lymph node metastases on the prognosis in patients with DTC.

The first issue to consider is that in our study, there was an intrinsic bias in the selection of patient candidates for pCLND: in fact, this treatment was reserved to cases in which preoperative evaluation including family history, physical examination, US features, FNAC findings, and intraoperative examination suggested a tumor with potentially aggressive behavior.

In our series, the patients who underwent pCLND more frequently had a cytologic diagnosis of PTC and, in addition, were younger than the patients who underwent TT alone. These aspects can be explained by the fact that the surgeon chooses to perform a pCLND in the case of certainty of a malignant nodule: in this case, the operator feels authorized to perform an aggressive intervention to achieve a radical excision of the tumor, mostly in younger patients with a longer life expectancy. On the other hand, when facing patients in whom preoperative diagnosis is uncertain, the surgeon seems inclined to more conservative surgery, preferring a prudent approach to prevent postoperative complications.

However, unlike what could be expected considering the inherent bias of our study in the selection of the surgical approach, at histopathological examination, the two groups appeared comparable: the nodule size and the presence of aggressive features including multicentricity, angioinvasivity, and extrathyroidal extension were similar between the two groups.

At this point, a consideration should be made with regard to the indication for pCLND. The ATA guidelines suggest this approach in cases of advanced primary tumors (T3 or T4). Even if our indications were larger than those purposed by the ATA, our work seems to indicate that preoperative and intraoperative evaluation have low reliability in establishing what tumors have pathologically aggressive features that could benefit from a pCLND.

The incidence of tall cell carcinoma, which has been largely described as an aggressive variant of PTC [29–31], was significantly higher in the pCLND group. This fact could be explained by the higher prevalence of the FNAC diagnostic for malignancy in the pCLND group: in fact, tall cell carcinoma is associated with considerable alterations of the cells that result in a higher incidence of Tir4 and Tir5. In contrast, the higher incidence of follicular variant of PTC in the TT group could be explained by the fact that this subtype of tumor presents less cellular abnormalities, thus is more often associated with inconclusive or negative FNAC, and consequently with a more conservative approach.

As expected, the incidence of lymph node metastases was higher in the pCLND group (25.3%) than in the TT group (4.7%). However, if we consider only the 99 patients in the TT group in which an evaluation of the N status was possible because at least one lymph node was excised, the real incidence of lymph node metastases was 15.2%, thus similar to the other group. Furthermore, this finding explains the fact that the lymph node ratio was significantly higher in the TT group, where the denominator of the fraction was smaller because a smaller number of lymph nodes was excised. These findings suggest that the incidence of lymph node metastases is higher when a larger number of lymph nodes is excised [24,28].

Considering the ATA risk stratification for structural disease recurrence, patients in the pCLND group were more often classified in the intermediate risk group. This could be explained by the fact that pCLND allows for more accurate staging of the tumor, ensuring a better assessment of the N status; in fact, the intermediate class of risk includes tumors in which more than five lymph nodes are involved. Thus, it is likely that pCLND allows to upstage tumors that otherwise would have been classified as low risk tumors, as already reported in the literature [28,32,33]. This fact also explains the higher incidence of patients who underwent RAI therapy after surgery in the pCNLD group.

Overall, our work failed to demonstrate an advantage on prognosis in patients who underwent pCLND. However, if we consider only patients at intermediate and high risk of recurrence, pCLND significantly improved the disease-free survival. We think that this is the key point because tumors at low risk of recurrence have a good prognosis, thus pCLND could be considered an overtreatment that does not modify the course of the disease; on the other hand, the real value of pCLND is expressed in tumors at intermediate and high risk of recurrence, which benefit from an aggressive surgery, with a reduction of recurrence rate.

These findings are in accordance with a recent meta-analysis by Zhao et al., which included 22 studies with over 6000 patients, where pCLND proved to be effective in reducing the risk of loco-regional recurrence [34]; another meta-analysis regarding pCNLD in patients who underwent hemithyroidectomy was consistent with this result [35].

The secondary outcome of our work was to assess whether pCLND was burdened by a higher incidence of postoperative complications. In our series, the occurrence of hypoparathyroidism and RLN injury was higher in the pCLND group, but this difference was not significant, suggesting that pCLND could be a safe procedure with an acceptable incidence of complications. However, this finding should be carefully considered and contextualized: in fact, the same meta-analysis of Zhao et al. that we previously reported, demonstrated a higher incidence of transient and permanent hypoparathyroidism and of transient RLN injury [34].

Furthermore, we must underline that the overall incidence of permanent hypoparathyroidism (9.8%) in our study was higher than the ones usually reported in the literature. As already stated in the Methods section, we defined hypoparathyroidism on the basis of PTH value; probably, this assessment overestimates the incidence of hypoparathyroidism compared to the centers that use only serum calcemia as a criterion, which can be easily influenced from oral calcium supplementation.

Finally, we considered the influence of lymph node metastases on prognosis. When excluding the patients in which the N status was not assessed because no lymph node was excised (pNx), the incidence of recurrent disease was considerably higher in patients with lymph node metastases (pN+), reaching up to 20% than in patients with uninvolved lymph nodes (pN0), with an incidence of 2.8%. It is also interesting to observe that in the group in which the N status was not assessed (pNx), the incidence of recurrences was almost twice (5%) that in patients in the pN0 group, perhaps suggesting that some of these recurrences could have been avoided if a lymphectomy had been performed.

As already mentioned, current guidelines are discordant regarding pCLND. In the ATA guidelines published in 2015, pCLND assumes a marginal role in the treatment of differentiated thyroid carcinoma [1]. The latest NCCN guidelines published in 2019 have eliminated, compared with the previous edition, pCLND in DTC [27]. Considering the negative impact on the prognosis and the high incidence of occult lymph node metastases, and taking into account the difficulties in establishing preoperatively and intraoperatively what tumors could have aggressive behavior, we think that indications for pCLND could be revised in order to achieve more efficacious treatment of aggressive tumors. Such considerations are in accordance with a recent meta-analysis of Zhao et al., which included over 4000 patients, reporting a poor sensitivity of US in detecting metastases of the central compartment (pooled sensitivity of 33%, range 10–57%) with an incidence of lymph node metastases of 48%, suggesting for these reasons that indications to pCLND should be extended to all patients with DTC [36].

This study has some limitations. First, this is a single center, retrospective study. The study was performed in an endemic iodine deficient region, with a high incidence of autoimmune thyroiditis; therefore, the generalization of our results to other populations should be made carefully. Finally, the real incidence of disease recurrence could be underestimated in our study, considering that the mean follow-up is 55.4 months, and that these kind of tumors are generally indolent, and recurrences can appear up to 10 years after surgery.

5. Conclusions

The selection of patients for prophylactic CLND is problematic due to the low accuracy of preoperative and intraoperative evaluation in establishing what tumors are aggressive and could benefit from aggressive surgery. Prophylactic CLND is a safe procedure, with an acceptable incidence of complications, comparable to that of patients who undergo thyroidectomy alone. Our study demonstrated that pCNLD allows for more accurate staging of the tumor and reduces the incidence of recurrent disease in patients with intermediate and high risk DTC. We think that indications for pCNLD should be revised by the main guidelines, in consideration with the latest evidence in the literature.

Author Contributions: Conceptualization, F.M. and P.G.C.; Methodology, F.M., G.L.C., G.C. and E.E.; Formal analysis, F.M., G.A. and F.C.; Investigation, G.C., E.E. and P.G.C.; Data curation, G.L.C., G.A. and F.C.; Writing—original draft preparation, F.M. and G.L.C.; Writing—review and editing, G.C. and F.C.; Visualization, G.A.; Supervision, E.E. and P.G.C. All authors have read and agreed to the published version of the manuscript.

Funding: This research received no external funding.

Conflicts of Interest: The authors declare no conflict of interest.

References

1. Haugen, B.R.; Alexander, E.K.; Bible, K.C.; Doherty, G.M.; Mandel, S.J.; Nikiforov, Y.E.; Pacini, F.; Randolph, G.W.; Sawka, A.M.; Schlumberger, M.; et al. 2015 American Thyroid Association Management Guidelines for Adult Patients with Thyroid Nodules and Differentiated Thyroid Cancer: The American Thyroid Association Guidelines Task Force on Thyroid Nodules and Differentiated Thyroid Cancer. *Thyroid* **2016**, *26*, 1–133. [CrossRef] [PubMed]
2. Barczyński, M.; Konturek, A.; Stopa, M.; Nowak, W. Prophylactic central neck dissection for papillary thyroid cancer. *BJS* **2013**, *100*, 410–418. [CrossRef] [PubMed]
3. Calò, P.G.; Conzo, G.; Raffaelli, M.; Medas, F.; Gambardella, C.; De Crea, C.; Gordini, L.; Patrone, R.; Sessa, L.; Erdas, E.; et al. Total thyroidectomy alone versus ipsilateral versus bilateral prophylactic central neck dissection in clinically node-negative differentiated thyroid carcinoma. A retrospective multicenter study. *Eur. J. Surg. Oncol. (EJSO)* **2017**, *43*, 126–132. [CrossRef] [PubMed]
4. Mazzaferri, E.L.; Jhiang, S.M. Long-term impact of initial surgical and medical therapy on papillary and follicular thyroid cancer. *Am. J. Med.* **1994**, *97*, 418–428. [CrossRef]

5. Otsuki, N.; Shimoda, H.; Morita, N.; Furukawa, T.; Teshima, M.; Shinomiya, H.; Nibu, K. Salvage surgery for structural local recurrence of papillary thyroid cancer: Recurrence patterns and surgical outcome. *Endocr. J.* **2020**. [CrossRef]
6. Kim, H.; Kim, T.H.; Choe, J.-H.; Kim, J.-H.; Kim, J.S.; Oh, Y.L.; Hahn, S.Y.; Shin, J.H.; Chi, S.A.; Jung, S.-H.; et al. Patterns of Initial Recurrence in Completely Resected Papillary Thyroid Carcinoma. *Thyroid* **2017**, *27*, 908–914. [CrossRef]
7. Wang, L.Y.; Migliacci, J.C.; Tuttle, R.M.; Shaha, A.R.; Shah, J.P.; Patel, S.G.; Ganly, I. Management and outcome of clinically evident neck recurrence in patients with papillary thyroid cancer. *Clin. Endocrinol.* **2017**, *87*, 566–571. [CrossRef]
8. Medas, F.; Canu, G.L.; Boi, F.; Lai, M.L.; Erdas, E.; Calò, P.G. Predictive Factors of Recurrence in Patients with Differentiated Thyroid Carcinoma: A Retrospective Analysis on 579 Patients. *Cancers (Basel)* **2019**, *11*, 1230. [CrossRef]
9. Enumah, S.; Fingeret, A.; Parangi, S.; Dias-Santagata, D.; Sadow, P.M.; Lubitz, C.C. BRAFV600E Mutation is Associated with an Increased Risk of Papillary Thyroid Cancer Recurrence. *World J. Surg.* **2020**. [CrossRef]
10. Alvarado, R.; Sywak, M.S.; Delbridge, L.; Sidhu, S.B. Central lymph node dissection as a secondary procedure for papillary thyroid cancer: Is there added morbidity? *Surgery* **2009**, *145*, 514–518. [CrossRef]
11. Calò, P.G.; Medas, F.; Pisano, G.; Boi, F.; Baghino, G.; Mariotti, S.; Nicolosi, A. Differentiated Thyroid Cancer: Indications and Extent of Central Neck Dissection—Our Experience. Available online: https://www.hindawi.com/journals/ijso/2013/625193/abs/ (accessed on 31 January 2019).
12. Moreno, M.A.; Edeiken-Monroe, B.S.; Siegel, E.R.; Sherman, S.I.; Clayman, G.L. In papillary thyroid cancer, preoperative central neck ultrasound detects only macroscopic surgical disease, but negative findings predict excellent long-term regional control and survival. *Thyroid* **2012**, *22*, 347–355. [CrossRef]
13. Ito, Y.; Tomoda, C.; Uruno, T.; Takamura, Y.; Miya, A.; Kobayashi, K.; Matsuzuka, F.; Kuma, K.; Miyauchi, A. Clinical significance of metastasis to the central compartment from papillary microcarcinoma of the thyroid. *World J. Surg.* **2006**, *30*, 91–99. [CrossRef]
14. Ito, Y.; Tomoda, C.; Uruno, T.; Takamura, Y.; Miya, A.; Kobayashi, K.; Matsuzuka, F.; Kuma, K.; Miyauchi, A. Ultrasonographically and anatomopathologically detectable node metastases in the lateral compartment as indicators of worse relapse-free survival in patients with papillary thyroid carcinoma. *World J. Surg.* **2005**, *29*, 917–920. [CrossRef] [PubMed]
15. Mazzaferri, E.L. Long-term outcome of patients with differentiated thyroid carcinoma: Effect of therapy. *Endocr. Pract.* **2000**, *6*, 469–476. [CrossRef]
16. Bhattacharyya, N. A population-based analysis of survival factors in differentiated and medullary thyroid carcinoma. *Otolaryngol. Head Neck Surg.* **2003**, *128*, 115–123. [CrossRef] [PubMed]
17. Steinmüller, T.; Klupp, J.; Rayes, N.; Ulrich, F.; Jonas, S.; Gräf, K.J.; Neuhaus, P. Prognostic factors in patients with differentiated thyroid carcinoma. *Eur. J. Surg.* **2000**, *166*, 29–33. [CrossRef]
18. Kim, B.Y.; Choi, N.; Kim, S.W.; Jeong, H.-S.; Chung, M.K.; Son, Y.-I. Randomized trial of prophylactic ipsilateral central lymph node dissection in patients with clinically node negative papillary thyroid microcarcinoma. *Eur. Arch. Otorhinolaryngol.* **2020**, *277*, 569–576. [CrossRef] [PubMed]
19. Shaha, A.R. Thyroid cancer: Extent of thyroidectomy. *Cancer Control* **2000**, *7*, 240–245. [CrossRef] [PubMed]
20. Beasley, N.J.P.; Lee, J.; Eski, S.; Walfish, P.; Witterick, I.; Freeman, J.L. Impact of nodal metastases on prognosis in patients with well-differentiated thyroid cancer. *Arch. Otolaryngol. Head Neck Surg.* **2002**, *128*, 825–828. [CrossRef] [PubMed]
21. Rotstein, L. The role of lymphadenectomy in the management of papillary carcinoma of the thyroid. *J. Surg. Oncol.* **2009**, *99*, 186–188. [CrossRef]
22. Yazıcı, D.; Çolakoğlu, B.; Sağlam, B.; Sezer, H.; Kapran, Y.; Aydın, Ö.; Demirkol, M.O.; Alagöl, F.; Terzioğlu, T. Effect of prophylactic central neck dissection on the surgical outcomes in papillary thyroid cancer: Experience in a single center. *Eur. Arch. Otorhinolaryngol.* **2020**, 1–7. [CrossRef] [PubMed]
23. Liu, H.; Li, Y.; Mao, Y. Local lymph node recurrence after central neck dissection in papillary thyroid cancers: A meta analysis. *Eur. Ann. Otorhinolaryngol. Head Neck Dis.* **2019**, *136*, 481–487. [CrossRef] [PubMed]
24. Conzo, G.; Calò, P.G.; Sinisi, A.A.; De Bellis, A.; Pasquali, D.; Iorio, S.; Tartaglia, E.; Mauriello, C.; Gambardella, C.; Cavallo, F.; et al. Impact of prophylactic central compartment neck dissection on locoregional recurrence of differentiated thyroid cancer in clinically node-negative patients: A retrospective study of a large clinical series. *Surgery* **2014**, *155*, 998–1005. [CrossRef]

25. Scherl, S.; Mehra, S.; Clain, J.; Dos Reis, L.L.; Persky, M.; Turk, A.; Wenig, B.; Husaini, H.; Urken, M.L. The effect of surgeon experience on the detection of metastatic lymph nodes in the central compartment and the pathologic features of clinically unapparent metastatic lymph nodes: What are we missing when we don't perform a prophylactic dissection of central compartment lymph nodes in papillary thyroid cancer? *Thyroid* **2014**, *24*, 1282–1288. [CrossRef]
26. Calò, P.; Pisano, G.; Medas, F.; Marcialis, J.; Gordini, L.; Erdas, E.; Nicolosi, A. Total thyroidectomy without prophylactic central neck dissection in clinically node-negative papillary thyroid cancer: Is it an adequate treatment? *World J. Surg. Oncol.* **2014**, *12*, 152. [CrossRef] [PubMed]
27. Haddad, R.I.; Kandeel, F.; Scheri, R.P. NCCN Guidelines Index Table of Contents Discussion. *J. Natl. Compr. Cancer Netw.* **2018**, *16*, 1429–1440. [CrossRef]
28. Takami, H.; Ito, Y.; Okamoto, T.; Onoda, N.; Noguchi, H.; Yoshida, A. Revisiting the Guidelines Issued by the Japanese Society of Thyroid Surgeons and Japan Association of Endocrine Surgeons: A Gradual Move Towards Consensus Between Japanese and Western Practice in the Management of Thyroid Carcinoma. *World J. Surg.* **2014**, *38*, 2002–2010. [CrossRef]
29. Ganly, I.; Ibrahimpasic, T.; Rivera, M.; Nixon, I.; Palmer, F.; Patel, S.G.; Tuttle, R.M.; Shah, J.P.; Ghossein, R. Prognostic implications of papillary thyroid carcinoma with tall-cell features. *Thyroid* **2014**, *24*, 662–670. [CrossRef]
30. Bernstein, J.; Virk, R.K.; Hui, P.; Prasad, A.; Westra, W.H.; Tallini, G.; Adeniran, A.J.; Udelsman, R.; Sasaki, C.T.; Roman, S.A.; et al. Tall cell variant of papillary thyroid microcarcinoma: Clinicopathologic features with BRAF(V600E) mutational analysis. *Thyroid* **2013**, *23*, 1525–1531. [CrossRef]
31. Axelsson, T.A.; Hrafnkelsson, J.; Olafsdottir, E.J.; Jonasson, J.G. Tall cell variant of papillary thyroid carcinoma: A population-based study in Iceland. *Thyroid* **2015**, *25*, 216–220. [CrossRef]
32. Raffaelli, M.; De Crea, C.; Sessa, L.; Giustacchini, P.; Revelli, L.; Bellantone, C.; Lombardi, C.P. Prospective evaluation of total thyroidectomy versus ipsilateral versus bilateral central neck dissection in patients with clinically node–negative papillary thyroid carcinoma. *Surgery* **2012**, *152*, 957–964. [CrossRef] [PubMed]
33. Sadowski, B.M.; Snyder, S.K.; Lairmore, T.C. Routine bilateral central lymph node clearance for papillary thyroid cancer. *Surgery* **2009**, *146*, 696–705. [CrossRef] [PubMed]
34. Zhao, W.; Luo, H.; Zhou, Y.; Dai, W.; Zhu, J. Evaluating the effectiveness of prophylactic central neck dissection with total thyroidectomy for cN0 papillary thyroid carcinoma: An updated meta-analysis. *Eur. J. Surg. Oncol.* **2017**, *43*, 1989–2000. [CrossRef] [PubMed]
35. Ahn, S.-H.; Kim, W.S. The effect of prophylactic central neck dissection during hemithyroidectomy on locoregional recurrence in patients with papillary thyroid carcinoma: A meta-analysis. *Clin. Exp. Otorhinolaryngol.* **2020**, *13*, 194. [CrossRef]
36. Zhao, H.; Li, H. Meta-analysis of ultrasound for cervical lymph nodes in papillary thyroid cancer: Diagnosis of central and lateral compartment nodal metastases. *Eur. J. Radiol.* **2019**, *112*, 14–21. [CrossRef]

cancers

MDPI

Review

Fluorescence Image-Guided Surgery for Thyroid Cancer: Utility for Preventing Hypoparathyroidism

Marco Stefano Demarchi [1,2], Barbara Seeliger [3,4,5,6], Jean-Christophe Lifante [2,7], Pier Francesco Alesina [6,8] and Frédéric Triponez [1,*]

1 Department of Thoracic and Endocrine Surgery and Faculty of Medicine, University Hospitals of Geneva, 4 Rue Gabrielle Perret-Gentil, 1211 Geneva, Switzerland; marcostefano.demarchi@hcuge.ch
2 Department of Endocrine Surgery, Lyon Sud University Hospitals, 69310 Pierre Benite, France; jean-christophe.lifante@chu-lyon.fr
3 IHU—Strasbourg, Institute of Image-Guided Surgery, 67091 Strasbourg CEDEX, France; barbara.seeliger@ihu-strasbourg.eu
4 IRCAD, Research Institute against Digestive Cancer, 67091 Strasbourg CEDEX, France
5 Department of General, Digestive, and Endocrine Surgery, Strasbourg University Hospitals, 67091 Strasbourg CEDEX, France
6 Department of Surgery and Center of Minimally Invasive Surgery, Evangelische Kliniken Essen-Mitte, Academic Teaching Hospital of the University of Duisburg-Essen, 45136 Essen, Germany; pieroalesina@yahoo.it
7 Health Services and Performance Research Lab (EA 7425 HESPER), Université Claude Bernard Lyon 1, 69622 Lyon, France
8 Department of Surgery, Gemelli Molise Hospital, Università Cattolica del Sacro Cuore, 86100 Campobasso, Italy
* Correspondence: frederic.triponez@hcuge.ch; Tel.: +41-(0)22-372-78-62

Simple Summary: The most frequent post-operative complication in thyroid surgery is hypoparathyroidism leading to temporary or definitive low blood calcium levels. This complication can result from intentional or inadvertent extirpation, trauma, or devascularization of the parathyroid glands. They are located right next to the thyroid, and are responsible for the blood calcium level regulation. Hypoparathyroidism is even more common when a lymph node dissection is needed in addition to thyroidectomy in case of thyroid cancer. The safeguarding of all four parathyroid glands with their vascularization can be extremely challenging, even for experienced surgeons. Fluorescence imaging is a relatively novel intraoperative tool to help identify, visualize, and preserve the parathyroid glands during thyroid surgery. In this review, we summarize the current scientific landscape and the potential benefits of fluorescence imaging to preserve the parathyroid glands and to prevent post-operative hypoparathyroidism in thyroid cancer surgery.

Abstract: Background: Hypoparathyroidism is one of the most frequent complications of thyroid surgery, especially when associated with lymph node dissection in cases of thyroid cancer. Fluorescence-guided surgery is an emerging tool that appears to help reduce the rate of this complication. The present review aims to highlight the utility of fluorescence imaging in preserving parathyroid glands during thyroid cancer surgery. **Methods:** We performed a systematic review of the literature according to PRISMA guidelines to identify published studies on fluorescence-guided thyroid surgery with a particular focus on thyroid cancer. Articles were selected and analyzed per indication and type of surgery, autofluorescence or exogenous dye usage, and outcomes. The Methodological Index for Non-Randomized Studies (MINORS) was used to assess the methodological quality of the included articles. **Results:** Twenty-five studies met the inclusion criteria, with three studies exclusively assessing patients with thyroid cancer. The remaining studies assessed mixed cohorts with thyroid cancer and other thyroid or parathyroid diseases. The majority of the papers support the potential benefit of fluorescence imaging in preserving parathyroid glands in thyroid surgery. **Conclusions:** Fluorescence-guided surgery is useful in the prevention of post-thyroidectomy hypoparathyroidism via enhanced early identification, visualization, and preservation of the parathyroid glands. These aspects are notably beneficial in cases of associated lymphadenectomy for thyroid cancer.

Citation: Demarchi, M.S.; Seeliger, B.; Lifante, J.-C.; Alesina, P.F.; Triponez, F. Fluorescence Image-Guided Surgery for Thyroid Cancer: Utility for Preventing Hypoparathyroidism. *Cancers* **2021**, *13*, 3792. https://doi.org/10.3390/cancers13153792

Academic Editor: Mary F. McMullin

Received: 25 May 2021
Accepted: 23 July 2021
Published: 28 July 2021

Keywords: thyroid surgery; thyroid cancer; hypoparathyroidism; fluorescence-guided surgery; near-infrared autofluorescence

1. Introduction

The global incidence of thyroid cancer has continuously increased over the past decades [1]. This upward trend has been attributed to improved diagnostic acumen owing to the availability of advanced technology, as well as to lifestyle and environmental changes. Thyroid cancer is currently the most common endocrine cancer worldwide [2,3]. Despite increases in incidence, mortality from thyroid cancer has remained stable over the past decades [1]. The life expectancy of many thyroid cancer patients, especially those younger than 45 years, is not reduced when compared with that of the general population [4]. The prevention of treatment-related morbidity is essential, including minimization of postoperative hypoparathyroidism rates, particularly for young patients with an overall excellent long-term prognosis. The majority of the thyroid cancer burden affects women [3], and the prevention of complications with repercussions on pregnancies is crucial for those of reproductive age.

The treatment of choice for thyroid cancer is surgical resection. Depending on the tumor extent, a total or near-total thyroidectomy with therapeutic or prophylactic lymph node dissection is indicated. Despite the significant benefits of total resection, including increased survival and reduced recurrence rates, extensive resections are typically accompanied by substantially increased complication rates [5]. Thus, the risks and benefits of thyroid cancer surgery must be balanced, targeting complete excision of malignant lesions while preserving critical structures such as the laryngeal nerves and parathyroid glands (PGs), particularly in thyroidectomy with lymphadenectomy. As these challenges are continuously encountered in thyroid cancer surgery, surgical innovations are targeted at minimizing procedure-related morbidity while maintaining therapeutic benefits.

One such innovation is intraoperative neuromonitoring (IONM) of the recurrent laryngeal nerve (RLN). Over the last two decades, IONM has gained popularity and has become the gold standard for thyroid surgeries in order to prevent injury to the RLN [6], despite initial controversial discussions regarding its benefit [7]. Another emerging technology is fluorescence image-guided surgery (FIGS), a real-time navigation modality based on optical imaging. The use of fluorescence imaging is relatively new in surgery, although it is a widely known method used in biomedical sciences for visualizing cells and tissues in vitro and in vivo [8]. The intraoperative use of light sources in the near-infrared (NIR) excitation range induces the emission of a fluorescent signal via a wavelength shift during tissue interaction [9].

In more detail, fluorescence is based on the property of certain substances to absorb external light at a given excitation wavelength and subsequently emit light at a different, longer wavelength with lower energy [10]. As a result, fluorescence imaging involves a sequence in which the tissue of interest is illuminated by a filtered light source at a specific excitation wavelength, light is absorbed by the target tissue, a longer wavelength is emitted, and the fluorescent band is detected by a specifically designed camera [11,12]. The advantage of light in the NIR range is a deeper tissue penetration (<1 cm, with a limited depth resolution beyond 5 mm) [13,14]; thus, NIR imaging devices enable the surgeon to see behind the tissue surface [15]. Other wavelengths (ultraviolet: 200–400 nm or visible: 400–650 nm) are limited for in vivo real-time imaging due to low light penetration into the tissues and autofluorescence from endogenous fluorophores in the body [16,17]. Current in vivo fluorescence imaging systems are thus optimized for the NIR range. This imaging modality provides the surgeon with real-time feedback during the surgical procedure to identify and differentiate surgical targets from normal tissue [12]. Two different modalities of detection of near-infrared autofluorescence (NIRAF) are actually used: a probe-based modality such as the PTeye (by AiBiomed, Santa Barbara, CA, USA) that provides a quantitative, and auditory feedback when the handheld fiber probe touches parathyroid tissue, and the imaging-based modality that uses an NIR light source in conjunction with a filtered camera to identify the autofluorescence of the tissue on a display monitor such as the Fluobeam-800/Fluobeam-LX (Fluoptics, France), PDE Neo II (Hamamatsu, Shizuoka Pref. Japan), and EleVision™ IR Platform (Medtronic, Minnesota, MN, USA), among others.

FIGS is gaining popularity and is being increasingly used in endocrine surgery, including adrenal [15,18], parathyroid, and thyroid surgery [19,20]. With the integration of specific contrast agents and advanced imaging systems, fluorescence guidance has the ability to bring about significant positive change in surgery, leading to better outcomes by improving the visualization of tissues for resection, such as tumors, or those to be preserved, such as nerves, blood vessels, and neighboring organs [12,21].

Two fluorescence imaging approaches are important in thyroid and parathyroid surgery, namely, contrast-enhanced fluorescence and autofluorescence imaging. The first technique is based on either intravascular or local administration of an exogenous contrast agent, whereas the second technique uses the intrinsic florescent properties of the target tissue via specific optical modalities [10,22].

1.1. Contrast-Enhanced Fluorescence and Autofluorescence

Exogenous contrast-enhanced fluorescence can be induced via the use of fluorescent dyes. For intraoperative imaging, indocyanine green (ICG), a sterile tricarbocyanine dye, is the most commonly utilized fluorophore. ICG absorbs light at excitation wavelengths of 790–805 nm and re-emits light at 835 nm [23]. Other NIR fluorescent agents, such as methylene blue, are used less frequently than ICG due to their potential toxicity [24].

In contrast, autofluorescence is based on intrinsic biomolecules that act as endogenous fluorophores. Light emission occurs in the ultraviolet, visible, or NIR spectral range when biological molecules are excited with light at an appropriate specific wavelength [25].

Intrinsic tissue fluorescence can be perceived as a background disturbance signal when cells and tissues are labeled with exogenous fluorophores. However, tissue autofluorescence alone has shown great promise when used for research and diagnostic purposes [25]. In particular, the PGs are characterized by exceptional autofluorescence in the NIR range, as discovered by tissue spectral analysis [26,27]. A research group at Vanderbilt University identified the ideal spectral range, with excitation light at 785 nm producing maximal autofluorescence from thyroid and parathyroid tissue within the NIR range (820 nm), with the parathyroid signal ranging from 1.2 to 25 times higher than thyroid, and all surrounding tissues [28] with brown fat and lymph nodes that are known false NIRAF positives in non-parathyroid tissues [13]. This group further explored real-time intraoperative autofluorescence imaging of the PGs [27,29]. The specific molecule acting as an intrinsic fluorophore has not yet been identified.

Multiple NIR imaging systems are commercially available for clinical use or for research purposes. Some of these devices are optimized for pure autofluorescence imaging, whereas others enable both autofluorescence and ICG contrast-enhanced fluorescence imaging. All autofluorescence devices can detect ICG, but the reverse is usually not true [29]. As the field of potential applications is expanding, customizable systems with a choice of different wavelengths and multispectral fluorescence imagers are being explored [30]. For example, hyperspectral imaging showed distinct spectral signatures of the thyroid glands and PGs compared with the surrounding tissue during neck exploration in a patient [12].

Postoperative complications after thyroid surgery may include temporary or permanent hypoparathyroidism, recurrent laryngeal nerve injury or palsy, chyle fistula, Horner's syndrome, injury to motor nerves in the neck, and hematoma or seroma formation [5,31]. Hypoparathyroidism is the most common complication after total or near-total thyroidectomy due to the accidental resection or devascularization of PGs. Fluorescence imaging has the potential to revolutionize thyroid surgery by significantly reducing hypoparathyroidism, especially for thyroid cancer necessitating an enlarged dissection.

1.2. Postoperative Hypoparathyroidism

Transient hypoparathyroidism has been reported in up to 20% of patients undergoing total thyroidectomy for thyroid cancer, with permanent hypoparathyroidism reported in up to 3% [32]. Transient hypoparathyroidism has been reported in up to 26.2% for cases of medullary thyroid carcinoma, with a clear association existing between the extent of lymph node dissection and the observation of four PGs [33]. A systematic review and meta-analysis on bilateral thyroid surgery demonstrated an even higher median rate of transient (27%, interquartile range—IQR: 19–38%) and permanent (1%, interquartile range—IQR: 0–3%) hypocalcemia [34]. The rates increase with the extent of surgery, with symptomatic hypoparathyroidism complications arising in 28.7% of thyroid cancer surgeries (28.4% temporary, 0.3% permanent), as reported from a single center [5]. The permanent hypoparathyroidism rate is reported as 0.4–13.8% [31] and can reach 37% in bilateral neck dissection for thyroid cancer [35].

Although the vast majority of postoperative hypoparathyroidism cases are transient and resolve within 6 months of surgery, a small percentage of patients require calcium and vitamin D supplementation for the rest of their lives. This situation is considered serious and negatively affects quality of life [5]. Women are significantly more likely than men to require permanent calcium replacement for postoperative hypoparathyroidism [36]. Consequently, women of child-bearing age require close monitoring during pregnancy, as they are at risk of hyper- and hypocalcemia. As both conditions have consequences to the fetus and the mother, calcium dose adjustments are frequent [37]. Other implications of postoperative hypoparathyroidism include the economic costs of prolonged hospital stay, additional investigations, procurement of medications, the medical burden associated with lifetime medication, and routine hospital visits for follow-ups. Moreover, there are considerable disease burdens related to chronic kidney failure, increased psychiatric complaints, and basal ganglia calcification, among other sequelae, and possible increases in mortality [38,39].

Surgical techniques that improve the preservation of the PGs and their blood supply are greatly needed. The present review highlights the utility of one such innovation, i.e., fluorescence imaging, in preserving the PGs during total or near-total thyroid resection ± lymph node dissection in the case of thyroid cancer.

The purpose of this review is to provide evidence on the utility of fluorescence-guided surgery for preserving the PGs and preventing hypoparathyroidism, with a particular focus on thyroid cancer surgery. The specific objectives of this review are (A) to determine the utility of the different fluorescence imaging techniques in preventing hypoparathyroidism as a complication of thyroid surgery; (B) to determine the feasibility of FIGS in thyroid cancer surgery, with an emphasis on ease of use, added surgical time, and complications related to the technique; and (C) to identify future directions in the use of fluorescence imaging to prevent postoperative hypoparathyroidism.

2. Materials and Methods

2.1. Search Strategy

This systematic literature review was conducted according to the Preferred Reporting in Systematic Review and Meta-Analysis (PRISMA) guidelines [40]. MEDLINE (PubMed), Science Direct, Google Scholar, Medline, Oxford Academic journals, and Cochrane library databases were searched, with MeSH terms and free-text key words used for studies investigating the role of fluorescence-guided surgery in preventing hypoparathyroidism as a complication of thyroidectomy for thyroid cancer. The following search string was then developed: (Fluorescence-guided surgery OR Fluorescence imaging OR Indocyanine green OR Near-infrared imaging OR Autofluorescence) AND (Thyroid cancer OR Thyroid malignancy) AND Thyroidectomy AND (Parathyroid glands OR Hypoparathyroidism). To complete the search, the references within the selected articles were searched as well. The search was conducted until May 2021 by the authors. No age or time limitations were used. After the titles and abstracts had been screened, full-text reports were assessed for eligibility, and references were screened within the selected articles.

A standard form for extracting the following data was used, addressing the characteristics of the selected studies (design, method of randomization), participants (baseline characteristics, tumor type, indication for surgery), and intervention (type of surgery, operative technique, lymph node dissection, type of fluorescence, type of fluorescent dye, dose, timing of administration during surgery, fluorescence system). Outcomes were influence on procedure duration, intra- and postoperative complications, and, particularly, presence of temporary and/or permanent hypoparathyroidism. These data were analyzed and are reported in tables and text. Outcome variables are reported as the absolute number and percentage, for all studies combined and separately for those studies with a control group.

2.2. Eligibility Criteria

The studies included in this review were original articles, written in English, published between 2000 and 2021, and reporting on the use of FIGS in preserving the PGs and their blood supply or preventing hypoparathyroidism during thyroid cancer surgery. Articles that report on the use of fluorescence imaging for other procedures or diseases other than thyroid cancer were excluded. Studies not presenting original patient data, animal studies, case reports, conference abstracts, technical notes, and articles written in languages other than English were also excluded.

2.3. Methodological Quality Assessment

The Methodological Index for Non-Randomized Studies (MINORS) was used to assess the methodological quality of the included articles [41]. MINORS is a valid instrument designed to assess the methodological quality of non-randomized surgical studies and is based on eight items for noncomparative studies and 12 items for studies with a control group.

3. Results

3.1. Data Extraction

The process of article selection is illustrated in Figure 1. The database searches retrieved 695 articles, and a reference list search retrieved 15 additional studies. After deduplication, 590 articles were screened, of which 67 full articles were retrieved. A total of 25 studies met the inclusion criteria. Overall, the outcomes of nearly 3000 patients were described. All included studies were published between 2016 and 2021, and the mean ages of the included participants ranged from 39.2 to 61.6 years for 22 studies, while three studies did not report the ages of their participants. Two studies reported age ranges (32–70 and 34–73 years, respectively) [42,43]. Five studies were retrospective, and seven studies had a control group. Three studies exclusively evaluated patients with thyroid cancer, whereas the remaining studies assessed patients with thyroid cancer and other thyroid or parathyroid diseases. The study characteristics of the included studies are presented in Table 1.

Table 1. Study characteristics of included studies. * Mean ± standard deviation unless otherwise stated.

s/n	Study	Number of Patients	Age (Years) *	Study Design	Indication for Surgery	Type of Surgery
1	(Jin et al., 2018) [44]	26	49.6 ± 14.7	Prospective cohort study	Thyroid cancer (23%) Benign thyroid disease (77%)	Open total thyroidectomy
2	(Benmiloud et al., 2020) [45]	241	53.6 ± 13.6	Prospective multicenter RCT	Thyroid cancer 56 (23.2%) Benign thyroid disease 185 (76.8%)	Open total thyroidectomy

Table 1. *Cont.*

s/n	Study	Number of Patients	Age (Years) *	Study Design	Indication for Surgery	Type of Surgery
3	(Kose et al., 2020) [46]	310 patients; 173 underwent thyroid surgery	55.6 ± 15.2	Prospective clinical study	Thyroid cancer 39 (13%) Benign thyroid nodule/multinodular goiter 115 (37%) Hyperthyroidism 19 (6%) Hyperparathyroidism 137 (44%)	Open total thyroidectomy 139 (45%) Thyroid lobectomy 34 (11%) Parathyroidectomy 137 (44%)
4	(Enny et al., 2020) [47]	72	39.2 ± 11.9	Prospective cohort study	Thyroid cancer 14 (18%) Benign thyroid disease 58 (69%)	Open total thyroidectomy
5	(Razavi et al., 2019) [48]	111 43—ICG 68—conventional	ICG: 50.51 ± 1.98 Conventional: 51.56 ± 1.46	Retrospective case–control study	**ICG**: Thyroid cancer (36.8%) Benign conditions (45.1%) **Conventional**: Thyroid cancer (34.9%) Benign conditions (44.6%)	Laparoscopic total or completion thyroidectomy
6	(McWade et al., 2019) [43]	30	Range: 32–70	Prospective clinical study	Thyroid diseases including cancer 12 (40%) Parathyroid diseases 15 (50%) Both 3 (10%)	Open thyroidectomy and parathyroidectomy
7	(Rudin et al., 2019) [49]	210 86—ICG 124—conventional	ICG: 47 Control: 49	Retrospective case–control study	**ICG**: Thyroid cancer (56%) Benign conditions (44%) **Control**: Thyroid cancer (65%) Benign conditions (35%)	Open total/near-total thyroidectomy
8	(van den Bos et al., 2019) [50]	30 surgeries in 26 patients	56.3 ± 16	Prospective clinical study	Suspected thyroid cancer 17 (56.7%) Proven thyroid cancer 7 (23.3%) Benign thyroid disease 6 (20.0%)	Open total thyroidectomy, completion thyroidectomy, and hemithyroidectomy
9	(Falco et al., 2017) [51]	74	48.4 ± 13.5	Retrospective clinical study	Thyroid cancer 35 (47%) Goiter 23 (31%) Primary hyperparathyroidism 13 (18%) Hyperthyroidism 3 (4%)	Not stated
10	(Lang et al., 2017) [52]	94	54.5 ± 15.0	Prospective clinical study	Thyroid cancer 12 (17.1%) Benign pathology 38 (54.3%) Graves' disease/toxic goiter 15 (21.4%) Indeterminate cytology 5 (7.1%)	Open total thyroidectomy

Table 1. *Cont.*

s/n	Study	Number of Patients	Age (Years) *	Study Design	Indication for Surgery	Type of Surgery
11	(Serra et al., 2020) [53]	105 45—study 65—control	Study group: 61.4 ± 15.5 Control: 61.6 ± 12.1	Prospective case–control study	**Study**: Malignant 20 (33.3%) Benign 40 (66.7%) **Control**: Malignant 8 (17.8%) Benign 37 (82.2%)	Open total thyroidectomy
12	(Lerchenberger et al., 2019) [54]	50	47.2	Prospective clinical study	Thyroid cancer 12 Benign thyroid disease 16 Parathyroidectomy 17	Open total thyroidectomy, hemithyroidectomy, and parathyroidectomy
13	(De Leeuw et al., 2016) [55]	35	40.9	Prospective clinical study	Benign and malignant thyroid diseases	Open total thyroidectomy, hemithyroidectomy, and parathyroidectomy
14	(Llorente et al., 2020) [56]	50	52 ± 12.9	Prospective cohort study	Thyroid cancer (70%) Multinodular goiter (26%) Graves' disease (4%)	Open total thyroidectomy
15	(S. W. Kim et al., 2016) [42]	8	Range: 34–73	Prospective clinical study	Papillary thyroid cancer	Open total thyroidectomy and hemithyroidectomy
16	(S. W. Kim et al., 2018) [57]	38	Not stated	Prospective clinical study	Papillary thyroid cancer	Open total thyroidectomy (44.7%) Unilateral lobectomy (55.3%)
17	(R. Ladurner et al., 2018) [58]	21	Not stated	Prospective clinical study	Thyroid diseases including thyroid cancer	Open thyroidectomy
18	(Roland Ladurner et al., 2019) [59]	117	49.9 Range: 19–81	Prospective clinical study	Thyroid cancer (21.3%) Thyroid benign (42.7%) Parathyroid disease (35.9%)	Total thyroidectomy, partial thyroidectomy, and parathyroidectomy
19	(Vidal Fortuny et al., 2016) [60]	36	49.8 ± 15.7	Prospective clinical study	Thyroid cancer (22.2%) Benign thyroid diseases (77.8%)	Total thyroidectomy
20	(Vidal Fortuny et al., 2018) [61]	196	Not stated	Prospective RCT	**Study group**: Malignancy 30 (41%) Benign 40 (59%) **Control**: Malignancy 17 (23%) Benign 56 (77%)	Completion thyroidectomy and total thyroidectomy
21	(Dip et al., 2019) [62]	170	47.3 ± 13.6	Prospective RCT	Thyroid cancer (48.2%) Benign conditions (51.8%)	Total thyroidectomy
22	(Zaidi et al., 2016) [63]	27	43.9 ± 1.0	Prospective feasibility study	Thyroid cancer (37.0%) Multinodular (48.2%) Graves' disease (14.8%)	Total thyroidectomy, completion thyroidectomy, and hemithyroidectomy

Table 1. *Cont.*

s/n	Study	Number of Patients	Age (Years) *	Study Design	Indication for Surgery	Type of Surgery
23	(Y. S. Kim et al., 2020) [64]	300 100—study 200—control	Study: 51.6 ± 15.2 Control: 50.2 ± 15.5	Retrospective case–control study	Thyroid cancer (55.3%) Benign thyroid disease (44.7%)	Total thyroidectomy
24	(Jin & Cui, 2020) [65]	56 28—test group 28—control group	42.68 ± 11.70	Randomized control trial	**Study group**: Malignancy 9 (32.1%) Benign thyroid disease 19 (67.9%) **Control**: Malignancy 9 (32.1%) Benign thyroid disease 19 (67.9%)	Total thyroidectomy
25	(D. H. Kim et al., 2021) [66]	542 261—NIRAF group 281—control group	NIRAF group: 51.30 ± 12.44 Control group: 52.83 ± 10.92	Retrospective study with historical control	All thyroid cancer patients	Total thyroidectomy with unilateral or bilateral central neck dissection

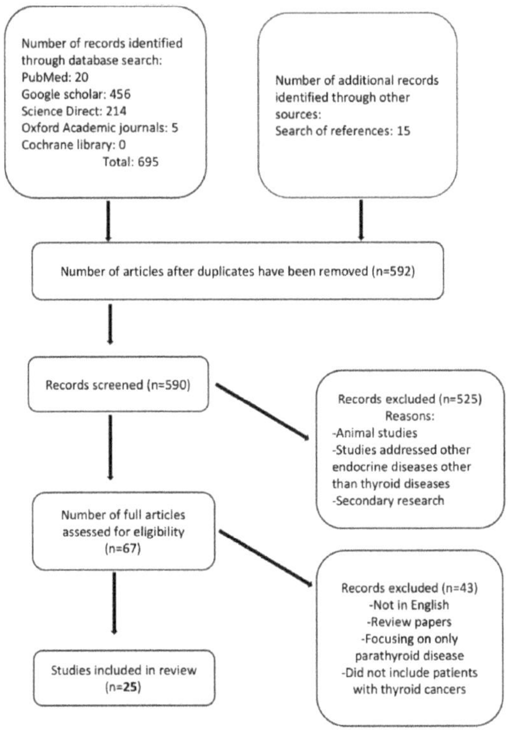

Figure 1. Flow diagram of study selection.

3.2. *Methodological Quality of Included Studies*

The risk of bias among the included studies was assessed using MINORS, as most of the studies were nonrandomized clinical studies. The maximum possible score was 16 for those without a control group and 24 for those with a control group. The mean quality score was 10.06 (range: 8–14) for noncomparative studies and 20 (range: 18–22) for comparative studies (Table 2). All but one study [53] clearly stated their aim. Nine studies adequately described the follow-up period, including the percentage lost to follow-up. No study included a prospective sample size calculation. All comparative studies had adequate control groups, and the study groups were contemporary with baseline equivalence of groups and adequate statistical analyses. In one study [49], the control group consisted of historical patients.

Table 2. Methodological Index for Non-Randomized Studies.

Study	A	B	C	D	E	F	G	H	I	J	K	L	Total
(Jin et al., 2018) [44]	2	2	2	2	2	2	2	0	X	X	X	X	14/16
(Benmiloud et al., 2020) [45]	2	2	2	2	2	2	2	0	2	2	2	2	22/24
(Kose et al., 2020) [46]	2	2	2	2	2	0	0	0	X	X	X	X	10/16
(Enny et al., 2020) [47]	2	2	2	1	2	1	0	0	X	X	X	X	10/16
(Razavi et al., 2019) [48]	2	2	2	2	2	2	2	0	2	2	2	2	22/24
(McWade et al., 2019) [43]	2	2	2	2	2	0	0	0	X	X	X	X	10/16
(Rudin et al., 2019) [49]	2	2	0	2	2	2	2	0	2	0	2	2	18/24
(van den Bos et al., 2019) [50]	2	2	2	2	2	1	0	0	X	X	X	X	11/16
(Falco et al., 2017) [51]	2	2	2	2	1	0	0	0	X	X	X	X	9/16
(Lang et al., 2017) [52]	2	2	2	2	2	0	0	0	X	X	X	X	10/16
(Serra et al., 2020) [53]	1	2	2	2	2	2	0	0	2	2	2	2	19/24
(Lerchenberger et al., 2019) [54]	2	2	2	1	1	0	0	0	X	X	X	X	8/16
(De Leeuw et al., 2016) [55]	2	2	2	2	0	0	0	0	X	X	X	X	8/16
(Llorente et al., 2020) [56]	2	2	2	2	0	2	0	0	X	X	X	X	10/16
(S. W. Kim et al., 2016) [42]	2	2	2	2	1	0	2	0	X	X	X	X	11/16
(S. W. Kim et al., 2018) [57]	2	2	2	2	1	0	2	0	X	X	X	X	11/16
(R. Ladurner et al., 2018) [58]	2	2	2	2	1	0	0	0	X	X	X	X	9/16
(Roland Ladurner et al., 2019) [54]	2	2	2	2	1	0	0	0	X	X	X	X	9/16
(Vidal Fortuny et al., 2016) [60]	2	2	2	2	2	0	0	0	X	X	X	X	10/16
(Vidal Fortuny et al., 2018) [61]	2	2	2	2	2	2	2	0	2	2	2	2	22/24
(Dip et al., 2019) [62]	2	2	2	2	2	2	2	0	2	2	2	2	22/24
(Zaidi et al., 2016) [63]	2	2	2	2	1	0	2	0	X	X	X	X	11/16
(Y. S. Kim et al., 2020) [64]	2	2	1	2	1	2	0	0	2	1	2	2	17/24
(Jin & Cui, 2020) [65]	2	2	2	2	1	2	0	0	2	2	2	2	19/24
(D. H. Kim et al., 2021) [66]	2	2	1	2	2	2	2	0	2	1	2	2	19/24

Items are scored as 0 (not reported), 1 (reported but inadequate), or 2 (reported and adequate). The maximum score is 16 for noncomparative studies and 24 for comparative studies. A—A clearly stated aim; B—Inclusion of consecutive patients; C—Prospective collection of data; D—Endpoints appropriate for the aim of the study; E—Unbiased assessment of study endpoint; F—Follow-up period appropriate for the aim of the study; G—Loss to follow-up less than 5%; H—Prospective calculation of the study size; I—Adequate control group; J—Contemporary groups; K—Baseline equivalence of groups; L—Adequate statistical analyses.

3.3. *Type of Fluorescence (Exogenous or Autofluorescence)*

NIR autofluorescence (NIRAF) alone was used in 11 studies, whereas an exogenous fluorophore was employed in 14 studies. Lerchenberger et al. [54] compared the usefulness of autofluorescence with an exogenous fluorophore, while Ladurner et al. assessed the utility of both autofluorescence and exogenous fluorophore, although not comparatively [59]. Dip et al. [62] compared the use of white light alone with the use of both autofluorescence and white light in the identification of PGs. ICG was used in all but one of the studies using exogenous fluorophores. Enny et al. used 500 mg of fluorescein dye to produce fluorescence in the PGs [47]. The ICG dose was 5 mg in five studies and 2.5 mg in two studies. Two studies reported the administration of repeat doses to a maximum of 5 mg/kg/day [60,61]. The fluorescence system varied from study to study, with the Fluobeam 800 system (Fluoptics, Grenoble, France) being the most common (five studies). The system was not specified in two studies [48,56] (Table 3). An image showing the autofluorescence of the PGs (Figure 2A) and the sequence of ICG angiography (ICGA) (Figure 2B,C) is provided in Figure 2.

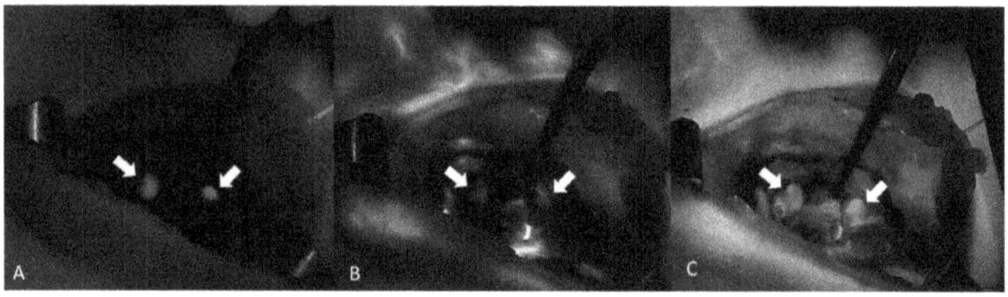

Figure 2. A sequence of images showing ICGA of two PGs (arrows) from A to C. (**A**) Autofluorescence of the PG before the injection of ICG. (**B**,**C**) Diffusion of the ICG contrast agent confirming a well-vascularized PG (Fluobeam LX®—Fluoptics©, Grenoble, France).

Table 3. Fluorescence type, dosage, timing, and fluorescence system.

Study	Autofluorescence or Exogenous Dye	Type of Exogenous Dye	Dose	Timing of Administration	Fluorescence System
(De Leeuw et al., 2016) [55]	AF	NA	NA	NA	Fluobeam 800 clinical system (Fluoptics, Grenoble, France)
(Serra et al., 2020) [53]	AF	NA	NA	NA	Custom NIRAF device (Thorlabs GmbH, Dachau, Deutschland and CCD Sony ICX254AL image detector)
(McWade et al., 2019) [43]	AF	NA	NA	NA	Overlay tissue imaging system (OTIS)
(Benmiloud et al., 2020) [45]	AF	NA	NA	NA	Fluobeam 800 system (Fluoptics)
(Kose et al., 2020) [46]	AF	NA	NA	NA	Fluobeam device (Fluoptics)
(S. W. Kim et al., 2016) [42]	AF	NA	NA	NA	Digital camera, NIR light-emitting diode (LED), and IR illuminating lights
(S. W. Kim et al., 2018) [57]	AF	NA	NA	NA	M780L3-C1, Thorlabs, Newton, NJ, USA and INFRALUX-300, Daekyung Electro Medical Co., Republic of Korea
(R. Ladurner et al., 2018) [58]	AF	NA	NA	NA	NIR/ICG endoscopic system (Karl Storz, Tuttlingen, Germany).
(Y. S. Kim et al., 2020) [64]	AF	NA	NA	NA	Fluobeam; Fluoptics, Grenoble, France
(D. H. Kim et al., 2021) [66]	AF	NA	NA	NA	Modified DSLR camera and LED (M780L3-C1, Thorlabs, New Jersey, USA) light source
(Dip et al., 2019) [62]	White light alone vs. AF + white light	NA	NA	NA	Fluobeam 800 system (Fluoptics)

Table 3. *Cont.*

Study	Autofluorescence or Exogenous Dye	Type of Exogenous Dye	Dose	Timing of Administration	Fluorescence System
(Lerchenberger et al., 2019) [54]	AF vs. exogenous	ICG	5 mg	After lateral mobilization of the thyroid and exposure of the RLN	NIR/ICG endoscopic system (Karl Storz, Tuttlingen, Germany).
(Roland Ladurner et al., 2019) [59]	AF and exogenous	ICG-Pulsion	5 mg	After lateral mobilization of the thyroid gland	Storz laparoscopic NIR/ICG imaging system
(Falco et al., 2017) [51]	Exogenous	ICG	0.5 mL	After exposure of the thyroid gland	NIRL (near infrared light) using a laser system
(Lang et al., 2017) [52]	Exogenous	ICG	2.5 mg	After resection of the thyroid gland	SPY fluorescent imaging system (Novadaq Technologies, Inc., Mississauga, ON, Canada)
(Jin et al., 2018) [44]	Exogenous	ICG	5 mg	After adequate exposure of each central neck compartment	Intraoperative navigation system (Digi-MIH-001-I, Digital Precision Medicine Technology Co., Ltd., Beijing, China); fluorescence imaging system
(Llorente et al., 2020) [56]	Exogenous	ICG	Not stated	After thyroid resection	Not specified
(Enny et al., 2020) [47]	Exogenous	Fluorescein dye	500 mg	After thyroid gland resection	LED blue light
(Razavi et al., 2019) [48]	Exogenous	ICG	5 mg	At the end of surgery	Not specified
(Rudin et al., 2019) [49]	Exogenous	ICG	6 mL (3 per side)	At the end of surgery	Laparoscopic PINPOINT camera (NOVADAQ, ON, Canada)
(van den Bos et al., 2019) [50]	Exogenous	ICG	7.5 mg twice, i.e., 15 mg	Before and after resection of the thyroid gland	Laparoscopic fluorescence imaging system (Karl Storz GmbH & Co., Tuttlingen, Germany)
(Vidal Fortuny et al., 2016) [60]	Exogenous	ICG	3 to 5 mL doses (75–150 mg) up to 5 mg/kg/day	After excision of the thyroid gland	Laparoscopic PINPOINT® camera (Novadaq, ON, Canada)
(Vidal Fortuny et al., 2018) [61]	Exogenous	ICG	2.5 mg doses up to 5 mg/kg/day	After excision of the thyroid gland	NIR camera (Pinpoint®; Novadaq, Toronto, ON, Canada
(Zaidi et al., 2016) [63]	Exogenous	ICG	5 mg	Before and after thyroid resection	Pinpoint video-assisted NIR system (Novadaq, Inc., Toronto, ON, Canada)
(Jin & Cui, 2020) [65]	Exogenous	ICG	5 mg/kg	After resection of thyroid lobes	Digi-MIH-I-001, Digital Precision Medicine Technology Co., Ltd, Beijing, China

AF—Autofluorescence; ICG—Indocyanine green; NA—not applicable.

3.4. Parathyroid Gland Visualization and Preservation

Twenty-three studies reported on the visualization and/or preservation of the PGs during thyroid surgery. Four of these studies [45,49,51,53] demonstrated improved visualization of the PGs using fluorescence imaging compared with conventional thyroid surgery. However, van den Bos et al. [23] showed better visualization with white light compared with NIR imaging. Lerchenberger et al. [54] reported that although autofluorescence demonstrated slightly better visualization of the PGs, it could not indicate whether the blood supply to the gland was still viable, in contrast to the use of ICG. Several studies also reported that fluorescence was used to identify PGs in resected segments or those whose blood supply had been disrupted, which were autotransplanted [57,60,62,67]. In the larger series of Kim et al. (542 patients), no statistical difference in PG visualization was observed between an NIRAF group and the control group (3.91 ± 0.36 vs. 3.90 ± 0.39; $p = 0.351$) [66]. Enny et al. [47] reported better visualization of the PGs using the naked eye than using fluorescein dye, although the difference was not significant. Corresponding data are shown in Table 4.

Table 4. Parathyroid gland visualization and preservation, postoperative serum parathyroid hormone levels, and postoperative serum calcium levels.

Study	PG Visualization and Preservation	Postoperative Serum PTH	Postoperative Serum Calcium
(Jin et al., 2018) [44]	Among 104 PGs, 86 were identified.	In the 22 patients with at least one PG with an ICG score of 2, postoperative PTH levels were normal. In four patients, ICG did not demonstrate a well-vascularized PG. Two of these patients developed transient hypoparathyroidism.	None of the patients developed hypocalcemia at the time of measurement.
(Benmiloud et al., 2020) [45]	The rate of patients with four identified PGs was higher in the NIRAF group (47.1% (95% CI, 38.5–56.4%)) than in the standard-care group (19.2% (95% CI, 12.1–26.2%); $p < 0.001$)	The PTH concentration at POD 1 was not significantly lower in the standard-care group (median (IQR), 28.6 (12.0–46.5) pg/mL) than in the NIRAF group (median (IQR), 33.2 (21.9–48.1) pg/mL).	The postoperative hypocalcemia rate was significantly lower in the NIRAF group (9.1% (95% CI, 4.0–14.2%)) than in the standard-care group (21.7% (95% CI, 14.3–29.0%); $p = 0.007$).
(Kose et al., 2020) [46]	For patients that underwent thyroidectomy, AF was demonstrated in 496 (98.6%) of the PGs; 33% had been first identified with NIRAF prior to visual recognition by the surgeon. In 5%, NIFI helped identify incidentally resected PGs.	Not measured	Not measured
(Enny et al., 2020) [47]	Two PGs in 30 (44.4%) patients, 0 PGs in 6 (6.9%) patients, and 4 PGs in 7 (9.7%) patients were visualized with fluorescein dye. With naked eye evaluation, 0 PGs in 1 patient, 2 PGs in 29 (41.7%) patients, and 4 PGs in 11 (15.3%) patients were visualized.	Not measured	Clinical hypocalcemia was observed in all patients in whom no PGs were visualized with fluorescein dye, whereas none of the patients in whom three or four PGs were visualized developed hypocalcemia. Among patients in whom three or four PGs were observed by the naked eye, 7 (28%) and 3 (23.7%) patients developed clinical hypocalcemia, respectively.
(Razavi et al., 2019) [48]	Not specified	Mean postoperative PTH decreased by 23.48 pg/mL for conventional care and 29.24 pg/mL for ICG.	Symptomatic hypocalcemia was observed in 3.90% of those who underwent conventional treatment and 7.90% of those in the ICG group.

Table 4. *Cont.*

Study	PG Visualization and Preservation	Postoperative Serum PTH	Postoperative Serum Calcium
(McWade et al., 2019) [43]	In total, 67 (97%) of exposed tissues of interest were correctly visualized as PGs.	Not measured	Not measured
(Rudin et al., 2019) [49]	Identification and autotransplantation were more common in the ICGA group at 36%, compared with 12% in the control group (p = 0.0001).	At POD 1, PTH was found to be low in 36% of controls and 37% of ICGA patients. An undetectable PTH level was present in 14% of control patients and 15% of ICGA patients. One patient in each group had permanent hypoparathyroidism.	Not measured
(van den Bos et al., 2019) [50]	In total, 41 PGs were visualized with white light in 25 patients, whereas 31 PGs were identified in 23 patients by NIRAF imaging.	Not measured	Three patients had transient hypocalcemia that resolved after 2 weeks.
(Falco et al., 2017) [51]	The mean number of identified PGs was 2.5 (±0.8) and 3.7 (±0.7) with WL (white light) and NIRAF respectively. In 86.5% (n = 64) of patients, four PGs were identified with NIFI, whereas four PGs were visualized with WL in only 12.2% (n = 9) of patients.	Not measured	Not stated
(Lang et al., 2017) [52]	A total of 340 PGs were identified, and 324 (95.3%) PGs were later confirmed to be PGs on histology.	Not measured	Nine (12.9%) patients developed transient hypocalcemia, while no patients had permanent hypocalcemia. There was a significant relationship between intensity of fluorescence image and the development of hypocalcemia. No patients with a greatest fluorescent light intensity developed postoperative hypocalcemia
(Serra et al., 2020) [53]	The mean number of PGs identified per patient was 3.47 in the study group and 2.33 in the control group (p < 0.0001).	Determinations of PTH 24 h after surgery showed a statistically significant difference favoring the study group.	In the study group, 24.4% presented 24-h postoperative hypocalcemia vs. 30% of the control group. At 6 months postoperation, three patients in the control group had permanent hypocalcemia, compared with no patients in the study group.
(Lerchenberger et al., 2019) [54]	A total of 64 (82%) PGs were visualized with AF; AF could not indicate whether the blood supply was still viable. On ICG administration, 63 PGs (81%) showed persistent fluorescence after a decrease in thyroid fluorescence.	Not measured	Only two patients developed transient hypocalcemia. No patients had permanent hypocalcemia
(De Leeuw et al., 2016) [55]	In total, 80 PGs were identified using the NIR system, and 81 glands were confirmed on frozen section to be PGs.	Not measured	Not measured
(Llorente et al., 2020) [56]	Not specified	Not measured	Eleven (22%) patients developed postoperative hypocalcemia. ICGA would allow immediate decision-making without the need to wait for intraoperative PTH measurements.
(S. W. Kim et al., 2016) [42]	All PGs were visualized.	No patient had postoperative hypoparathyroidism.	Not measured
(S. W. Kim et al., 2018) [57]	All but one PG were identified in vivo and preserved. The excised PG was autotransplanted	Not measured	Only one patient had transient hypocalcemia.

Table 4. *Cont.*

Study	PG Visualization and Preservation	Postoperative Serum PTH	Postoperative Serum Calcium
(R. Ladurner et al., 2018) [58]	Of the 41 PGs examined, 37 were identified by AF. AF assisted the preservation and autotransplantation of PGs in two patients	Not measured	Not measured
(Roland Ladurner et al., 2019) [59]	In total, 179 PGs (87.3%) displayed NIRAF showing a typical bluish violet color.	Not measured	Not measured
(Vidal Fortuny et al., 2016) [60]	Of the 36 patients who underwent ICGA, 30 had an ICG score of 2 for at least one PG. Autotransplantation was performed for those with poor ICG scores.	In the 30 patients with at least one PG with an ICG score of 2, postoperative PTH levels were in the normal range.	The postoperative adjusted calcium levels were within the normal range in 29 (80.6%) patients.
(Vidal Fortuny et al., 2018) [61]	In 146 patients, at least one preserved PG had an ICG score of 2.	Hypoparathyroidism was not observed in either group.	Hypocalcemia was not observed in either group.
(Dip et al., 2019) [62]	With NIRI, an average of 2.6 (0.85) PGs were detected prior to dissection. In four patients, PGs were transplanted after identification with NIRI.	Not measured	Significantly higher mean serum calcium levels were observed in the study group, with 8.2% having serum calcium <8 mg/dL compared with 16.5% in the control group. However, 1.2% in both groups required long-term calcium replacement, which was resolved by 6 months.
(Zaidi et al., 2016) [63]	A total of 71 (84%) PGs were identified on fluorescence.	The mean POD-1 PTH level of patients with at least two glands exhibiting <30% fluorescence at completion of thyroidectomy was 9 pg/dL, whereas those with fewer than two glands demonstrating <30% fluorescence had a POD-1 PTH of 19.5 pg/dL (p = 0.05).	Postoperatively, three patients (11%) had a serum calcium value <8 mg/dL, and one patient was symptomatic.
(Y. S. Kim et al., 2020) [64]	The mean number of PGs identified intraoperatively was similar between the two groups. The rate of incidental parathyroidectomy reported by pathology was higher in the conventional group (14%) than in the NIFI group (6%) (p = 0.039).	The POD-1 value was 23.9 pg/mL (17.6) in the NIRI group and 23.0 pg/mL (22.4) in the control group. The POD-14 level was 38.9 pg/mL (35.5) in the NIRI group and 35.8 pg/mL (26.1) in the control group.	At POD 1, the NIFI group had a level of 9.0 mg/dL (0.6) compared with 8.8 mg/dL (0.6) for the control group (p = 0.004). At POD 14, the NIFI group had a value of 8.8 mg/dL (0.6), compared with 8.6 mg/dL (0.6) for the control group (p = 0.008). All 5 patients with postoperative hypocalcemia in the NIFI group recovered within 2 weeks, while 1 of 14 patients with postoperative hypocalcemia in the conventional group had persistent hypocalcemia beyond 6 months.
Jin & Cui, 2020) [65]	In total, 186 PGs were visualized in 56 patients.	No patient in either group developed hypoparathyroidism.	No patient in either group developed hypocalcemia.
(D. H. Kim et al., 2021) [66]	PGs were found in 244 cases (93.5%) in the NIRAF group and in 260 cases (92.5%) in the control group. The mean count of identified PGs was 3.91 ± 0.36 in the NIRAF group vs. 3.90 ± 0.39 in the control group (p = 0.351).	The incidence of transient postoperative hypoparathyroidism was significantly lower in the NIRAF group than in the control group during hospitalization (33.7% vs. 46.6%; p = 0.002) and at 1 month (8.8% vs. 18.9%; p = 0.001)	The incidence of hypocalcemia during hospitalization was 6.5% in the NIRAF group and 10.0% in the control group. There was no significant difference in the rate of hypocalcemia between the two groups for any follow-up period.

PG—Parathyroid gland; ICG—Indocyanine green; NIRI—Near-infrared imaging; POD—postoperative day; AF—autofluorescence; NIRAF—near-infrared autofluorescence.

3.5. Postoperative Serum Parathyroid Hormone

Thirteen of the 25 studies reported on postoperative parathyroid hormone (PTH) levels. Some studies using ICG reported that having at least one well-perfused PG (with an ICG score of 2) after thyroid gland resection predicted normal postoperative PTH [44,60,65]. None of the comparative studies found a statistically significant relationship for postoperative PTH levels between study and control groups, except for [66], which found a statistically significant lower incidence of transient hypoparathyroidism in the NIRAF group (33.7% vs. 46.6%; $p = 0.002$). Three studies [45,48,49] demonstrated better PTH levels for fluorescence-guided surgery (Table 4).

3.6. Effects on the Autotransplantation Rate

DiMarco et al. [68] stated that NIRAF imaging might detect inadvertent parathyroidectomy and allow autotransplantation, even though no difference between the NIRAF imaging and control groups was found. Similarly, Ladurner et al. [58] stated that NIRAF imaging assisted in identifying several inferior parathyroid glands that otherwise would have been lost for autotransplantation. Bellier et al. [69] found that NIRAF imaging can help detect the accidental removal of parathyroid glands and that 60% of these glands can be spared and autotransplanted during the surgery. In the controlled study of Benmiloud et al. [70], NIRAF imaging appeared to reduce the autotransplantation rate (from 15% to 2.1%) and the inadvertent parathyroid resection rate (from 7.2% to 1.1%) thanks to improved parathyroid gland identification. These findings were confirmed later by the same author [45] in a study utilizing NIRAF imaging to detect a reduction in the inadvertent resection rate (from 11.7 to 2.5; $p = 0.006$) and the autotransplantation rate (from 13.3 to 3.3; $p = 0.009$).

Kim et al. [64] found that the rate of incidental parathyroidectomy was higher in the conventional (14%) versus NIRAF imaging group (6%) ($p = 0.039$) despite similar autotransplantation rates (4% vs 6%, respectively; $p = 0.562$). This was in line with another study [66] reporting that the number of inadvertently resected PGs (in the pathologic specimen) was significantly lower in the NIRAF group (12.8% vs 6.9%; $p = 0.021$), but that the number of autotransplanted PGs in both groups was similar.

The autotransplantation rate based on ICG angiography was approximately 17% [52]; however, some authors [49] found it significantly increased not only in the ICG group compared to the control group (36% vs. 12%; $p = 0.0001$), but also comparing the ICG group with the NIRAF group [54].

Several authors [49,71] have stated that ICG angiography can guide more appropriate autotransplantation without compromising postoperative parathyroid function. This is in contrast with Razavi et al. [48], who assert that ICG angiography may lead to unnecessary parathyroid autotransplantation because low-flow ICG patterns are not associated with postoperative PTH changes or transient hypocalcemia.

3.7. Postoperative Serum Calcium

As shown in Table 4, 17 studies reported on postoperative hypocalcemia among their patients. Some demonstrated an absence of postoperative hypocalcemia [44,60,66].

Benmiloud et al. reported a significantly lower rate of hypocalcemia in the NIRAF group compared with the standard group (14.3% vs. 21.7%; $p = 0.007$) [45]. Permanent hypocalcemia was reported in only one study, where three patients in the control group (conventional surgery) required calcium supplementation over 6 months, as opposed to no patients in the study group (autofluorescence) [53]. Razavi et al. [48] observed hypocalcemia in 7.9% of the ICG group versus 3.9% of the conventional group. Dip et al. [62] reported higher mean serum calcium levels in the study group compared with the control group, although this finding did not reach a level of statistical significance. In a study in which patients with an ICG score of at least 2 in one PG were randomized into two groups, of which one group received calcium supplementation and the other did not [65], none of the participants in either group had hypocalcemia. Moreover, there were no significant differences in serum calcium levels between the two groups.

3.8. Additional Duration of Surgery

The duration of surgery or additional time spent on NIR imaging during surgery was given in 10 of the 25 studies, with an additional time of 3–10 min for the procedure. In one study [45], the procedures in the NIRAF group required an additional time of 8 min compared with those in the standard group, which is in contrast with another study [64]. The total operating time was not significantly affected by NIRAF imaging in another study [57]. In contrast, a different study reported that NIRAF added 5–8 min to the operating time, with ICG use adding another 3 min [54]. Four other studies [57,59,60,62] also reported that NIR imaging required an additional time of 3–10 min.

The average durations of the entire procedure were 92 $\pm$ 32 min and 109.1 $\pm$ 49.8 min in two studies [50,52], with 5 min spent on NIR imaging in [50].

3.9. Complications Related to Technique

No complications attributed to the technique were reported in any of the articles.

3.10. Cost

None of the included studies described the cost implication of using NIR imaging.

4. Discussion

An increasing number of scientific reports have investigated the utility of fluorescence-guided surgery in preserving the PGs and preventing hypoparathyroidism as a complication of thyroid surgery. However, only three studies have addressed thyroid cancer patients alone. In contrast, in the majority of reports, the patient cohorts are mixed, including both benign and malignant indications and thyroid as well as parathyroid diseases. According to the available literature, NIRAF imaging improves the visualization and preservation of the PGs during thyroidectomy. This technique is feasible and safe, as NIRAF imaging is non-invasive. Moreover, no NIR imaging-related complications were reported in any of the studies, including the studies with ICG injection.

Among the included reports, NIRAF was used in 11 studies, and an exogenous fluorophore was employed in 14 studies. Because NIRAF exploits the endogenous fluorophore of the PGs, no additional time is required to administer an exogenous dye [42]. Consequently, the only equipment required for NIRAF imaging is a fluorescence camera system. A comparative study of NIRAF and ICG imaging found only a minimal difference in the usefulness of both techniques for identifying the PGs [54]. However, preserved perfusion can be visualized only by the introduction of a contrast agent (e.g., ICG) via the blood stream. Therefore, NIRAF is technically inappropriate for assessing the integrity of arterial supply and venous outflow. In contrast to ICG, NIRAF cannot determine the vascular integrity of the PG. ICG has a short half-life of 3–5 min and is eliminated by the hepatic system after approximately 15 min [19]. Hence, repeated doses can be required and safely administered [50,60,61]. The toxic dose in adults is 5 mg/kg circulating per time point [19]. All doses administered in the included studies were well below this threshold. ICG was administered intravenously in all cases, and a duration of 1–3 min was required for the PG to take up the ICG [44,48,52,72]. Upon excitation with NIR light, the fluorescence produced by the gland was scored as 0, 1, or 2 if the gland appeared black (not vascular), grey (partially vascular), or white (vascular), respectively [48,60,61].

The prevailing causes of hypoparathyroidism after thyroidectomy are disruption of the blood supply to the glands and their incidental removal. These complications are more frequently seen in thyroidectomy for thyroid cancer [19], especially with accompanying lymph node resection. Because of the ability of NIR imaging to visualize the PGs and to detect impaired blood supply to the glands during thyroid cancer surgery, this technique is invaluable in averting hypoparathyroidism. In a randomized controlled trial, there was a significant difference between the number of PGs identified with NIRAF compared with conventional surgery. The percentage of patients with four identified PGs was higher in the NIRAF group than in the standard-care group (47.1% vs. 19.2%, respectively; $p < 0.001$). Consequently, the number of incidentally resected PGs was significantly lower in the NIRAF group [45]. In another controlled study, visual and ICGA assessment of vascularity showed agreement in 87% of cases. ICGA prevented autotransplantation of 19 (6.8%) glands that were shown to be adequately perfused on ICGA, but would have been transplanted if visual inspection alone had been used. Interestingly, autotransplantation of the PGs was significantly more common among the ICGA group than the control group (36% vs. 12%, $p = 0.0001$) [49].

In a retrospective study [51], the use of white light and the use of ICG and NIR imaging were compared for identifying the PGs at an early dissection stage. The surgeons documented the number of PGs that were visualized with the naked eye using white light. Next, the operating room's light was turned off, and the surgical field was illuminated with NIR light. The number of PGs visualized with NIR light was significantly higher than in white light. Furthermore, the integrity of the blood supply to the PGs was assessed via ICGA in cases of ambiguity. Perfusion was intact in all cases; hence, no autotransplantation was performed. While the majority of the studies in this review reported improved visualization of the PGs in favor of NIR fluorescence imaging, one study [50] reported slightly better visualization of the glands in white light. It is possible that the bright background signal of highly vascularized malignant tissue may have interfered with visualization on fluorescence imaging. In the same study, the majority of surgeons considered NIR fluorescence imaging to be advantageous. The reduction in both the autotransplantation rate and the inadvertent parathyroid resection rate, which are both risk factors for postoperative hypocalcemia, reported by studies in this review is corroborated by Fanaropoulou et al. [19].

The largest series reported in the literature included 542 patients [66] and focused exclusively on thyroid cancer. This study found no significant differences in the number of visualized PGs between the NIRAF group and the conventional group. This finding could be due to the substantial experience of the surgeon. The same article still reported a significantly lower incidence of transient hypoparathyroidism in the NIRAF group compared with the control group. Based on the large series included in this study and the quality of the study, this statement seems to be well supported.

Visualization of the PGs alone may not be sufficient to prevent postoperative sequelae. Dissection may lead to inadvertent damage to the end arteries that supply the PGs. Hence, some studies addressed the assessment of PGs after resection of the thyroid gland to ensure its viability and/or the need for autotransplantation [47,48,52]. Enny et al. [47] found that the identification of PG viability by NIR imaging visualization of intact vascularity at the end of the procedure is associated with a reduced need for routine postoperative calcium and vitamin D supplementation, along with reductions in accompanying costs and duration of hospital stay. However, some authors [48] recommend that surgeons interpret these results with caution, as their study on the use of ICGA did not show a significant improvement in thyroid surgery outcomes. In particular, poor vascular perfusion on ICGA did not correlate with a postoperative reduction in PTH levels or transient hypocalcemia. The ability of ICGA to detect impaired perfusion and to induce a change in surgical strategy was demonstrated in colorectal surgery with a positive outcome [23].

Thirteen studies reported on postoperative PTH levels, whereas 17 studies reported serum calcium levels. Jin et al. [73] performed a small study assessing PG perfusion via ICGA after resection of the first thyroid lobe, with serum PTH and calcium levels assayed on postoperative day (POD) 1, 7, and 14, and 6 months after operation. PGs that had been accidentally devascularized during the surgery were identified using ICGA and were autotransplanted. Their findings showed that the ICGA score was predictive of postoperative PTH levels, as all of the 22 patients with at least one PG having an ICG score of 2 (84.6%) had normal postoperative PTH levels, while half of those with poor vascularization on ICGA developed transient hypoparathyroidism. Similar findings were reported in another study [60], where all patients with at least one well-vascularized gland as detected by ICGA (83.3%) had normal serum PTH levels. One of these patients had asymptomatic hypocalcemia at POD 10. In contrast, two out of six patients with poor vascularization on ICGA developed transient hypoparathyroidism. Overall, postoperative supplementation with calcium or vitamin D was averted in all patients. Thus, ICGA can be used intraoperatively to determine whether at least one PG remains vascularized and functional, in order to predict the absence of postoperative hypoparathyroidism.

The use of fluorescein dye to visualize the PGs was found to be superior to naked eye assessment with regard to preventing hypocalcemia. Among patients with >3 PGs visualized via fluorescein dye, none suffered clinical hypocalcemia, as opposed to more than 20% with clinical hypocalcemia when >3 PGs were visualized with the naked eye only [47].

Several comparative studies [45,53,64] reported better postoperative PTH and calcium levels among NIR imaging groups compared with conventional surgery groups, but the opposite trend was observed by others [48,49]. Among the latter, Razavi et al. suggested that intraoperative monitoring of PTH levels should remain, which they suggest as a better method than ICGA for predicting PG vascularization. Rudin et al. opined that the potential of ICGA to quickly identify PGs and to positively alter surgical strategy cannot be ignored, but that more research should be conducted to determine whether this practice reduces the risk of postoperative hypoparathyroidism.

This controversy is fueled by a lack of standardization among NIR fluorescence techniques, such as in the timing of assessment and the quantification of fluorescent signal intensity. PG visualization can be enhanced with NIR imaging prior to any dissection or during thyroid dissection. Early identification can prevent inadvertent resection or impairment of vascular supply. In this way, NIR imaging can contribute to the preservation of all PGs. The distinction between the more intense fluorescence of the PGs compared with that of the lymph nodes can provide guidance during lymphadenectomy. Late detection, such as that performed on the specimen, can allow functional recovery of the PG with autotransplantation. Contrast-enhanced fluorescence imaging with intravenous ICG or fluorescein injection can visualize preserved versus impaired perfusion (e.g., congruent results shown intraoperatively for adrenal perfusion) [9]. However, except for quantitative contrast-enhanced NIR imaging research protocols [74], fluorescent signals and ICG scores are generally assessed subjectively. For ICG injections, the rate at which the fluorescence signal intensity increases, as well as the added signal intensity produced by reinjections, can only be objectively assessed with a quantitative approach, which has not yet been integrated into commercially available NIR imaging systems.

Furthermore, it can be concluded from this review that the use of NIR imaging is safe and feasible. No study reported any complication arising from this technique. Rare allergic reactions to ICG have been previously reported [75]. These reactions are particularly attributable to iodine or sodium iodide, which is often added to improve fluorophore solubility [19]. Therefore, patients with iodine allergy are not eligible for ICG administration. However, ICG solutions without iodine are commercially available (e.g., INFRACYANINE, SERB S.à.r.l.); thus, this categorical exclusion of patients for iodine allergy or hyperthyroid status might be lifted in the future.

Several studies in this review reported minimal added time (3–10 min) for NIR imaging but this was shown as not statistically significative [45,54,62]; anyway, this added time would be negligible, considering the benefits of the technique. Similar findings were reported by van den Bos et al. [50]. Interestingly, and in contrast to the observation of a longer duration with the use of fluorescence imaging, two studies reported that more time was spent during conventional surgery [45,64]. Although this trend was not elucidated, it may have been due to a more rapid identification of the glands using autofluorescence, without the added duration needed for the administration and uptake of an exogenous fluorophore.

Concerning ICGA, among the authors who analyzed this factor, the procedure required an additional operative time of 2–5 min; however, this approach has the benefit of eliminating any doubt on the viability of the explored PGs. Moreover, according to some authors [47,61], ICGA can also prevent systematical postoperative calcium supplementation, thus eventually reducing the hospital stay. The use of fluorescence imaging in surgery has been reported as cost-effective [44,76]. However, no study in the present review stated the cost implication of NIR imaging, which is mainly associated with equipment purchase. The camera systems required for NIR imaging can be expensive. However, once a fluorescence system is installed, autofluorescence creates no further cost. Hence, the additional cost is limited to the price of the exogenous fluorophore used per patient [77] and the sterile cover. When assessed in light of the deleterious health effects and economic burden of hypoparathyroidism and hypocalcemia, NIR imaging can be viewed as very cost-effective, as demonstrated by its positive impact.

In a cost–benefit analysis on the usefulness of routine intraoperative intact parathyroid hormone (IOPTH) assay in parathyroid surgery, it was recommended to reserve the use of IOPTH assays for select cases due to its high cost (EUR 170 for five rapid IOPTH assays vs. EUR 125 for five delayed PTH assays, plus added OR time amounting to EUR 15/min in the authors' institution) [78].

The NIR fluorescence equipment cost is amortized more rapidly when it is used by several disciplines within a hospital environment, as abovementioned NIRAF use then generates no additional cost, and a 25 mg bottle of ICG costs around USD 80 and could, in appropriate sterile conditions, be used for 3 to 5 patients in the same day.

The majority of the analyzed articles appear to agree that NIRAF imaging allows a better identification of PGs but that its impact on autotransplantation rate is difficult to determine. Notably, some authors state that NIRAF imaging allows the identification and autotransplantation of accidentally resected glands (e.g., found on the specimen or in central neck dissection) and that the better early identification of PGs in an expert surgeon's hands will be able to spare these PGs from vascular disruption, thereby reducing the need for autotransplantation [45,70].

ICG angiography is commonly accepted to assist in decision-making on autotransplantation. However, it appears to lead to an increase in the autotransplantation rate, and some authors have mentioned the risk of unnecessary parathyroid autotransplantation on the basis of low-flow ICG patterns [48]. They suggested limiting autotransplantation only to clearly devascularized glands that cannot be preserved.

Moreover, metastatic lymph nodes from papillary thyroid cancer are known false positives presenting an high autofluorescence pattern similar to the one of PGs [55], and reimplantation of an autofluorescent nodule found in the central neck dissection should be done with caution if not clearly a PG or confirmed with an intraoperative frozen biopsy analysis [79].

Limitations

The present review has several limitations. First, only three studies addressed thyroid cancer exclusively, and findings in the other studies were not separated according to the indication for surgery. Hence, there are insufficient data to draw any conclusions regarding the impact of fluorescence imaging on the outcome of thyroid cancer surgery in particular. Further studies should include a more detailed investigation of the observations of a potentially increased benefit of NIR imaging for extended oncological surgery, including neck dissection. Second, the majority of the available and included studies were of limited quality, with only three RCTs (randomized controlled trials). The retrospective nature of some studies [48,49,64] hinders correction for confounders between the study and control groups. However, this aspect could enhance the comparability of both groups by allowing the selection of similar controls for each case. Third, the majority of included studies were small studies with a lack of prospective sample size calculation, which may have affected the observed outcomes.

Another limitation is the variability in NIR imaging use among the reports. In most studies, not all four PGs were visualized. Therefore, the vascularization and viability of the unidentified glands remained unknown, which may have affected the outcome of the surgery. Furthermore, the subjective nature of estimating the fluorescence level in a gland is a limitation, as the available systems only allow qualitative assessments. This limitation leads to subjective interpretation and interobserver differences in scoring the fluorescence intensity of a gland. To eliminate this limitation, future studies should integrate computer-assisted quantitative contrast-enhanced NIR imaging evaluations [12] or pixel/color-analyzing computer programs, as suggested by Fanaropoulou et al. [19].

5. Conclusions

Fluorescence-guided surgery is useful for preventing post-thyroidectomy hypoparathyroidism and is also feasible and safe. As this review has shown, fluorescence-guided surgery enhances early identification, visualization, and preservation of the PGs and may reduce the incidence of postoperative hypoparathyroidism and hypocalcemia. Moreover, this technique assists in the identification of accidentally resected glands on the specimen for subsequent autotransplantation. In thyroid cancer surgery, such intraoperative guidance is particularly beneficial for extended dissection and lymphadenectomy. Further studies are needed to focus on thyroid cancer surgery, as current data are scarce. Moreover, standard-of-practice guidelines are needed to identify the ideal timepoint(s) for NIRAF and ICG imaging during thyroid cancer surgery to optimize the beneficial influence of NIR imaging and proper adoption of the technique.

Most authors highlighted the potential of fluorescence imaging to curtail the need for postoperative supplementation with calcium and vitamin D, especially when paired with the surgeon's critical decision-making skills. However, the articles published thus far have analyzed outcomes for highly experienced/high-volume surgeons. Thus, more high-quality research is required to validate the long-term advantages of these techniques over use of the naked eye, especially in the case of less-experienced surgeons, who will most likely benefit more from NIR imaging techniques.

Author Contributions: Conceptualization, M.S.D., B.S., P.F.A. and F.T.; methodology, M.S.D. and B.S.; validation, M.S.D., B.S., J.-C.L., P.F.A. and F.T.; formal analysis, M.S.D.; investigation, M.S.D.; data curation, M.S.D.; writing—original draft preparation, M.S.D. and B.S.; writing—review and editing, M.S.D., B.S., P.F.A. and F.T.; visualization: M.S.D., B.S., J.-C.L., P.F.A. and F.T.; supervision: M.S.D., B.S., J.-C.L. and P.F.A. All authors have read and agreed to the published version of the manuscript.

Funding: This work was supported by French state funds managed within the "Plan Investissements d'Avenir" and by the ANR (reference ANR-10-IAHU-02).

Institutional Review Board Statement: Not applicable.

Informed Consent Statement: Not applicable.

Data Availability Statement: No new data were created or analyzed in this study. Data sharing is not applicable to this article.

Conflicts of Interest: The authors declare no conflict of interest.

References

1. Pellegriti, G.; Frasca, F.; Regalbuto, C.; Squatrito, S.; Vigneri, R. Worldwide increasing incidence of thyroid cancer: Update on epidemiology and risk factors. *J. Cancer Epidemiol.* **2013**, *2013*, 1–10. [CrossRef] [PubMed]
2. Du, L.; Wang, Y.; Sun, X.; Li, H.; Geng, X.; Ge, M.; Zhu, Y. Thyroid cancer: Trends in incidence, mortality and clinical-pathological patterns in Zhejiang Province, Southeast China. *BMC Cancer* **2018**, *18*, 291. [CrossRef] [PubMed]
3. Deng, Y.; Li, H.; Wang, M.; Li, N.; Tian, T.; Wu, Y.; Xu, P.; Yang, S.; Zhai, Z.; Zhou, L.; et al. Global burden of thyroid cancer from 1990 to 2017. *JAMA Netw. Open* **2020**, *3*, e208759. [CrossRef]
4. Links, T.P.; van Tol, K.M.; Jager, P.L.; Plukker, J.T.M.; Piers, D.A.; Boezen, H.M.; Dullaart, R.P.F.; de Vries, E.G.E.; Sluiter, W.J. Life expectancy in differentiated thyroid cancer: A novel approach to survival analysis. *Endocr. Relat. Cancer* **2005**, *12*, 273–280. [CrossRef]

5. Lee, Y.S.; Nam, K.-H.; Chung, W.Y.; Chang, H.-S.; Park, C.S. Postoperative complications of thyroid cancer in a single center experience. *J. Korean Med. Sci.* **2010**, *25*, 541–545. [CrossRef]
6. Medas, F.; Canu, G.L.; Erdas, E.; Giorgio, P. Intraoperative neuromonitoring in thyroid surgery. In *Knowledges on Thyroid Cancer*; Canu, G.L., Ed.; IntechOpen: Rijeka, Croatia, 2019; Chapter 6; ISBN 978-1-78923-984-3.
7. Bai, B.; Chen, W. Protective effects of intraoperative nerve monitoring (IONM) for recurrent laryngeal nerve injury in thyroidectomy: Meta-analysis. *Sci. Rep.* **2018**, *8*, 7761. [CrossRef] [PubMed]
8. Alander, J.T.; Kaartinen, I.; Laakso, A.; Pätilä, T.; Spillmann, T.; Tuchin, V.V.; Venermo, M.; Välisuo, P. A Review of indocyanine green fluorescent imaging in surgery. *Int. J. Biomed. Imaging* **2012**, *2012*, 940585. [CrossRef] [PubMed]
9. Seeliger, B.; Alesina, P.F.; Walz, M.K.; Pop, R.; Charles, A.-L.; Geny, B.; Messaddeq, N.; Kontogeorgos, G.; Mascagni, P.; Seyller, E.; et al. Intraoperative imaging for remnant viability assessment in bilateral posterior retroperitoneoscopic partial adrenalectomy in an experimental model. *Br. J. Surg.* **2020**, *107*, 1780–1790. [CrossRef] [PubMed]
10. Demarchi, M.S.; Karenovics, W.; Bédat, B.; Triponez, F. Intraoperative autofluorescence and indocyanine green angiography for the detection and preservation of parathyroid glands. *JCM* **2020**, *9*, 830. [CrossRef]
11. De Boer, E.; Harlaar, N.J.; Taruttis, A.; Nagengast, W.B.; Rosenthal, E.L.; Ntziachristos, V.; Van Dam, G.M. Optical innovations in surgery. *Br. J. Surg.* **2015**, *102*, 56–72. [CrossRef]
12. Mascagni, P.; Longo, F.; Barberio, M.; Seeliger, B.; Agnus, V.; Saccomandi, P.; Hostettler, A.; Marescaux, J.; Diana, M. New intraoperative imaging technologies: Innovating the surgeon's eye toward surgical precision. *J. Surg. Oncol.* **2018**, *118*, 265–282. [CrossRef] [PubMed]
13. Solórzano, C.C.; Thomas, G.; Baregamian, N.; Mahadevan-Jansen, A. Detecting the near infrared autofluorescence of the human parathyroid: Hype or opportunity? *Ann. Surg.* **2019**. [CrossRef] [PubMed]
14. Weissleder, R.; Pittet, M.J. Imaging in the era of molecular oncology. *Nature* **2008**, *452*, 580–589. [CrossRef]
15. Seeliger, B.; Walz, M.K.; Alesina, P.F.; Agnus, V.; Pop, R.; Barberio, M.; Saadi, A.; Worreth, M.; Marescaux, J.; Diana, M. Fluorescence-enabled assessment of adrenal gland localization and perfusion in posterior retroperitoneoscopic adrenal surgery in a preclinical model. *Surg. Endosc.* **2020**, *34*, 1401–1411. [CrossRef] [PubMed]
16. Sajedi, S.; Sabet, H.; Choi, H.S. Intraoperative biophotonic imaging systems for image-guided interventions. *Nanophotonics* **2018**, *8*, 99–116. [CrossRef] [PubMed]
17. Van Manen, L.; Handgraaf, H.J.M.; Diana, M.; Dijkstra, J.; Ishizawa, T.; Vahrmeijer, A.L.; Mieog, J.S.D. A practical guide for the use of indocyanine green and methylene blue in fluorescence-guided abdominal surgery. *J. Surg. Oncol.* **2018**, *118*, 283–300. [CrossRef] [PubMed]
18. Kahramangil, B.; Kose, E.; Berber, E. Characterization of fluorescence patterns exhibited by different adrenal tumors: Determining the indications for indocyanine green use in adrenalectomy. *Surgery* **2018**, *164*, 972–977. [CrossRef] [PubMed]
19. Fanaropoulou, N.M.; Chorti, A.; Markakis, M.; Papaioannou, M.; Michalopoulos, A.; Papavramidis, T. The use of indocyanine green in endocrine surgery of the neck: A systematic review. *Medicine* **2019**, *98*, e14765. [CrossRef] [PubMed]
20. Solórzano, C.C.; Thomas, G.; Berber, E.; Wang, T.S.; Randolph, G.W.; Duh, Q.-Y.; Triponez, F. Current state of intraoperative use of near infrared fluorescence for parathyroid identification and preservation. *Surgery* **2021**, *169*, 868–878. [CrossRef] [PubMed]
21. Barth, C.W.; Gibbs, S. Fluorescence image-guided surgery: A perspective on contrast agent development. In *Molecular-Guided Surgery: Molecules, Devices, and Applications VI*; SPIE: Bellingham, WA, USA, 2020.
22. Orosco, R.K.; Tsien, R.Y.; Nguyen, Q.T. Fluorescence imaging in surgery. *IEEE Rev. Biomed. Eng.* **2013**, *6*, 178–187. [CrossRef] [PubMed]
23. Van den Bos, J.; Al-Taher, M.; Schols, R.M.; van Kuijk, S.; Bouvy, N.D.; Stassen, L.P.S. Near-infrared fluorescence imaging for real-time intraoperative guidance in anastomotic colorectal surgery: A systematic review of literature. *J. Laparoendosc. Adv. Surg. Tech.* **2018**, *28*, 157–167. [CrossRef] [PubMed]
24. Vutskits, L.; Briner, A.; Klauser, P.; Gascon, E.; Dayer, A.G.; Kiss, J.Z.; Muller, D.; Licker, M.J.; Morel, D.R. Adverse effects of methylene blue on the central nervous system. *Anesthesiology* **2008**, *108*, 684–692. [CrossRef] [PubMed]
25. Croce, A.C.; Bottiroli, G. Autofluorescence spectroscopy and imaging: A tool for biomedical research and diagnosis. *Eur. J. Histochem. EJH* **2014**, *58*, 2461. [CrossRef]
26. Das, K.; Stone, N.; Kendall, C.; Fowler, C.; Christie-Brown, J. Raman spectroscopy of parathyroid tissue pathology. *Lasers Med. Sci.* **2006**, *21*, 192–197. [CrossRef] [PubMed]
27. Paras, C.; Keller, M.; White, L.; Phay, J.; Mahadevan-Jansen, A. Near-infrared autofluorescence for the detection of parathyroid glands. *J. Biomed. Opt.* **2011**, *16*, 067012. [CrossRef]
28. McWade, M.A.; Paras, C.; White, L.M.; Phay, J.E.; Solórzano, C.C.; Broome, J.T.; Mahadevan-Jansen, A. Label-free intraoperative parathyroid localization with near-infrared autofluorescence imaging. *J. Clin. Endocrinol. Metab.* **2014**, *99*, 4574–4580. [CrossRef] [PubMed]
29. Di Marco, A.N.; Palazzo, F.F. Near-infrared autofluorescence in thyroid and parathyroid surgery. *Gland Surg.* **2020**, *9*, S136–S146. [CrossRef]
30. DSouza, A.V.; Lin, H.; Henderson, E.R.; Samkoe, K.S.; Pogue, B.W. Review of fluorescence guided surgery systems: Identification of key performance capabilities beyond indocyanine green imaging. *J. Biomed. Opt.* **2016**, *21*, 080901. [CrossRef] [PubMed]

31. Chahardahmasumi, E.; Salehidoost, R.; Amini, M.; Aminorroaya, A.; Rezvanian, H.; Kachooei, A.; Iraj, B.; Nazem, M.; Kolahdoozan, M. Assessment of the early and late complication after thyroidectomy. *Adv. Biomed. Res.* **2019**, *8*, 14. [CrossRef] [PubMed]
32. Tuttle, M.R. Differentiated Thyroid Cancer: Overview of Management. 2021. Available online: https://www.uptodate.com/contents/differentiated-thyroid-cancer-overview-of-management (accessed on 4 January 2021).
33. Van Beek, D.-J.; Almquist, M.; Bergenfelz, A.O.; Musholt, T.J.; Nordenström, E. Complications after medullary thyroid carcinoma surgery: Multicentre study of the SQRTPA and EUROCRINE® databases. *Br. J. Surg.* **2020**. [CrossRef]
34. Edafe, O.; Antakia, R.; Laskar, N.; Uttley, L.; Balasubramanian, S.P. Systematic review and meta-analysis of predictors of post-thyroidectomy hypocalcaemia. *Br. J. Surg.* **2014**, *101*, 307–320. [CrossRef] [PubMed]
35. McMullen, C.; Rocke, D.; Freeman, J. Complications of bilateral neck dissection in thyroid cancer from a single high-volume center. *JAMA Otolaryngol. Head Neck Surg.* **2017**, *143*, 376–381. [CrossRef] [PubMed]
36. Ritter, K.; Elfenbein, D.; Schneider, D.F.; Chen, H.; Sippel, R.S. Hypoparathyroidism after total thyroidectomy: Incidence and resolution. *J. Surg. Res.* **2015**, *197*, 348–353. [CrossRef]
37. Khan, A.A.; Clarke, B.; Rejnmark, L.; Brandi, M.L. Hypoparathyroidism in pregnancy: Review and evidence-based recommendations for management. *Eur. J. Endocrinol.* **2019**, *180*, R37–R44. [CrossRef]
38. Hicks, G.; George, R.; Sywak, M. Short and long-term impact of parathyroid autotransplantation on parathyroid function after total thyroidectomy. *Gland Surg.* **2017**, *6* (Suppl. 1), S75–S85. [CrossRef] [PubMed]
39. Almquist, M.; Ivarsson, K.; Nordenström, E.; Bergenfelz, A. Mortality in patients with permanent hypoparathyroidism after total thyroidectomy. *Br. J. Surg.* **2018**, *105*, 1313–1318. [CrossRef] [PubMed]
40. Page, M.J.; McKenzie, J.E.; Bossuyt, P.M.; Boutron, I.; Hoffmann, T.C.; Mulrow, C.D.; Shamseer, L.; Tetzlaff, J.M.; Akl, E.A.; Brennan, S.E.; et al. The PRISMA 2020 statement: An updated guideline for reporting systematic reviews. *BMJ* **2021**, *372*, n71. [CrossRef] [PubMed]
41. Slim, K.; Nini, E.; Forestier, D.; Kwiatkowski, F.; Panis, Y.; Chipponi, J. Methodological index for non-randomized studies (minors): Development and validation of a new instrument. *ANZ J. Surg.* **2003**, *73*, 712–716. [CrossRef]
42. Kim, S.W.; Song, S.H.; Lee, H.S.; Noh, W.J.; Oak, C.; Ahn, Y.C.; Lee, K.D. Intraoperative real-time localization of normal parathyroid glands with autofluorescence imaging. *J. Clin. Endocrinol. Metab.* **2016**, *101*, 4646–4652. [CrossRef]
43. McWade, M.A.; Thomas, G.; Nguyen, J.Q.; Sanders, M.E.; Solórzano, C.C.; Mahadevan-Jansen, A. Enhancing parathyroid gland visualization using a near infrared fluorescence-based overlay imaging system. *J. Am. Coll. Surg.* **2019**, *228*, 730–743. [CrossRef]
44. Jin, H.; Dong, Q.; He, Z.; Fan, J.; Liao, K.; Cui, M. Application of a fluorescence imaging system with indocyanine green to protect the parathyroid gland intraoperatively and to predict postoperative parathyroidism. *Adv. Ther.* **2018**, *35*, 2167–2175. [CrossRef] [PubMed]
45. Benmiloud, F.; Godiris-Petit, G.; Gras, R.; Gillot, J.-C.; Turrin, N.; Penaranda, G.; Noullet, S.; Chéreau, N.; Gaudart, J.; Chiche, L.; et al. Association of autofluorescence-based detection of the parathyroid glands during total thyroidectomy with postoperative hypocalcemia risk: Results of the PARAFLUO multicenter randomized clinical trial. *JAMA Surg.* **2020**, *155*, 106. [CrossRef] [PubMed]
46. Kose, E.; Rudin, A.V.; Kahramangil, B.; Moore, E.; Aydin, H.; Donmez, M.; Krishnamurthy, V.; Siperstein, A.; Berber, E. Autofluorescence imaging of parathyroid glands: An assessment of potential indications. *Surgery* **2020**, *167*, 173–179. [CrossRef] [PubMed]
47. Enny, L.; Ramakant, P.; Singh, K.R.; Rana, C.; Garg, S.; Mishra, A.K. Efficacy of fluorescein green dye in assessing intra-operative parathyroid gland vascularity and predicting post-thyroidectomy hypocalcaemia—A novel prospective cohort study. *Indian J. Endocrinol. Metab.* **2020**, *24*, 446. [PubMed]
48. Razavi, A.C.; Ibraheem, K.; Haddad, A.; Saparova, L.; Shalaby, H.; Abdelgawad, M.; Kandil, E. Efficacy of indocyanine green fluorescence in predicting parathyroid vascularization during thyroid surgery. *Head Neck* **2019**, *41*, 3276–3281. [CrossRef] [PubMed]
49. Rudin, A.V.; McKenzie, T.J.; Thompson, G.B.; Farley, D.R.; Lyden, M.L. Evaluation of parathyroid glands with indocyanine green fluorescence angiography after thyroidectomy. *World J. Surg.* **2019**, *43*, 1538–1543. [CrossRef]
50. Van den Bos, J.; van Kooten, L.; Engelen, S.M.E.; Lubbers, T.; Stassen, L.P.S.; Bouvy, N.D. Feasibility of indocyanine green fluorescence imaging for intraoperative identification of parathyroid glands during thyroid surgery. *Head Neck* **2019**, *41*, 340–348. [CrossRef] [PubMed]
51. Falco, J.; Dip, F.; Quadri, P.; de la Fuente, M.; Prunello, M.; Rosenthal, R.J. Increased identification of parathyroid glands using near infrared light during thyroid and parathyroid surgery. *Surg. Endosc.* **2017**, *31*, 3737–3742. [CrossRef] [PubMed]
52. Lang, B.H.-H.; Wong, C.K.H.; Hung, H.T.; Wong, K.P.; Mak, K.L.; Au, K.B. Indocyanine green fluorescence angiography for quantitative evaluation of in situ parathyroid gland perfusion and function after total thyroidectomy. *Surgery* **2017**, *161*, 87–95. [CrossRef] [PubMed]
53. Serra, C.; Canudo, A.; Silveira, L. Intraoperative identification of parathyroid glands by autofluorescence on total thyroidectomy—Does it really reduces post-operative hypocalcemia? *Surg. Pract. Sci.* **2020**, *2*, 100011. [CrossRef]
54. Lerchenberger, M.; Al Arabi, N.; Gallwas, J.K.S.; Stepp, H.; Hallfeldt, K.K.J.; Ladurner, R. Intraoperative near-infrared autofluorescence and indocyanine green imaging to identify parathyroid glands: A comparison. *Int. J. Endocrinol.* **2019**, *2019*. [CrossRef] [PubMed]

55. De Leeuw, F.; Breuskin, I.; Abbaci, M.; Casiraghi, O.; Mirghani, H.; Lakhdar, A.B.; Laplace-Builhé, C.; Hartl, D. Intraoperative near-infrared imaging for parathyroid gland identification by auto-fluorescence: A feasibility study. *World J. Surg.* **2016**, *40*, 2131–2138. [CrossRef] [PubMed]
56. Llorente, P.M.; Martínez, J.M.F.; Barrasa, A.G. Intraoperative parathyroid hormone measurement vs indocyanine green angiography of parathyroid glands in prediction of early postthyroidectomy hypocalcemia. *JAMA Surg.* **2020**, *155*, 84–85. [CrossRef] [PubMed]
57. Kim, S.W.; Lee, H.S.; Ahn, Y.C.; Park, C.W.; Jeon, S.W.; Kim, C.H.; Ko, J.B.; Oak, C.; Kim, Y.; Lee, K.D. Near-infrared autofluorescence image-guided parathyroid gland mapping in thyroidectomy. *J. Am. Coll. Surg.* **2018**, *226*, 165–172. [CrossRef]
58. Ladurner, R.; Al Arabi, N.; Guendogar, U.; Hallfeldt, K.; Stepp, H.; Gallwas, J. Near-infrared autofluorescence imaging to detect parathyroid glands in thyroid surgery. *Ann. R. Coll. Surg. Engl.* **2018**, *100*, 33–36. [CrossRef]
59. Ladurner, R.; Lerchenberger, M.; Al Arabi, N.; Gallwas, J.K.S.; Stepp, H.; Hallfeldt, K.K.J. Parathyroid autofluorescence—How does it affect parathyroid and thyroid surgery? A 5 year experience. *Molecules* **2019**, *24*, 2560. [CrossRef]
60. Vidal Fortuny, J.; Belfontali, V.; Sadowski, S.M.; Karenovics, W.; Guigard, S.; Triponez, F. Parathyroid gland angiography with indocyanine green fluorescence to predict parathyroid function after thyroid surgery. *Br. J. Surg.* **2016**, *103*, 537–543. [CrossRef] [PubMed]
61. Vidal Fortuny, J.; Sadowski, S.M.; Belfontali, V.; Guigard, S.; Poncet, A.; Ris, F.; Karenovics, W.; Triponez, F. Randomized clinical trial of intraoperative parathyroid gland angiography with indocyanine green fluorescence predicting parathyroid function after thyroid surgery. *Br. J. Surg.* **2018**, *105*, 350–357. [CrossRef]
62. Dip, F.; Falco, J.; Verna, S.; Prunello, M.; Loccisano, M.; Quadri, P.; White, K.; Rosenthal, R. Randomized controlled trial comparing white light with near-infrared autofluorescence for parathyroid gland identification during total thyroidectomy. *J. Am. Coll. Surg.* **2019**, *228*, 744–751. [CrossRef] [PubMed]
63. Zaidi, N.; Bucak, E.; Yazici, P.; Soundararajan, S.; Okoh, A.; Yigitbas, H.; Dural, C.; Berber, E. The feasibility of indocyanine green fluorescence imaging for identifying and assessing the perfusion of parathyroid glands during total thyroidectomy. *J. Surg. Oncol.* **2016**, *113*, 775–778. [CrossRef]
64. Kim, Y.S.; Erten, O.; Kahramangil, B.; Aydin, H.; Donmez, M.; Berber, E. The impact of near infrared fluorescence imaging on parathyroid function after total thyroidectomy. *J. Surg. Oncol.* **2020**. [CrossRef]
65. Jin, H.; Cui, M. Research on intra-operative indocyanine green angiography of the parathyroid for predicting postoperative hypoparathyroidism: A noninferior randomized controlled trial. *Endocr. Pract.* **2020**, *26*, 1469–1476. [CrossRef] [PubMed]
66. Kim, D.H.; Kim, S.W.; Kang, P.; Choi, J.; Lee, H.S.; Park, S.Y.; Kim, Y.; Ahn, Y.-C.; Lee, K.D. Near-infrared autofluorescence imaging may reduce temporary hypoparathyroidism in patients undergoing total thyroidectomy and central neck dissection. *Thyroid* **2021**. [CrossRef] [PubMed]
67. Kose, E.; Kahramangil, B.; Aydin, H.; Donmez, M.; Berber, E. Heterogeneous and low-intensity parathyroid autofluorescence: Patterns suggesting hyperfunction at parathyroid exploration. *Surgery* **2019**, *165*, 431–437. [CrossRef] [PubMed]
68. DiMarco, A.; Chotalia, R.; Bloxham, R.; McIntyre, C.; Tolley, N.; Palazzo, F.F. Does fluoroscopy prevent inadvertent parathyroidectomy in thyroid surgery? *Ann. R. Coll. Surg. Engl.* **2019**, *101*, 508–513. [CrossRef] [PubMed]
69. Bellier, A.; Wazne, Y.; Chollier, T.; Sturm, N.; Chaffanjon, P. Spare parathyroid glands during thyroid surgery with perioperative autofluorescence imaging: A diagnostic study. *World J. Surg.* **2021**. [CrossRef] [PubMed]
70. Benmiloud, F.; Rebaudet, S.; Varoquaux, A.; Penaranda, G.; Bannier, M.; Denizot, A. Impact of autofluorescence-based identification of parathyroids during total thyroidectomy on postoperative hypocalcemia: A before and after controlled study. *Surgery* **2018**, *163*, 23–30. [CrossRef] [PubMed]
71. Kim, S.W.; Lee, H.S.; Lee, K.D. Intraoperative real-time localization of parathyroid gland with near infrared fluorescence imaging. *Gland Surg.* **2017**, *6*, 516–524. [CrossRef] [PubMed]
72. Rudin, A.V.; Berber, E. Impact of fluorescence and autofluorescence on surgical strategy in benign and malignant neck endocrine diseases. *Best Pract. Res. Clin. Endocrinol. Metab.* **2019**, *33*, 101311. [CrossRef] [PubMed]
73. Jin, H.; Dong, Q.; He, Z.; Fan, J.; Liao, K.; Cui, M. Research on indocyanine green angiography for predicting postoperative hypoparathyroidism. *Clin. Endocrinol.* **2019**, *90*, 487–493. [CrossRef]
74. Lütken, C.D.; Achiam, M.P.; Osterkamp, J.; Svendsen, M.B.; Nerup, N. Quantification of fluorescence angiography: Toward a reliable intraoperative assessment of tissue perfusion—A narrative review. *Langenbecks Arch. Surg.* **2021**, *406*, 251–259. [CrossRef] [PubMed]
75. Meira, J.; Marques, M.L.; Falcão-Reis, F.; Rebelo Gomes, E.; Carneiro, Â. Immediate reactions to fluorescein and indocyanine green in retinal angiography: Review of literature and proposal for patient's evaluation. *Clin. Ophthalmol.* **2020**, *14*, 171–178. [CrossRef] [PubMed]
76. Lorente-Poch, L.; Sancho, J.J.; Ruiz, S.; Sitges-Serra, A. Importance of In Situ preservation of parathyroid glands during total thyroidectomy. *Br. J. Surg.* **2015**, *102*. [CrossRef]
77. Baiocchi, G.L.; Diana, M.; Boni, L. Indocyanine green-based fluorescence imaging in visceral and hepatobiliary and pancreatic surgery: State of the art and future directions. *World J. Gastroenterol.* **2018**, *24*, 2921–2930. [CrossRef] [PubMed]

78. Badii, B.; Staderini, F.; Foppa, C.; Tofani, L.; Skalamera, I.; Fiorenza, G.; Qirici, E.; Cianchi, F.; Perigli, G. Cost-benefit analysis of the intraoperative parathyroid hormone assay in primary hyperparathyroidism: Cost-benefit analysis of intraoperative PTH assay. *Head Neck* **2017**, *39*, 241–246. [CrossRef] [PubMed]
79. Thomas, G.; McWade, M.A.; Paras, C.; Mannoh, E.A.; Sanders, M.E.; White, L.M.; Broome, J.T.; Phay, J.E.; Baregamian, N.; Solórzano, C.C.; et al. Developing a clinical prototype to guide surgeons for intraoperative label-free identification of parathyroid glands in real time. *Thyroid* **2018**, *28*, 1517–1531. [CrossRef] [PubMed]

cancers

MDPI

Article

CONUT Score: A New Tool for Predicting Prognosis in Patients with Advanced Thyroid Cancer Treated with TKI

Cristina Dalmiglio [1], Lucia Brilli [1], Michele Campanile [1], Cristina Ciuoli [1], Alessandra Cartocci [2] and Maria Grazia Castagna [1,*]

[1] Department of Medical, Surgical and Neurological Sciences, University of Siena, 53100 Siena, Italy; cristina.dalmiglio@student.unisi.it (C.D.); lucia.brilli@ao-siena.toscana.it (L.B.); michele.campanile@student.unisi.it (M.C.); c.ciuoli@ao-siena.toscana.it (C.C.)
[2] Department of Medical Biotechnologies, University of Siena, 53100 Siena, Italy; alessandra.cartocci@dbm.unisi.it
* Correspondence: mariagrazia.castagna@unisi.it; Tel.: +39-0577585406

Simple Summary: Many studies have shown that an impaired nutritional status correlated with a worse prognosis in cancer patients. The aim of our retrospective study was to evaluate the potential role of baseline Controlling Nutritional Status (CONUT score) in predicting prognosis of advanced thyroid cancer treated with tyrosine kinase inhibitors (TKI). We were able to confirm that baseline CONUT score significantly correlated with progression free survival (PFS) and overall survival (OS) and was the only independent prognostic factor for both outcomes. In particular, a CONUT score ≥3 was associated with a worse PFS and OS. The CONUT score represents a relatively new screening tool that is useful in predicting prognosis in thyroid cancer patients before the beginning of anti-tumoral treatment.

Abstract: (1) Background: The Controlling Nutritional Status (CONUT) score is an immuno-nutritional screening tool based on serum albumin, total cholesterol, and lymphocyte count. The aim of the study was to assess the CONUT score as a potential prognostic factor of response to therapy in patients with advanced thyroid cancer treated with tyrosine kinase inhibitors (TKIs). (2) Methods: We retrospectively evaluated 42 metastatic thyroid cancer patients (54.8% female). The median age at the time of TKI treatment was 69 years. Histological diagnosis was differentiated thyroid cancer in 66.7%, poorly differentiated thyroid cancer in 21.4%, and medullary thyroid cancer in 11.9% of patients. CONUT score was assessed before starting TKI therapy. (3) Results: Progression-free survival (PFS) and overall survival (OS) were significantly influenced by baseline CONUT score. The best CONUT cut-off able to predict the response to treatment was 3. Both PFS and OS were better in patients with CONUT score <3 than in those with CONUT score ≥3 ($p < 0.0001$). CONUT score was the only independent prognostic factor associated with PFS ($p = 0.021$) and OS ($p = 0.007$). (4) Conclusions: CONUT score represents a relatively new screening tool, easily applicable in clinical practice and potentially useful in predicting prognosis in thyroid cancer patients treated with TKIs.

Keywords: CONUT score; thyroid cancer; tyrosine kinase inhibitors

Citation: Dalmiglio, C.; Brilli, L.; Campanile, M.; Ciuoli, C.; Cartocci, A.; Castagna, M.G. CONUT Score: A New Tool for Predicting Prognosis in Patients with Advanced Thyroid Cancer Treated with TKI. *Cancers* **2022**, *14*, 724. https://doi.org/10.3390/cancers14030724

Academic Editor: Fabio Medas

Received: 13 December 2021
Accepted: 28 January 2022
Published: 30 January 2022

1. Introduction

Tyrosine kinase inhibitors (TKIs) are a new class of oncological drugs with activity against receptors of different growth factors and able to inhibit pathways involved in tumor cell proliferation and neoangiogenesis [1]. They have been approved in many tumors including thyroid cancer as they play a crucial therapeutic role when conventional treatments are no longer effective [2]. To date, different TKIs have been approved by the Food and Drug Administration (FDA) and European Medical Agency (EMA) for RAI-refractory differentiated thyroid cancer (sorafenib and lenvatinib) and medullary thyroid cancer (vandetanib and cabozantinib), while dabrafenib/trametinib combination has obtained regulatory approval by the FDA for anaplastic thyroid cancer with a *BRAF* V600 mutation [3–7].

It has been demonstrated that TKIs significantly improved the progression free survival of patients with advanced disease; on the other hand, they are frequently associated with adverse events, which may affect the quality of life or request a permanent drug withdrawal in about 20% of cases [3–8]. TKIs are often associated with weight loss, anorexia, fatigue, and gastrointestinal side effects that may contribute to a malnutrition state.

Malnutrition is a common finding in cancer patients with advanced disease. It is associated with a reduction in physical function, it may negatively affect the prognosis and interfere with the anti-cancer treatment [9]. The energy deficit and the loss of lean body mass are related to the reduced food intake and metabolic disorders (increased basal metabolic rate, insulin-resistance, catabolic processes induced by cytokines and inflammatory factors), but anti-cancer therapy itself can also promote malnutrition.

Recent studies have shown the importance of single nutritional indices such as serum albumin in predicting poor outcomes in cancer patients [10–12]. Additionally, more complex indices have been developed and validated in order to evaluate the nutritional status [13,14]. The Controlling Nutritional Status (CONUT) score has recently been introduced as a nutritional screening tool [15]. Moreover, it has been recognized as a prognostic factor in patients affected by several chronic or malignant diseases [16–26].

Its utility has been demonstrated in the assessment of the prognosis of patients with end-stage liver disease and acute heart failure [16,17]; it has also been correlated with the disease activity in patients with lupus nephritis [27]. The impact of CONUT score on survival has also been reported in hospitalized elderly people [28] and in patients with hypertension [18] or in peritoneal dialysis [19]. Moreover, the prognostic role of CONUT score has been widely investigated in the context of several types of neoplasms. Many studies have demonstrated how a low CONUT score at the baseline correlates with a better prognosis in patients with small cell lung cancer, gastrointestinal, pancreatic, ovarian, breast, and urological cancers [20–26]. It has also been shown to be a parameter that correlates with prognosis and response to treatment in oncology [29].

To date, there are no studies in the literature that have investigated the relationship between CONUT score and thyroid cancer.

The aim of our study was to assess the CONUT score as a potential prognostic factor of response to therapy in patients with advanced thyroid cancer (differentiated, medullary, or poorly differentiated thyroid cancer) treated with TKIs.

2. Materials and Methods

2.1. Study Population

We retrospectively evaluated 71 patients with locally advanced or metastatic thyroid carcinoma treated with at least one TKI at our institution between November 2004 and October 2020.

The data collected included age at diagnosis, gender, histological findings, stage at diagnosis, numbers of anatomical site involved, information on treatment with TKIs (type of TKI, time-lapse between diagnosis and treatment start, duration of treatment, reason for discontinuation), tumor response, and data on last follow-up/death.

Patients without available complete biochemical data and those receiving statin treatment for cholesterol control with a serum total cholesterol <180 mg/dl were excluded from our study.

The final population was made of 42 patients (54.8% female). The mean age at the time of TKI treatment was 67.5 ± 13.8 years (median 69 years, 30–96 years). All patients had metastatic disease. In detail, the number of anatomical sites involved by metastatic disease was one in five patients (11.9%), two in 10 patients (23.8%), three in 18 patients (42.8%), four in four patients (9.5%), and five in five patients (11.9%). Histological diagnosis was differentiated thyroid cancer (DTC) in 28 patients (66.7%), poorly differentiated thyroid cancer (PDTC) in nine patients (21.4%), and medullary thyroid cancer (MTC) in five (11.9%).

Time-lapse between cancer diagnosis and TKI treatment start ranged from 0.06 to 15.4 years (mean 5.4 ± 4.4, median 5.4 years) and ranged from 0 to 14.2 years (mean 3.43 ± 3.5, median 2.8 years) between the appearance of metastases and TKI treatment beginning.

The TKI used as first-line therapy was: lenvatinib in 16 patients (38.1%), sorafenib in 18 patients (42.8%), vandetanib in four patients (9.5%), and motesanib in four patients (9.5%). Ten out of the 42 patients (23.8%) were treated with other TKI.

The median body mass index (BMI) at baseline was 26.5 kg/m^2 (mean 27.2 ± 6.0 range 18.1–47.0 kg/m^2). The performance status at baseline, according to the Eastern Cooperative Oncology Group (ECOG) scale, was 0 in 36 patients (85.7%), one in four patients (9.5%), and two in two patients (4.8%).

All data are summarized in Table 1.

Table 1. Baseline clinical-pathological features in the whole population and according to histological diagnosis.

	All Patients (*n* = 42)	DTC (*n* = 28)	PDTC (*n* = 9)	MTC (*n* = 5)
Gender *n* (%)				
F	23 (54.8%)	18 (64.3%)	3 (33.3%)	2 (40%)
M	19 (45.2%)	10 (35.7%)	6 (66.7%)	3 (60%)
Age at the time of TKI treatment (years) Median (range)	69 (30–9)	71.6 (43–87)	67.2 (51.2–96.2)	51.4 (30–80)
Time-lapse between cancer diagnosis and TKI treatment (years) Median (range)	5.4 (0.06–15.4)	5.71 (0.09–15.4)	1.96 (0.06–12)	7.7 (1.1–9.9)
Time-lapse between appearance of metastases and TKI treatment (years) Median (range)	2.8 (0–14.2)	3.2 (0.03–14.2)	1.2 (0–12)	1.1 (0.6–4.9)
Numbers of anatomical site involved *n* (%)				
1	5 (11.9%)	4 (14.3%)	1 (11.1%)	0 (0%)
2	10 (23.8%)	8 (28.6%)	1 (11.1%)	1 (20%)
≥3	27 (64.3%)	16 (57.1%)	7 (77.8%)	4 (80%)
Patients with bone metastasis *n* (%)	15 (35.7%)	9 (32.1%)	3 (33.3%)	3 (60%)
Type of first-line TKI *n* (%)				
Lenvatinib	16 (38.1%)	10 (35.7%)	6 (66.7%)	0 (0%)
Sorafenib	18 (42.8%)	14 (50%)	3 (33.3%)	1 (20%)
Vandetanib	4 (9.5%)	2 (7.1%)	0 (0%)	2 (40%)
Motesanib	4 (9.5%)	2 (7.1%)	0 (0%)	2 (40%)
BMI (kg/m^2) Median (range)	26.5 (18.1–47)	26.9 (18.7–44.1)	24.6 (18–46.9)	24.8 (22.7–34.4)
ECOG PS *n* (%) [1]				
0	31 (86.1%)	20 (83.33%)	7 (87.5%)	4 (100%)
1	3 (8.3%)	2 (8.33%)	1 (12.5%)	0 (0%)
2	2 (5.6%)	2 (8.33%)	0 (0%)	0 (0%)

[1] ECOG PS was evaluated in 36 patients.

2.2. Assessments and Definitions

We evaluated in all patients the following anthropometric parameters: weight, height, and body mass index (BMI). The weight (kilograms) and height (meters) were measured using a scale with an altimeter (Seca-Intermed, Milan, Italy). The BMI was calculated as 'weight over height square'.

At baseline (before starting TKI treatment), fasting venous blood sample was collected for biochemical tests including albumin, total cholesterol, and total lymphocyte count. The concentration of such parameters was measured with standard colorimetric methods using the Cobas c 701/702 analyzer (Roche/Hitachi, Mannheim, Germany). The CONUT score was defined as the sum of the following parameters, as described below:

- for serum albumin levels >3.5, between 3.0 and 3.49, between 2.5 and 2.99 and <2.5 g/dl, 0, 2, 4, and 6 points were assigned, respectively.
- for serum total cholesterol levels >180, between 140 and 179, between 100 and 139 and <100 mg/dl, 0, 1, 2, and 3 points were assigned, respectively.
- for serum total lymphocyte count >1600, between 1200 and 1599, between 800 and 1199 and <800 / mm^3, 0, 1, 2, and 3 points were assigned, respectively.

Radiological evaluation was performed at baseline (before treatment) and on average every 3–6 months thereafter with computed tomography (CT) scanning with contrast medium or magnetic resonance imaging (MRI).

The time from TKI administration to the first evidence of tumor progression or until death defines the progression free survival (PFS). Tumor progression was documented by CT or MRI examination according to Response Evaluation Criteria in Solid Tumors (RECIST) v 1.1. Best response (BR) was defined as the best response recorded from the start of the treatment until disease progression. The time from the start date of the TKI treatment to the time of death from any cause defines the overall survival (OS).

2.3. Statistical Analysis

A preliminary descriptive analysis was performed: quantitative variables were summarized by mean ± standard deviation, median and minimum–maximum range, and qualitative variables by absolute frequencies and percentages. Kruskal test and the post hoc Dunn test were performed to compare the differences of OS and PFS among the three CONUT score ranges (0–2, 3–4, 5–7). Multiple chi-squared test with Bonferroni correction was performed to compare the response (partial response/stable disease and progressive disease) among the three CONUT score levels. ROC curve was performed to obtain a CONUT score cut-off for the most accurate prevision of PFS and OS at 12 months.

The associations with the dichotomous CONUT score (0–2 and 3–7) were evaluated with the chi-squared test or Fisher exact test. The differences between low and high CONUT were evaluated with the t-test or the Mann–Whitney test based on the Kolmogorov–Smirnov test for the normality distribution.

Kaplan–Meier and Cox regression analyses were used to assess progression free survival and overall survival. Hazard ratio and their 95% confidence interval (CI) were estimated. Stepwise Cox regression was performed. A p-value < 0.05 was considered statistically significant. The analyses were performed with SPSS statistics version 27.

3. Results

3.1. Baseline CONUT Score (before TKI Treatment)

The median baseline CONUT score was 2 (range 0–7). In detail, it was 0 in 9/42 patients (21.4%), one in 10/42 patients (23.8%), two in 9/42 patients (21.4%), three in 5/42 patients (11.9%), four in 4/42 patients (9.5%), five in 3/42 patients (7.1%), six in 1/42 patients (2.4%), and seven in 1/42 patients (2.4%).

3.2. TKI Treatment

The median duration of first TKI therapy was 15.7 months (mean 23.4 ± 19.3 months, range 0.9–76.2 months). At the last follow-up, 9/42 (21.4%) patients were still being treated, 27/42 (64.3%) patients discontinued therapy due to disease progression [20/27 (74.1%)] or other reasons (adverse events, patient decision) [7/27 (25.9%)], while 6/42 (14.3%) patients died.

The median PFS was 12.9 months (mean 16.6 ± 15.1, range 0.9–71.7 months). The best response, evaluable in 40/42 patients (95.2%), was partial response (PR) in 14/40 patients

(35%), stable disease (SD) in 21/40 patients (52.5%), and progressive disease (PD) in 5/40 patients (12.5%).

The OS was assessed in a sub-population of 32 patients treated with only one TKI to avoid the potential bias due to those patients treated with more than one TKI. The median OS in this group was 16.8 months (mean 19.1 ± 13.4, range 0.9–56.1 months).

3.3. Correlation between Baseline CONUT Score and Response to TKI Treatment

In order to evaluate a possible correlation between nutritional status and the response to first TKI treatment, patients were stratified into three groups according to CONUT score value. We observed that patients with a CONUT score 0–2 (Group A) had a significantly better PFS and OS than patients with a CONUT score 3–4 (Group B) (p = 0.001 for PFS and p = 0.006 for OS) and with a CONUT score 5–7 (Group C) (p = 0.02 for PFS, p = 0.002 for OS). Accordingly, we also observed that patients with a CONUT score 0–2 had a significantly better response, according to RECIST criteria, than the other two groups (p = 0.002 and p = 0.003, respectively). In contrast, PFS, OS, and radiological response were not significantly different between patients with a CONUT score 3–4 (Group B) and 5–6 (Group C) (Table 2).

Table 2. Response to TKIs according to baseline CONUT score (Group A score 0–2, Group B score 3–4, Group C score 5–7).

	Patients (*n*; %)	BR1 (*n*; %)	PFS [1] Median (Months) Range	OS [2] Median (Months) Range
Group A (CONUT score 0–2)	28 (66.7%)	PR 10/27 (37%) SD 17/27 (63%) PD 0/27 (0%)	17.9 (2.4–71.7)	23.5 (3.1–56.1)
Group B (CONUT score 3–4)	9 (21.4%)	PR 3/8 (37.5%) SD 2/8 (25%) PD 3/8 (37.5%)	3.6 (0.9–11.8)	8.9 (0.9–19.0)
Group C (CONUT score 5–7)	5 (11.9%)	PR 1/5 (20%) SD 2/5 (40%) PD 2/5 (40%)	7.9 (2.2–10.9)	9.6 (2.2–15.4)
		p A vs. B = 0.002 p A vs. C = 0.003 p B vs. C = 0.759	p A vs. B = 0.001 p A vs. C = 0.0224 p B vs. C = 0.737	p A vs. B = 0.0006 p A vs. C = 0.0028 p B vs. C = 0.923

[1] BR and PFS were assessed in 40 patients. [2] OS was evaluated in 32 patients treated with only one TKI.

3.4. ROC Analysis for 12 Months—PFS and OS

By ROC curves analysis, we found that the best CONUT score cut-off able to predict the response to TKI treatment was 3 (Table S1). This cut-off had a specificity of 100% and 93.7% and a sensitivity of 70% and 68.8% for PFS and OS, respectively, with an Area Under the Curve (AUC) of 0.980 for mPFS, (p < 0.0001) and of 0.846 for mOS (p = 0.0001), as showed in Figure 1.

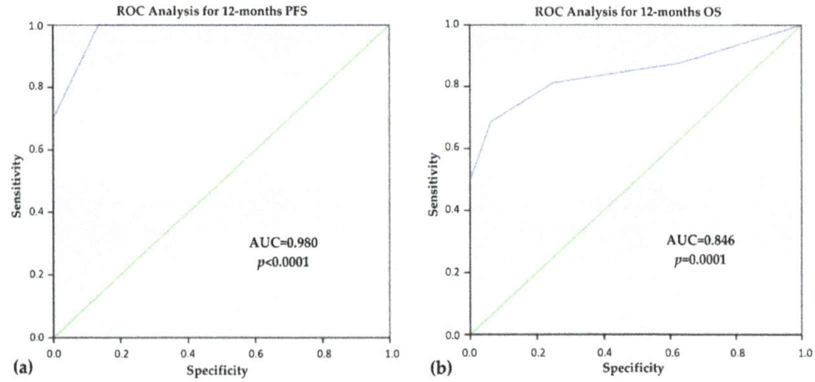

Figure 1. ROC curve analysis for 12-month progression free survival (PFS) (**a**) and 12-month overall survival (OS) (**b**).

3.5. Clinical-Pathological Features in Thyroid Cancer Patients with CONUT Score <3 (Group 1) and ≥3 (Group 2)

According to the cut-off obtained by ROC analysis, the study population was divided into two groups: Group 1 (CONUT score <3) and Group 2 (CONUT score ≥3). No significant differences between the two groups regarding all clinical-pathological data collected (gender, age at beginning of treatment, time-lapse between cancer diagnosis and treatment, time-lapse between appearance of metastasis and treatment, tumor histotype, numbers of anatomical site involved, rate of bone metastasis, type of TKI, BMI, and ECOG PS) were observed in Group 1 compared to Group 2 (Table S2).

3.6. Clinical Outcomes According to CONUT Score

Using Kaplan–Meier curves, a significant better PFS was observed in Group 1 patients when compared to Group 2 (22.5 vs. 5.0 months, $p < 0.0001$, Figure 2a). Similarly, the OS was longer in Group 1 than Group 2 (35.1 vs. 9.2 months, $p < 0.0001$, Figure 2b). All but one patient died for thyroid disease, confirming a better disease specific survival in Group 1 than in Group 2.

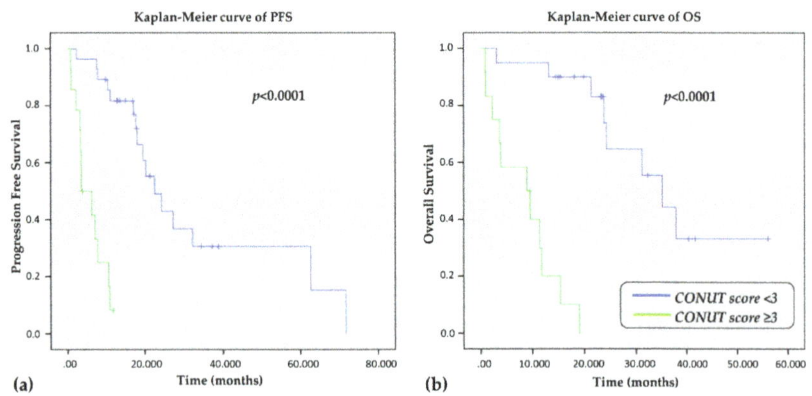

Figure 2. Kaplan–Meier curve for PFS (**a**) and OS (**b**) according to the CONUT cut-off of 3.

We also performed a sub-analysis of PFS and OS according to the histology. Prognostic power of the CONUT score was still valid in DTC patients (OS: HR 1609, 95% CI 1.232–2.12, $p < 0.0001$; PFS: HR 1.505, 95% CI 1.186–1.908, $p = 0.001$), but not in MTC and PDTC patients, probably due to the small cohort of patients in these two groups.

3.7. Univariate and Multivariate Analysis for PFS and OS

At univariate Cox-regression analysis, serum albumin level [HR 0.408 (95% CI 0.168–0.991), $p = 0.048$], total lymphocyte count [HR 0.999 (95% CI 0.999–1.00), $p = 0.035$], and baseline CONUT score [HR 12.211 (95% CI 4.084–36.512), $p < 0.0001$] were prognostic factors for PFS as well as serum albumin level [HR 0.224 (95% CI 0.083–0.604), $p = 0.003$], serum total cholesterol [HR 0.982 (95% CI 0.969–0.995), $p = 0.007$], and CONUT score [HR 23.551 (95% CI 4.949–112.060), $p < 0.0001$] were prognostic factors for OS. According to stepwise Cox-regression analysis, the CONUT score was the only independent prognostic factor associated with PFS ($p < 0.0001$) and OS ($p < 0.0001$), whose HRs were confirmed to be 12.211 (95% CI 4.084–36.512) for PFS and 23.551 (95% CI 4.949–112.060) for OS.

4. Discussion

Recently, the prognostic value of nutritional status and inflammation has been de-bated in cancer patients [30,31]. Many studies have demonstrated that an impaired nutritional status and an increased inflammatory response are related to a worse prognosis in patients with different types of human cancer [32,33]. Different biochemical parameters have been proposed to evaluate the immune-nutritional status such as blood neutrophil, lymphocyte, monocyte, platelet count, neutrophil–lymphocyte ratio (NLR), lymphocyte–monocyte ratio (LMR), and platelet–lymphocyte ratio (PLR) [34–36]. Immune-nutritional scores such as the Prognostic Nutritional Index (PNI) and the Controlling Nutritional Status (CONUT) have also recently been evaluated in human cancer [20–26,37]. The latter has recently been implemented as a tool of nutritional screening, emerging as an independent prognostic factor for OS in several types of solid tumors [38] as well as in hematological cancer [39,40].

To our knowledge, our study is the first to investigate the potential role of the baseline CONUT score as a prognostic factor for PFS and OS in patients with advanced thyroid cancer (differentiated, medullary, or poorly differentiated thyroid cancer) treated with TKIs. In recent years, TKIs have become a pivotal therapy in many types of cancer [2]. These drugs are scheduled for chronic administration and are often associated with systemic side effects favoring malnutrition (i.e., diarrhea, nausea, mucositis), if not properly managed [8].

Our cohort of patients showed an overall baseline good nutritional status, with a CONUT score suggestive of moderate malnutrition only in 5/42 (11.9%) patients, while none had severe grade of malnutrition (highest CONUT score recorded equal to 7). Nevertheless, a significant correlation between immuno-nutritional status and clinical outcome was observed. Using ROC curve analysis, we found that a cut-off of 3 was able to predict the response to treatment with 100% of specificity and 70% of sensitivity for PFS (AUC 0.980, $p < 0.0001$), and 93.7% of specificity and 68.8% of sensitivity for OS (AUC 0.840, $p = 0.001$). It is important to underline that the two groups of patients (CONUT score <3 and ≥ 3) were similar for clinical and pathological features that could have an impact on the clinical outcome. Nevertheless, the number of patients that took the full dosage did not differ between the two groups at the beginning of TKI treatment as well as at the last follow-up. Since TKI dosage is mostly related to the adverse events, we can assume that the tolerance to therapy was also similar in the two groups of patients.

The optimal cut-off of the CONUT score varied across different studies [38]; in our study, it was higher compared to that found in patients with small cell lung cancer [20], but lower compared to that calculated in other cancer studies [21–23,29]. This difference is probably due to the different nutritional status and pathogenic mechanisms underlying the various types of cancer.

Multiple potential mechanisms underlying the relationship between parameters included in the CONUT score and cancer prognosis have been widely analyzed. The serum albumin reflects both the nutritional and the inflammatory status and is considered as a prognostic factor in several cancers [10–12]. It has been postulated that pro-inflammatory cytokines such as interleukin 6 (IL-6) and tumor necrosis factor alpha (TNF-α), which modulate albumin hepatic synthesis, are associated with lower serum concentrations of this protein [41,42]. TNF-α induces gluconeogenesis and the lipid and muscle protein catabolism. It also stimulates the production of reactive oxygen species (ROS) in tissues, leading to the activation of ubiquitin-proteasome pathway and inducing muscle protein catabolism [43]. Moreover, in preclinical studies, it has been demonstrated that TNF-α and interleukin 1 (IL-1) penetrate the hematoencephalic barrier, causing an anorexigenic effect [44]. The protein deficit causes a downregulation of hormonal and antibody synthesis, leading to a suppression in B-cell differentiation and T-cell activation [45].

There are many assumptions about the relationship between serum cholesterol and prognosis in cancer [46–48]. Okuyama et al. [49] and many other authors have demonstrated a correlation between hypocholesterolemia and worse prognosis in non-small cell lung cancer, gastric cancer, and localized renal cell carcinoma [50–52]. It seems that tumoral cells can determine a reduction in serum cholesterol through many mechanisms. such as an increased uptake into the cells caused by the exposition of low-density lipoprotein (LDL)-cholesterol receptors on the cell membrane [53].

The lymphocyte count is widely used in prognostic scores since the immune response against cancer largely depends on lymphocytes. CD4+ and CD8+ lymphocytes are implied in the prevention of neoplastic proliferation and invasion, CD8+ T cell counts are consistently associated with better survival in many types of cancer [54–56].

Interestingly, the CONUT score cut-off found in our study was the only independent parameter associated with PFS (HR 12.2, $p < 0.0001$) and OS (HR 23.55, $p < 0.0001$) by multivariate stepwise Cox-regression analysis, suggesting a possible role of nutritional status in the clinical outcome of thyroid cancer patients with advanced disease treated with anticancer therapy.

The study has a few limitations such as the presence of multiple histotypes of thyroid cancer, the use of different TKIs, the small sample size, and the retrospective design of the study.

However, the study has several strengths such as standardized management in the same institution with detailed information regarding diagnosis, treatment, and follow-up. Finally, to our knowledge, this is the first study to have evaluated the role of CONUT score as an immuno-nutritional tool in the clinical outcome of advanced thyroid carcinoma treated with TKIs.

5. Conclusions

The CONUT score represents a relatively new screening tool, easily applicable in clinical practice with a possible prognostic role in the management of patients with advanced thyroid cancer treated with TKIs.

Based on this evidence, the nutritional status should be taken into account in metastatic thyroid cancer patients, since the efficacy of anticancer treatments could potentially be impaired by malnutrition. The improvement in the nutritional status of cancer patients before starting and/or during TKI treatment could be one of the strategies to obtain the maximum efficacy of anticancer therapy. This study shows promising and innovative results, opening the way to future prospective studies on a larger sample size to strengthen the correlation between the nutritional status, evaluated at baseline and during cancer treatment, and the response to TKI treatment in patients with advanced thyroid cancer.

Supplementary Materials: The following supporting information can be downloaded at: https://www.mdpi.com/article/10.3390/cancers14030724/s1, Table S1: CONUT score cut-offs according to ROC analysis for Progression Free Survival (a) and Overall Survival (b); Table S2: Clinical-pathological features in thyroid cancer patients with CONUT score <3 (Group 1) and $\geq$3 (Group 2).

Author Contributions: Conceptualization, C.C., M.G.C., L.B. and C.D.; Methodology, M.G.C. and L.B.; Validation, M.G.C. and L.B.; Resources L.B. and C.D.; Formal analysis, A.C., M.G.C., L.B., C.D. and M.C.; Investigation, M.G.C. and L.B.; Data curation C.D., M.C. and L.B.; Writing—original draft preparation, M.G.C., L.B., C.D. and M.C.; Visualization, C.D. and M.C.; Supervision, M.G.C. All authors have read and agreed to the published version of the manuscript.

Funding: This research received no external funding.

Institutional Review Board Statement: The study was conducted in accordance with the Declaration of Helsinki, and approved by the local Ethics Committee of Azienda Ospedaliera Universitaria Senese, Siena, Italy (protocol code # 10167/2016, 17 October 2016).

Informed Consent Statement: The patients provided their written informed consent to participate in this study.

Data Availability Statement: Data are contained within the article.

Conflicts of Interest: The authors declare no conflict of interest.

References

1. Gotink, K.J.; Verheul, H.M. Anti-angiogenic tyrosine kinase inhibitors: What is their mechanism of action? *Angiogenesis* **2010**, *13*, 1–14. [CrossRef] [PubMed]
2. Roskoski, R., Jr. Properties of FDA-approved small molecule protein kinase inhibitors: A 2021 update. *Pharmacol. Res.* **2021**, *165*, 105463. [CrossRef] [PubMed]
3. Wells, S.A., Jr.; Robinson, B.G.; Gagel, R.F.; Dralle, H.; Fagin, J.A.; Santoro, M.; Schlumberger, M.J.; Read, J.; Langmuir, P.; Ryan, A.J.; et al. Vandetanib in patients with locally advanced or metastatic medullary thyroid cancer: A randomized, double-blind phase III trial. *J. Clin. Oncol.* **2012**, *30*, 134–141. [CrossRef] [PubMed]
4. Elisei, R.; Schlumberger, M.; Müller, S.P.; Schöffski, P.; Brose, M.S.; Shah, M.H.; Sherman, S.I.; Yaron, Y.; Ball, D.; Nelkin, B.; et al. Cabozantinib in progressive medullary thyroid cancer. *J. Clin. Oncol.* **2013**, *31*, 3639–3646. [CrossRef] [PubMed]
5. Brose, M.S.; Nutting, C.M.; Jarzab, B.; Elisei, R.; Siena, S.; Bastholt, L.; Schlumberger, M.J.; Kappeler, C.; Peña, C.; Molnár, I.; et al. Sorafenib in radioactive iodine-refractory, locally advanced or metastatic differentiated thyroid cancer: A randomized, double-blind, phase 3 trial. *Lancet* **2014**, *384*, 319–328. [CrossRef]
6. Schlumberger, M.; Tahara, M.; Wirth, L.J.; Robinson, B.; Brose, M.S.; Elisei, R.; Sherman, S.I.; Dutcus, C.E.; de las Heras, B.; Zhu, J.; et al. Lenvatinib versus placebo in radioiodine-refractory thyroid cancer. *N. Engl. J. Med.* **2015**, *372*, 621–630. [CrossRef] [PubMed]
7. Subbiah, V.; Kreitman, R.J.; Wainberg, Z.A.; Cho, J.Y.; Schellens, J.H.M.; Soria, J.C.; Wen, P.Y.; Zielinski, C.; Cabanillas, M.E.; Urbanowitz, G.; et al. Dabrafenib and Trametinib Treatment in Patients With Locally Advanced or Metastatic BRAF V600-Mutant Anaplastic Thyroid Cancer. *J. Clin. Oncol.* **2018**, *36*, 7–13. [CrossRef]
8. Cabanillas, M.E.; Ryder, M.; Jimenez, C. Targeted Therapy for Advanced Thyroid Cancer: Kinase Inhibitors and Beyond. *Endocr. Rev.* **2019**, *40*, 1573–1604. [CrossRef]
9. Reber, E.; Schönenberger, K.A.; Vasiloglou, M.F.; Stanga, Z. Nutritional Risk Screening in Cancer Patients: The First Step Toward Better Clinical Outcome. *Front. Nutr.* **2021**, *8*, 152. [CrossRef]
10. Wu, N.; Chen, G.; Hu, H.; Pang, L.; Chen, Z. Low pretherapeutic serum albumin as a risk factor for poor outcome in esophageal squamous cell carcinomas. *Nutr. Cancer* **2015**, *67*, 481–485. [CrossRef]
11. Cengiz, O.; Kocer, B.; Surmeli, S.; Santicky, M.J.; Soran, A. Are pretreatment serum albumin and cholesterol levels prognostic tools in patients with colorectal carcinoma? *Med. Sci. Monit. Basic Res.* **2006**, *12*, 240–247.
12. Onate-Ocana, L.F.; Aiello-Crocifoglio, V.; Gallardo-Rincon, D.; Herrera-Goepfert, R.; Brom-Valladares, R.; Carrillo, J.F.; Cervera, E.; Mohar-Betancourt, A. Serum albumin as a significant prognostic factor for patients with gastric carcinoma. *Ann. Surg. Oncol.* **2007**, *14*, 381–389. [CrossRef] [PubMed]
13. Sun, K.; Chen, S.; Xu, J.; Li, G.; He, Y. The prognostic significance of the prognostic nutritional index in cancer: A systematic review and meta-analysis. *J. Cancer Res. Clin. Oncol.* **2014**, *140*, 1537–1549. [CrossRef] [PubMed]
14. Arfsten, H.; Cho, A.; Prausmüller, S.; Spinka, G.; Novak, J.; Goliasch, G.; Pavo, N.; Preusser, M.; Hengstenberg, C.; Hülsmann, M.; et al. Inflammation-Based Scores as a Common Tool for Prognostic Assessment in Heart Failure or Cancer. *Front. Cardiovasc. Med.* **2021**, *8*, 725903. [CrossRef] [PubMed]
15. Ignacio de Ulíbarri, J.; González-Madroño, A.; De Villar, N.G.; González, P.; Gonzalez, B.; Mancha, A.; Rodriguez, F.; Fernandez, G. CONUT: A tool for Controlling Nutritional Status. First validation in a hospital population. *Nutr. Hosp.* **2005**, *20*, 38–45. [PubMed]
16. Shirakabe, A.; Hata, N.; Kobayashi, N.; Okazaki, H.; Matsushita, M.; Shibata, Y.; Nishigoori, S.; Uchiyama, S.; Asai, K.; Shimizu, W. The prognostic impact of malnutrition in patients with severely decompensated acute heart failure, as assessed using the Prognostic Nutritional Index (PNI) and Controlling Nutritional Status (CONUT) score. *Heart Vessel.* **2018**, *33*, 134–144. [CrossRef]
17. Fukushima, K.; Ueno, Y.; Kawagishi, N.; Kondo, Y.; Inoue, J.; Kakazu, E.; Ninomiya, M.; Wakui, Y.; Saito, N.; Satomi, S.; et al. The nutritional index 'CONUT' is useful for predicting long-term prognosis of patients with end-stage liver diseases. *Tohoku J. Exp. Med.* **2011**, *224*, 215–219. [CrossRef]
18. Sun, X.; Luo, L.; Zhao, X.; Ye, P. Controlling Nutritional Status (CONUT) score as a predictor of all-cause mortality in elderly hypertensive patients: A prospective follow-up study. *BMJ Open* **2017**, *7*, 015649. [CrossRef] [PubMed]
19. Zhou, H.; Chao, W.; Cui, L.; Li, M.; Zou, Y.; Yang, M. Controlling Nutritional Status (CONUT) score as immune-nutritional predictor of outcomes in patients undergoing peritoneal dialysis. *Clin. Nutr.* **2020**, *39*, 2564–2570. [CrossRef]

20. Yılmaz, A.; Tekin, S.B.; Bilici, M.; Yılmaz, H. The Significance of Controlling Nutritional Status (CONUT) Score as a Novel Prognostic Parameter in Small Cell Lung Cancer. *Lung* **2020**, *198*, 695–704. [CrossRef]
21. Zhang, Y.; Zhang, X. Controlling nutritional status score, a promising prognostic marker in patients with gastrointestinal cancers after surgery: A systematic review and meta-analysis. *Int. J. Surg.* **2018**, *55*, 39–45. [CrossRef] [PubMed]
22. Takagi, K.; Buettner, S.; Ijzermans, J.N.M. Prognostic significance of the controlling nutritional status (CONUT) score in patients with colorectal cancer: A systematic review and meta-analysis. *Int. J. Surg.* **2020**, *78*, 91–96. [CrossRef] [PubMed]
23. Terasaki, F.; Sugiura, T.; Okamura, Y.; Ito, T.; Yamamoto, Y.; Ashida, R.; Uesaka, K.; Ohgi, K. The preoperative controlling nutritional status (CONUT) score is an independent prognostic marker for pancreatic ductal adenocarcinoma. *Updates Surg.* **2021**, *73*, 251–259. [CrossRef] [PubMed]
24. Li, Y.; Zhang, C.; Ji, R.; Lu, H.; Zhang, W.; Li, L.L.; He, A.; Liu, R.; Qian, H. Prognostic significance of the controlling nutritional status (CONUT) score in epithelial ovarian cancer. *Int. J. Gynecol. Cancer* **2020**, *30*, 74–82. [CrossRef] [PubMed]
25. Li, W.; Li, M.; Wang, T.; Ma, G.; Deng, Y.; Pu, D.; Zhou, Q.; Liu, Z.; Wu, Q.; Liuet, X. Controlling Nutritional Status (CONUT) score is a prognostic factor in patients with resected breast cancer. *Sci. Rep.* **2020**, *10*, 6633. [CrossRef]
26. Niu, X.; Zhu, Z.; Bao, J. Prognostic significance of pretreatment controlling nutritional status score in urological cancers: A systematic review and meta-analysis. *Cancer Cell Int.* **2021**, *21*, 126. [CrossRef]
27. Ahn, S.S.; Yoo, J.; Jung, S.M.; Song, J.J.; Park, Y.B.; Lee, S.W. Comparison of the Clinical Implications among Five Different Nutritional Indices in Patients with Lupus Nephritis. *Nutrients* **2019**, *11*, 1456. [CrossRef]
28. Cabré, M.; Ferreiro, C.; Arus, M.; Roca, M.; Palomera, E.; Serra-Prat, M. Evaluation of CONUT for clinical malnutrition detection and shorttermprognostic assessment in hospitalized elderly people. *J. Nutr. Health Aging* **2015**, *19*, 729–733. [CrossRef]
29. Shimose, S.; Kawaguchi, T.; Iwamoto, H.; Tanaka, M.; Miyazaki, K.; Ono, M.; Torimura, T.; Koga, H.; Noguchi, K.; Yokokura, Y.; et al. Controlling Nutritional Status (CONUT) Score is Associated with Overall Survival in Patients with Unresectable Hepatocellular Carcinoma Treated with Lenvatinib: A Multicenter Cohort Study. *Nutrients* **2020**, *12*, 1076. [CrossRef]
30. Coussens, L.M.; Werb, Z. Inflammation and cancer. *Nature* **2002**, *420*, 860–867. [CrossRef]
31. Zitvogel, L.; Pietrocola, F.; Kroemer, G. Nutrition, inflammation and cancer. *Nat. Immunol.* **2017**, *18*, 843–850. [CrossRef] [PubMed]
32. Diakos, C.I.; Charles, K.A.; McMillan, D.C.; Clarke, S.J. Cancer-related inflammation and treatment effectiveness. *Lancet Oncol.* **2014**, *15*, 493–503. [CrossRef]
33. Mantzorou, M.; Koutelidakis, A.; Theocharis, S.; Giaginis, C. Clinical Value of Nutritional Status in Cancer: What is its Impact and how it Affects Disease Progression and Prognosis? *Nutr. Cancer* **2017**, *69*, 1151–1176. [CrossRef] [PubMed]
34. Trinh, H.; Dzul, S.P.; Hyder, J.; Hyejeong, J.; Jang, H.; Kim, S.; Flowers, J.; Miller, S.; Chen, J.; Winer, I. Prognostic value of changes in neutrophil-to-lymphocyte ratio (NLR), platelet-to-lymphocyte ratio (PLR) and lymphocyte-to-monocyte ratio (LMR) for patients with cervical cancer undergoing definitive chemoradiotherapy (dCRT). *Clin. Chim. Acta* **2020**, *510*, 711–716. [CrossRef] [PubMed]
35. Chen, Y.; Wang, W.; Zhang, X.; Xiangyang, Y.; Xi, K.; Wen, Y.; Zhang, L.; Wang, G.; Feng, X. Prognostic significance of combined preoperative platelet-to-lymphocyte ratio and lymphocyte-to-monocyte ratio in patients undergoing surgery with stage IB non-small-cell lung cancer. *Cancer Manag. Res.* **2018**, *10*, 5411–5422. [CrossRef]
36. Lee, S.M.; Russell, A.; Hellawell, G. Predictive value of pretreatment inflammation-based prognostic scores (neutrophil-to-lymphocyte ratio, platelet-to-lymphocyte ratio, and lymphocyte-to-monocyte ratio) for invasive bladder carcinoma. *Korean J. Urol.* **2015**, *56*, 749–755. [CrossRef]
37. Yan, L.; Nakamura, T.; Casadei-Gardini, A.; Bruixola, G.; Huang, Y.L.; Hu, Z.D. Long-term and short-term prognostic value of the prognostic nutritional index in cancer: A narrative review. *Ann. Transl. Med.* **2021**, *9*, 1630. [CrossRef]
38. Kheirouri, S.; Alizadeh, M. Prognostic Potential of the Preoperative Controlling Nutritional Status (CONUT) Score in Predicting Survival of Patients with Cancer: A Systematic Review. *Adv. Nutr.* **2021**, *12*, 234–250. [CrossRef]
39. Matsukawa, T.; Suto, K.; Kanaya, M.; Izumiyama, K. North Japan Hematology Study Group (NJHSG). Validation and comparison of prognostic values of GNRI, PNI, and CONUT in newly diagnosed diffuse large B cell lymphoma. *Ann. Hematol.* **2020**, *99*, 2859–2868. [CrossRef]
40. Okamoto, S.; Ureshino, H.; Kidoguchi, K.; Kusaba, K.; Kizuka-Sano, H.; Sano, H.; Kimura, S.; Kojima, K.; Kawaguchi, A.; Sueoka, E.; et al. Clinical impact of the CONUT score in patients with multiple myeloma. *Ann. Hematol.* **2020**, *99*, 113–119. [CrossRef]
41. Peters, S.J.; Vanhaecke, T.; Papeleu, P.; Rogiers, V.; Haagsman, H.P.; van Norren, K. Co-culture of primary rat hepatocytes with rat liver epithelial cells enhances interleukin-6-induced acute-phase protein response. *Cell Tissue Res.* **2010**, *340*, 451–457. [CrossRef] [PubMed]
42. Honda, H.; Qureshi, A.R.; Heimburger, O.; Barany, P.; Wang, K.; Pecoits-Filho, R.; Lindholm, B.; Stenvinkel, P. Serum albumin, C-reactive protein, interleukin 6, and fetuin a as predictors of malnutrition, cardiovascular disease, and mortality in patients with ESRD. *Am. J. Kidney Dis.* **2006**, *47*, 139–148. [CrossRef] [PubMed]
43. Op den Kamp, C.M.; Langen, R.C.; Snepvangers, F.J.; de Theije, C.C.; Schellekens, J.M.; Laugs, F.; Schols, A.M.; Dingemans, A.-M.C. Nuclear transcription factor κ B activation and protein turnover adaptations in skeletal muscle of patients with progressive stages of lung cancer cachexia. *Am. J. Clin. Nutr.* **2013**, *98*, 738–748. [CrossRef] [PubMed]
44. Banks, W.A. Anorectic effects of circulating cytokines: Role of the vascular blood-brain barrier. *Nutrition* **2001**, *17*, 434–437. [CrossRef]

45. Law, D.K.; Dudrick, S.J.; Abdou, N.I. Immunocompetence of patients with protein-calorie malnutrition. The effects of nutritional repletion. *Ann. Intern. Med.* **1973**, *79*, 545–550. [CrossRef] [PubMed]
46. Menendez, J.A.; Lupu, R. Fatty acid synthase and the lipogenic phenotype in cancer pathogenesis. *Nat. Rev. Cancer* **2007**, *7*, 763–777. [CrossRef] [PubMed]
47. Vitols, S.; Gahrton, G.; Björkholm, M.; Peterson, C. Hypocholesterolaemia in malignancy due to elevated low-density-lipoprotein-receptor activity in tumour cells: Evidence from studies in patients with leukaemia. *Lancet* **1985**, *2*, 1150–1154. [CrossRef]
48. Henriksson, P.; Eriksson, M.; Ericsson, S.; Rudling, M.; Berglund, L.; Angelin, B. Hypocholesterolaemia and increased elimination of low-density lipoproteins in metastatic cancer of the prostate. *Lancet* **1989**, *2*, 1178–1180. [CrossRef]
49. Okuyama, H.; Ichikawa, Y.; Sun, Y.; Hamazaki, T.; Lands, W.E. Cancer and all-cause mortalities are lower in the higher total cholesterol groups among general populations. *World Rev. Nutr. Diet.* **2007**, *96*, 37–54.
50. Li, J.R.; Zhang, Y.; Zheng, J.L. Decreased pretreatment serum cholesterol level is related with poor prognosis in resectable non-small cell lung cancer. *Int. J. Clin. Exp. Pathol.* **2015**, *8*, 11877–11883.
51. Shin, H.J.; Roh, C.K.; Son, S.Y.; Hoon, H.; Han, S.U. Prognostic value of hypocholesterolemia in patients with gastric cancer. *Asian J. Surg.* **2021**, *44*, 72–79. [CrossRef] [PubMed]
52. Lee, H.; Jeong, C.W.; Kwak, C.; Kim, H.H.; Seo, S.I.; Lee, H.M.; Byun, S.S.; Lee, S.C.; Hong, S.K.; Lee, S.E.; et al. Preoperative Cholesterol Level Is Associated With Worse Pathological Outcomes and Postoperative Survival in Localized Renal Cell Carcinoma Patients: A Propensity Score-Matched Study. *Clin. Genitourin. Cancer* **2017**, *15*, 935–941. [CrossRef] [PubMed]
53. Kang, R.; Li, P.; Wang, T.; Li, X.; Wei, Z.; Zhang, Z.; Chen, X.F.; Xu, H.; Huang, C.; Bu, G.; et al. Apolipoprotein E epsilon 2 allele and low serum cholesterol as risk factors for gastric cancer in a Chinese Han population. *Sci. Rep.* **2016**, *6*, 19930. [CrossRef] [PubMed]
54. Chiba, T.; Ohtani, H.; Mizoi, T.; Naito, Y.; Sato, E.; Nagura, H.; Satomi, S.; Ohuchi, K.; Shiiba, K.; Kurokawa, Y.; et al. Intraepithelial CD8+ T-cell-count becomes a prognostic factor after a longer follow-up period in human colorectal carcinoma: Possible association with suppression of micrometastasis. *Br. J. Cancer* **2004**, *91*, 1711–1717. [CrossRef]
55. Nakano, O.; Sato, M.; Naito, Y.; Suzuki, K.; Orikasa, S.; Aizawa, M.; Ohtani, H.; Suzuki, Y.; Shintaku, I.; Nagura, H. Proliferative activity of intratumoral CD8(+) T-lymphocytes as a prognostic factor in human renal cell carcinoma: Clinicopathologic demonstration of antitumor immunity. *Cancer Res.* **2001**, *61*, 5132–5136.
56. Schumacher, K.; Haensch, W.; Röefzaad, C.; Schlag, P.M. Prognostic significance of activated CD8(+) T cell infiltrations within esophageal carcinomas. *Cancer Res.* **2001**, *61*, 3932–3936.

cancers

MDPI

Article

Optimal Surgical Extent in Patients with Unilateral Multifocal Papillary Thyroid Carcinoma

Joohyun Woo and Hyungju Kwon *

Department of Surgery, Ewha Womans University Medical Center, Seoul 07985, Korea; jwoo@ewha.ac.kr
* Correspondence: hkwon@ewha.ac.kr; Tel.: +82-2-2650-5025

Simple Summary: Around 30% of patients with papillary thyroid cancer (PTC) have multifocality. As tumor multifocality could increase the risk of recurrence in patients with PTC, more aggressive treatments, including total thyroidectomy and higher-dose radioiodine, are commonly used to treat patients with multifocal PTC. However, it is unclear whether aggressive treatment can decrease the risk of recurrence. Our study of 718 patients demonstrated that thyroid lobectomy showed comparable recurrence-free survival to that of total thyroidectomy. Moreover, our findings indicated that thyroid lobectomy could be safely performed on multifocal PTC patients with high-risk factors, such as large tumor size or lymph node metastasis. In conclusion, thyroid lobectomy was not associated with the risk of recurrence in patients with multifocal PTCs. Multifocality in PTC may not always require aggressive surgery.

Abstract: Multifocality increases the risk of recurrence in patients with papillary thyroid carcinoma (PTC); however, it is unclear whether multifocality justifies more extensive or aggressive surgical treatment. Here, we evaluated the effect of the operative extent on the recurrence-free survival (RFS) of patients with multifocal PTC. Between 2010 and 2019, 718 patients with unilateral multifocal PTC were enrolled; 115 patients (16.0%) underwent ipsilateral thyroid lobectomy, and 606 patients (84.0%) underwent total thyroidectomy. With a mean follow up of 5.2 years, RFS was comparable between the total thyroidectomy and lobectomy groups (p = 0.647) after adjusting for potential confounders. Multivariable Cox regression analysis also demonstrated that the operative extent was not an independent predictor of recurrence (HR 1.686, 95% CI: 0.321–8.852). Subgroup analyses further indicated that both total thyroidectomy and thyroid lobectomy resulted in comparable RFS for multifocal PTC patients with other high-risk factors, including tumor size > 1 cm (p = 0.711), lymph node metastasis (p = 0.536), and intermediate ATA risk of recurrence (p = 0.682). In conclusion, thyroid lobectomy was not associated with the risk of recurrence in patients with multifocal PTCs. Multifocality in PTC may not always require aggressive surgery.

Keywords: papillary thyroid carcinoma; multifocality; lobectomy; operative extent

Citation: Woo, J.; Kwon, H. Optimal Surgical Extent in Patients with Unilateral Multifocal Papillary Thyroid Carcinoma. *Cancers* **2022**, *14*, 432. https://doi.org/10.3390/cancers14020432

Academic Editors: Fabio Medas and Pier Francesco Alesina

Received: 13 December 2021
Accepted: 13 January 2022
Published: 15 January 2022

1. Introduction

Thyroid cancer is the ninth most prevalent cancer worldwide, and its incidence has dramatically increased over the last four decades [1]. There were 586,202 new cases of thyroid cancer in 2020, and papillary thyroid carcinoma (PTC) represented over 80% of all thyroid cancers [1]. Surgery for thyroid cancer is the most important element of a multi-faceted treatment approach [2]. Earlier guidelines recommended total thyroidectomy as the initial surgical treatment option, whereas the latest 2015 American Thyroid Association (ATA) guidelines have endorsed that thyroid lobectomy is safe and sufficient in selected patients with a low to intermediate risk of recurrence [2–4]. The optimal surgical extent can be determined by several clinicopathological factors, including personal history of radiation treatment to the head and neck, familial history of thyroid cancer, tumor size, extrathyroidal extension (ETE), regional or distant metastases, and multifocality [2].

Multifocality is defined as the simultaneous presence of two or more tumor foci within the thyroid gland [5]. Tumor multifocality is a common finding in PTC, with a prevalence of 18–87% of cases in the literature [6]. Multifocality is considered as a prognostic marker for the progression of PTC [7]. Multifocality has been associated with the high-risk features of PTC, including aggressive histology, ETE, lymph node (LN) involvement, and distant metastasis [7,8]. A recent meta-analysis also indicated that multifocality was an independent predictor of recurrence [9]. Some researchers further suggested that multifocal PTC could increase the risk of cancer-specific and overall mortality [10]. Therefore, more aggressive treatments, including total thyroidectomy and higher-dose radioiodine, are commonly used to treat patients with multifocal PTC [9,11–13].

There is a controversy about the optimal operative extent for patients with multifocal PTC. Several studies demonstrated that total thyroidectomy decreased the risk of recurrence compared with thyroid lobectomy [14–16]. On the contrary, other studies have suggested that lobectomy could be a feasible and valid option for patients with unilateral multifocal PTC [17–20]. These conflicting results are because, at least in part, all previous studies except one investigated the impact of operative extent without adjustment of other risk factors. Only Jeon et al. evaluated the significance of the surgical extent using a multivariable Cox proportional hazards model; however, this study only included patients with tumor size $\leq$ 1 cm, absence of gross ETE, and node-negative PTC (pT1aN0M0) [19].

Therefore, in the present study, we investigated the effect of the operative extent on the recurrence of multifocal PTC patients with various risk factors.

2. Materials and Methods

2.1. Study Design

This was a retrospective cohort study of patients aged 20 years or older with a diagnosis of unilateral multifocal PTC from 2010 to 2019 at the Ewha University Medical Center Mokdong Hospital. Institutional Review Board approval (Approval No. 2021-07-015) was obtained, and the need for written informed consent was waived.

2.2. Participant Selection

Patients were included in the present study if they were 20 years or older, had a pathologic diagnosis of unilateral multifocal PTC, and underwent curative-intent surgical treatment, including thyroid lobectomy or total thyroidectomy. The medical record of each patient was reviewed for clinicopathological data. Patients were excluded if they had high-risk histologic subtypes (including diffuse sclerosing, tall cell, and hobnail variants), gross ETE, or distant metastasis. Patients with incomplete data were also excluded. Data on patient demographics and tumor characteristics, including tumor size, microscopic ETE, LN metastasis, resection margin involvement, and coexisting Hashimoto thyroiditis, as well as recurrence status, were collected. The American Joint Committee on Cancer 7th edition was used for pathologic tumor, node, metastasis (TNM) staging.

2.3. Study End Points

The primary outcome measure was recurrence-free survival (RFS), which was defined as the time from initial surgery to the first event of recurrence. Recurrence was defined as newly found malignant lesions on the operative bed or metastatic LNs after 1 year from initial surgery, which were proven to be malignant by cytologic or histologic examination.

2.4. Statistical Analysis

SPSS Statistics version 23.0 (IBM Corp., Armonk, NY, USA) and R 3.5.3 (R Development Core Team, Vienna, Austria) were used for statistical analyses. Continuous data were compared by Student's t-tests. The comparison of dichotomous data was performed by Pearson chi-squared tests. To minimize potential confounding effects and selection bias, we performed 3:1 propensity score matching [21]. We selected 4 factors that could affect the recurrence as follows: tumor size, microscopic ETE, LN metastasis, and coexisting

Hashimoto thyroiditis. RFS was assessed by Kaplan–Meier survival analysis and log-rank test. As the RFS curves for lobectomy met those for total thyroidectomy, we checked the proportionality of the hazards to use a Cox proportional hazards regression model. The log(-log(survival)) plot and the scaled Schoenfeld residuals test for assessment of proportionality of hazards were used to verify the proportional hazards assumption [22]. The log(-log(survival)) plot for operative extent gave rise to reasonably parallel lines and suggested proportionality (Figure S1). The scaled Schoenfeld residuals test also produced no evidence of a poor fit ($p = 0.42$). Univariable and multivariable Cox proportional hazards regression models, therefore, were used to identify risk factors that could affect recurrence. A p-value < 0.05 was considered to indicate a statistically significant difference.

3. Results

3.1. Clinicopathological Characteristics of Included Patients

The baseline characteristics of 718 patients are summarized in Table 1. The mean age was 46.8 ± 11.3 years at the time of surgery, and 603 of the patients (83.6%) were women. The mean follow-up period was 5.2 ± 2.6 years. Of the 718 enrolled patients, 115 patients (16.0%) underwent ipsilateral thyroid lobectomy, and 606 patients (84.0%) underwent total thyroidectomy. Patients in the total thyroidectomy group had a larger tumor size (0.8 ± 0.5 cm vs. 0.7 ± 0.4 cm; $p = 0.047$), a higher rate of ETE (55.6% vs. 40.0%; $p = 0.002$), and an increased risk of LN metastasis (33.0% vs. 22.6%; $p = 0.028$) compared with those in the lobectomy group. Coexisting Hashimoto thyroiditis was also more common in the total thyroidectomy group than in the lobectomy group (33.7% vs. 21.7%; $p = 0.012$). Other clinicopathological factors, including age, sex, and margin involvement, showed no significant differences between the groups.

Table 1. Comparison of clinicopathological characteristics between lobectomy and total thyroidectomy groups.

Characteristics	Total Thyroidectomy (n = 603)	Thyroid Lobectomy (n = 115)	p-Value
Age (years)	47.1 ± 11.1	46.3 ± 11.1	0.489
Female sex	509 (84.4%)	91 (79.1%)	0.161
Pathologic characteristics			
Tumor size			
Mean (cm)	0.8 ± 0.5	0.7 ± 0.4	0.047
Microcarcinoma (%)	476 (78.9%)	99 (86.1%)	0.079
Microscopic ETE	335 (55.6%)	46 (40.0%)	0.002
LN metastasis	199 (33.0%)	26 (22.6%)	0.028
Margin involvement	32 (5.3%)	5 (4.3%)	0.670
Coexisting Hashimoto thyroiditis	203 (33.7%)	25 (21.7%)	0.012
Postoperative management			NA
^{131}I remnant ablation	353 (58.5%)		
^{131}I dose (mCi)	131.3 ± 33.3		
Follow-up period (years)	5.4 ± 2.4	4.4 ± 3.3	0.005
Recurrence	8 (1.3%)	2 (1.7%)	0.729

ETE, extrathyroidal extension; LN, lymph node; NA, not applicable.

Recurrences were observed in 8 patients (1.3%) in the total thyroidectomy group and 2 patients (1.7%) in the lobectomy group ($p = 0.729$). In the total thyroidectomy group, 7 patients developed ipsilateral neck LN recurrences, and thyroid bed recurrence was observed in the remaining patient. All recurrences in the lobectomy group were found in the ipsilateral lateral neck LN. The log-rank test indicated that the RFS of the total thyroidectomy group ($p = 0.515$) was comparable to that of the lobectomy group (Figure 1a).

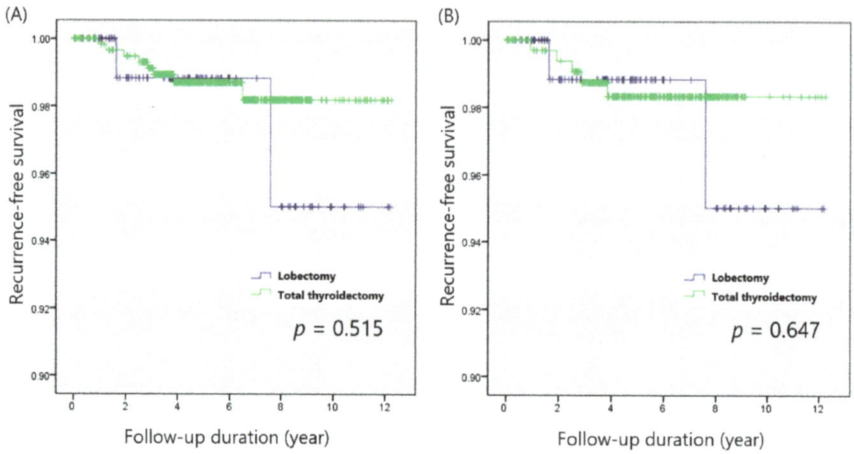

Figure 1. Recurrence-free survival according to the operative extent in patients with multifocal PTCs, (**A**) before and (**B**) after propensity score matching.

3.2. Recurrence-Free Survival in the 3:1 Matched Patient Group

As tumor size, microscopic ETE, or LN metastasis could affect recurrence, we performed 3:1 propensity score matching and yielded 115 matched pairs. Table 2 shows the clinicopathological comparison between the 3:1 matched total thyroidectomy and ipsilateral thyroid lobectomy groups. The matched cohorts did not differ in terms of clinicopathological features, including tumor size, microscopic ETE, and LN metastasis.

Table 2. Comparison of clinicopathological characteristics between lobectomy and total thyroidectomy groups after matching.

Characteristics	Total Thyroidectomy (n = 345)	Thyroid Lobectomy (n = 115)	p-Value
Age (years)	46.2 ± 11.0	46.3 ± 11.1	0.938
Female sex	276 (80.0%)	91 (79.1%)	0.841
Pathologic characteristics			
Tumor size			
Mean (cm)	0.7 ± 0.5	0.7 ± 0.4	0.523
Microcarcinoma (%)	283 (82.0%)	99 (86.1%)	0.315
Microscopic ETE	136 (39.4%)	46 (40.0%)	0.912
LN metastasis	87 (25.2%)	26 (22.6%)	0.574
Margin involvement	12 (3.5%)	5 (4.3%)	0.669
Coexisting Hashimoto thyroiditis	89 (25.8%)	25 (21.7%)	0.383
Postoperative management			NA
^{131}I remnant ablation	171 (49.6%)		
^{131}I dose (mCi)	128.1 ± 38.6		
Follow-up period (years)	5.3 ± 2.5	4.4 ± 3.3	0.014
Recurrence	5 (1.4%)	2 (1.7%)	0.826

ETE, extrathyroidal extension; LN, lymph node; NA, not applicable.

After adjusting for potential confounders, the overall recurrence rate was still comparable between the groups (1.4% vs. 1.7%; $p = 0.826$). RFS of the total thyroidectomy group ($p = 0.647$) also showed no significant difference from that of the lobectomy group (Figure 1b).

3.3. Predictive Factors of Poor RFS in Patients with Multifocal PTCs

The univariable Cox proportional hazards model indicated that only LN metastasis (hazards ratio [HR]: 5.370, 95% confidence interval [CI]: 1.388–20.785) was significantly associated with recurrence, and the operative extent (HR of thyroid lobectomy: 1.666, 95% CI: 0.353–7.870) was not predictive of the risk of recurrence (Table 3). LN metastasis (HR: 4.863, 95% CI: 1.179–20.056) retained statistical significance in multivariable analysis.

Table 3. Univariable and multivariable analysis for predictive factors of recurrence in patients with multifocal PTCs.

Covariates	Univariable Analysis		Multivariable Analysis	
	HR (95% CI)	*p*-Value	HR (95% CI)	*p*-Value
Age (years)	0.958 (0.902–1.017)	0.157	0.958 (0.899–1.021)	0.189
Male sex	2.289 (0.592–8.854)	0.230	1.637 (0.403–6.641)	0.490
Tumor size (cm)	1.027 (0.349–3.022)	0.962	0.805 (0.192–3.377)	0.767
Microscopic ETE	1.270 (0.358–4.503)	0.711	1.137 (0.290–4.457)	0.853
LN metastasis	5.370 (1.388–20.785)	0.015	4.863 (1.179–20.056)	0.029
Margin involvement	0.046 (0.000–6959.675)	0.612	0.000 (0.000-infinite)	0.982
Hashimoto thyroiditis	0.253 (0.032–2.002)	0.193	0.288 (0.035–2.402)	0.250
Operative extent	1.666 (0.353–7.870)	0.519	1.686 (0.321–8.852)	0.537

HR, hazard ratio; CI, confidence interval; ETE, extrathyroidal extension; LN, lymph node.

3.4. Lack of an Independent Role of Operative Extent in Patients with Other Risk Factors

Subgroup analyses were performed to assess the impact of the operative extent in multifocal PTC patients with several risk factors. We examined 3 factors that might influence the recurrence of PTC: primary tumor size (≤1 cm or >1 cm), LN metastasis (node-negative or node-positive), and ATA risk of recurrence (low or intermediate).

Papillary thyroid microcarcinoma (PTMC; defined as PTC $\leq$ 1 cm) was found in 476 patients, and 143 patients had PTC larger than 1 cm (non-PTMC). The recurrence rates of the total thyroidectomy and lobectomy groups were 6 of 476 (1.1%) and 2 of 99 (2.0%; $p = 0.469$), respectively, for PTMC patients and 2 of 127 (3.2%) and 0 of 16 (0.0%; $p = 0.467$), respectively, for non-PTMC patients. Kaplan–Meier analysis also indicated that total thyroidectomy showed comparable RFS to that of thyroid lobectomy in both the PTMC ($p = 0.443$) and non-PTMC ($p = 0.711$) groups (Figure 2A,B).

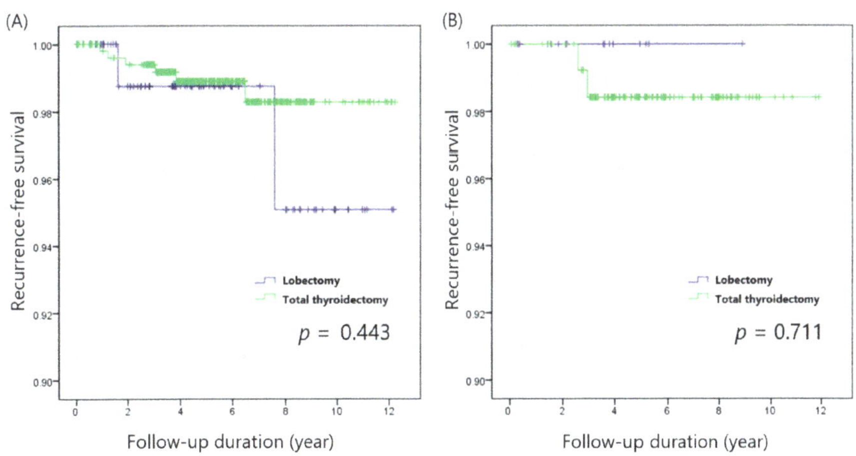

Figure 2. Recurrence-free survival in patients with (**A**) PTMC and (**B**) non-PTMC.

There were 490 patients with node-negative PTC, and LN metastasis was diagnosed in 225 patients. In the node-negative group, recurrences were observed in 2 of 404 patients (0.5%) after total thyroidectomy and 1 of 89 patients (1.1%) after thyroid lobectomy (p = 0.490). In the node-positive group, 6 of 199 patients (3.0%) with total thyroidectomy and 1 of 26 patients (3.8%) with thyroid lobectomy developed recurrences (p = 0.818). RFS was not considerably different between total thyroidectomy and thyroid lobectomy in both the node-negative (p = 0.447) and node-positive (p = 0.536) groups (Figure 3A,B).

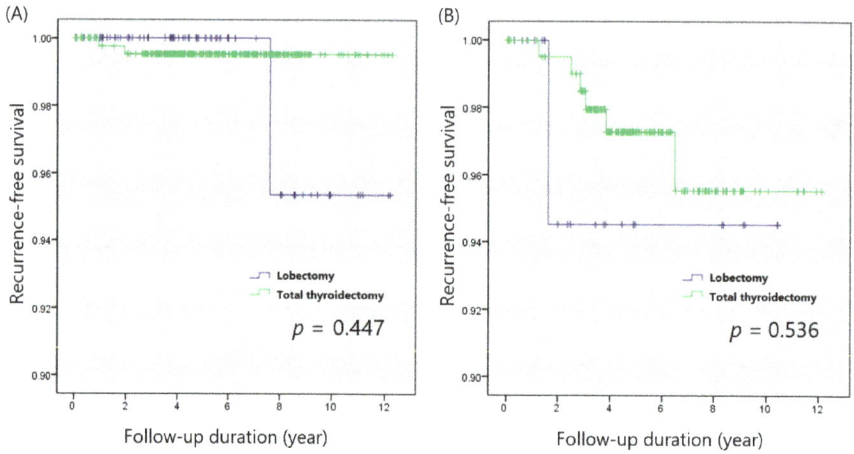

Figure 3. Recurrence-free survival in patients with (**A**) node-negative and (**B**) node-positive PTC.

When we stratified patients according to the ATA risk of recurrence categories, 324 and 394 patients were classified as low risk and intermediate risk, respectively. In ATA low-risk patients, recurrence rates were comparable between the total thyroidectomy and lobectomy groups (0.4% vs. 1.5%; p = 0.297). Patients with ATA intermediate risk also showed no difference in the recurrence rates be-tween groups (2.0% vs. 2.0%; p = 0.996). Total thyroidectomy and lobectomy demonstrated similar RFS in the ATA low-risk (p = 0.411) and ATA intermediate-risk (p = 0.682) groups (Figure 4A,B).

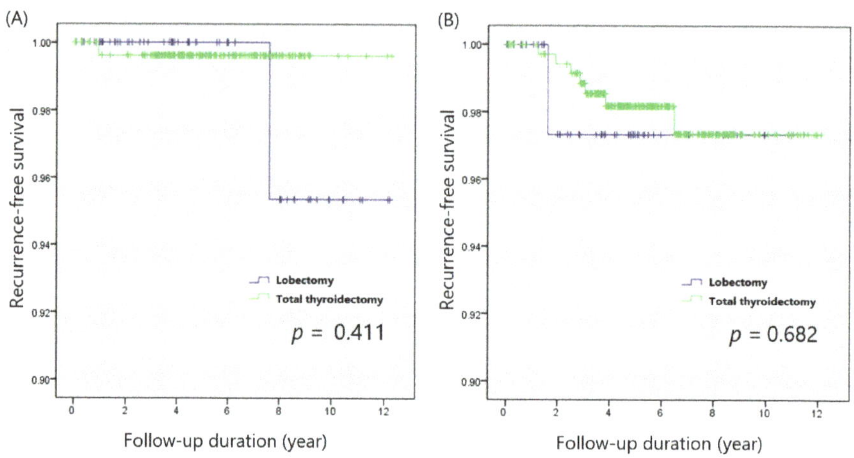

Figure 4. Recurrence-free survival in patients with (**A**) ATA low risk and (**B**) intermediate risk.

4. Discussion

The present study demonstrated that the operative extent of patients with unilateral multifocal PTC was not associated with risk of recurrence. Various guidelines and recent publications have promoted a "less is more" approach for the treatment of low-risk PTC, which represents the vast majority of thyroid cancers; this involves less extensive operation, less radioiodine, and less or no thyroid hormone suppression [23]. A global trend toward less radical surgical procedures, including thyroid lobectomy, has also gained traction in recent years [24]. Thyroid lobectomy has several advantages, including lowering the risk of complications and possibly avoiding a lifelong need for thyroid hormone supplements; however, concerns about oncological safety remain for patients with specific risk factors, including multifocality [25].

Determining the optimal surgical extent for patients with multifocal PTC has been a long-standing problem [26–28]. A consensus report of the European Society of Endocrine Surgeons recommended total or near-total thyroidectomy for multifocal PTC patients to reduce local recurrence [12]. A meta-analysis further indicated that patients with multifocal PTC should undergo central LN dissection [29]. On the contrary, recent studies demonstrated comparable RFS between total thyroidectomy and lobectomy for patients with node-negative multifocal PTC [18,19]. This inconsistency may be partly attributed to multifocality-associated risk factors, including large tumor size and LN metastasis, which can affect the operative extent decision [7]. These factors should also be considered to determine the optimal surgical extent for multifocal PTC.

Total thyroidectomy is usually performed instead of lobectomy for patients with more aggressive clinicopathological characteristics [30]. In the present study, compared with the thyroid lobectomy group, the total thyroidectomy group was also found to have a larger tumor size, a higher rate of microscopic ETE, and an increased risk of LN metastasis. As these high-risk features could affect the development of recurrence, propensity score matching was performed to minimize potential biases [21]. After adjusting for possible confounding factors, including tumor size, microscopic ETE, LN metastasis, and coexisting Hashimoto thyroiditis, our matched cohorts showed no difference in RFS between the total thyroidectomy and lobectomy groups. Our results further confirmed the overall oncologic safety of thyroid lobectomy for patients with multifocal PTC.

Subgroup analyses were performed to determine whether thyroid lobectomy is feasible for multifocal PTC patients with various risk factors. Total thyroidectomy showed comparable RFS to that of thyroid lobectomy for patients with non-PTMC (p = 0.711), node-positive PTC (p = 0.536), and ATA intermediate risk of recurrence (p = 0.682). Our findings suggest that multifocal PTC patients with tumor size > 1 cm, LN involvement, or intermediate ATA risk of recurrence do not always require a more extensive operation. Multivariable Cox proportional hazards analysis also indicated that the operative extent was not associated with the risk of recurrence, regardless of other risk factors. Therefore, we believe that thyroid lobectomy is suitable for all multifocal PTC patients without high-risk factors that require total thyroidectomy.

Our study has some limitations. First, this study was a retrospective cohort study, which is prone to selection bias. Patient selection for total thyroidectomy might be influenced by various factors, and the assignment of thyroid lobectomy and total thyroidectomy was not randomized. Although we performed propensity score matching, the results might be influenced by selection bias. Second, we did not evaluate long-term outcomes such as cancer-specific survival. During the mean follow-up period of 5.2 years, there was no cancer-specific mortality in the present study. Third, the number of patients with other risk factors of recurrence was relatively small. When we calculated the sample size for survival analysis using the data from Table 3, more than 255 recurrences were required to determine the statistical significance with HR of 1.686, 90% of power, and 2.5% of significance. Further validation studies with a larger cohort and long-term follow-up are warranted.

5. Conclusions

Thyroid lobectomy was not associated with the risk of recurrence in patients with multifocal PTCs. Multifocality in PTC may not always require aggressive surgery.

Supplementary Materials: The following is available online at https://www.mdpi.com/article/10.3390/cancers14020432/s1: Figure S1. Comparison of survival analysis by the operative extent: log(-log(survival)) plot.

Author Contributions: Conceptualization, J.W. and H.K.; methodology, J.W.; validation, H.K.; formal analysis, J.W. and H.K.; resources, H.K.; data curation, H.K.; writing—original draft preparation, J.W.; writing—review and editing, J.W. and H.K.; project administration, H.K. All authors have read and agreed to the published version of the manuscript.

Funding: This research received no external funding.

Institutional Review Board Statement: The study was conducted according to the guidelines of the Declaration of Helsinki and approved by the Institutional Review Board of Ewha University Medical Center Mokdong Hospital (approval number: 2021-07-015 and date of approval: 30 July 2021).

Informed Consent Statement: Patient consent was waived by the institutional review board, because (1) this research involved no more than minimal risk to subjects and (2) this research could be carried out practicably without the waiver.

Data Availability Statement: The data presented in this study are available on request from the corresponding author. The data are not publicly available due to institutional policy.

Conflicts of Interest: The authors declare no conflict of interest.

References

1. Sung, H.; Ferlay, J.; Siegel, R.L.; Laversanne, M.; Soerjomataram, I.; Jemal, A.; Bray, F. Global Cancer Statistics 2020: GLOBOCAN Estimates of Incidence and Mortality Worldwide for 36 Cancers in 185 Countries. *CA Cancer J. Clin.* **2021**, *71*, 209–249. [CrossRef]
2. Haugen, B.R.; Alexander, E.K.; Bible, K.C.; Doherty, G.M.; Mandel, S.J.; Nikiforov, Y.E.; Pacini, F.; Randolph, G.W.; Sawka, A.M.; Schlumberger, M.; Schuff, K.G.; Sherman, S.I.; Sosa, J.A.; Steward, D.L.; Tuttle, R.M.; Wartofsky, L. 2015 American Thyroid Association Management Guidelines for Adult Patients with Thyroid Nodules and Differentiated Thyroid Cancer: The American Thyroid Association Guidelines Task Force on Thyroid Nodules and Differentiated Thyroid Cancer. *Thyroid* **2016**, *26*, 1–133. [CrossRef] [PubMed]
3. Cooper, D.S.; Doherty, G.M.; Haugen, B.R.; Kloos, R.T.; Lee, S.L.; Mandel, S.J.; Mazzaferri, E.L.; McIver, B.; Sherman, S.I.; Tuttle, R.M.; American Thyroid Association Guidelines, T. Management guidelines for patients with thyroid nodules and differentiated thyroid cancer. *Thyroid* **2006**, *16*, 109–142. [CrossRef] [PubMed]
4. Cooper, D.S.; Doherty, G.M.; Haugen, B.R.; Kloos, R.T.; Lee, S.L.; Mandel, S.J.; Mazzaferri, E.L.; McIver, B.; Pacini, F.; Schlumberger, M.; et al. Revised American Thyroid Association management guidelines for patients with thyroid nodules and differentiated thyroid cancer. *Thyroid* **2009**, *19*, 1167–1214. [CrossRef] [PubMed]
5. Kuhn, E.; Teller, L.; Piana, S.; Rosai, J.; Merino, M.J. Different clonal origin of bilateral papillary thyroid carcinoma, with a review of the literature. *Endocr Pathol.* **2012**, *23*, 101–107. [CrossRef] [PubMed]
6. Qu, N.; Zhang, L.; Ji, Q.H.; Zhu, Y.X.; Wang, Z.Y.; Shen, Q.; Wang, Y.; Li, D.S. Number of tumor foci predicts prognosis in papillary thyroid cancer. *BMC Cancer.* **2014**, *14*, 914. [CrossRef] [PubMed]
7. Joseph, K.R.; Edirimanne, S.; Eslick, G.D. Multifocality as a prognostic factor in thyroid cancer: A meta-analysis. *Int J. Surg.* **2018**, *50*, 121–125. [CrossRef]
8. Vuong, H.G.; Duong, U.N.P.; Pham, T.Q.; Tran, H.M.; Oishi, N.; Mochizuki, K.; Nakazawa, T.; Hassell, L.; Katoh, R.; Kondo, T. Clinicopathological Risk Factors for Distant Metastasis in Differentiated Thyroid Carcinoma: A Meta-analysis. *World J. Surg.* **2018**, *42*, 1005–1017. [CrossRef]
9. Kim, H.; Kwon, H.; Moon, B.I. Association of Multifocality With Prognosis of Papillary Thyroid Carcinoma: A Systematic Review and Meta-analysis. *JAMA Otolaryngol. Head Neck Surg.* **2021**, *147*, 847–854. [CrossRef] [PubMed]
10. Markovic, I.; Goran, M.; Besic, N.; Buta, M.; Djurisic, I.; Stojiljkovic, D.; Zegarac, M.; Pupic, G.; Inic, Z.; Dzodic, R. Multifocality as independent prognostic factor in papillary thyroid cancer - A multivariate analysis. *J. BUON.* **2018**, *23*, 1049–1054.
11. Kim, K.J.; Kim, S.M.; Lee, Y.S.; Chung, W.Y.; Chang, H.S.; Park, C.S. Prognostic significance of tumor multifocality in papillary thyroid carcinoma and its relationship with primary tumor size: A retrospective study of 2,309 consecutive patients. *Ann. Surg. Oncol.* **2015**, *22*, 125–131. [CrossRef]
12. Iacobone, M.; Jansson, S.; Barczynski, M.; Goretzki, P. Multifocal papillary thyroid carcinoma–a consensus report of the European Society of Endocrine Surgeons (ESES). *Langenbecks Arch. Surg.* **2014**, *399*, 141–154. [CrossRef]
13. Kim, H.J.; Sohn, S.Y.; Jang, H.W.; Kim, S.W.; Chung, J.H. Multifocality, but not bilaterality, is a predictor of disease recurrence/persistence of papillary thyroid carcinoma. *World J. Surg.* **2013**, *37*, 376–384. [CrossRef]
14. Xue, S.; Wang, P.; Liu, J.; Chen, G. Total thyroidectomy may be more reasonable as initial surgery in unilateral multifocal papillary thyroid microcarcinoma: A single-center experience. *World J. Surg. Oncol.* **2017**, *15*, 62. [CrossRef]

15. Li, X.; Zhao, C.; Hu, D.; Yu, Y.; Gao, J.; Zhao, W.; Gao, M. Hemithyroidectomy increases the risk of disease recurrence in patients with ipsilateral multifocal papillary thyroid carcinoma. *Oncol. Lett.* **2013**, *5*, 1412–1416. [CrossRef]
16. Ross, D.S.; Litofsky, D.; Ain, K.B.; Bigos, T.; Brierley, J.D.; Cooper, D.S.; Haugen, B.R.; Jonklaas, J.; Ladenson, P.W.; Magner, J.; Robbins, J.; Skarulis, M.C.; Steward, D.L.; Maxon, H.R.; Sherman, S.I. Recurrence after treatment of micropapillary thyroid cancer. *Thyroid* **2009**, *19*, 1043–1048. [CrossRef] [PubMed]
17. Albinsaad, L.S.; Kim, W.W.; Lee, Y.M.; Sung, T.Y.; Chung, K.W.; Hong, S.J. The appropriateness of thyroid lobectomy as an initial surgery for preoperatively detected unilateral multifocal papillary carcinoma. *Asian J. Surg.* **2021**, *44*, 1050–1055. [CrossRef] [PubMed]
18. Harries, V.; Wang, L.Y.; McGill, M.; Xu, B.; Tuttle, R.M.; Wong, R.J.; Shaha, A.R.; Shah, J.P.; Ghossein, R.; Patel, S.G.; Ganly, I. Should multifocality be an indication for completion thyroidectomy in papillary thyroid carcinoma? *Surgery* **2020**, *167*, 10–17. [CrossRef]
19. Jeon, Y.W.; Gwak, H.G.; Lim, S.T.; Schneider, J.; Suh, Y.J. Long-Term Prognosis of Unilateral and Multifocal Papillary Thyroid Microcarcinoma After Unilateral Lobectomy Versus Total Thyroidectomy. *Ann. Surg. Oncol.* **2019**, *26*, 2952–2958. [CrossRef] [PubMed]
20. Huang, H.; Liu, S.; Xu, Z.; Ni, S.; Zhang, Z.; Wang, X. Long-term outcome of thyroid lobectomy for unilateral multifocal papillary carcinoma. *Medicine* **2017**, *96*, e7461. [CrossRef]
21. Woo, J.; Kim, H.; Kwon, H. Impact of Multifocality on the Recurrence of Papillary Thyroid Carcinoma. *J. Clin. Med.* **2021**, 10. [CrossRef]
22. Bradburn, M.J.; Clark, T.G.; Altman, D.G. Survival analysis Part III: Multivariate data analysis – choosing a model and assessing its adequacy and fit. *Br. J. Cancer* **2003**, *89*, 605–611. [CrossRef] [PubMed]
23. Hartl, D.M.; Guerlain, J.; Breuskin, I.; Hadoux, J.; Baudin, E.; Al Ghuzlan, A.; Terroir-Cassou-Mounat, M.; Lamartina, L.; Leboulleux, S. Thyroid Lobectomy for Low to Intermediate Risk Differentiated Thyroid Cancer. *Cancers* **2020**, *12*, 3282. [CrossRef] [PubMed]
24. Marciniak, C.; Lenne, X.; Clement, G.; Bruandet, A.; Lifante, J.C.; Sebag, F.; Mirallie, E.; Mathonnet, M.; Brunaud, L.; Donatini, G.; et al. Partial Versus Total Thyroidectomy: What Influences Most Surgeons' Decision? Analysis of a Nationwide Cohort of 375,810 Patients Over 10 Years. *Ann. Surg.* **2021**, *274*, 829–835. [CrossRef] [PubMed]
25. Raffaelli, M.; Tempera, S.E.; Sessa, L.; Lombardi, C.P.; De Crea, C.; Bellantone, R. Total thyroidectomy versus thyroid lobectomy in the treatment of papillary carcinoma. *Gland. Surg.* **2020**, *9*, S18–s27. [CrossRef] [PubMed]
26. Feng, J.W.; Pan, H.; Wang, L.; Ye, J.; Jiang, Y.; Qu, Z. Determine the Optimal Extent of Thyroidectomy and Lymphadenectomy for Patients With Papillary Thyroid Microcarcinoma. *Front. Endocrinol. (Lausanne)* **2019**, *10*, 363. [CrossRef]
27. Wang, Z.; Xiang, J.; Gui, Z.; Qin, Y.; Sun, W.; Huang, J.; He, L.; Dong, W.; Zhang, D.; Zhang, T.; Shao, L.; Lv, C.; Zhang, P.; Zhang, H. Unilateral Tnm T1 And T2 Papillary Thyroid Carcinoma With Lateral Cervical Lymph Node Metastasis: Total Thyroidectomy or Lobectomy? *Endocr. Pract.* **2020**, *26*, 1085–1092. [CrossRef]
28. Jiang, L.H.; Yin, K.X.; Wen, Q.L.; Chen, C.; Ge, M.H.; Tan, Z. Predictive Risk-scoring Model For Central Lymph Node Metastasis and Predictors of Recurrence in Papillary Thyroid Carcinoma. *Sci. Rep.* **2020**, *10*, 710. [CrossRef] [PubMed]
29. Zhang, T.; He, L.; Wang, Z.; Dong, W.; Sun, W.; Zhang, P.; Zhang, H. The Differences Between Multifocal and Unifocal Papillary Thyroid Carcinoma in Unilateral Lobe: A Meta-Analysis. *Front. Oncol.* **2021**, *11*, 657237. [CrossRef] [PubMed]
30. Filetti, S.; Durante, C.; Hartl, D.; Leboulleux, S.; Locati, L.D.; Newbold, K.; Papotti, M.G.; Berruti, A.; ESMO Guidelines Committee. Thyroid cancer: ESMO Clinical Practice Guidelines for diagnosis, treatment and follow-up. *Ann. Oncol.* **2019**, *30*, 1856–1883. [CrossRef] [PubMed]

cancers

MDPI

Article

Use of Diagnostic Criteria from ACR and EU-TIRADS Systems to Improve the Performance of Cytology in Thyroid Nodule Triage

Davide Seminati [1], Giulia Capitoli [2], Davide Leni [3], Davide Fior [3], Francesco Vacirca [3], Camillo Di Bella [1], Stefania Galimberti [2], Vincenzo L'Imperio [1] and Fabio Pagni [1,*]

1 Department of Medicine and Surgery, University of Milano-Bicocca, Pathology, 20900 Monza, Italy; d.seminati@campus.unimib.it (D.S.); camillo.dibella@asst-monza.it (C.D.B.); vincenzo.limperio@gmail.com (V.L.)
2 Bicocca Bioinformatics Biostatistics and Bioimaging B4 Center, School of Medicine and Surgery, University of Milano-Bicocca, 20900 Monza, Italy; giulia.capitoli@unimib.it (G.C.); stefania.galimberti@unimib.it (S.G.)
3 Department of Radiology, ASST Monza, 20900 Monza, Italy; davide.leni@asst-monza.it (D.L.); davide.fior@asst-monza.it (D.F.); franscesco.vacirca@asst-monza.it (F.V.)
* Correspondence: fabio.pagni@unimib.it

Simple Summary: From a prospective series of 480 thyroid nodules, we compared the performances of the American College of Radiology (ACR) and the European Thyroid Association (EU) scoring systems in triaging thyroid nodules for fine-needle aspiration (FNA). FNA was recommended on 46.5% and 51.9% of the nodules using the ACR and EU-TIRADS scores, respectively. The ACR system demonstrated a higher specificity as compared to the EU-TIRADS (59.0% vs. 52.4%, $p = 0.0012$) in predicting ≥TIR3A/III (SIAPEC/Bethesda) nodules. Moreover, specific radiological features (i.e., echogenic foci and margins), combined with the cytological classes improved the specificity (97.5% vs. 91%, $p < 0.0001$) and positive predictive value (77.5% vs. 50.7%, $p < 0.0001$) of the cytology alone, maintaining an excellent sensitivity and negative predictive value.

Abstract: Objective: The American College of Radiology (ACR) and the European Thyroid Association (EU) have proposed two scoring systems for thyroid nodule classification. Here, we compared the ability of the two systems in triaging thyroid nodules for fine-needle aspiration (FNA) and tested the putative role of an approach that combines ultrasound features and cytology for the detection of malignant nodules. **Design and Methods:** The scores obtained with the ACR and EU Thyroid Imaging Reporting and Data Systems (TIRADS) from a prospective series of 480 thyroid nodules acquired from 435 subjects were compared to assess their performances in FNA triaging on the final cytological diagnosis. The US features that showed the highest contribution in discriminating benign nodules from malignancies were combined with cytology to improve its diagnostic performance. **Results:** FNA was recommended on 46.5% and 51.9% of the nodules using the ACR and EU TIRADS scores, respectively. The ACR system demonstrated a higher specificity as compared to the EU-TIRADS (59.0% vs. 52.4%, $p = 0.0012$) in predicting ≥ TIR3A/III (SIAPEC/Bethesda) nodules. Moreover, specific radiological features (i.e., echogenic foci and margins), combined with the cytological classes improved the specificity (97.5% vs. 91%, $p < 0.0001$) and positive predictive values (77.5% vs. 50.7%, $p < 0.0001$) compared to cytology alone, especially in the setting of indeterminate nodules (TIR3A/III and TIR3B/IV), maintaining an excellent sensitivity and negative predictive value. **Conclusions:** The ACR-TIRADS system showed a higher specificity compared to the EU-TIRADS in triaging thyroid nodules. The use of specific radiological features improved the diagnostic ability of cytology.

Keywords: ultrasound imaging; thyroid nodule; thyroid carcinoma; fine-needle aspiration

Citation: Seminati, D.; Capitoli, G.; Leni, D.; Fior, D.; Vacirca, F.; Di Bella, C.; Galimberti, S.; L'Imperio, V.; Pagni, F. Use of Diagnostic Criteria from ACR and EU-TIRADS Systems to Improve the Performance of Cytology in Thyroid Nodule Triage. *Cancers* **2021**, *13*, 5439. https://doi.org/10.3390/cancers13215439

Academic Editor: Fabio Medas

Received: 5 October 2021
Accepted: 26 October 2021
Published: 29 October 2021

1. Introduction

In the international scenario, different alternative ultrasound (US) algorithms have been proposed for characterizing thyroid nodules [1]. The American College of Radiology (ACR) Thyroid Imaging Reporting and Data Systems (TIRADS) consists of a scale with increasing scores for specific US features of thyroid nodules and is able to stratify lesions with a progressively higher risk of malignancy (ROM) [2–4]. On this side of the Atlantic ocean, the European Thyroid Association (EU-TIRADS) proposed in 2017 a US pattern recognition method that combines high-risk criteria, such as nodule composition, echogenicity, margins, shape, and calcifications [5]. The main purpose of these scoring systems is the reduction in inappropriate fine-needle aspirations (FNAs), triaging thyroid nodules at their best. However, the final FNA results do not always match the pre-biopsy risk class assigned by these two systems. Indeed, the indication of a biopsy is influenced by subjectivity in US interpretation, different ROMs in the screened populations, and personalized clinical decisions [6,7]. On the other hand, defensive medicine, excessive scrupulousness, or limited experience could induce clinicians to perform FNA regardless of the TIRADS score, especially in large nodules, still depending on cytology for the final answer regarding the nature of a thyroid lesion and thus reducing the practical utility of TIRADS [8]. Although the most recent reports in the literature stress the recommendation to implement these algorithms in the clinical setting, the selection of more impactful radiological criteria may improve the contribution of these systems to risk assessments [6,9–11]. In this work, we present a comparative analysis of the most widely employed US classifications to support their systematic application in a first-level general hospital for the bioptic triage of thyroid nodules [8]. Moreover, the present paper supports the hypothesis that specific US features, coupled with cytological classes, might be better able predict the final malignant nature of a thyroid nodule.

2. Materials and Methods

2.1. Patients Selection

This prospective study included 448 consecutive patients who underwent 493 US-guided FNA from January to June 2019 at the interventional radiology clinic, ASST Monza, Italy, during an Italian Association for Research on Cancer (AIRC)-granted project for the diagnosis of thyroid carcinoma [8]. All nodules were subjected to FNA, regardless of their ACR/EU-TIRADS scores, after an endocrinological clinical indication. Thirteen lesions with an unsatisfactory cytology and no FNA repetition were excluded for a final set of 480 nodules and 435 subjects. Histology was available in 49 resected nodules. US was performed at the 12-month follow-up visit in 352 patients, while 79 cases, corresponding to 70 TIR3A/III, 8 TIR3B/IV, and 1 TIR4/V, were lost to follow-up. This study was approved by the ASST Monza Ethical Board (October 2016, 27102016) and appropriate informed consent was obtained from all patients.

2.2. Ultrasound Evaluation

Patients were placed in supine position with their neck in hyperextension. The US was performed with the Philips Epiq Elite machine. For each nodule, the radiologists used real-time clips to measure the major axis and analyzed its composition, echogenicity, shape, margins, and the presence of calcifications, as previously described [3]. The final theoretical indication for FNA execution was formulated according to the ACR and EU-TIRADS algorithms [3,5]. US was performed by three different radiologists (DL, DF, FV) who were experts in thyroid imaging and who contributed equally to the evaluation of the case series.

2.3. Cytopathology and Histopathology

Aspiration was performed by two pathologists (FP and CDB) with 10 years of experience in thyroid FNA under US guidance with 22–25 gauge diameter needles. The aspirated material was smeared onto 3–4 traditional slides per nodule. The slides were fixed with spray alcohol (Cytofix, propan-2-ol) and then stained with Papanicolau, or air-dried and stained with May–Grunwald Giemsa. Cases were diagnosed according to two standard systems for reporting thyroid cytopathology: the Italian Society of Pathology classification (SIAPEC) and the Bethesda System [12,13]. The TIRADS indication of FNA was considered correct in the presence of a cytology ≥TIR3A/III (SIAPEC/Bethesda). TIR1c-TIR2 patients and those with TIR3 who did not undergo surgery, underwent a US examination 12 months after the first US-guided FNA performed by the same radiologist [14]. Nodules were considered benign in the absence of the following conditions:

- new echographic suspicious features—i.e., US features with ≥2 ACR-TIRADS points;
- >20% increase in size;
- enlarged lymph nodes;
- appearance of new suspicious nodules—i.e., with ACR or EU-TIRADS class ≥ 3.

A histological evaluation was performed on the surgical specimens of total or hemithyroidectomy [15]. The tissue was formalin-fixed, paraffin-embedded, and stained with haematoxylin and eosin. The ROM was estimated according to histological evaluation or US follow-up examination.

2.4. Statistical Analysis

Mean and standard deviation or quartiles were used for descriptive purposes, as appropriate. The diagnostic ability of the TIRADS systems in distinguishing thyroid nodules that required or not FNA was evaluated using cytology as reference standard (<TIR3A/III vs. ≥TIR3A/III) in all 480 nodules. The results of the TIRADS classifications and cytology were also compared to the histopathological/follow-up findings on 401 nodules. Sensitivity, specificity, and positive and negative predictive values (PPV and NPV) were calculated alongside their 95% confidence intervals (CI). The McNemar test was considered for the comparison of the performances (two-sided test, $\alpha = 0.05$). A decision tree was applied to the cytological classes and to the single TIRADS ecographic components of each thyroid nodule to explore whether and which US features were relevant in malignancy detection. The risk of malignancy was calculated as the rate of prevalence. All of the statistical analyses were performed using the open-source R software v.3.6.0 (R Foundation for Statistical Computing, Vienna, Austria).

3. Results

3.1. ACR vs. EU-TIRADS

The comparison between the ACR and EU systems in classifying the 480 nodules is shown in Table 1.

Table 1. Comparison between the ACR and EU-TIRADS systems in the indication to perform FNA.

	ACR-TIRADS								
	No Indication of FNA					Indication of FNA			
EU-TIRADS	ACR1	ACR2	ACR3 <2.5 cm	ACR4 <1.5 cm	ACR5 <1.0 cm	ACR3 ≥2.5 cm	ACR4 ≥1.5 cm	ACR5 ≥1.0 cm	Total
No indication of FNA									
EU 1	0	0	0	0	0	0	0	0	0
EU 2	30	2	0	0	0	0	0	0	32
EU 3 ≤ 2.0 cm	0	15	50	3	0	0	1	0	69
EU 4 ≤ 1.5 cm	0	0	19	81	0	0	11	0	111
EU 5 ≤ 1.0 cm	0	0	0	10	3	0	0	6	19
Indication of FNA									
EU 3 > 2.0 cm	0	22	4	0	0	39	9	0	74
EU 4 > 1.5 cm	0	0	8	0	0	16	69	0	93
EU 5 > 1.0 cm	0	0	0	10	0	0	27	45	82
Total	30	39	81	104	3	55	117	51	480

Considering the nodules requiring FNA as per the ACR (n = 223, 46.5%) and EU-TIRADS (n = 249, 51.9%) criteria, 86 (38.6%) and 90 (36.1%) were deemed to be ≥TIR3A/III after cytological assessment. Overall, a good agreement between the two systems was noted, reaching an accordance for FNA indication in 87.1% (418/480) of the nodules. The major discrepancies on the execution of cytology were observed in the setting of EU-TIRADS class 3, with 26 cases that would not be submitted to biopsy as per ACR, either for different US scores (n = 22) or size cut-off (n = 4). Similarly, 12 cases that received FNA following the ACR-TIRADS criteria did not reach the indication in the EU-TIRADS system, either for different US scores (n = 1) or size cut-offs (n = 11). Finally, 11.1% (6/54) of the cases labeled as class 5 in both the systems would be biopsied only following ACR due to the presence of a size "grey-zone" of exactly 1 cm in the classifications [3,5]. The assessment of the performances of these systems in the final FNA indication showed a significantly higher specificity for the ACR as compared to the EU-TIRADS (59.0% vs. 52.4%, p = 0.0012), with a similar sensitivity (58.9% vs. 61.6%, p = 0.3173), PPV (38.6% vs. 36.1%, p = 0.1116), and NPV (76.7% vs. 75.8%, p = 0.5288) (Tables 2 and 3). The difference noted in terms of the specificity was mainly due to the discordances of the two systems in terms of the size cutoff and the US feature "echogenicity".

Table 2. ACR-TIRADS vs. SIAPEC/Bethesda system cytological classifications. False negative cases are in bold. False positive cases are in italics.

	SIAPEC/Bethesda System						
ACR-TIRADS	**TIR1c/I**	**TIR2/II**	**TIR3A/III**	**TIR3B/IV**	**TIR4/V**	**TIR5/VI**	**Total**
No indication of FNA							
ACR 1	12	16	**2**	**0**	**0**	**0**	30
ACR 2	1	33	**5**	**0**	**0**	**0**	39
ACR 3 < 2.5 cm	0	63	**13**	**2**	**2**	**1**	81
ACR 4 < 1.5 cm	0	72	**21**	**4**	**3**	**4**	104
ACR 5 < 1.0 cm	0	0	**2**	**0**	**1**	**0**	3
Indication of FNA							
ACR 3 ≥ 2.5 cm	*1*	35	15	3	1	0	55
ACR 4 ≥ 1.5 cm	*1*	77	29	7	3	0	117
ACR 5 ≥ 1.0 cm	*0*	23	9	5	2	12	51
Total	15	319	96	21	12	17	480

Table 3. EU-TIRADS vs. SIAPEC/Bethesda system cytological classifications. False negative cases are in bold. False positive cases are in italics.

	SIAPEC/Bethesda System						
EU-TIRADS	**TIR1c/I**	**TIR2/II**	**TIR3A/III**	**TIR3B/IV**	**TIR4/V**	**TIR5/VI**	**Total**
No indication of FNA							
EU 1	0	0	**0**	**0**	**0**	**0**	0
EU 2	12	18	**2**	**0**	**0**	**0**	32
EU 3 ≤ 2.0 cm	0	54	**11**	**1**	**2**	**1**	69
EU 4 ≤ 1.5 cm	0	84	**21**	**3**	**2**	**1**	111
EU 5 ≤ 1.0 cm	0	7	**7**	**2**	**2**	**1**	19
Indication of FNA							
EU 3 > 2.0 cm	*2*	*47*	20	4	1	0	74
EU 4 > 1.5 cm	*1*	*67*	20	3	2	0	93
EU 5 > 1.0 cm	*0*	*42*	15	8	3	14	82
Total	15	319	96	21	12	17	480

Histological evaluation was performed on 10.2% (49/480) of the nodules, 81.6% (40/49) of which had an FNA result ≥ TIR3B/IV. A total of 34 out of the 49 (69.3%) nodules showed malignancy (27 PTC, 3 EFVPTC, 1 Hurthle cell carcinoma, 1 medullary carcinoma, 1 anaplastic carcinoma, and 1 metastasis of the melanoma). The ACR-TIRADS confirmed a significantly higher specificity (57.2% vs. 51.2%, $p = 0.0019$), with a similar sensitivity (67.6% vs. 70.6%, $p = 0.6547$), PPV (12.8% vs. 11.8%, $p = 0.4030$), and NPV (95% vs. 94.9%, $p = 0.9435$) in the diagnosis of malignancy (Table 4). As reported for the analysis of FNA indication, the difference in terms of the specificity between the two systems was mainly driven by the size cutoff and US feature "echogenicity".

Table 4. Diagnostic performances of TIRADS systems, cytology, and combination of US features and cytology in the diagnosis of malignant nodules ($n = 401$).

	TP	FP	TN	FN	Sensitivity (%)	Specificity (%)	PPV (%)	NPV (%)
ACR	23	157	210	11	67.6 (23/34) [49.5–82.6]	57.2 (210/367) [52.0–62.3]	12.8 (23/180) [8.3–18.6]	95.0 (210/221) [91.3–97.5]
EU	24	179	188	10	70.6 (24/34) [52.5–84.9]	51.2 (188/367) [46.0–56.4]	11.8 (24/203) [7.7–17.1]	94.9 (188/198) [90.9–97.6]
Cytology	34	33	334	0	**100** (34/34) [89.7–100]	91.0 (334/367) [87.6–93.7]	50.7 (34/67) [38.2–63.2]	**100** (334/334) [98.9–100]
Cytology +EF/M	31	9	358	3	91.2 (31/34) [76.3–98.1]	**97.5** (358/367) [95.4–98.9]	**77.5** (31/40) [61.5–89.2]	99.2 (358/361) [97.6–99.8]

The best performances are in bold, 95% confidence intervals in brackets. TP: true positive; FP: false negative; TN: true negative; FN: false negative; PPV: positive predictive value; NPV: negative predictive value; EF/M: echogenic foci/margins.

3.2. Combining US Features with Cytology for Diagnostication

The diagnostic performance of cytology alone, using the TIR3A/III class as the threshold, showed a sensitivity of 100% (34/34, 95% CI = 89.7–100%), a specificity of 91% (334/367, 95% CI = 87.6–93.7%), a PPV of 50.7% (34/67, 95% CI = 38.2–63.2%), and an NPV of 100% (334/334, 95% CI = 98.9–100%) (Table 4).

As expected, combining the TIRADS and cytology classes did not improve their performance. However, a decision tree applied to cytology and single US features of the two TIRADS systems identified two independent characteristics, i.e., echogenic foci and irregular margins, able to contribute to diagnostication, especially in the setting of undetermined nodules (Figure 1).

Indeed, this approach adequately detected four cases of carcinoma, otherwise classified as TIR3A/III ($n = 1$) and TIR3B/IV ($n = 3$). Moreover, three indeterminate nodules (one TIR3A/III and two TIR3B/IV) were wrongly classified as benign by the application of this approach and corresponded to an encapsulated follicular variant of papillary thyroid carcinoma (EFVPTC), whose malignant potential is still debated. Similarly, among the eight cases misclassified as malignant by the decision tree, four were diagnosed as follicular adenomas on the final histology (two TIR3A/III and two TIR3B/IV), and, although these lesions are benign, they usually require the complete histological assessment of the final surgical specimen for the exclusion of carcinoma. Finally, the adoption of this combined US/cytology approach led to a significant increase in the specificity (97.5% vs. 91%, $p < 0.0001$) and PPV (77.5% vs. 50.8%, $p < 0.0001$), with still excellent values of sensitivity (91.2% vs. 100%, $p = 0.0833$) and NPV (99.2% vs. 100%, $p = 0.0820$), as compared to cytology alone (Table 4).

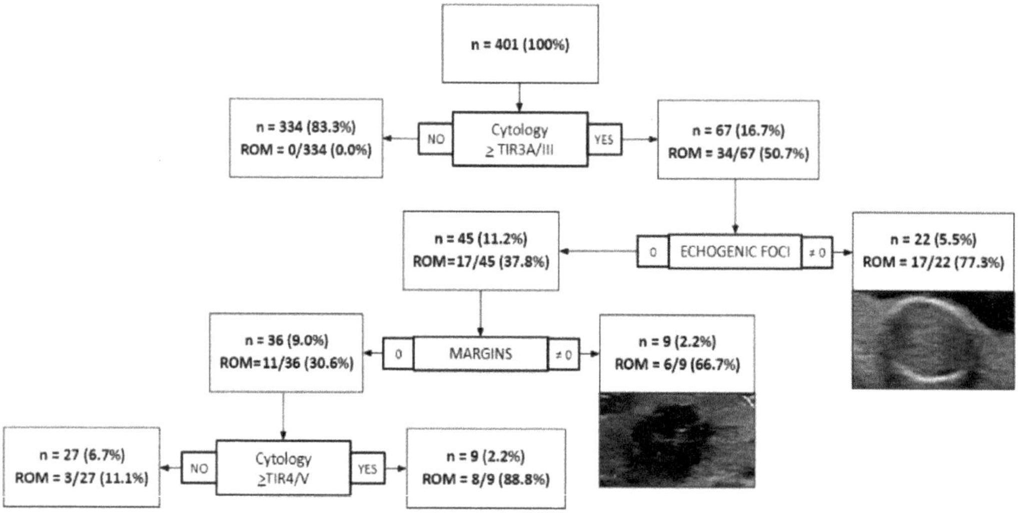

Figure 1. Nodules' risk of malignancy (ROM, based on histology or follow-up) using a combination of cytology with ultrasound ACR features of the echogenic foci and margins.

4. Discussion

Various studies have shown the good performance of ACR-TIRADS in selecting thyroid nodules deserving FNA, stressing its high "rule-out" role, as confirmed by our group here and previous experience [1,6,8,16–18]. In the present work, the ACR and EU-TIRADS systems recommended FNA in 46.5% (223/480) and 51.9% (249/480) of the nodules, respectively. The rate of correct FNA indication as per ACR and EU (i.e., nodules with indication for FNA and with a cytology result ≥TIR3A), was 38.6% (86/223) and 36.1% (90/249), respectively, without statistical significance ($p = 0.5872$), in accordance with the literature [1,19]. On the other hand, in this experiment, the proportions of cytological tests that could be avoided as per ACR-TIRADS and EU-TIRADS were 28.5% (137/480) and 33.1% (159/480), close to what has been recently reported in a meta-analysis (25% and 38%, respectively) [19]. Moreover, some studies have also found no statistically significant differences in the pooled diagnostic performances between the two scores [20].

A meta-analysis showed a pooled sensitivity and specificity of 95% and 55% for TIR4/V and TIR5/VI classes in the ACR system, respectively, and a pooled sensitivity and specificity of 96% and 52% for the same classes in the EU-TIRADS [21]. Another recent meta-analysis showed better overall diagnostic performances for ACR than for EU (sensitivity 74% vs. 54%, specificity 64% vs. 53%, PPV 43% vs. 29%, NPV 84% vs. 81%, respectively) [22]. Other reports indicate that the ACR-TIRADS had significantly higher specificity and PPV but a lower sensitivity and similar NPV when compared to the EU-TIRADS system [1,10,23]. Our findings are in line with those of the latter studies, showing a slightly lower sensitivity (58.9% vs. 61.6%, $p = 0.3173$) but a significantly higher specificity (59.0% vs. 52.4%, $p = 0.0012$) for ACR, with similar PPV (38.6% vs. 36.1%, $p = 0.1116$) and NPV (76.7% vs. 75.8%, $p = 0.5288$). Although the cytological classes already help in the stratification of patients through a predicted ROM known for every single class, other ancillary tests/criteria might help in the distinction of lesions with malignant behavior, especially in indeterminate categories [12,13,24,25]. According to the routine cytopathological classifications, the expected rates of malignancy for classes TIR3A/III and TIR3B/IV are <10%/5–15% and 15–30%, respectively [12,13]. The results of an Italian study showed a malignancy rate estimated based on surgical outcomes of 17% and 40% for TIR3A/III and TIR3B/IV, respectively [26]. In our series, based on the cases with available surgical excision, the risk of malignancy was 22% (2/9) and 38% (5/13) in the

TIR3A/III and TIR3B/IV classes, respectively, which is slightly lower compared to those reported in a recent meta-analyses (TIR3A/III 10%, TIR3B/IV 52%) [27]. Wu et al. tried to better stratify the indeterminate nodules through a KRAS mutation assessment by polymerase chain reaction (PCR), assuming that this genetic alteration is usually associated with a moderate risk of malignancy, mainly represented by follicular tumors with a good prognosis [24]. However, this approach failed to improve the diagnostic performances of the sole ACR-TIRADS, and the KRAS mutation was exclusively found in tumors classified as TIR3B/IV, with no malignant mutated cases in the TIR3A/III class. In this setting, the combination of the existing radiological scales (e.g., ACR and EU-TIRADS) with the routinely used cytological systems has been previously investigated in challenging nodules. Hong et al. combined ultrasound patterns with cytology, finding a lower risk of malignancy for TIR3A/III class nodules with a Korean TIRADS 3 score [28]. A meta-analysis evaluated the putative role of thyroid US in predicting the malignancy of TIR3A/III nodules, finding a high variability in terms of the sensitivity and specificity among the studies analyzed, probably due to the heterogeneity of the different US criteria employed to detect malignant nodules and due to the variable prevalence of malignancies in the different cohorts [7]. However, the only feature with a significant influence on diagnostic accuracy was the increased vascularization of the nodules, which is not taken into account by both the ACR and EU-TIRADS systems. Other recent studies investigated the impact of different dimensional cutoffs, e.g., $\leq$2 and >2 cm, on the final performances of the available US systems, showing a range of values quite close to the ones obtained in the present cohort with the ACR and EU-TIRADS systems [8,29]. An innovative approach was proposed in 2017 by He et al., creating a new algorithm that significantly increased the predictive performance of US features [30]. In our case series, we found no improvement in diagnostic accuracy by combining either ACR or EU-TIRADS and the cytology class. Nevertheless, the combination of the cytological classes with specific US features extracted from the ACR system—namely, echogenic foci and margins with a not-zero score—led to a significant increase in specificity and PPV, with a slight reduction in sensitivity and NPV as compared to cytology alone (Table 4). The introduction of this new combined US-cytological approach allowed the correct identification of nodules with a ROM > 60%, which could certainly benefit from surgery, as well as those with a low ROM (<10%), still amenable for clinical follow-up as per SIAPEC and Bethesda operative indications (Figure 1) [12,13]. Although these promising results might represent a starting point for the improvement of the actual diagnostic performances of cytological classifications, we recognize some limitations in the present study: the limited number of cases with indeterminate cytology, i.e., TIR3A/III and TIR3B/IV, the short US follow-up period (12 months) for nodules who did not undergo surgery, the low number of cases that underwent surgery, and the high prevalence of benign nodules. This latter situation reflects the target population of multinodular hyperplastic goiters typical of a first-level general hospital population, which only partly reflects the settings encountered in highly specialized centers with a large proportion of malignant cases and where molecular testing may be more easily performed [31]. However, as a description of a real-life practice in first-level general hospitals, this could be of help in validating the proposed combined approach in larger cohorts to further verify the reported diagnostic performances, eventually leading to their implementation for the clinical assessment of thyroid nodules.

5. Conclusions

In this study, we compared the performances of the ACR and EU-TIRADS systems, showing the statistically significant higher specificity of the ACR and a comparable sensitivity, PPV, and NPV. The coupled use of the ACR or EU-TIRADS with the cytological class did not improve the diagnostic performance in identifying malignant nodules. However, the combination of specific ultrasound features with cytological class might help in the diagnosis of malignant nodules, especially with an indeterminate for the malignancy pathological report.

Author Contributions: Conceptualization, D.S., G.C., S.G., V.L. and F.P.; Data curation, D.S., G.C., D.L., D.F., F.V., C.D.B., S.G., V.L. and F.P.; Formal analysis, D.S., G.C., S.G., V.L. and F.P.; Funding acquisition, F.P.; Methodology, F.P.; Writing—original draft, D.S., G.C., S.G., V.L. and F.P.; Writing—review and editing, D.S., G.C., S.G., V.L. and F.P. All authors have read and agreed to the published version of the manuscript.

Funding: This work was funded by the grant Ricerca Finalizzata 2019-GR-2019-12368592 (Italian Minister of Health, Ministero della Salute).

Institutional Review Board Statement: The study was conducted according to the guidelines of the Declaration of Helsinki and approved by the ASST Monza Ethical Board (October 2016, 27102016).

Informed Consent Statement: Informed consent was obtained from all subjects involved in the study.

Data Availability Statement: The data presented in this study are more extensively available in Leni, D.; Seminati, D.; Fior, D.; Vacirca, F.; Capitoli, G.; Cazzaniga, L.; Di Bella, C.; L'Imperio, V.; Galimberti, S.; Pagni, F. Diagnostic Performances of the ACR-TIRADS System in Thyroid Nodules Triage: A Prospective Single Center Study. Cancers 2021, 13, 2230. https://doi.org/10.3390/cancers13092230.

Conflicts of Interest: The authors do not have any conflicts of interest to declare.

Abbreviations

US	ultrasound
FNA	fine-needle aspiration
TIRADS	Thyroid Imaging Reporting and Data Systems
ACR	American College of Radiology
EU	European Thyroid Association
AIRC	Italian Association for Research on Cancer
SIAPEC	Società Italiana di Anatomia Patologica e Citologia
ROM	risk of malignancy
PTC	papillary thyroid carcinoma
EFVPTC	encapsulated follicular variant of papillary thyroid carcinoma

References

1. Huh, S.; Lee, H.S.; Yoon, J.; Kim, E.-K.; Moon, H.J.; Yoon, J.H.; Park, V.Y.; Kwak, J.Y. Diagnostic Performances and Unnecessary US-FNA Rates of Various TIRADS after Application of Equal Size Thresholds. *Sci. Rep.* **2020**, *10*, 10632. [CrossRef]
2. Haugen, B.R.; Alexander, E.K.; Bible, K.C.; Doherty, G.M.; Mandel, S.J.; Nikiforov, Y.E.; Pacini, F.; Randolph, G.W.; Sawka, A.M.; Schlumberger, M.; et al. 2015 American Thyroid Association Management Guidelines for Adult Patients with Thyroid Nodules and Differentiated Thyroid Cancer: The American Thyroid Association Guidelines Task Force on Thyroid Nodules and Differentiated Thyroid Cancer. *Thyroid* **2016**, *26*, 1–133. [CrossRef]
3. Tessler, F.N.; Middleton, W.D.; Grant, E.G.; Hoang, J.K.; Berland, L.L.; Teefey, S.A.; Cronan, J.J.; Beland, M.D.; Desser, T.S.; Frates, M.C.; et al. ACR Thyroid Imaging, Reporting and Data System (TI-RADS): White Paper of the ACR TI-RADS Committee. *J. Am. Coll. Radiol.* **2017**, *14*, 587–595. [CrossRef]
4. Horvath, E.; Majlis, S.; Rossi, R.; Franco, C.; Niedmann, J.P.; Castro, A.; Dominguez, M. An Ultrasonogram Reporting System for Thyroid Nodules Stratifying Cancer Risk for Clinical Management. *J. Clin. Endocrinol. Metab.* **2009**, *94*, 1748–1751. [CrossRef]
5. Russ, G.; Bonnema, S.J.; Erdogan, M.F.; Durante, C.; Ngu, R.; Leenhardt, L. European Thyroid Association Guidelines for Ultrasound Malignancy Risk Stratification of Thyroid Nodules in Adults: The EU-TIRADS. *Eur. Thyroid. J.* **2017**, *6*, 225–237. [CrossRef] [PubMed]
6. Ha, S.M.; Baek, J.H.; Na, D.G.; Suh, C.H.; Chung, S.R.; Choi, Y.J.; Lee, J.H. Diagnostic Performance of Practice Guidelines for Thyroid Nodules: Thyroid Nodule Size versus Biopsy Rates. *Radiology* **2019**, *291*, 92–99. [CrossRef] [PubMed]
7. Gao, L.-Y.; Wang, Y.; Jiang, Y.-X.; Yang, X.; Liu, R.-Y.; Xi, X.-H.; Zhu, S.-L.; Zhao, R.-N.; Lai, X.-J.; Zhang, X.-Y.; et al. Ultrasound Is Helpful to Differentiate Bethesda Class III Thyroid Nodules: A PRISMA-Compliant Systematic Review and Meta-Analysis. *Medicine* **2017**, *96*, e6564. [CrossRef]
8. Leni, D.; Seminati, D.; Fior, D.; Vacirca, F.; Capitoli, G.; Cazzaniga, L.; Di Bella, C.; L'Imperio, V.; Galimberti, S.; Pagni, F. Diagnostic Performances of the ACR-TIRADS System in Thyroid Nodules Triage: A Prospective Single Center Study. *Cancers* **2021**, *13*, 2230. [CrossRef]
9. Xu, T.; Wu, Y.; Wu, R.-X.; Zhang, Y.-Z.; Gu, J.-Y.; Ye, X.-H.; Tang, W.; Xu, S.-H.; Liu, C.; Wu, X.-H. Validation and Comparison of Three Newly-Released Thyroid Imaging Reporting and Data Systems for Cancer Risk Determination. *Endocrine* **2019**, *64*, 299–307. [CrossRef]
10. Shen, Y.; Liu, M.; He, J.; Wu, S.; Chen, M.; Wan, Y.; Gao, L.; Cai, X.; Ding, J.; Fu, X. Comparison of Different Risk-Stratification Systems for the Diagnosis of Benign and Malignant Thyroid Nodules. *Front. Oncol.* **2019**, *9*, 378. [CrossRef]

11. Ahmadi, S.; Oyekunle, T.; Jiang, X.; Scheri, R.; Perkins, J.; Stang, M.; Roman, S.; Sosa, J.A. A direct comparison of the ata and ti-rads ultrasound scoring systems. *Endocr. Pract.* **2019**, *25*, 413–422. [CrossRef]
12. Nardi, F.; Basolo, F.; Crescenzi, A.; Fadda, G.; Frasoldati, A.; Orlandi, F.; Palombini, L.; Papini, E.; Zini, M.; Pontecorvi, A.; et al. Italian Consensus for the Classification and Reporting of Thyroid Cytology. *J. Endocrinol. Investig.* **2014**, *37*, 593–599. [CrossRef]
13. Ali, S.Z.; Cibas, E.S. *The Bethesda System for Reporting Thyroid Cytopathology: Definitions, Criteria, and Explanatory Notes*; Springer: Berlin/Heidelberg, Germany, 2017; ISBN 9783319605708.
14. Gharib, H.; Papini, E.; Garber, J.R.; Duick, D.S.; Harrell, R.M.; Hegedus, L.; Paschke, R.; Valcavi, R.; Vitti, P. American Association of Clinical Endocrinologists, American College of Endocrinology, and Associazione Medici Endocrinologi Medical Guidelines for Clinical Practice for the Diagnosis and Management of Thyroid Nodules—2016 Update Appendix. *Endocr. Pract.* **2016**, *22*, 1–60. [CrossRef] [PubMed]
15. Pacini, F.; Basolo, F.; Bellantone, R.; Boni, G.; Cannizzaro, M.A.; De Palma, M.; Durante, C.; Elisei, R.; Fadda, G.; Frasoldati, A.; et al. Italian Consensus on Diagnosis and Treatment of Differentiated Thyroid Cancer: Joint Statements of Six Italian Societies. *J. Endocrinol. Investig.* **2018**, *41*, 849–876. [CrossRef]
16. Grani, G.; Lamartina, L.; Ascoli, V.; Bosco, D.; Biffoni, M.; Giacomelli, L.; Maranghi, M.; Falcone, R.; Ramundo, V.; Cantisani, V.; et al. Reducing the Number of Unnecessary Thyroid Biopsies While Improving Diagnostic Accuracy: Toward the "Right" TIRADS. *J. Clin. Endocrinol. Metab.* **2018**, *104*, 95–102. [CrossRef] [PubMed]
17. Ruan, J.-L.; Yang, H.-Y.; Liu, R.-B.; Liang, M.; Han, P.; Xu, X.-L.; Luo, B.-M. Fine Needle Aspiration Biopsy Indications for Thyroid Nodules: Compare a Point-Based Risk Stratification System with a Pattern-Based Risk Stratification System. *Eur. Radiol.* **2019**, *29*, 4871–4878. [CrossRef]
18. Middleton, W.D.; Teefey, S.A.; Reading, C.C.; Langer, J.E.; Beland, M.D.; Szabunio, M.M.; Desser, T.S. Comparison of Performance Characteristics of American College of Radiology TI-RADS, Korean Society of Thyroid Radiology TIRADS, and American Thyroid Association Guidelines. *Am. J. Roentgenol.* **2018**, *210*, 1148–1154. [CrossRef]
19. Kim, P.H.; Suh, C.H.; Baek, J.H.; Chung, S.R.; Choi, Y.J.; Lee, J.H. Unnecessary Thyroid Nodule Biopsy Rates under Four Ultrasound Risk Stratification Systems: A Systematic Review and Meta-Analysis. *Eur. Radiol.* **2021**, *31*, 2877–2885. [CrossRef]
20. Magri, F.; Chytiris, S.; Croce, L.; Molteni, M.; Bendotti, G.; Gruosso, G.; Tata Ngnitejeu, S.; Agozzino, M.; Rotondi, M.; Chiovato, L. Performance of the ACR TI-RADS and EU TI-RADS Scoring Systems in the Diagnostic Work-up of Thyroid Nodules in a Real-Life Series Using Histology as Reference Standard. *Eur. J. Endocrinol.* **2020**, *183*, 521–528. [CrossRef]
21. Kim, P.H.; Suh, C.H.; Baek, J.H.; Chung, S.R.; Choi, Y.J.; Lee, J.H. Diagnostic Performance of Four Ultrasound Risk Stratification Systems: A Systematic Review and Meta-Analysis. *Thyroid* **2020**, *30*, 1159–1168. [CrossRef]
22. Castellana, M.; Castellana, C.; Treglia, G.; Giorgino, F.; Giovanella, L.; Russ, G.; Trimboli, P. Performance of Five Ultrasound Risk Stratification Systems in Selecting Thyroid Nodules for FNA. *J. Clin. Endocrinol. Metab.* **2020**, *105*, 1659–1669. [CrossRef] [PubMed]
23. Yang, R.; Zou, X.; Zeng, H.; Zhao, Y.; Ma, X. Comparison of Diagnostic Performance of Five Different Ultrasound TI-RADS Classification Guidelines for Thyroid Nodules. *Front. Oncol.* **2020**, *10*, 598225. [CrossRef] [PubMed]
24. Wu, H.; Zhang, B.; Cai, G.; Li, J.; Gu, X. American College of Radiology Thyroid Imaging Report and Data System Combined with K-RAS Mutation Improves the Management of Cytologically Indeterminate Thyroid Nodules. *PLoS ONE* **2019**, *14*, e0219383. [CrossRef] [PubMed]
25. Marina, M.; Zatelli, M.C.; Goldoni, M.; Del Rio, P.; Corcione, L.; Martorana, D.; Percesepe, A.; Bonatti, F.; Mozzoni, P.; Crociara, A.; et al. Combination of Ultrasound and Molecular Testing in Malignancy Risk Estimate of Bethesda Category IV Thyroid Nodules: Results from a Single-Institution Prospective Study. *J. Endocrinol. Investig.* **2021**. [CrossRef] [PubMed]
26. Massa, F.; Caraci, P.; Sapino, A.; De Rosa, G.; Volante, M.; Papotti, M. Outcome and Diagnostic Reproducibility of the Thyroid Cytology "indeterminate Categories" SIAPEC/SIE 2014 in a Consecutive Series of 302 Cases. *J. Endocrinol. Investig.* **2020**, *44*, 803–809. [CrossRef]
27. Trimboli, P.; Crescenzi, A.; Giovanella, L. Performance of Italian Consensus for the Classification and Reporting of Thyroid Cytology (ICCRTC) in Discriminating Indeterminate Lesions at Low and High Risk of Malignancy. A Systematic Review and Meta-Analysis. *Endocrine* **2018**, *60*, 31–35. [CrossRef]
28. Hong, M.J.; Na, D.G.; Baek, J.H.; Sung, J.Y.; Kim, J.-H. Cytology-Ultrasonography Risk-Stratification Scoring System Based on Fine-Needle Aspiration Cytology and the Korean-Thyroid Imaging Reporting and Data System. *Thyroid* **2017**, *27*, 953–959. [CrossRef]
29. Na, D.G.; Paik, W.; Cha, J.; Gwon, H.Y.; Kim, S.Y.; Yoo, R.-E. Diagnostic Performance of the Modified Korean Thyroid Imaging Reporting and Data System for Thyroid Malignancy according to Nodule Size: A Comparison with Five Society Guidelines. *Ultrasonography* **2021**, *40*, 474–485. [CrossRef] [PubMed]
30. He, Y.-P.; Xu, H.-X.; Zhao, C.-K.; Sun, L.-P.; Li, X.-L.; Yue, W.-W.; Guo, L.-H.; Wang, D.; Ren, W.-W.; Wang, Q.; et al. Cytologically Indeterminate Thyroid Nodules: Increased Diagnostic Performance with Combination of US TI-RADS and a New Scoring System. *Sci. Rep.* **2017**, *7*, 6906. [CrossRef]
31. Kuru, B.; Kefeli, M.; Danaci, M. Comparison of Five Thyroid Ultrasound Stratification Systems for Differentiation of Benign and Malignant Nodules and to Avoid Biopsy Using Histology as Reference Standard. *Endocr. Pract.* **2021**. [CrossRef]

cancers MDPI

Review

Current Management of Bone Metastases from Differentiated Thyroid Cancer

Satoshi Kato *, Satoru Demura, Kazuya Shinmura, Noriaki Yokogawa, Takaki Shimizu and Hiroyuki Tsuchiya

Department of Orthopaedic Surgery, Graduate School of Medical Sciences, Kanazawa University 13-1 Takara-machi, Kanazawa 920-8641, Japan; msdemura@gmail.com (S.D.); kazuyashinmura@yahoo.co.jp (K.S.); chakkun1981chakkun@yahoo.co.jp (N.Y.); takaki.shimizu0928@gmail.com (T.S.); tsuchi@med.kanazawa-u.ac.jp (H.T.)

* Correspondence: skato323@gmail.com; Tel.: +81-76-265-2374

Simple Summary: Patients with bone metastases (BMs) from differentiated thyroid carcinoma (DTC) can live longer than those with BMs from other cancers. BMs from DTC create destructive lesions and easily cause intractable pain and neurological symptoms, including paralysis. These symptoms related to BMs affect mortality directly and indirectly by hampering the application of systemic therapies. Therefore, long-term local control of BMs in patients with DTC is desired, especially in patients with single or a small number of metastases. Local treatments for BMs have recently become advanced and sophisticated in surgery, radiotherapy, and percutaneous procedures. These therapies, either alone or in combination with other treatments, can effectively improve, or prevent the deterioration of, the performance status and quality of life of patients with DTC-BM. Among local therapies, complete surgical resection and stereotactic radiosurgery are the mainstay for achieving long-term control of DTC-BM.

Abstract: After the lung, the skeleton is the second most common site of distant metastases in differentiated thyroid carcinoma (DTC). Patients with osteolytic bone metastases (BMs) from thyroid carcinoma often have significantly reduced performance status and quality of life. Recent advancements in cancer therapy have improved overall survival in multiple cancer subtypes, including thyroid cancer. Therefore, long-term local control of thyroid BMs is desired, especially in patients with a single metastasis or oligometastases. Here, we reviewed the current management options for DTC-BMs and especially focused on local treatments for long-term local tumor control from an orthopedic tumor surgeon's point of view. Metastasectomy and stereotactic radiosurgery can be performed either alone or in combination with radioiodine therapy and kinase inhibitors to cure skeletal lesions in selected patients. Percutaneous procedures have been developed in recent years, and they can also have a curative role in small BMs. Recent advancements in local therapies have the potential to provide not only long-term local tumor control but also a better prognosis.

Keywords: differentiated thyroid cancer; bone metastasis; metastasectomy; stereotactic radiosurgery

Citation: Kato, S.; Demura, S.; Shinmura, K.; Yokogawa, N.; Shimizu, T.; Tsuchiya, H. Current Management of Bone Metastases from Differentiated Thyroid Cancer. *Cancers* **2021**, *13*, 4429. https://doi.org/10.3390/cancers13174429

Academic Editors: Fabio Medas and Pier Francesco Alesina

Received: 6 August 2021
Accepted: 24 August 2021
Published: 2 September 2021

1. Introduction

Differentiated thyroid carcinoma (DTC) is the most common endocrine malignancy [1]. The prognosis of DTC is generally favorable, with a 10-year survival rate of over 95% [2,3]. However, in 5% to 25% of patients, distant metastases are detected at the time of diagnosis or during the disease's course. In patients with DTC, bone metastases (BMs) occur in 2% to 13% of all patients and in nearly half of the patients with distant metastases [2]. In patients with DTC, the bone is the second most common site for distant metastases after the lung [2,4]. The spine is the site where DTC-BMs are most likely to occur, and it is affected in almost half of patients with DTC-BM [5]. BM from DTC is associated with a worse overall prognosis than lung metastasis [6–9]. However, the prognosis of patients with BM from DTC is still favorable, with a 10-year overall survival (OS) rate of

35% to 47% [10,11], compared with that of patients with BM from other cancers. Despite this relatively favorable prognosis, patients with osteolytic BMs from DTC often have a significantly reduced performance status (PS) and quality of life (QOL), with intractable pain, neurological symptoms, and increased mortality [12–14]. Farooki et al. have reported a 78% occurrence of at least one clinical skeletal-related event (SRE) with a median of 5 months from the identification of BM to the first SRE in patients with DTC with BM. After a median of 10.7 months, 65% of patients sustained a second SRE [12]. Importantly, mortality is significantly higher in patients with BM who develop SREs [12]. The goals of treatment for BMs remain palliative, striving toward symptom palliation, and improved PS and QOL, besides the long-term local control of the tumor. Recent advancements in cancer therapy have dramatically improved OS across multiple cancer subtypes. Therefore, long-term local control of thyroid BMs is desired, especially in patients with a single metastasis or oligometastases, who are expected to live longer.

Here, we reviewed the current management options for DTC-BMs and especially focused on local treatment for long-term local tumor control, including surgical metastasectomy, from the orthopedic tumor surgeon's point of view.

2. Systemic Therapy

2.1. Radioiodine Therapy

Radioactive iodine (RAI) therapy is the first-line treatment in patients with DTC and RAI-avid metastases [1]. However, RAI is ineffective for larger metastases, although it can extirpate small lesions [15]. RAI refractoriness in DTC metastases has a negative effect on prognosis [7,16].

In treating DTC-BM, RAI therapy is effective for patients with RAI-avid lesions [17], and such patients have a better prognosis than patients with non-RAI-avid lesions [11]. A recent retrospective study reported that RAI therapy in combination with one or more local or systemic therapies was associated with a better prognosis compared with RAI therapy alone [18]. However, this therapy was less effective for BM than for metastases in other organs. It was reported that patients with lung metastases had higher remission rates (50% to 74%) than those with BM (10% to 17%) [4,19]. Moreover, more than 20% of BMs do not show any RAI uptake [4,20].

Patients with small BMs that are undetectable on ordinary image inspections but that are detected on ^{131}I diagnostic scans have a better prognosis than patients with large and symptomatic BMs [21]. Generally, large BMs are refractory to ^{131}I and cause the occurrence or impending occurrence of SREs. Therapy is insufficient for multiple BMs; other treatment approaches are required [2,21]. RAI therapy may be contraindicated in patients with large BMs in the cranium or spine. This is because the enlargement of the tumor lesions can be induced by increased thyroid-stimulating hormone (TSH) levels, following either the administration of recombinant human TSH or hormone withdrawal, which can lead to compressive symptoms [22]. Specifically, in patients with BMs of the spine, pathological fractures and spinal cord compression from spinal lesions severely compromise PS. A reduced PS in patients with metastatic disease affects mortality directly and indirectly by hindering the delivery of systemic therapies, including radioiodine therapy. For patients with oligometastases, long-term control of large and symptomatic BMs by other treatment options, including metastasectomy, is ideal for prolonged survival and the future application of RAI therapy for other, newly-developed organ lesions. For patients with coexisting vital organ metastases and a large BM, the efficacy of RAI therapy for vital organ metastases can significantly increase after metastasectomy for BM by decreasing the total volume of the tumors.

2.2. Kinase Inhibitors

Kinase inhibitors (KIs) were recently applied in the treatment of progressive RAI-refractory DTC with distant metastases, and they offered a favorable outcome [23]. The latest guidelines recommend systemic treatment for patients with progressive RAI-refractory disease and greater tumor burden [1,16,24].

In contrast, in cases of BM, several studies have reported a worse response to treatment and a shorter progression-free survival (PFS) rate among patients treated with sorafenib and sunitinib [25–28]. In a retrospective study to evaluate KI therapies for DMs from DTC, bone and pleural lesions were the most refractory to therapies [28]. A prospective study showed that the absence of BM independently predicted superior PFS and OS in patients with RAI-refractory DTC who were treated with sorafenib [29]. The BMs that had received external beam radiotherapy (EBRT) before the onset of KI therapy were more susceptible, whereas non-irradiated BMs showed progression despite the response to KI that was shown in non-BM lesions [25]. The progression of BM while on KI may occur despite the sustained benefit of KI at other metastatic sites. These findings indicate that KI therapies alone play a limited role in the treatment of BMs from DTC. The findings also suggest that, for patients with DTC-BM, a multimodal approach should be combined with local and systemic therapies, including KI therapy, which should be used for reducing systemic tumor burden.

2.3. Antiresorptive Therapies

Bisphosphonate therapy is the current standard of care for preventing SREs in patients with BM [30,31]. Bisphosphonates inhibit osteoclast-mediated bone resorption and have antitumor effects by inhibiting tumor cell proliferation, adhesion, and invasion; by inhibiting angiogenesis; and by inducing apoptosis [31]. Recently, denosumab, a monoclonal antibody to the receptor activator of nuclear factor-kappa B ligand (RANKL) that inhibits osteoclast activity. It has been frequently used in cases of BM, and it has proven superior to bisphosphonate zoledronic acid in the prevention of SREs [32].

The number of studies that examine the effects of antiresorptive therapy in patients with DTC-BM is still limited. Recent studies have reported that in patients with multiple thyroid BMs, treatment with bisphosphonates can improve QOL and reduce SREs [33–35]. Despite the occurrence of BMs, OS in DTC is often significantly better than in other cancers. The potential benefit of antiresorptive therapy in reducing SRE should be weighed against the adverse events associated with its long-term use, such as osteonecrosis of the jaw (ONJ) and atypical femoral fractures. There are no differences between the incidence rates of these adverse events in patients using bisphosphonates and those using denosumab [36,37]. Because patients with malignancies treated with chemotherapy or head and neck EBRT have a higher risk of ONJ, these patients have to undergo a careful dental evaluation before the start of antiresorptive therapies [30]. The potential harm and benefits of combination therapy with antiresorptive drugs and KIs should be verified because anti-angiogenic KI therapies have also been associated with ONJ without antiresorptive therapy in a patient with DTC [38].

3. Local Therapy

3.1. Surgery

BMs from DTC tend to be highly destructive, resulting in pathological fractures and spinal cord compression from lesions in the spine. These SREs, including intractable pain and neurological symptoms, severely compromise the PS and QOL of patients. Local tumor control without SREs is important for patients with DTC-BMs because the prognosis of these patients is more favorable compared with that of patients with BMs from other cancers. Therefore, surgery for BMs is indicated more often than that for other organ metastases. For BMs, there are palliative and excisional surgery (metastasectomy) categories. Palliative surgery is performed to prevent symptomatic SREs, including pathological fractures and spinal cord compression, or to alleviate symptoms due to SREs. Metastasectomy is the complete excision of the tumor, aimed at achieving long term local tumor control.

3.1.1. Palliative Surgery (Stabilization with or without Partial Tumor Resection)

Osteolytic BMs from DTC easily cause SREs, especially in the spine and lower limb bones, which require weight bearing in daily activities [12]. Palliative surgery is mainly indicated in the presence of pathological or impending fracture risk and spinal cord compression with or without vertebral fracture [2]. In palliative surgery, reconstruction or fixation of the diseased lesion is the main procedure, and spinal cord decompression with partial resection of the tumor is also applied to the spinal lesion.

To aid clinicians in the diagnosis of neoplastic instability, an 18-point Spinal Instability Neoplastic Score (SINS) [39] for spinal lesions and a 12-point Mirels score [40] for upper and lower extremity lesions have recently been the most widely-used systems. The SINS system for the spine includes six parameters: location, pain, alignment, osteolysis, vertebral body collapse, and posterior element involvement. A high score, from 13 to 18, indicates the need for surgical stabilization to restore spinal stability from the affected lesion. The Mirels system for the extremities includes four parameters: location, pain, osteolysis, and tumor size. A high score, from 9 to 12, indicates the need for surgical intervention. These criteria have been shown to be valid, reliable, and reproducible [41,42].

3.1.2. Metastasectomy (Complete Resection of the Tumor)

Generally, BMs from DTC are more resistant to radiotherapy and systemic therapy than other metastases [2,43]. A significant proportion of patients with DTC-BM in the spine, which is the site most affected by DTC-BM, have a solitary spinal lesion without non-spinal BMs or other organ metastases [5]. Based on these factors, skeletal lesions from DTC have the best indication for metastasectomy, if feasible. Surgery is intended to improve or maintain the QOL and PS over a long-term period and to prolong survival [5]. Since the 2000s, metastasectomy for DTC-BM has been reported to be a significant factor associated with improved survival rates [20,44,45]. The guidelines state that complete resection of BMs can prolong survival and is particularly appropriate for younger patients [1,46]. Moreover, the declining performance of daily activities and neurological deficits caused by BMs make it difficult for patients to undergo RAI therapy, which is the mainstay of treatment for metastases, especially in vital organ lesions, from DTC. Thus, metastasectomy of skeletal lesions, if achievable, should be considered. This aggressive surgery can be applied to patients with metastases from DTC because of its unique characteristics, mentioned above, and its favorable prognosis. The treatment strategy for thyroid BMs is therefore different from that for BMs from other malignancies.

Table 1 presents studies of surgery for BM from thyroid carcinoma, mainly DTC, with detailed clinical results, including information about postoperative survival and/or local tumor control in the operated lesions [9,47–52]. To reflect the most contemporary practice, only studies published in the last 10 years are included. However, there are few comparative studies on complete and incomplete excision of DTC-BM [9,47,48]. The postoperative survival rate of patients undergoing metastasectomy was more favorable, with lower local recurrence rates, than that of patients who underwent incomplete excision [47,48]. Kato et al. examined the minimum 4-year postoperative outcomes for patients who underwent surgery for spinal lesions and reported that only one patient who underwent complete excision experienced local tumor recurrence in the operated spine, whereas all long-term survivors (>18 months after surgery) in the incomplete excision group experienced local tumor recurrence and a consequent deterioration of PS [48]. Satcher et al. examined the clinical outcomes for patients who underwent surgery for appendicular skeletal lesions; after adjusting for age and sex, they reported that patients who had their tumor excised or presented with solitary bone involvement had a lower risk of death [49]. Yin et al. examined the clinical outcomes for patients with BMs in the cervical spine, which severely compromised the PS of the patients; they reported that the strongest factor in improved survival rates after the diagnosis of cervical spine metastasis was local disease control of the lesion, and that surgical intervention was significantly associated with improved survival [52].

Table 1. Clinical outcomes of surgery for thyroid cancer BMs published in the last 10 years.

Study [Ref. No.] (Year of Pub.)	No. of Patients (M/F)	PTC/ FTC/ Others	Mean Age (Years; Range)	Location	Surgery (No.)	Mean Follow-Up after Surgery (Mos; Range)	5-Year Survival Rate after Surgery (Median Survival)	Local Tumor Control in the Operated Spine
Three studies including the detailed outcomes of complete excision (metastasectomy for BM from thyroid carcinoma)								
Demura S [47] (2011)	24	8/15/1	60.7 (39–77)	Spine: 24	Complete Ex: 10 Incomplete Ex: 14	55 mos (12–180)	All: 74%, Complete Ex: 90%, Incomplete Ex: 63%	[LR rate] Complete Ex: 10% Incomplete Ex: 57%
Nakayama R [9] (2014)	40 (16/24)	12/28/0	40.6 (23–64)	Spine: 18 Nonspinal bone: 34	Complete Ex: 35 Incomplete Ex: 17	46 mos [median] (4–233)	All: 64%	[5-year LC rate] Complete Ex: 84% Incomplete Ex: 55%
Kato S [48] (2016)	32	10/21/1	60.5 (N/A)	Spine: 32	Complete Ex: 20 Incomplete Ex: 12	N/A (>4-year post-op FU)	All: 71%, Complete Ex: 84%, Incomplete Ex: 50%	[LR rate] Complete Ex: 5% Incomplete Ex: 75%
Four studies detailing the outcomes of surgery for BM from thyroid carcinoma								
Satcher RL [49] (2012)	41 (19/22)	21/6/14	59 (12–82)	Nonspinal bone: 41	Complete Ex: 15 Incomplete Ex: 19 No Ex: 7	60 mos [median] (10–102)	29% (22.8 months)	LR rate: 20%
Sellin JN [50] (2015)	43	9/20/14	59 (36–79)	Spine: 43	Incomplete Ex: 43	39 mos (2–63) for 4 patients who were alive at last FU	N/A (15.4 months)	N/A
Zhang D [51] (2019)	52 (17/35)	7/43/2	57.6 (26–82)	Spine: 52	Complete Ex: 8 Incomplete Ex: 44	47 mos (12–126)	79%	N/A
Yin LX [52] (2020)	16	8/4/4	66 (at last FU)	Cervical spine: 16	Incomplete Ex: 16	30 mos (after diagnosis of BM)	45% (after diagnosis of BM)	N/A

BM, bone metastasis; Ex, excision; F, female; FTC, follicular thyroid carcinoma; FU, follow-up; LC, local control; LR, local recurrence; M, male; N/A, not available; No., number; PTC, papillary thyroid carcinoma; pub., publication.

Excisional surgery for BMs, especially in the spine, is a remarkable and technically demanding surgery for general orthopedic and spine surgeons because the metastases are hypervascular and destructive, and reconstruction to support the operated lesion against load is required after tumor resection in most cases. Although it is not always feasible, complete resection of macroscopically identified bone tumor is recommended, and a favorable outcome has been reported even in patients with coexisting controlled lung metastases (Figure 1) [48]. Isolated and resectable BMs from kidney cancer are also indicated for metastasectomy. A simple and tailored treatment algorithm for spinal metastases from these two cancers has been reported [53], and it can be adapted for nonspinal BMs.

3.2. *Radiotherapy*

The main treatment goals for patients with BMs are symptom palliation and maintenance or improvement of PS and QOL. Conventional EBRT has been used as the primary and adjuvant treatment for BMs for decades. Recently, the demand for long-term local control of solitary or oligometastatic bone lesions, stereotactic radiosurgery (SRS), has become popular as the mainstay of treatment for long-term BM control.

3.2.1. Conventional Radiation Therapy

EBRT is widely used as a local treatment for BMs. It can be used to complement surgery or alone in cases with intractable bone pain to reduce the pain and/or prevent pathological fractures, or in cases with spinal cord compression [54]. However, it is likely that conventional EBRT is related to a higher rate of relapse in patients who live longer. Although patients with mechanical instability in skeletal lesions require surgical stabilization, patients with low SINS or Mirels scores typically experience resolution of pain after radiotherapy [55,56]. EBRT generally delivers wide-field radiation in small additive doses, such as 30 Gy in 10 fractions. The dose is delivered to the tumor, although it is limited by the amount that can be tolerated by the surrounding organs at risk, such as the spinal cord.

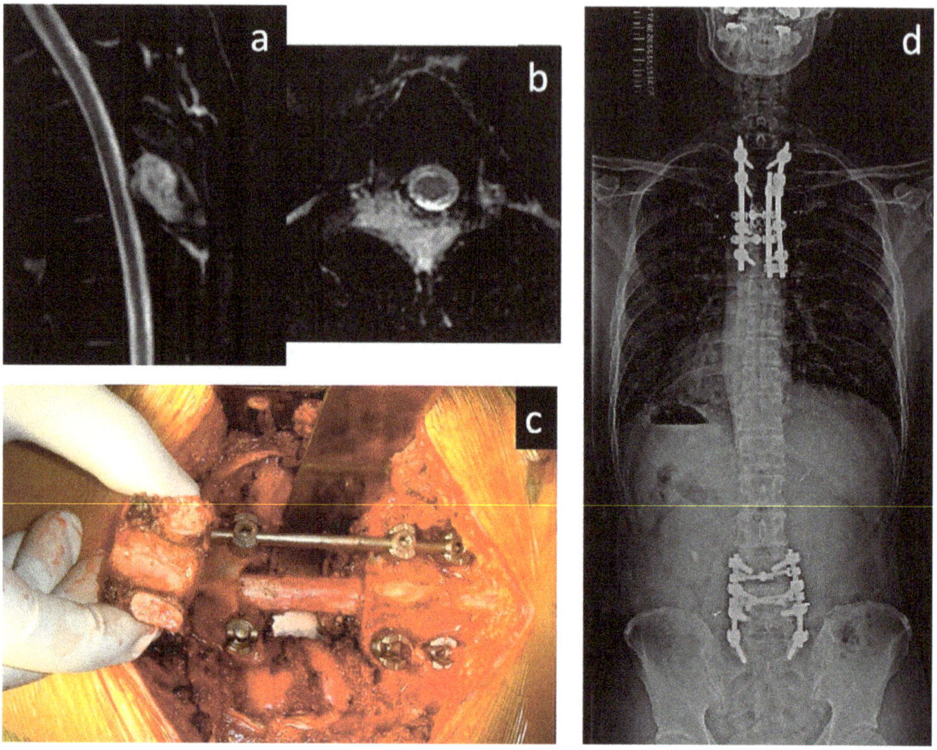

Figure 1. A 39-year-old man diagnosed with multiple lung and spinal metastases of T4 and L4. He underwent metastasectomies for spinal lesions. He also underwent radioactive iodine (RAI) therapy after the spinal metastasectomies and other metastasectomies for BMs, which subsequently appeared in the sacrum, left ilium, and humerus after RAI therapy. Eleven years after the first metastasectomy, he had no local tumor recurrences in the operated lesions; he still performed his normal daily activities and worked without any difficulties. (**a**) Sagittal and (**b**) axial T2-weighted magnetic resonance imaging of the thoracic spine, showing metastasis of T4. (**c**) Spondylectomy of T4 (complete resection of the tumor-affected vertebra) without any significant perioperative complications. (**d**) A recent full-spine radiography showing good maintenance of the reconstructed spine.

Despite the relative radioresistance of DTC [57], EBRT is the main and standard treatment option for patients with symptomatic or asymptomatic BMs at a higher risk of fracture and/or neurological symptoms.

3.2.2. Stereotactic Radiosurgery

The development of SRS, which can be used to deliver significantly high radiation doses with submillimeter accuracy, has changed the treatment paradigm, especially for patients with oligometastases, including BMs. It can deliver high-dose radiation (14–16 Gy in a single fraction) to the target volume, while sparing adjacent at-risk critical organs [58]. Owing to these characteristics, SRS can offer favorable outcomes and allow the re-irradiation of previously treated sites if necessary.

Recently, several studies have reported the efficacy of SRS for DTC-BM, although treatment protocols of SRS are different [59–63]. Table 2 presents studies of SRS for BM from thyroid carcinoma, mainly DTC, with detailed clinical results, including information about post-treatment survival rates and/or local tumor control in the treated lesions [59–61,63]. Bernstein et al. prospectively evaluated the efficacy of frame-based SRS in 23 patients with thyroid cancer, with 27 spinal lesions, as primary or adjuvant/salvage therapy. They reported that the local tumor control rates were 88% and 79% at 2 and 3 years, respectively.

Pain flare was observed in 30% of patients in the median follow-up of 29 months [59]. Ishigaki et al. retrospectively evaluated the efficacy of SRS using the Cyberknife system and reported the local control rate of 97% at 1 year in 13 patients with DTC with 60 skeletal lesions, including only 7 symptomatic lesions [60]. Meanwhile, a recent retrospective study of 12 patients with 32 spinal lesions treated with Cyberknife reported a lower local tumor control rate of 67% at 1 year [61]. This difference between clinical outcomes could be due to the baseline characteristics of the BM lesions (a proportion of large and/or spinal lesions associated with significant symptoms and local tumor control). Another retrospective study reported that the use of Cyberknife SRS for DTC-BM was considered successful [62]. The largest series, including 67 patients and 133 skeletal lesions, reported excellent outcomes of 96% and 82% in 1- and 5-year local control rates, respectively [63].

Table 2. Four studies that included detailed outcomes of SRS for BM from thyroid carcinoma.

Study [Ref. No.] (Year of Pub.)	No. of Patients (M/F)	PTC/ FTC/ Others	Median Age (Years; Range)	Location	SRS Characteristics	Median Follow-Up after SRS (Mos; Range)	Survival Rate after SRS (Median Survival)	Local Tumor Control Rate in the Treated Lesions
Bernstain MB [59] (2016)	23 (13/10)	9/6/8	58 (33–79)	Spine: 27	16–18 Gy in 1 fr 27–30 Gy in 3 to 5 fr	29 mos (5–93)	85% and 67% at 1 and 2 years, respectively	88% and 79% at 2 and 3 years, respectively
Ishigaki T [60] (2019)	13 (3/10)	3/9/1	69 (42–87)	Spine: 28 Nonspinal bone: 32	8–48 Gy in 1–10 fr (median; 27 Gy, 3 fr)	11 mos (2–56) in 40 lesions that were assessable for effectiveness	75% and 38% at 3 and 4 years, respectively	97% at 1 year
Hariri O [61] (2019)	12 (8/4)	5/6/1	71 (48–87)	Spine: 32	Mean dose: 20 Gy given in 1 to 4 fr	29 mos (0.5–140) 17 mos for imaging evaluation	55%, 44%, and 33% at 1, 2, and 3 years, respectively	67%, 56%, and 34% at 1, 2, and 3 years, respectively
Boyce-Fappiano D [63] (2020)	67 (34/33)	22/24/21	60 (28–80)	Spine: 133	18–24 Gy in 1 fr 27–30 Gy in 3–5 fr	31 mos for patients who were alive at last FU	86%, 74%, and 44% at 1, 2, and 5 years, respectively (43 mos)	96%, 89%, and 82% at 1, 2, and 5 years, respectively

BM, bone metastasis; DTC, differentiated thyroid carcinoma; F, female; Fr, fraction; FTC, follicular thyroid carcinoma; FU, follow-up; Gy, gray; LC, local control; LR, local recurrence; M, male; N/A, not available; No., number; PTC, papillary thyroid carcinoma; pub., publication; SRS, stereotactic radiosurgery.

In all the previously cited studies, SRS was effective and safe without the occurrence of spinal cord injury. However, a potential risk of vertebral compression fractures after treatment has been reported. Risk factors for fractures include older age, baseline fracture or pain, osteolytic lesion, higher tumor burden, higher radiation dose, and spinal deformity [64,65]. In patients with these risk factors and high SINS or Mirels scores, prophylactic stabilization should be considered before applying SRS to avoid the complication [64,65]. For patients with epidural disease, separation surgery focused on circumferential spinal cord decompression is performed to create an adequate distance (typically 1–2 mm) between the tumor and the spinal cord to safely provide optimal dosing in the following SRS [66,67].

SRS treatment is reported as showing a trend toward a significant improvement in PFS and OS rates in patients with oligometastatic disease from other cancers [68]. However, the effect of this treatment on survival rates among patients with DTC-BM remains unclear, in contrast to the effect of metastasectomy. A recent nationwide multicenter study has reported no significant effect of EBRT in decreasing the overall mortality of patients with DTC-BM [17]. Future studies are required to identify patients amenable to SRS and its effect on survival.

3.3. Percutaneous Procedures

Percutaneous procedures play an important role in the management of oligometastatic BMs from DTC. They are less invasive alternatives to surgery, especially in patients with decreased PS that is not suitable for surgery or with local tumor recurrence at the previously operated site. They can be applied in combination with systemic therapy in cases of symptomatic BM at a higher risk of local complications. The available percutaneous techniques for BMs from DTC are categorized into ablative, vascular, and consolidative treatment, which can be applied alone or combined and tailored according to the specific needs of the patient [69]. Cazzato et al. published their experience with percutaneous procedures including cementoplasty (77.5%) and ablation techniques (22.5%) for BMs from DTC. They reported a complete local remission rate of 56% at a median follow-up after treatment of 4.6 years, and an OS rate after treatment of 72%, 67%, and 60% at 1, 2, and 3 years, respectively [70]. However, well-designed studies of these techniques are scarce; most are retrospective, reliant on small sample sizes, and often conducted without a long-term follow-up. Future studies that compare the efficacy and tolerability of different procedures are required.

3.3.1. Ablation Techniques

Thermal ablation techniques, including radiofrequency ablation and cryoablation, are minimally invasive treatments that create local tissue necrosis around the tip of a needle by heating or freezing the tissue, respectively. These therapies have also been applied in patients with DTC-BM [70,71]. Another ablation technique is microwave ablation, which uses electromagnetic waves to increase the intra-tumoral temperature. After the application of these ablation therapies for BM, consolidation with surgical or percutaneous techniques is required for the sites exposed to mechanical stress to avoid secondary pathological fractures [69]. Ablation techniques, which are available either alone or in combination with cementoplasty, are found to be effective and safe treatments for painful metastases [70]. Although thermal ablation techniques are usually used for palliation or for the prevention of symptoms from BM, in the selected patients they have a potentially curative role, which should be further explored and which can be advanced in the future [72].

3.3.2. Cementoplasty

Percutaneous cementoplasty (vertebroplasty in the spine) is a minimally invasive procedure that involves the injection of bone cement (polymethylmethacrylate) into BMs with structural weakness, to provide pain relief and mechanical stability [73,74]. This procedure is usually applied to patients experiencing significant pain due to osteolytic and destructive BMs, especially in weight-bearing bones, including the spine and pelvis, which are common sites for DTC-BM [70,74,75]. Cementoplasty can be used in combination with other procedures, such as radiofrequency ablation and RAI therapy [75]. A careful indication of cementoplasty is required in patients with solitary or oligometastatic lesions because the procedure can theoretically increase the number of circulating tumor cells from the treated BMs [76]. A case report has demonstrated that pulmonary intravascular metastases developed as a result of vertebroplasty for prostate cancer spinal metastases [77].

3.3.3. Embolization

Percutaneous transarterial embolization has been widely applied for the treatment of BMs from DTC alone or in combination with other treatments [69]. This technique aims to provide devascularization and size reduction of the tumor tissue through vascular occlusion by several embolic materials, causing ischemia and subsequent necrosis. The efficacy of the procedure for BMs from DTC is related to the hypervascularity's characteristics. The procedure alone can provide palliation or the prevention of symptoms and reduce tumor burden for more than half of patients [78]. However, its efficacy is usually rapid, but transient. The procedure is often performed just before surgery to reduce operative bleeding, shrink tumor size, and allow a clearer separation between the tumor and the surrounding tissues [79,80]. The combination of EBRT and RAI therapy has a potential effect on the prolonged duration of symptom control without tumor progression [81].

4. Conclusions

Patients with BMs, especially those who have them in the spine, have a worse prognosis than those with lung metastasis in multiple cancer subtypes. However, the prognosis of patients with BM from DTC is still favorable compared to that of patients with other cancers. Patients with osteolytic BMs from thyroid carcinoma often have a significantly reduced PS.

The PS affects mortality directly and indirectly by hampering the application of systemic therapies using RAI and/or KIs, which are the mainstay of treatment for patients with metastatic DTC. Therefore, long-term local control of BMs from DTC is desirable, especially in patients with single or oligometastases. Along with systemic therapies, local therapies, including metastasectomy and SRS, can be valuable as treatment options, and even as curative measures of BM in selected patients. Recent advancements in local therapies have the potential to provide not only long-term local tumor control but also a better prognosis.

Author Contributions: Writing the original draft, S.K.; writing the review and editing, S.D., K.S., N.Y., T.S. and H.T. All authors have read and agreed to the published version of the manuscript.

Funding: This research received no external funding.

Conflicts of Interest: The authors declare no conflict of interest.

References

1. Haugen, B.R.; Alexander, E.K.; Bible, K.C.; Doherty, G.M.; Mandel, S.J.; Nikiforov, Y.E.; Pacini, F.; Randolph, G.W.; Sawka, A.M.; Schlumberger, M.; et al. American Thyroid Association Management guidelines for adult patients with thyroid nodules and differentiated thyroid cancer: The AMERICAN Thyroid Association guidelines task force on thyroid nodules and differentiated thyroid cancer. *Thyroid* **2016**, *26*, 1–133. [CrossRef]
2. Muresan, M.M.; Olivier, P.; Leclère, J.; Sirveaux, F.; Brunaud, L.; Klein, M.; Zarnegar, R.; Weryha, G. Bone metastases from differentiated thyroid carcinoma. *Endocr. Relat. Cancer* **2008**, *15*, 37–49. [CrossRef]
3. Schlumberger, M.J. Papillary and follicular thyroid carcinoma. *N. Engl. J. Med.* **1998**, *338*, 297–306. [CrossRef] [PubMed]
4. Durante, C.; Haddy, N.; Baudin, E.; Leboulleux, S.; Hartl, D.; Travagli, J.P.; Caillou, B.; Ricard, M.; Lumbroso, J.D.; De Vathaire, F.; et al. Long-term outcome of 444 patients with distant metastases from papillary and follicular thyroid carcinoma: Benefits and limits of radioiodine therapy. *J. Clin. Endocrinol. Metab.* **2006**, *91*, 2892–2899. [CrossRef]
5. Kushchayeva, Y.S.; Kushchayev, S.V.; Carroll, N.M.; Felger, E.A.; Links, T.P.; Teytelboym, O.M.; Bonichon, F.; Preul, M.C.; Sonntag, V.K.; Van Nostrand, D.; et al. Spinal metastases due to thyroid carcinoma: An analysis of 202 patients. *Thyroid* **2014**, *24*, 1488–1500. [CrossRef] [PubMed]
6. Choi, Y.M.; Kim, W.G.; Kwon, H.; Jeon, M.J.; Lee, J.J.; Ryu, J.S.; Hong, E.G.; Kim, T.Y.; Shong, Y.K.; Kim, W.B. Early prognostic factors at the time of diagnosis of bone metastasis in patients with bone metastases of differentiated thyroid carcinoma. *Eur. J. Endocrinol.* **2016**, *175*, 165–172. [CrossRef]
7. Lang, B.H.-H.; Wong, K.P.; Cheung, C.Y.; Wan, K.Y.; Lo, C.-Y. Evaluating the prognostic factors associated with cancer-specific survival of differentiated thyroid carcinoma presenting with distant metastasis. *Ann. Surg. Oncol.* **2013**, *20*, 1329–1335. [CrossRef] [PubMed]
8. Lin, J.-D.; Lin, S.-F.; Chen, S.-T.; Hsueh, C.; Li, C.-L., Chao, T.-C. Long-term follow-up of papillary and follicular thyroid carcinomas with bone metastasis. *PLoS ONE* **2017**, *12*, e0173354.
9. Nakayama, R.; Horiuchi, K.; Susa, M.; Watanabe, I.; Watanabe, K.; Tsuji, T.; Matsumoto, M.; Toyama, Y.; Morioka, H. Clinical outcome after bone metastasis (BM) surgery in patients with differentiated thyroid carcinoma (DTC): A retrospective study of 40 cases. *Jpn. J. Clin. Oncol.* **2014**, *44*, 918–925. [CrossRef]
10. Slook, O.; Levy, S.; Slutzky-Shraga, I.; Tsvetov, G.; Robenshtok, E.; Shimon, I.; Benbassat, C.; Hirsch, D. Long-term outcomes and prognostic factors in patients with differentiated thyroid carcinoma and bone metastases. *Endocr. Pract.* **2019**, *25*, 427–437. [CrossRef]
11. Pittas, A.G.; Adler, M.; Fazzari, M.; Larson, S.M.; Robbins, R.J.; Rosai, J. Bone metastases from thyroid carcinoma: Clinical characteristics and prognostic variables in one hundred forty-six patients. *Thyroid* **2000**, *10*, 261–268. [CrossRef] [PubMed]
12. Farooki, A.; Leung, V.; Tala, H.; Tuttle, R.M. Skeletal-related events due to bone metastases from differentiated thyroid cancer. *J. Clin. Endocrinol. Metab.* **2012**, *97*, 2433–2439. [CrossRef] [PubMed]
13. Quan, G.M.; Pointillart, V.; Palussière, J.; Bonichonet, F. Multidisciplinary treatment ad survival of patients with vertebral metastases from thyroid carcinoma. *Thyroid* **2012**, *22*, 125–130. [CrossRef]
14. Georgy, B.A. Metastatic spinal lesions: State-of-the-art treatment options and future trend. *Am. J. Neuroradiol.* **2008**, *29*, 1605–1611. [CrossRef]
15. Robenshtok, E.; Farooki, A.; Grewal, R.K.; Tuttle, R.M. Natural history of small radioiodine-avid bone metastases that have no structural correlate on imaging studies. *Endocrine* **2014**, *47*, 266–272. [CrossRef]
16. Fugazzola, L.; Elisei, R.; Fuhrer, D.; Jarzab, B.; Leboulleux, S.; Newbold, K.; Smit, J. European Thyroid Association guidelines for the treatment and follow-up of advanced radioiodine-refractory thyroid cancer. *Eur. Thyroid J.* **2019**, *8*, 227–245. [CrossRef] [PubMed]
17. Mazziotti, G.; Formenti, A.M.; Panarotto, M.B.; Arvat, E.; Chiti, A.; Cuocolo, A.; Dottorini, M.E.; Durante, C., Agate, L., Filetti, S.; et al. Real-life management and outcome of thyroid carcinoma-related bone metastases: Results from a nationwide multicenter experience. *Endocrine* **2018**, *59*, 90–101. [CrossRef] [PubMed]

18. Wu, D.; Gomes Lima, C.J.; Moreau, S.L.; Kulkarni, K.; Zeymo, A.; Burman, K.D.; Wartofsky, L.; Van Nostrand, D. Improved survival after multimodal approach with 131I treatment in patients with bone metastases secondary to differentiated thyroid cancer. *Thyroid* **2019**, *29*, 971–978. [CrossRef] [PubMed]
19. Schlumberger, M.; Challeton, C.; De Vathaire, F.; Travagli, J.P.; Gardet, P.; Lumbroso, J.D.; Francese, C.; Fontaine, F.; Ricard, M.; Parmentier, C. Radioactive iodine treatment and external radiotherapy for lung and bone metastases from thyroid carcinoma. *J. Nucl. Med.* **1996**, *37*, 598–605. [PubMed]
20. Bernier, M.O.; Leenhardt, L.; Hoang, C.; Aurengo, A.; Mary, J.Y.; Menegaux, F.; Enkaoua, E.; Turpin, G.; Chiras, J.; Saillant, G.; et al. Survival and therapeutic modalities in patients with bone metastases of differentiated thyroid carcinomas. *J. Clin. Endocrinol. Metab.* **2001**, *86*, 1568–1573. [CrossRef]
21. Hindié, E.; Zanotti-Fregonara, P.; Keller, I.; Duron, F.; Devaux, J.Y.; Calzada-Nocaudie, M.; Sarfati, E.; Moretti, J.L.; Bouchard, P.; Toubert, M.E. Bone metastases of differentiated thyroid cancer: Impact of early 131I-based detection on outcome. *Endocr. Relat. Cancer* **2007**, *14*, 799–807. [CrossRef] [PubMed]
22. Choudhury, P.S.; Gupta, M. Differentiated thyroid cancer theranostics: Radioiodine and beyond. *Br. J. Radiol.* **2018**, *91*, 20180136. [CrossRef]
23. Schlumberger, M.; Tahara, M.; Wirth, L.J.; Robinson, B.; Brose, M.S.; Elisei, R.; Habra, M.A.; Newbold, K.; Shah, M.H.; Hoff, A.O.; et al. Lenvatinib versus placebo in radioiodine-refractory thyroid cancer. *N. Engl. J. Med.* **2015**, *372*, 621–630. [CrossRef] [PubMed]
24. Pacini, F.; Basolo, F.; Bellantone, R.; Boni, G.; Cannizzaro, M.A.; De Palma, M.; Durante, C.; Elisei, R.; Fadda, G.; Frasoldati, A.; et al. Italian consensus on diagnosis and treatment of differentiated thyroid cancer: Joint statements of six Italian societies. *J. Endocrinol. Investig.* **2018**, *41*, 849–876. [CrossRef] [PubMed]
25. Cabanillas, M.E.; Waguespack, S.G.; Bronstein, Y.; Williams, M.D.; Feng, L.; Hernandez, M.; Lopez, A.; Sherman, S.I.; Busaidy, N.L. Treatment with tyrosine kinase inhibitors for patients with differentiated thyroid cancer: The M. D. Anderson experience. *J. Clin. Endocrinol. Metab.* **2010**, *95*, 2588–2595. [CrossRef]
26. Hoftijzer, H.; Heemstra, K.A.; Morreau, H.; Stokkel, M.P.; Corssmit, E.P.; Gelderblom, H.; Weijers, K.; Pereira, A.M.; Huijberts, M.; Kapiteijn, E.; et al. Beneficial effects of sorafenib on tumor progression, but not on radioiodine uptake, in patients with differentiated thyroid carcinoma. *Eur. J. Endocrinol.* **2009**, *161*, 923–931. [CrossRef]
27. Schneider, T.C.; Abdulrahman, R.M.; Corssmit, E.P.; Morreau, H.; Smit, J.W.; Kapiteijn, E. Long-term analysis of the efficacy and tolerability of sorafenib in advanced radio-iodine refractory differentiated thyroid carcinoma: Final results of a phase II trial. *Eur. J. Endocrinol.* **2012**, *167*, 643–650. [CrossRef]
28. Massicotte, M.H.; Brassard, M.; Claude-Desroches, M.; Borget, I.; Bonichon, F.; Giraudette, A.L.; Do Cao, C.; Chougnet, C.N.; Leboulleux, S.; Baudin, E.; et al. Tyrosine kinase inhibitor treatments in patients with metastatic thyroid carcinomas: A retrospective study of the TUTHYREF network. *Eur. J. Endocrinol.* **2014**, *170*, 575–582. [CrossRef]
29. Cheng, L.; Fu, H.; Jin, Y.; Sa, R.; Chen, L. Clinicopathological features predict outcomes in patients with radioiodine-refractory differentiated thyroid cancer treated with sorafenib: A real-world study. *Oncologist* **2020**, *25*, e668–e678. [CrossRef]
30. Wexler, J.A. Approach to the thyroid cancer patients with bone metastases. *J. Clin. Endocrinol. Metab.* **2011**, *96*, 2296–2307. [CrossRef]
31. Lüftner, D.; Henschke, P.; Possinger, K. Clinical value of bisphosphonates in cancer therapy. *Anticancer Res.* **2007**, *27*, 1759–1768. [PubMed]
32. Zheng, G.Z.; Chang, B.; Lin, F.X.; Xie, D.; Hu, Q.X.; Yu, G.Y.; Du, S.X.; Li, X.D. Meta-analysis comparing denosumab and zoledronic acid for treatment of bone metastases in patients with advanced solid tumours. *Eur. J. Cancer Care* **2017**, *26*, e12541. [CrossRef] [PubMed]
33. Vitale, G.; Fonderico, F.; Martignetti, A.; Caraglia, M.; Ciccarelli, A.; Nuzzo, V.; Abbruzzese, A.; Lupoli, G. Pamidronate improves the quality of life and induces clinical remission of bone metastases in patients with thyroid cancer. *Br. J. Cancer* **2001**, *84*, 1586–1590. [CrossRef] [PubMed]
34. Orita, Y.; Sugitani, I.; Toda, K.; Manabe, J.; Fujimoto, Y. Zoledronic acid in the treatment of bone metastases from differentiated thyroid carcinoma. *Thyroid* **2011**, *21*, 31–35. [CrossRef] [PubMed]
35. Orita, Y.; Sugitani, I.; Takao, S.; Toda, K.; Manabe, J.; Miyata, S. Prospective evaluation of zoledronic acid in the treatment of bone metastases from differentiated thyroid carcinoma. *Ann. Surg. Oncol.* **2015**, *22*, 4008–4013. [CrossRef] [PubMed]
36. Chen, F.; Pu, F. Safety of denosumab versus zoledronic acid in patients with bone metastases: A meta-analysis of randomized controlled trials. *Oncol. Res. Treat.* **2016**, *39*, 453–459. [CrossRef]
37. Menshawy, A.; Mattar, O.; Abdulkarim, A.; Kasem, S.; Nasreldin, N.; Menshawy, E.; Mohammed, S.; Abdel-Maboud, M.; Gadelkarim, M.; El Ashal, G.G.; et al. Denosumab versus bisphosphonates in patients with advanced cancers-related bone metastasis: Systematic review and meta-analysis of randomized controlled trials. *Support. Care Cancer* **2018**, *26*, 1029–1038. [CrossRef]
38. Mauceri, R.; Panzarella, V.; Morreale, I.; Campisi, G. Medication-related osteonecrosis of the jaw in a cancer patient receiving lenvatinib. *Int. J. Oral Maxillofac. Surg.* **2019**, *48*, 1530–1532. [CrossRef]
39. Fisher, C.G.; DiPaola, C.P.; Ryken, T.C.; Bilsky, M.K.; Shaffrey, C.I.; Berven, S.H.; Harrop, J.S.; Fehlings, M.G.; Boriani, S.; Chou, D.; et al. A novel classification system for spinal instability in neoplastic disease: An evidence-based approach and expert consensus from the Spine Oncology Study Group. *Spine* **2010**, *35*, E1221–E1229. [CrossRef]

40. Mirels, H. Metastatic disease in long bones: A proposed scoring system for diagnosing impending pathologic fracture. *Clin. Orthop. Relat. Res.* **1989**, *249*, 256–264. [CrossRef]
41. Fourney, D.R.; Frangou, E.M.; Ryken, T.C.; Dipaola, C.P.; Shaffrey, C.I.; Berven, S.H.; Bilsky, M.H.; Harrop, J.S.; Fehlings, M.G.; Boriani, S.; et al. Spinal instability neoplastic score: An analysis of reliability and validity from the spine oncology study group. *J. Clin. Oncol.* **2011**, *29*, 3072–3077. [CrossRef]
42. Damron, T.A.; Morgan, H.; Prakash, D.; Grant, W.; Aronowitz, J.; Heiner, J. Critical evaluation of Mirels' rating system for impending pathologic fractures. *Clin. Orthop. Relat. Res.* **2003**, *415*, S201–S207. [CrossRef] [PubMed]
43. Nervo, A.; Ragni, A.; Retta, F.; Gallo, M.; Piovesan, A.; Liberini, V.; Gatti, M.; Ricardi, U.; Deandreis, D.; Arvat, E. Bone metastases from differentiated thyroid carcinoma: Current knowledge and open issues. *J. Endocrinol. Investig.* **2021**, *44*, 403–419. [CrossRef]
44. Zettinig, G.; Fueger, B.J.; Passler, C.; Kaserer, K.; Pirich, C.; Dudczak, R.; Niederle, B. Long-term follow-up of patients with bone metastases from differentiated thyroid carcinoma—Surgery or conventional therapy? *Clin. Endocrinol.* **2002**, *56*, 377–382. [CrossRef] [PubMed]
45. Stojadinovic, A.; Shoup, M.; Ghossein, R.A.; Nissan, A.; Brennan, M.F.; Shah, J.P.; Shaha, A.R. The role of operations for distantly metastatic well-differentiated thyroid carcinoma. *Surgery* **2002**, *131*, 636–643. [CrossRef] [PubMed]
46. Kushchayeva, Y.S.; Kushchayev, S.V.; Wexler, J.A.; Carroll, N.M.; Preul, M.C.; Teytelboym, O.M.; Sonntag, V.K.; Van Nostrand, D.; Burman, K.D.; Boyle, L.M. Current treatment modalities for spinal metastases secondary to thyroid carcinoma. *Thyroid* **2014**, *24*, 1442–1455. [CrossRef]
47. Demura, S.; Kawahara, N.; Murakami, H.; Abdel-Wanis, M.E.; Kato, S.; Yoshioka, K.; Tomita, K.; Tsuchiya, H. Total en bloc spondylectomy for spinal metastasis in thyroid carcinoma. *J. Neurosurg. Spine* **2011**, *14*, 172–176. [CrossRef]
48. Kato, S.; Murakami, H.; Demura, S.; Fujimaki, Y.; Yoshioka, K.; Yokogawa, N.; Tsuchiya, H. The impact of complete surgical resection of spinal metastases on the survival of patients with thyroid cancer. *Cancer Med.* **2016**, *5*, 2343–2349. [CrossRef]
49. Satcher, R.L.; Lin, P.; Harun, N.; Feng, L.; Moon, B.S.; Lewis, V.O. Surgical management of appendicular skeletal metastases in thyroid carcinoma. *Int. J. Surg. Oncol.* **2012**, *2012*, 417086. [CrossRef]
50. Sellin, J.N.; Suki, D.; Harsh, V.; Elder, B.D.; Fahim, D.K.; McCutcheon, I.E.; Rao, G.; Rhines, L.D.; Tatsui, C.E. Factors affecting survival in 43 consecutive patients after surgery for spinal metastases from thyroid carcinoma. *J. Neurosurg. Spine* **2015**, *23*, 419–428. [CrossRef] [PubMed]
51. Zhang, D.; Yin, H.; Wu, Z.; Yang, X.; Liu, T.; Xiao, J. Surgery and survival outcomes of 22 patients with epidural spinal cord compression caused by thyroid tumor spinal metastases. *Eur. Spine J.* **2013**, *22*, 569–576. [CrossRef]
52. Yin, L.X.; Puccinelli, C.L.; Van Abel, K.; Kasperbauer, J.L.; Price, D.L.; Janus, J.R.; Ryder, M.; Moore, E.J. Prognostic Factors in Patients with Differentiated Thyroid Cancers Metastatic to the Cervical Spine. *Laryngoscope* **2021**, *131*, E1741–E1747. [CrossRef] [PubMed]
53. Kato, S.; Murakami, H.; Demura, S.; Yoshioka, K.; Yokogawa, N.; Yonezawa, N.; Shimizu, T.; Oku, N.; Kitagawa, R.; Tsuchiya, H. Kidney and Thyroid Cancer-Specific Treatment Algorithm for Spinal Metastases: A Validation Study. *World Neurosurg.* **2019**, *122*, e1305–e1311. [CrossRef] [PubMed]
54. Gerszten, P.C.; Mendel, E.; Yamada, Y. Radiotherapy and radiosurgery for metastatic spine disease: What are the options, indications and outcomes? *Spine* **2009**, *34*, S78–S92. [CrossRef] [PubMed]
55. Huisman, M.; van der Velden, J.M.; van Vulpen, M.; van den Bosch, M.A.; Chow, E.; Öner, F.C.; Yee, A.; Verkooijen, H.M.; Verlaan, J.J. Spinal instability as defined by the spinal instability neoplastic score is associated with radiotherapy failure in metastatic spinal disease. *Spine J.* **2014**, *14*, 2835–2840. [CrossRef] [PubMed]
56. Tatar, Z.; Soubrier, M.; Dillies, A.F.; Verrelle, P.; Boisgard, S.; Lapeyre, M. Assessment of the risk factors for impending fractures following radiotherapy for long bone metastases using CT scan-based virtual simulation: A retrospective study. *Radiat. Oncol.* **2014**, *9*, 227. [CrossRef]
57. Simpson, W.J. Radioiodine and radiotherapy in the management of thyroid cancers. *Otolaryngol. Clin. N. Am.* **1990**, *23*, 509–521. [CrossRef]
58. Gerszten, P.C.; Burton, S.A.; Ozhasglu, C.; Welch, W.C. Radiosurgery for spinal metastases: Clinical experience in 500 cases from a single institution. *Spine* **2007**, *32*, 193–199. [CrossRef]
59. Bernstein, M.B.; Chang, E.L.; Amini, B.; Pan, H.; Cabanillas, M.; Wang, X.A.; Allen, P.K.; Rhines, L.D.; Tatsui, C.; Li, J.; et al. Spine stereotactic radiosurgery for patients with metastatic thyroid cancer: Secondary analysis of phase I/II trials. *Thyroid* **2016**, *26*, 1269–1275. [CrossRef] [PubMed]
60. Ishigaki, T.; Uruno, T.; Sugino, K.; Masaki, C.; Akaishi, J.; Hames, K.Y.; Suzuki, A.; Tomoda, C.; Matsuzu, K.; Ohkuwa, K.; et al. Stereotactic radiotherapy using the CyberKnife is effective for local control of bone metastases from differentiated thyroid cancer. *J. Radiat. Res.* **2019**, *60*, 831–836. [CrossRef]
61. Hariri, O.; Takayanagi, A.; Lischalk, J.; Desai, K.; Florence, T.J.; Yazdian, P.; Chang, S.D.; Vrionis, F.; Adler, J.R.; Quadri, S.A.; et al. Clinical efficacy of frameless stereotactic radiosurgery in the management of spinal metastases from thyroid carcinoma. *Spine* **2019**, *44*, E1188–E1195. [CrossRef]
62. Harada, Y.; Miyazaki, S. Multisession CyberKnife radiosurgery for advanced follicular thyroid cancer. *Cureus* **2019**, *11*, e6159. [CrossRef]

63. Boyce-Fappiano, D.; Gjyshi, O.; Pezzi, T.A.; Allen, P.K.; Solimman, M.; Taku, N.; Bernstein, M.B.; Cabanillas, M.E.; Amini, B.; Tatsui, C.E.; et al. Spine stereotactic radiosurgery for metastatic thyroid cancer: A single-institution experience. *J. Neurosurg. Spine* **2020**, *14*, 1–9. [CrossRef] [PubMed]
64. Boehling, N.S.; Grosshans, D.R.; Allen, P.K.; McAleer, M.F.; Burton, A.W.; Azeem, S.; Rhines, L.D.; Chang, E.L. Vertebral compression fracture risk after stereotactic body radiotherapy for spinal metastases. *J. Neurosurg. Spine* **2012**, *16*, 379–386. [CrossRef] [PubMed]
65. Faruqi, S.; Tseng, C.L.; Whyne, C.; Alghamdi, M.; Wilson, J.; Myrehaug, S.; Soliman, H.; Lee, Y.; Maralani, P.; Yang, V.; et al. Vertebral compression fracture after spine stereotactic body radiation therapy: A review of the pathophysiology and risk factors. *Neurosurgery* **2018**, *83*, 314–322. [CrossRef]
66. Barzilai, O.; Laufer, I.; Robin, A.; Xu, R.; Yamada, Y.; Bilsky, M.H. Hybrid Therapy for Metastatic Epidural Spinal Cord Compression: Technique for Separation Surgery and Spine Radiosurgery. *Oper. Neurosurg.* **2019**, *16*, 310–318. [CrossRef]
67. Rothrock, R.; Pennington, Z.; Ehresman, J.; Bilsky, M.H.; Barzilai, O.; Szerlip, N.J.; Sciubba, D.M. Hybrid Therapy for Spinal Metastases. Neurosurg. *Clin. N. Am.* **2020**, *31*, 191–200.
68. Ricardi, U.; Badellino, S.; Filippi, A.R. Clinical applications of stereotactic radiation therapy for oligometastatic cancer patients: A disease-oriented approach. *J. Radiat. Res.* **2016**, *57*, i58–i68. [CrossRef]
69. Cazzato, R.L.; Garnon, J.; Koch, G.; Shaygi, B.; Tsoumakidou, G.; Caudrelier, J.; Boatta, E.; Buy, X.; Palussiere, J.; Gangi, A. Current role of interventional radiology in the management of visceral and bone metastases from thyroid cancer. *Gland Surg.* **2018**, *7*, 80–88. [CrossRef]
70. Cazzato, R.L.; Bonichon, F.; Buy, X.; Godbert, Y.; de Figuereido, B.H.; Pointillart, V.; Palussière, J. Over ten years of single-institution experience in percutaneous image-guided treatment of bone metastases from differentiated thyroid cancer. *Eur. J. Surg. Oncol.* **2015**, *41*, 1247–1255. [CrossRef] [PubMed]
71. Barat, M.; Tselikas, L.; de Baère, T.; Gravel, G.; Yevich, S.; Delpla, A.; Magand, N.; Louvel, G.; Hadoux, J.; Berdelou, A.; et al. Thermal-ablation of vertebral metastases prevents adverse events in patients with differentiated thyroid carcinoma. *Eur. J. Radiol.* **2019**, *119*, 108650. [CrossRef]
72. Deschamps, F.; Farouil, G.; Ternes, N.; Gaudin, A.; Hakime, A.; Tselikas, L.; Teriitehau, C.; Baudin, E.; Auperin, A.; de Baere, T. Thermal ablation techniques: A curative treatment of bone metastases in selected patients? *Eur. Radiol.* **2014**, *24*, 1971–1980. [CrossRef]
73. Murphy, K.J.; Deramond, H. Percutaneous vertebroplasty in benign and malignant disease. *Neuroimag. Clin. N. Am.* **2000**, *10*, 535–545.
74. Kushchayev, S.; Kushchayeva, Y.; Theodore, N.; Preul, M.C.; Clark, O.H. Percutaneous vertebroplasty for thyroid cancer metastases to the spine. *Thyroid* **2010**, *20*, 555–560. [CrossRef]
75. Song, H.J.; Wu, C.G.; Xue, Y.L.; Xu, Y.H.; Qiu, Z.L.; Luo, Q.Y. Percutaneous osteoplasty combined with radioiodine therapy as a treatment for bone metastasis developing after differentiated thyroid carcinoma. *Clin. Nucl. Med.* **2012**, *37*, e129–e133. [CrossRef] [PubMed]
76. Mohme, M.; Riethdorf, S.; Dreimann, M.; Werner, S.; Maire, C.L.; Joosse, S.A.; Bludau, F.; Mueller, V.; Neves, R.P.L.; Stoecklein, N.H.; et al. Circulating Tumour Cell Release after Cement Augmentation of Vertebral Metastases. *Sci. Rep.* **2017**, *7*, 7196. [CrossRef] [PubMed]
77. Mercer, J.; Lam, A.C.L.; Smith, R.; Fallah-Rad, N.; Kavanagh, J. Development of pulmonary endovascular metastases following vertebroplasty: Case report. *J. Neurosurg. Spine* **2019**, *29*, 1–4.
78. De Vries, M.M.; Persoon, A.C.; Jager, P.L.; Gravendeel, J.; Plukker, J.T.; Sluiter, W.J.; Links, T.P. Embolization therapy of bone metastases from epithelial thyroid carcinoma: Effect on symptoms and serum thyroglobulin. *Thyroid* **2008**, *18*, 1277–1284. [CrossRef]
79. Smit, J.W.; Vielvoye, G.J.; Goslings, B.M. Embolization for vertebral metastases of follicular thyroid carcinoma. *J. Clin. Endocrinol. Metab.* **2000**, *85*, 989–994. [CrossRef]
80. Son, H.Y.; An, S.Y.; Kim, E.Y.; Ahn, S.B.; Lee, B.C. Selective embolization for hypervascular metastasis from differentiated thyroid cancer: A case series. *J. Med. Case. Rep.* **2014**, *8*, 405. [CrossRef]
81. Eustatia-Rutten, C.F.; Romijn, J.A.; Guijt, M.J.; Vielvoye, G.J.; van den Berg, R.; Corssmit, E.P.; Pereira, A.M.; Smit, J.W. Outcome of palliative embolization of bone metastases in differentiated thyroid carcinoma. *J. Clin. Endocrinol. Metab.* **2003**, *88*, 3184–3189. [CrossRef] [PubMed]

cancers

MDPI

Review

PRKAR1A and Thyroid Tumors

Georgia Pitsava [1,2], Constantine A. Stratakis [2] and Fabio R. Faucz [2,*]

[1] Division of Intramural Population Health Research, Eunice Kennedy Shriver National Institutes of Child Health and Human Development, National Institutes of Health, Bethesda, MD 20892, USA; georgia.pitsava@nih.gov

[2] Section on Endocrinology and Genetics, Eunice Kennedy Shriver National Institute of Child Health and Human Development, National Institutes of Health, Bethesda, MD 20892, USA; stratakc@mail.nih.gov

* Correspondence: fabio.faucz@nih.gov; Tel.: +1-301-451-7177

Simple Summary: In 2021 it is estimated that there will be 44,280 new cases of thyroid cancer in the United States and the incidence rate is higher in women than in men by almost 3 times. Well-differentiated thyroid cancer is the most common subtype of thyroid cancer and includes follicular (FTC) and papillary (PTC) carcinomas. Over the last decade, researchers have been able to better understand the molecular mechanisms involved in thyroid carcinogenesis, identifying genes including but not limited to *RAS*, *BRAF*, *PAX8/PPAR*γ chromosomal rearrangements and others, as well as several tumor genes involved in major signaling pathways regulating cell cycle, differentiation, growth, or proliferation. Patients with Carney complex (CNC) have increased incidence of thyroid tumors, including cancer, yet little is known about this association. CNC is a familial multiple neoplasia and lentiginosis syndrome cause by inactivating mutations in the *PRKAR1A* gene which encodes the regulatory subunit type 1α of protein kinase A. This work summarizes what we know today about *PRKAR1A* defects in humans and mice and their role in thyroid tumor development, as the first such review on this issue.

Citation: Pitsava, G.; Stratakis, C.A.; Faucz, F.R. *PRKAR1A* and Thyroid Tumors. *Cancers* **2021**, *13*, 3834. https://doi.org/10.3390/cancers13153834

Academic Editors: Fabio Medas and Pier Francesco Alesina

Received: 16 June 2021
Accepted: 27 July 2021
Published: 30 July 2021

Abstract: Thyroid cancer is the most common type of endocrine malignancy and the incidence is rapidly increasing. Follicular (FTC) and papillary thyroid (PTC) carcinomas comprise the well-differentiated subtype and they are the two most common thyroid carcinomas. Multiple molecular genetic and epigenetic alterations have been identified in various types of thyroid tumors over the years. Point mutations in *BRAF*, *RAS* as well as *RET/PTC* and *PAX8/PPAR*γ chromosomal rearrangements are common. Thyroid cancer, including both FTC and PTC, has been observed in patients with Carney Complex (CNC), a syndrome that is inherited in an autosomal dominant manner and predisposes to various tumors. CNC is caused by inactivating mutations in the tumor-suppressor gene encoding the cyclic AMP (cAMP)-dependent protein kinase A (PKA) type 1α regulatory subunit (*PRKAR1A*) mapped in chromosome 17 (17q22–24). Growth of the thyroid is driven by the TSH/cAMP/PKA signaling pathway and it has been shown in mouse models that PKA activation through genetic ablation of the regulatory subunit *Prkar1a* can cause FTC. In this review, we provide an overview of the molecular mechanisms contributing to thyroid tumorigenesis associated with inactivation of the *RRKAR1A* gene.

Keywords: thyroid carcinoma; *PRKAR1A*; PKA; Carney complex; cAMP

1. Introduction

1.1. Incidence of Thyroid Cancer

Thyroid cancer is the most common endocrine tumor in the general population and the incidence continues to rise in the United States [1]. The American Cancer Society estimates that there will be 44,280 new cases of thyroid cancer (12,150 in men and 32,130 in women) and about 2200 deaths (1050 in men and 1150 in women) in the United States in 2021 [2]. The increased incidence could be possibly attributed to the increased detection of these tumors with imaging technics (like ultrasound and computed tomography (CT)) that better characterize incidental findings of small thyroid nodules [3].

1.2. Subtypes of Thyroid Cancer

In the majority of patients (about 90%), well-differentiated epithelial thyroid cancer is present; this is further categorized into papillary thyroid cancer (PTC) and follicular thyroid cancer (FTC), based on histological criteria [3,4]. The long-term survival of those patients is excellent, with 5-year relative survival rate (as of 2010–2016) being as high as 98% in all stages (>99% for local tumors and 55% for tumors with distant metastases) [2]. However, FTC tends to behave more aggressively with distant metastases and vascular invasion [5,6] being more common and thus its prognosis is poorer than PTC [7]. The rest of the thyroid carcinomas (~2–3%) include medullary thyroid carcinomas (MTCs) that originate from the calcitonin-producing parafollicular C cells, while anaplastic carcinomas (ATCs) and poorly differentiated carcinomas account for the remaining 7–8% [4]. In addition to the above tumors, benign thyroid tumors that usually present as thyroid nodules as well, include benign hyperplasia or benign follicular adenomas [3].

1.3. Evaluation of a Thyroid Nodule

Thyroid nodules are quite common and are found either clinically or as an incidental finding on imaging studies [8]. The majority of them are benign [9]; only a small percentage harbors thyroid cancer [8]. The initial steps in the evaluation of a thyroid nodule consist of medical history including symptoms (recent onset of hoarseness, neck discomfort or dysphagia), history of head/neck radiation and personal/family history of cancer, followed by physical examination and measurement of serum thyrotropin levels. Ultrasonography (US) is the next step in order to determine the size of the nodule, its characteristics and to assess for cervical lymphadenopathy [10]. If thyrotropin levels are normal or elevated and the nodule size is >1 cm, then fine needle aspiration (FNA) is indicated, according to the American Thyroid Association guidelines [11,12]. If thyrotropin levels are low, then Iodine-123 or technetium-99m thyroid scanning is recommended. In the case that the nodule is nonfunctioning and bigger than 1cm, FNA is the next step. If the cytological interpretation is benign, then repeated FNA is not required unless suspicious features appear in the follow up [12,13]. Currently, US-guided FNA is the gold standard in the diagnosis; however, in about 25% of the cases, the diagnosis remains indeterminate [9,14–20]. If cytologic results are interpreted as atypia of underdetermined significance or follicular lesion of underdetermined significance, then in the case of high suspicion, assessment of the aspirate for molecular abnormalities (e.g., mutations or rearrangements) is indicated [21].

1.4. Thyroid Cancer as Part of Genetic Syndromes

Thyroid malignancies are also associated with at least two syndromes with inherited tumor predisposition, Cowden syndrome (CS, OMIM# 158350) and Carney Complex (CNC, OMIM #160980). CS is a multiple hamartoma syndrome, including FTC, brain and breast cancer. It is caused by inactivating mutations in the *PTEN* gene, a dual-specificity phosphatase that negatively regulates PI3 Kinase/AKT pathway; mutations in this gene have been detected in 5% of FTCs [22]; however, a mouse harboring a deletion of *Pten* in the thyroid developed thyroid hyperplasia and not FTC [23].

In this review, we will focus on CNC, which is a multiple neoplasia syndrome that presents as the complex of myxomas, spotty skin pigmentation and endocrine tumors (Table 1) [24]. CNC is caused by inactivating mutations in the *PRKAR1A* gene (mapped in 17q22–24) [25]; somatic mutations in this gene have been reported in sporadic cases of thyroid cancer [26]. In tumors associated with CNC as well as in thyroid and adrenal tumors with downregulation of *PRKAR1A*, allelic losses of the 17q22–24 *PRKAR1A* chromosomal locus are frequently identified and are associated with changes in PKA activity [26–29].

Table 1. Diagnostic criteria for Carney Complex [24].

Main Diagnostic Criteria	
1.	Spotty skin pigmentation with a typical distribution (lips, conjunctiva and inner or outer canthi, vaginal and penile mucosa)
2.	Myxoma (cutaneous and mucosal) [a]
3.	Cardiac myxoma [a]
4.	Breast myxomatosis [a] or fat-suppressed magnetic resonance imaging findings suggestive of this diagnosis
5.	PPNAD [a] or paradoxical positive response of urinary glucocorticosteroids to dexamethasone administration during 6-day modified Liddle test
6.	Acromegaly due to GH-producing adenoma [a]
7.	LCCSCT [a] or characteristic calcification on testicular ultrasonography
8.	Thyroid carcinoma [a] or multiple, hypoechoic nodules on thyroid ultrasonography
9.	Psammomatous melanotic schwannoma [a]
10.	Blue nevus, epithelioid blue nevus (multiple) [a]
11.	Breast ductal adenoma (multiple)
12.	Osteochondroma of bone [a]
Supplementary Criteria	
1.	Affected 1st-degree relative
2.	Inactivating mutation of the *PRKAR1A* gene

[a] with histologic confirmation; *LCCSCT* large cell calcifying Sertoli cell tumor, *PPNAD* primary pigmented nodular adrenocortical disease; To make a diagnosis of CNC, a patient must either: (1) exhibit two of the manifestations of the disease listed, or (2) exhibit one of these manifestations and meet one of the supplemental criteria.

2. *PRKAR1A* Structure and Function

Cyclic adenosine monophosphate (cAMP)-dependent protein kinase type 1-alpha regulatory subunit is encoded by the *PRKAR1A* gene. *PRKAR1A* consists of 11 exons; ten of them (2–11) are coding. Protein kinase A (PKA) (Figure 1), a serine/threonine kinase, is a second messenger-dependent enzyme and it is involved in G-protein coupled intracellular pathways. It is the main mediator of cAMP actions for various cellular processes in mammals, including cell differentiation, proliferation, and apoptosis [30–32].

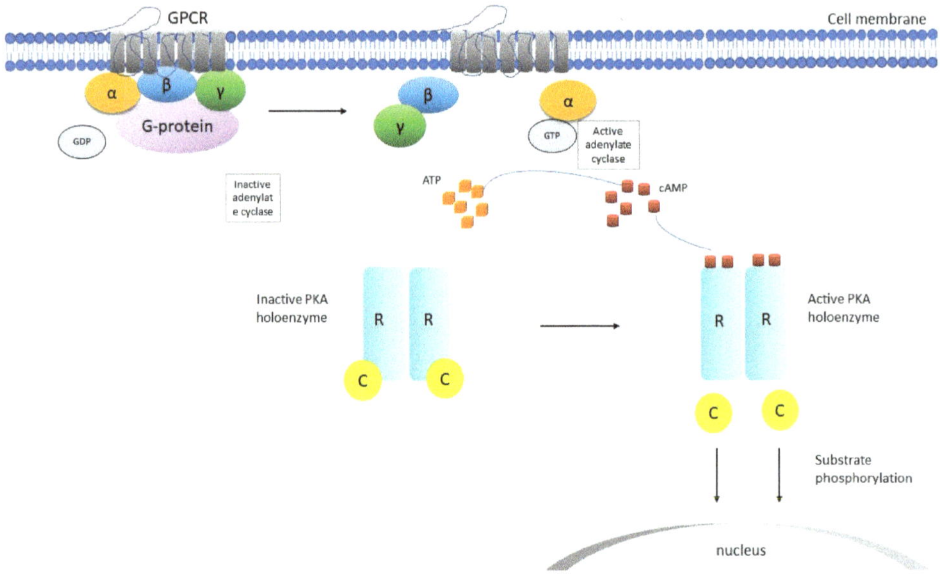

Figure 1. Schematic representation of cyclic adenosine monophosphate (cAMP) signaling pathway. *C* catalytic subunit of PKA, *GDP* guanosine diphosphate, *GPCR* G-protein coupled receptor, *GTP* guanosine triphosphate, *PKA* protein kinase, *R* regulatory subunit of PKA, α, β, γ subunits. After the GPCR is activated, adenylate cyclase is activated and produces cAMP, which binds to the R subunit and activates PKA. Then, conformational changes ensue and the C subunits are released and phosphorylate cytoplasmic targets.

The PKA holoenzyme is a hetero-tetramer composed of two regulatory (R) subunits and each is bound to one catalytic (C) subunit [33]. Four subtypes of R (RIα, RIβ, RIIα, RIIβ) and four subtypes of C (Cα, Cβ, Cγ and Prkx) subunits have been identified so far. A gene is coding each R (*PRKR1A*, *PRKR1B*, *PRKR2A*, *PRKR2B*) and each C (*PRKACA*, *PRKACB*, *PRKACG*, *PRKX*) subunit, respectively [33,34]. Two major isozymes have been identified, type I and type II PKA, based on their chromatographic elution patterns [32]; they are comprised of homodimers of either RIα and RIβ or RIIα and RIIβ, respectively [31,35]. In the basal state, the catalytic subunits bind mostly to type II subunits [31,35–37]. When cAMP binds to the R subunits, it alters their conformation; this causes the dissociation of each active C subunit from the dimer with the corresponding R subunit. Following that, the free C subunits phosphorylate threonine and serine residues of proteins that are critical to the activation of downstream processes [38–40].

RIα haploinsufficiency, as shown by mice and human studies, predisposes to the development of tumors [29,41]. The majority of *PRKAR1A* mutations result in premature stop codons with unstable mRNAs undergoing nonsense-mediated decay [25,42]. In the thyroid, PKA through the production of cAMP, signals downstream of thyrotropin (TSH) on cell proliferation and differentiation; increased levels of TSH in humans have been associated with thyroid tumors [43]. In addition, in a series of thyroid tumors, the Cα subunit was investigated but no mutations were detected [44].

3. Role of *PRKAR1A* in Thyroid Cancer

3.1. Mouse Studies

3.1.1. Mouse Models

In 2004, Griffin et al. generated a mouse model carrying an antisense transgene for *Prkar1a* exon 2 (X2AS) under the control of a tetracycline responsive promoter (the Tg(Prakr1a*x2as)1Stra, Tg(tTAhCMV)3Uh, or tTA/X2AS) [45]. Increased cAMP signaling was demonstrated due to significant *Prkar1a* downregulation and the mice exhibited a more severe phenotype with high incidence of thyroid lesions (thyroid follicular hyperplasia and adenomas). This was an extremely rare finding in wild type animals but quite common in those with the genetic defect (as it is common among patients with CNC). Furthermore, the lesions were associated with allelic loss of the *Prkar1a* locus on chromosome 11 as it happens in thyroid tumors with *PRKAR1A* mutations. Moreover, tumor tissues demonstrated an increase in the activity of type II PKA and higher RIIβ levels, an abnormal cAMP response.

In a later study, *Prkar1a* haploinsufficiency in mice was investigated. It was shown that *Prkar1a* haploinsufficiency leads to tumor development arising in cAMP-responsive tissues, including among others, benign and malignant thyroid neoplasms [41]. Mice heterozygous for a conventional null allele of *Prkar1a* (*Prkar1a*$^{\Delta 2/+}$ mice) were generated. These mice developed tumors in the same spectrum as CNC patients. Thyroid neoplasms were present in 10% of *Prkar1a*$^{\Delta 2/+}$ mice [41]. In addition, allelic loss occurred in a portion of tumor cells, as indicated by genetic analysis, suggesting that complete loss of *Prkar1a* plays a vital role in tumor formation.

A different mouse model, carrying a thyroid-specific deletion of *Prkar1a* (Tpo-R1αKO) was studied [46]. In 43% of mice, FTC was observed by 1 year of age. However, distant hematogenous metastases were not present, which is a key feature of FTC in humans [46]; this could potentially suggest that metastases may be triggered by another genetic mutation in the case of *Prkar1a* mutation in the thyroid. An interesting observation by the authors was that thyroid ablation of *PRKAR1A/Prkar1a* is the only genetic change that has been described that results in FTC in both mice and humans.

3.1.2. Activation of mTOR Pathway

The role of PKA as a key regulator of FTC has also been suggested by a recent study demonstrating a concurrent activation of PKA and mTOR. In this study a double *Prkar1a-Pten* knockout mouse (*DRP-Tpo*KO mice) with thyroid-specific deletion of both genes was generated and was compared to signaling alterations to human FTCs [1]; they found that mice developed aggressive FTC that exhibited 100% penetrance by 8 weeks of age. In addition, well-differentiated lung metastases appeared to be common in these mice (approximately one third of them), mimicking the human disease. The signaling pathways were analyzed and it was shown that PKA and the mammalian target of rapamycin (mTOR) pathways were consistently activated. mTOR has an essential role in promoting the metabolic changes that occur during tumorigenesis and is regulated by the AMP-dependent protein kinase (AMPK) [47]. AMPK is activated under nutrition restriction or increase in the AMP/ATP ration in order to increase energy production [48].

It has been suggested before that mTOR could be activated by *Prkar1a* deletion and that it could possibly interact with Prkar1a directly [49], but the data remain controversial [50]. Furthermore, activation of mTOR by TSH has been suggested to be partly due to PKA phosphorylation of the target of rapamycin complex 1 complex member PRAS40 [51]. Mouse models have been developed over the years that recapitulate how human FTCs progress from benign follicular adenoma (at one year of age) in the *Pten-TpoKO* [23] to locally invasive FTC as in the *R1a-TpoKO* [46] and subsequently to invasive and distantly metastatic FTC. The authors identified PKA and mTOR as essential signaling pathways and showed that activation of mTOR can occur independently of Akt [1]. Further, the concurrent activation of PKA and mTOR that was observed in human FTCs led to the conclusion that PKA activates mTOR/p70S6K that results in thyroid cancer, indicating that PKA is a vital component regulating FTC in both mice and humans [1].

The same group reported that, in FTCs, both in mice and humans, AMPK and mTOR pathways are activated concomitantly [52]. They showed that the tumor suppressor that causes Peutz–Jeghers syndrome, LKB1, mediates the signaling from PKA to AMPK in driving tumorigenesis [53,54]. The role of AMPK in the development of cancer has not been determined yet; according to the literature, it can act either as tumor promoter or tumor suppressor [55,56]. LKB1, like AMPK, can act as tumor promoter/suppressor as well, depending on the context [55,57–61]. Even though it typically suppresses the activity of mTOR [56,62], there is evidence that it can also act as a tumor promoter [63–65], which means that its functions depend on the type of tissue and other intracellular signals that may be present.

3.1.3. Targeting Downstream Effectors of cAMP

Because of the various effects of cAMP in physiological responses, therapies targeting cAMP signaling result in side effects; thus, understanding downstream targets of cAMP signaling has been attempted in a number of studies [66,67]. The roles of Rap1 and Epac1 in *Prkar1a*-associated thyroid carcinogenesis have been studied [68]. *Rap1* is a small GTPase essential for effective signal transduction. There are two isoforms and each one is encoded by a separate gene, *Rap1a* and *Rap1b*, respectively. The activity of Rap1 has been shown to be regulated by both PKA and cAMP though signaling by TSH [69]. Increased Rap activity has been linked to various cancers, including thyroid cancer, while dysregulation of Rap1 has been postulated to contribute to the development of malignancy [70–74]. Epac (Exchange protein directly activated by cAMP) proteins are intracellular sensors for cAMP and mediate its effects to activate Rap1 [75,76]. The two isoforms include Epac1 which is ubiquitously expressed, with particularly high levels in the thyroid, among other tissues, and Epac2 which is not detected in the thyroid; however, it is expressed in a limited number of other tissues [76,77]. Epac regulates Rap activity in concert with and independently of PKA, and the effects—either stimulatory or inhibitory—seem to depend on the cellular context and the type of stimuli [69,75,78,79]. In addition, it has been shown that Epac1 plays a role in cell migration and invasion in other types of cancer [78,80]. Loss of *Rap*, specifically of the Rap1b isoform, in *Prkar1a* KO thyroids in the setting of overactivation of the PKA pathway, resulted in reduced risk of developing thyroid cancer by 65%; this occurred independently of Epac1 as its deletion did not have any effect in PKA-Rap1 associated thyroid tumorigenesis, underlying the essential role of PKA-Rap1 signaling in the development of FTC [68]. However, even though tumor suppression happened to a significant extent, the carcinogenic phenotype was not completely rescued, which led to the speculation that more complex signaling interactions may be involved [68].

These findings were further supported by other studies that showed that Rap proteins can be directly regulated by PKA using a specific phosphorylation site at serine 180 on Rap1a and serine 179 on Rap1b [81]. When PKA phosphorylates Rap, it regulates its subcellular localization, and its downstream effectors such as ERK and Rap-dependent regulation of cell migration [82,83]. These previous studies indicate that PKA can control Rap action and downstream cellular processes directly suggesting that PKA-Rap1 pathway is independent of Epac1 in thyroid cancer. On the other hand, previous studies have shown, that both PKA and Epac signal to Rap1 downstream of TSH [69,75], but it seems to be tissue-dependent [78,79].

In combination, these studies demonstrated that cAMP or PKA signaling or both play an important role in tumor development and that additional factors may contribute to *Prkar1a* haploinsufficiency in causing those tumors. *Trp53*+/− mice and other animal models for diseases like CNC, including Peutz–Jeghers and neurofibromatosis type 1, did not exhibit the same phenotype as in humans; it only occurred when one or more tumor suppressor genes were knocked out as well [84–86]. *Prkar1a* haploinsufficiency in addition to either *Trp53* or *Rb1* haploinsufficiency resulted in more tumors and decreased survival compared to *Trp53*+/− or *Rb1*+/− mice [87]. Specifically, *Rb1*+/− *Prkar1a*+/− mice developed more MTCs than *Rb1*+/− mice [87].

3.2. Studies in Humans

Further evidence to support the involvement of PKA in thyroid tumors was demonstrated by studying the *PRKAR1A* gene in thyroid tissue from patients with CNC [29]. The involvement of the thyroid in the syndrome was reported for the first time twelve years after CNC was first described [88], in 1997 [89]. In a cohort of 53 individuals with familial

CNC, thyroid disease was identified in 11% of patients; of them, three were studied in detail, two with thyroid carcinomas (one PTC, one FTC) and one patient with a benign follicular adenoma. [89]. In addition, 60% of patients with the sporadic form of the complex exhibited thyroid gland lesions of follicular origin [89]. The authors concluded that thyroid carcinomas may develop in situ from precursor benign lesions in these patients. It is important to note that patients' ethnicity does not seem to play a role in CNC phenotype that include thyroid carcinomas.

Since the *PRKAR1A* gene was identified as causal in CNC, many disease-causing mutations have been identified [24,90]. Sandrini et al. showed that in thyroid cancer the activity of PKA is greater than in adenomas, partly due to genetic defects in the *PRKAR1A* gene and/or locus [26]. The region 17q22–24 was frequently lost in cancer but not in benign tumors. In addition, it was shown that RIα, the most abundant regulatory subunit of cAMP-dependent PKA [91], in thyroid cells, possibly exhibits a tumor-suppressor function, as indicated by decreased expression of the RIα subunit in carcinomas and by the losses of *PRKAR1A* 17q22–24 locus in about 50% of all informative cancers. It has been known that the activation of cAMP/PKA pathway is involved in normal thyroid cell growth [92]; the same appears to be true for thyroid adenomas, while in the case of PTCs inhibition is induced [93]. The results suggested that *PRKAR1A* is indeed involved in sporadic thyroid tumors, along with other genes [94–97], some of which could be associated with the PKA pathway [91]. Any disruption of that, because of deficiency of the RIα subunit, could lead to cAMP-dependent PKA mediated cell proliferation and/or stimulation of other pathways linked to proliferation of thyroid cells [91,98].

In a recent series of 353 CNC patients from 185 families, patients from various ethnicities and with a wide range of clinical manifestations were studied [99]. More than 60% of them harbored mutations in the *PRKAR1A* gene. In 25% of patients, thyroid tumors were present while thyroid cancer (either FTC or PTC or both) was present in 2.5% of cases. In addition, thyroid tumors ($p = 0.016$) were more frequent in *PRKAR1A* carriers and presented at a younger age ($p = 0.03$). Moreover, they were more commonly associated with the 'hot spot' c.491–492delTG mutation in comparison with all other *PRKAR1A* defects. It was also observed that patients with no mutations of the *PRKAR1A* gene or its genomic locus 17q22–24, were less likely to develop thyroid tumors. In a review of 26 patients, in 61% of them benign lesions (including follicular adenoma, follicular hyperplasia or nodular hyperplasia) were detected, while 38% of them had thyroid carcinomas (seven with FTC and three with PTC). The majority of patients presented with an asymptomatic thyroid nodule and included middle-aged women [100].

4. Other Molecular Events in Thyroid Cancer

A significant number of mutations in thyroid cancer involves encoding genes of the MAPK and PI3K/AKT pathways. Mutated genes that affect these pathways encode the signal transduction molecules RAS, BRAF and NTRK1 and RET receptor tyrosine kinases. These mutations are present in approximately 70% of patients with PTCs and they exhibit particular clinical manifestations as well as specific histopathological characteristics in the tumor level [101–104]. Among FTCs, *RAS* mutations and *PAX8/PPARγ* rearrangements are common [105]. Because PAX8 is important for the development of the thyroid, it has been speculated that the fusion of *PPARγ* and *PAX8* can lead to cancer by activation of aberrant gene transcription [3]. *PAX8/PPARγ* is found in FTCs with a frequency of 30–35% and in a very small percentage of the follicular variant PTCs and follicular adenomas [106–109]. Thyroid tumors harboring *RAS* mutations, most commonly *NRAS* and *HRAS* mutations, include FTCs in 40–50%, PTCs in 10–20% and 20–40% of anaplastic and poorly differentiated carcinomas [110–116]. Because PTCs that harbor *RAS* mutations form neoplastic follicles and no papillary structures, they are known as follicular variant of PTC [101,117]. Benign follicular adenomas have also been found to harbor *RAS* mutations in 20–40%, indicating that they may be precursors of *RAS*-positive FTCs and follicular variant of PTCs [118–121]. Furthermore, $BRAF^{V600E}$ mutation represents 98–99% of all BRAF mutations in thyroid cancer [122–124]. It accounts for 40–45% of classic PTCs, 30–40% of ATCs, and 20–40% of poorly differentiated thyroid carcinomas [125–128].

Mutations in *BRAF* and *RAS* are thought to represent an early event in the progression of thyroid cancer, given that they are present in poorly and well-differentiated thyroid cancer, as well as in ATCs. On the other hand, additional genetic alterations are usually present in poorly differentiated carcinomas and ATCs; these constitute late events that may be necessary for tumor dedifferentiation. These genetic alterations include mutations in the *TP53* and *CTNNB1* genes and encoding genes of the PI3K/AKT signaling pathway [105]. In 50–80% of ATCs, point mutations that lead to loss-of-function of *TP53* have been identified; these are very rare in well-differentiated thyroid cancer [129,130]. *CTNNB1* mutations occur in approximately 60% of ATCs [131,132].

5. Medullary Thyroid Cancer as Part of MEN2 Syndromes

About one-third of MTCs are hereditary, presenting as multicentric and bilateral, in contrast with sporadic cases that are a single unilateral tumor [133,134]. They present as part of MEN2A (70–80%), MEN2B (5%), or familial MTC (FMTC) (10–20%). The first inherited subtype of MTC, MEN2A, consists of primary hyperparathyroidism, pheochromocytoma and MTC in which it can occur early in life (approximately 5 years of age) in contrast with sporadic cases that presents between 15 and 20 years [134,135]. MEN2B is characterized by pheochromocytoma, MTC and non-endocrine diseases such as mucosal neuromas, intestinal tumors (most commonly ganglioneuromas) and Marfanoid habitus [135]. In the case of FMTC, only the thyroid gland is affected, but in a significant number of relatives in the same family, usually between the ages of 20 and 40 [135–137]. Activating germline *RET* mutations have been identified as the main cause of up to 98% of hereditary MTCs and up to half of sporadic cases [138]. Depending on the mutated residue within the RET protein, the phenotype may differ [139–142]. Families with two or more members with MTC are referred for genetic counseling and screening, if positive they undergo further testing for hyperparathyroidism and pheochromocytoma [2,143,144]. In the case of sporadic MTCs, somatic *RET* mutations, particularly M918T, has been shown to be associated with more aggressive disease and worse prognosis [144,145].

6. Anaplastic Thyroid Carcinoma

ATC is a rare (1–2%) but very aggressive type of thyroid cancer [146] with average age at diagnosis over 70 years [147]. It is considered to evolve from dedifferentiation of a pre-existing DTC caused by accumulation of several genetic alterations that lead to disruption of two signaling pathways that are involved in cell proliferation, PI3K-AKT and MAPK [148–150]. The most common mutations include *TP53*, which is considered a genetic hallmark of ATC, as well as *RAS*, *BRAF*, *PIK3CA* [151,152], mutations that have also been identified in DTC [153]. Median survival is usually less than 6 months after diagnosis and the mortality rate is >90% [154,155]. Due to its extremely aggressive nature, it is critical to be diagnosed promptly. Clinical symptoms are usually used for the diagnosis, in contrast with DTC in which diagnosis is made by FNA of a suspicious nodule [147]. The symptoms can last from 4 weeks to 11 months and usually consist of a rapidly enlarging neck mass along with vocal cord paralysis and dyspnea [147].

7. Systemic Treatments for Thyroid Cancer

Two multikinase inhibitors (MKI), lenvatinib and sorafenib, are currently approved by the US Food and Drug Administration (FDA) for the treatment of advanced DTC. Sorafenib was approved based on the favorable results of a placebo-controlled phase 3 clinical trial (DECISION) [156]. The positive results of the lenvatinib phase 3 SELECT trial [157] as well as a phase 2 study led to the approval of that drug [158]. Cabozatinib and vandetanib are approved by the FDA for the treatment of MTC. Vandetanib is approved for symptomatic, unresectable, locally advanced, or metastatic MTC in patients based on a phase 3 trial (ZETA) [159]. Cabozantinib was studied in a phase 3 clinical trial

(EXAM) [160] and showed good results while another clinical trial in MTC patients is still active (EXAMINER, NCT01896479). RET-inhibitors have been studied as well for thyroid cancers that harbor *RET* mutations (NCT03157128, NCT04211337, NCT03906331, NCT04280081, NCT03037385).

7.1. Immunotherapy

In the recent years, immunotherapy has emerged as a new transformative approach into the body's natural antitumor defenses. To date, there is no approved immunotherapy for advanced thyroid cancer. A few clinical trials using novel immunotherapy agents like programmed cell death protein 1 (PD-1) checkpoint inhibitors are ongoing. Pembrolizumab in an Ib phase trial (KEYNOTE) showed a tumor size reduction of 35–50% in PTC and FTC. The use of another anti-PD1 agent (spartalizumab) was evaluated in progressive ATC that responded to therapy [161]. In an ongoing phase 2 clinical trial (NCT03246958), the efficacy of the combination of nivolumab (anti-PD1-1) and ipilimumab (anti-CTLA-4-cytotoxic T-lymphocyte-associated protein 4) was evaluated in patients with aggressive thyroid cancer. In addition, multiple clinical trials with VEGF and/or VEGF inhibitor and immune checkpoint inhibitors have been designed. Pemproblizumab plus lenvatinib was investigated in a phase 2 trial for unresectable ATC (NCT04171622) as well as in a randomized study in a small group of advanced ATC and PDTC [162]. The same combination is under study in DTC and PDTC naïve or progressing after lenvatinib patients (NCT02973997). Triple combined therapy (cabozantinib plus nivolumab and ipilimumab) is under evaluation for DTC and PDTC (NCT03914300).

7.2. Treatment for PRKAR1A-Associated Thyroid Tumors

To date, there is no medical treatment targeting cAMP/PKA signaling in CNC. Surgical treatment is the treatment of choice in patients with PRKAR1A-associated thyroid tumor [163].

8. Clinical Surveillance in Patients with PRKAR1A-Associated Thyroid Tumors

Human studies in CNC underly the importance of investigating thyroid nodules in these patients. Multiple thyroid nodules are present in up to 75% of patients with CNC on thyroid ultrasound; the majority of them are non-functioning follicular adenomas [164]. However, thyroid carcinomas are common as well. Early detection is vital and CNC patients should be followed with long-term clinical and/or ultrasound surveillance with biopsy of suspicious nodules, for early detection of carcinomas [164].

Because CNC is inherited in an autosomal dominant manner, each child of an affected individual has a 50% chance of inheriting the pathogenic variant. Most of the affected patients (approximately 70%) have an affected parent. In the case that the pathogenic variant is known in a family, prenatal testing may be recommended [164].

9. Conclusions

In summary, recent advances in molecular mechanisms of thyroid cancer have improved cancer prognosis and detection. *PRKAR1A*, a regulator of PKA activity, is possibly involved in the molecular events that contribute to thyroid cancer. Identifying the genetic basis of *PRKAR1A*-associated thyroid tumors is important as it will provide better clinical management to these patients.

Funding: This work was supported by the project Z01-HD008920 (Principal Investigator: C.A.S.) of the Intramural Research Program of the *Eunice Kennedy Shriver* National Institute of Child Health & Human Development (NICHD), National Institutes of Health (NIH), Bethesda, MD, USA.

Conflicts of Interest: C.A.S. holds patent on the *PRKAR1A*, *PDE11A*, and *GPR101* genes and/or their function and his laboratory has received research funding from Pfizer, Inc. F.R.F. holds patent on the *GPR101* gene and/or its function. C.A.S. is receiving compensation by ELPEN, Inc. Neither

Pfizer, Inc. nor ELPEN, Inc. had any role in the study design, data collection and analysis, decision to publish, or preparation of the manuscript. All authors declare no conflict of interest.

References

1. Pringle, D.R.; Vasko, V.V.; Yu, L.; Manchanda, P.K.; Lee, A.A.; Zhang, X.; Kirschner, J.M.; Parlow, A.F.; Saji, M.; Jarjoura, D.; et al. Follicular thyroid cancers demonstrate dual activation of PKA and mTOR as modeled by thyroid-specific deletion of Prkar1a and Pten in mice. *J. Clin. Endocrinol. Metab.* **2014**, *99*, E804–E812. [CrossRef]
2. Eng, C.; Mulligan, L.M.; Smith, D.P.; Healey, C.S.; Frilling, A.; Raue, F.; Neumann, H.P.; Ponder, M.A.; Ponder, B.A. Low frequency of germline mutations in the RET proto-oncogene in patients with apparently sporadic medullary thyroid carcinoma. *Clin. Endocrinol.* **1995**, *43*, 123–127. [CrossRef] [PubMed]
3. Raman, P.; Koenig, R.J. Pax-8-PPAR-gamma fusion protein in thyroid carcinoma. *Nat. Rev. Endocrinol.* **2014**, *10*, 616–623. [CrossRef] [PubMed]
4. Younis, E. Oncogenesis of Thyroid Cancer. *Asian Pac. J. Cancer Prev.* **2017**, *18*, 1191–1199. [CrossRef] [PubMed]
5. Besic, N.; Auersperg, M.; Golouh, R. Prognostic factors in follicular carcinoma of the thyroid—A multivariate survival analysis. *Eur. J. Surg. Oncol.* **1999**, *25*, 599–605. [CrossRef]
6. Nguyen, X.V.; Roy Choudhury, K.; Tessler, F.N.; Hoang, J.K. Effect of Tumor Size on Risk of Metastatic Disease and Survival for Thyroid Cancer: Implications for Biopsy Guidelines. *Thyroid* **2018**, *28*, 295–300. [CrossRef]
7. Sugino, K.; Ito, K.; Nagahama, M.; Kitagawa, W.; Shibuya, H.; Ohkuwa, K.; Yano, Y.; Uruno, T.; Akaishi, J.; Kameyama, K.; et al. Prognosis and prognostic factors for distant metastases and tumor mortality in follicular thyroid carcinoma. *Thyroid* **2011**, *21*, 751–757. [CrossRef]
8. Burman, K.D.; Wartofsky, L. Clinical Practice. Thyroid Nodules. *N. Engl. J. Med.* **2015**, *373*, 2347–2356. [CrossRef]
9. Yassa, L.; Cibas, E.S.; Benson, C.B.; Frates, M.C.; Doubilet, P.M.; Gawande, A.A.; Moore, F.D., Jr.; Kim, B.W.; Nose, V.; Marqusee, E.; et al. Long-term assessment of a multidisciplinary approach to thyroid nodule diagnostic evaluation. *Cancer* **2007**, *111*, 508–516. [CrossRef] [PubMed]
10. Cooper, D.S. American Thyroid Association Guidelines Taskforce on Thyroid Nodules and Differentiated Thyroid Cancer. Revised American Thyroid Association management guidelines for patients with thyroid nodules and differentiated thyroid cancer. *Thyroid* **2009**, *19*, 1167–1214. [CrossRef]
11. Frates, M.C.; Benson, C.B.; Charboneau, J.W.; Cibas, E.S.; Clark, O.H.; Coleman, B.G.; Cronan, J.J.; Doubilet, P.M.; Evans, D.B.; Goellner, J.R.; et al. Management of thyroid nodules detected at US: Society of Radiologists in Ultrasound consensus conference statement. *Radiology* **2005**, *237*, 794–800. [CrossRef] [PubMed]
12. Haugen, B.R.; Alexander, E.K.; Bible, K.C.; Doherty, G.M.; Mandel, S.J.; Nikiforov, Y.E.; Pacini, F.; Randolph, G.W.; Sawka, A.M.; Schlumberger, M.; et al. 2015 American Thyroid Association Management Guidelines for Adult Patients with Thyroid Nodules and Differentiated Thyroid Cancer: The American Thyroid Association Guidelines Task Force on Thyroid Nodules and Differentiated Thyroid Cancer. *Thyroid* **2016**, *26*, 1–133. [CrossRef] [PubMed]
13. Oertel, Y.C.; Miyahara-Felipe, L.; Mendoza, M.G.; Yu, K. Value of repeated fine needle aspirations of the thyroid: An analysis of over ten thousand FNAs. *Thyroid* **2007**, *17*, 1061–1066. [CrossRef]
14. Brander, A.; Viikinkoski, P.; Nickels, J.; Kivisaari, L. Thyroid gland: US screening in a random adult population. *Radiology* **1991**, *181*, 683–687. [CrossRef] [PubMed]
15. Papini, E.; Guglielmi, R.; Bianchini, A.; Crescenzi, A.; Taccogna, S.; Nardi, F.; Panunzi, C.; Rinaldi, R.; Toscano, V.; Pacella, C.M. Risk of malignancy in nonpalpable thyroid nodules: Predictive value of ultrasound and color-Doppler features. *J. Clin. Endocrinol. Metab.* **2002**, *87*, 1941–1946. [CrossRef]
16. Carroll, B.A. Asymptomatic thyroid nodules: Incidental sonographic detection. *AJR Am. J. Roentgenol.* **1982**, *138*, 499–501. [CrossRef]
17. Sclabas, G.M.; Staerkel, G.A.; Shapiro, S.E.; Fornage, B.D.; Sherman, S.I.; Vassillopoulou-Sellin, R.; Lee, J.E.; Evans, D.B. Fine-needle aspiration of the thyroid and correlation with histopathology in a contemporary series of 240 patients. *Am. J. Surg.* **2003**, *186*, 702–710. [CrossRef] [PubMed]
18. Greaves, T.S.; Olvera, M.; Florentine, B.D.; Raza, A.S.; Cobb, C.J.; Tsao-Wei, D.D.; Groshen, S.; Singer, P.; Lopresti, J.; Martin, S.E. Follicular lesions of thyroid: A 5-year fine-needle aspiration experience. *Cancer* **2000**, *90*, 335–341. [CrossRef]
19. Tomimori, E.; Pedrinola, F.; Cavaliere, H.; Knobel, M.; Medeiros-Neto, G. Prevalence of incidental thyroid disease in a relatively low iodine intake area. *Thyroid* **1995**, *5*, 273–276. [CrossRef]
20. Wiest, P.W.; Hartshorne, M.F.; Inskip, P.D.; Crooks, L.A.; Vela, B.S.; Telepak, R.J.; Williamson, M.R.; Blumhardt, R.; Bauman, J.M.; Tekkel, M. Thyroid palpation versus high-resolution thyroid ultrasonography in the detection of nodules. *J. Ultrasound Med.* **1998**, *17*, 487–496. [CrossRef]
21. Burman, K.D.; Wartofsky, L. Thyroid Nodules. *N. Engl. J. Med.* **2016**, *374*, 1294–1295. [CrossRef] [PubMed]
22. Nagy, R.; Ganapathi, S.; Comeras, I.; Peterson, C.; Orloff, M.; Porter, K.; Eng, C.; Ringel, M.D.; Kloos, R.T. Frequency of germline PTEN mutations in differentiated thyroid cancer. *Thyroid* **2011**, *21*, 505–510. [CrossRef] [PubMed]
23. Yeager, N.; Klein-Szanto, A.; Kimura, S.; Di Cristofano, A. Pten loss in the mouse thyroid causes goiter and follicular adenomas: Insights into thyroid function and Cowden disease pathogenesis. *Cancer Res.* **2007**, *67*, 959–966. [CrossRef] [PubMed]

24. Stratakis, C.A.; Kirschner, L.S.; Carney, J.A. Clinical and molecular features of the Carney complex: Diagnostic criteria and recommendations for patient evaluation. *J. Clin. Endocrinol. Metab.* **2001**, *86*, 4041–4046. [CrossRef] [PubMed]
25. Kirschner, L.S.; Sandrini, F.; Monbo, J.; Lin, J.P.; Carney, J.A.; Stratakis, C.A. Genetic heterogeneity and spectrum of mutations of the PRKAR1A gene in patients with the carney complex. *Hum. Mol. Genet.* **2000**, *9*, 3037–3046. [CrossRef]
26. Sandrini, F.; Matyakhina, L.; Sarlis, N.J.; Kirschner, L.S.; Farmakidis, C.; Gimm, O.; Stratakis, C.A. Regulatory subunit type I-alpha of protein kinase A (PRKAR1A): A tumor-suppressor gene for sporadic thyroid cancer. *Genes Chromosomes Cancer* **2002**, *35*, 182–192. [CrossRef]
27. Bertherat, J.; Groussin, L.; Sandrini, F.; Matyakhina, L.; Bei, T.; Stergiopoulos, S.; Papageorgiou, T.; Bourdeau, I.; Kirschner, L.S.; Vincent-Dejean, C.; et al. Molecular and functional analysis of PRKAR1A and its locus (17q22-24) in sporadic adrenocortical tumors: 17q losses, somatic mutations, and protein kinase A expression and activity. *Cancer Res.* **2003**, *63*, 5308–5319.
28. Bossis, I.; Voutetakis, A.; Bei, T.; Sandrini, F.; Griffin, K.J.; Stratakis, C.A. Protein kinase A and its role in human neoplasia: The Carney complex paradigm. *Endocr. Relat. Cancer* **2004**, *11*, 265–280. [CrossRef]
29. Kirschner, L.S.; Carney, J.A.; Pack, S.D.; Taymans, S.E.; Giatzakis, C.; Cho, Y.S.; Cho-Chung, Y.S.; Stratakis, C.A. Mutations of the gene encoding the protein kinase A type I-alpha regulatory subunit in patients with the Carney complex. *Nat. Genet.* **2000**, *26*, 89–92. [CrossRef]
30. McKnight, G.S.; Clegg, C.H.; Uhler, M.D.; Chrivia, J.C.; Cadd, G.G.; Correll, L.A.; Otten, A.D. Analysis of the cAMP-dependent protein kinase system using molecular genetic approaches. *Recent Prog. Horm. Res.* **1988**, *44*, 307–335. [CrossRef]
31. Cho-Chung, Y.S.; Pepe, S.; Clair, T.; Budillon, A.; Nesterova, M. cAMP-dependent protein kinase: Role in normal and malignant growth. *Crit. Rev. Oncol. Hematol.* **1995**, *21*, 33–61. [CrossRef]
32. Skalhegg, B.S.; Tasken, K. Specificity in the cAMP/PKA signaling pathway. Differential expression, regulation, and subcellular localization of subunits of PKA. *Front. Biosci.* **2000**, *5*, D678–D693. [CrossRef] [PubMed]
33. Bossis, I.; Stratakis, C.A. Minireview: PRKAR1A: Normal and abnormal functions. *Endocrinology* **2004**, *145*, 5452–5458. [CrossRef] [PubMed]
34. Almeida, M.Q.; Stratakis, C.A. How does cAMP/protein kinase A signaling lead to tumors in the adrenal cortex and other tissues? *Mol. Cell Endocrinol.* **2011**, *336*, 162–168. [CrossRef]
35. Amieux, P.S.; McKnight, G.S. The essential role of RI alpha in the maintenance of regulated PKA activity. *Ann. N. Y. Acad. Sci.* **2002**, *968*, 75–95. [CrossRef]
36. Cho-Chung, Y.S.; Nesterova, M.; Pepe, S.; Lee, G.R.; Noguchi, K.; Srivastava, R.K.; Srivastava, A.R.; Alper, O.; Park, Y.G.; Lee, Y.N. Antisense DNA-targeting protein kinase A-RIA subunit: A novel approach to cancer treatment. *Front. Biosci.* **1999**, *4*, D898–D907. [CrossRef]
37. Scott, J.D. Cyclic nucleotide-dependent protein kinases. *Pharmacol. Ther.* **1991**, *50*, 123–145. [CrossRef]
38. Griffioen, G.; Thevelein, J.M. Molecular mechanisms controlling the localisation of protein kinase A. *Curr. Genet.* **2002**, *41*, 199–207. [CrossRef] [PubMed]
39. Colledge, M.; Scott, J.D. AKAPs: From structure to function. *Trends Cell Biol.* **1999**, *9*, 216–221. [CrossRef]
40. Wang, L.; Sunahara, R.K.; Krumins, A.; Perkins, G.; Crochiere, M.L.; Mackey, M.; Bell, S.; Ellisman, M.H.; Taylor, S.S. Cloning and mitochondrial localization of full-length D-AKAP2, a protein kinase A anchoring protein. *Proc. Natl. Acad. Sci. USA* **2001**, *98*, 3220–3225. [CrossRef]
41. Kirschner, L.S.; Kusewitt, D.F.; Matyakhina, L.; Towns, W.H., 2nd; Carney, J.A.; Westphal, H.; Stratakis, C.A. A mouse model for the Carney complex tumor syndrome develops neoplasia in cyclic AMP-responsive tissues. *Cancer Res.* **2005**, *65*, 4506–4514. [CrossRef]
42. Robinson-White, A.; Hundley, T.R.; Shiferaw, M.; Bertherat, J.; Sandrini, F.; Stratakis, C.A. Protein kinase-A activity in PRKAR1A-mutant cells, and regulation of mitogen-activated protein kinases ERK1/2. *Hum. Mol. Genet.* **2003**, *12*, 1475–1484. [CrossRef]
43. Haymart, M.R.; Repplinger, D.J.; Leverson, G.E.; Elson, D.F.; Sippel, R.S.; Jaume, J.C.; Chen, H. Higher serum thyroid stimulating hormone level in thyroid nodule patients is associated with greater risks of differentiated thyroid cancer and advanced tumor stage. *J. Clin. Endocrinol. Metab.* **2008**, *93*, 809–814. [CrossRef]
44. Esapa, C.T.; Harris, P.E. Mutation analysis of protein kinase A catalytic subunit in thyroid adenomas and pituitary tumours. *Eur. J. Endocrinol.* **1999**, *141*, 409–412. [CrossRef] [PubMed]
45. Griffin, K.J.; Kirschner, L.S.; Matyakhina, L.; Stergiopoulos, S.G.; Robinson-White, A.; Lenherr, S.M.; Weinberg, F.D.; Claflin, E.S.; Batista, D.; Bourdeau, I.; et al. A transgenic mouse bearing an antisense construct of regulatory subunit type 1A of protein kinase A develops endocrine and other tumours: Comparison with Carney complex and other PRKAR1A induced lesions. *J. Med. Genet.* **2004**, *41*, 923–931. [CrossRef]
46. Pringle, D.R.; Yin, Z.; Lee, A.A.; Manchanda, P.K.; Yu, L.; Parlow, A.F.; Jarjoura, D.; La Perle, K.M.; Kirschner, L.S. Thyroid-specific ablation of the Carney complex gene, PRKAR1A, results in hyperthyroidism and follicular thyroid cancer. *Endocr. Relat. Cancer* **2012**, *19*, 435–446. [CrossRef]
47. Zoncu, R.; Efeyan, A.; Sabatini, D.M. mTOR: From growth signal integration to cancer, diabetes and ageing. *Nat. Rev. Mol. Cell Biol.* **2011**, *12*, 21–35. [CrossRef] [PubMed]
48. Lin, S.C.; Hardie, D.G. AMPK: Sensing Glucose as well as Cellular Energy Status. *Cell Metab.* **2018**, *27*, 299–313. [CrossRef] [PubMed]

49. Mavrakis, M.; Lippincott-Schwartz, J.; Stratakis, C.A.; Bossis, I. mTOR kinase and the regulatory subunit of protein kinase A (PRKAR1A) spatially and functionally interact during autophagosome maturation. *Autophagy* **2007**, *3*, 151–153. [CrossRef]
50. Day, M.E.; Gaietta, G.M.; Sastri, M.; Koller, A.; Mackey, M.R.; Scott, J.D.; Perkins, G.A.; Ellisman, M.H.; Taylor, S.S. Isoform-specific targeting of PKA to multivesicular bodies. *J. Cell Biol.* **2011**, *193*, 347–363. [CrossRef] [PubMed]
51. Blancquaert, S.; Wang, L.; Paternot, S.; Coulonval, K.; Dumont, J.E.; Harris, T.E.; Roger, P.P. cAMP-dependent activation of mammalian target of rapamycin (mTOR) in thyroid cells. Implication in mitogenesis and activation of CDK4. *Mol. Endocrinol.* **2010**, *24*, 1453–1468. [CrossRef]
52. Kari, S.; Vasko, V.V.; Priya, S.; Kirschner, L.S. PKA Activates AMPK Through LKB1 Signaling in Follicular Thyroid Cancer. *Front. Endocrinol.* **2019**, *10*, 769. [CrossRef] [PubMed]
53. Jenne, D.E.; Reimann, H.; Nezu, J.; Friedel, W.; Loff, S.; Jeschke, R.; Muller, O.; Back, W.; Zimmer, M. Peutz-Jeghers syndrome is caused by mutations in a novel serine threonine kinase. *Nat. Genet.* **1998**, *18*, 38–43. [CrossRef] [PubMed]
54. Hemminki, A.; Markie, D.; Tomlinson, I.; Avizienyte, E.; Roth, S.; Loukola, A.; Bignell, G.; Warren, W.; Aminoff, M.; Hoglund, P.; et al. A serine/threonine kinase gene defective in Peutz-Jeghers syndrome. *Nature* **1998**, *391*, 184–187. [CrossRef]
55. Monteverde, T.; Muthalagu, N.; Port, J.; Murphy, D.J. Evidence of cancer-promoting roles for AMPK and related kinases. *FEBS J.* **2015**, *282*, 4658–4671. [CrossRef] [PubMed]
56. Brunton, J.; Steele, S.; Ziehr, B.; Moorman, N.; Kawula, T. Feeding uninvited guests: mTOR and AMPK set the table for intracellular pathogens. *PLoS Pathog.* **2013**, *9*, e1003552. [CrossRef] [PubMed]
57. Fu, T.G.; Wang, L.; Li, W.; Li, J.Z.; Li, J. miR-143 inhibits oncogenic traits by degrading NUAK2 in glioblastoma. *Int. J. Mol. Med.* **2016**, *37*, 1627–1635. [CrossRef]
58. Tang, L.; Tong, S.J.; Zhan, Z.; Wang, Q.; Tian, Y.; Chen, F. Expression of NUAK2 in gastric cancer tissue and its effects on the proliferation of gastric cancer cells. *Exp. Ther. Med.* **2017**, *13*, 676–680. [CrossRef] [PubMed]
59. Miranda, F.; Mannion, D.; Liu, S.; Zheng, Y.; Mangala, L.S.; Redondo, C.; Herrero-Gonzalez, S.; Xu, R.; Taylor, C.; Chedom, D.F.; et al. Salt-Inducible Kinase 2 Couples Ovarian Cancer Cell Metabolism with Survival at the Adipocyte-Rich Metastatic Niche. *Cancer Cell* **2016**, *30*, 273–289. [CrossRef]
60. Hubaux, R.; Thu, K.L.; Vucic, E.A.; Pikor, L.A.; Kung, S.H.; Martinez, V.D.; Mosslemi, M.; Becker-Santos, D.D.; Gazdar, A.F.; Lam, S.; et al. Microtubule affinity-regulating kinase 2 is associated with DNA damage response and cisplatin resistance in non-small cell lung cancer. *Int. J. Cancer* **2015**, *137*, 2072–2082. [CrossRef]
61. Lizcano, J.M.; Goransson, O.; Toth, R.; Deak, M.; Morrice, N.A.; Boudeau, J.; Hawley, S.A.; Udd, L.; Makela, T.P.; Hardie, D.G.; et al. LKB1 is a master kinase that activates 13 kinases of the AMPK subfamily, including MARK/PAR-1. *EMBO J.* **2004**, *23*, 833–843. [CrossRef]
62. Luo, Z.; Zang, M.; Guo, W. AMPK as a metabolic tumor suppressor: Control of metabolism and cell growth. *Future Oncol.* **2010**, *6*, 457–470. [CrossRef]
63. Dasgupta, B.; Chhipa, R.R. Evolving Lessons on the Complex Role of AMPK in Normal Physiology and Cancer. *Trends Pharmacol. Sci.* **2016**, *37*, 192–206. [CrossRef] [PubMed]
64. Jeon, S.M.; Chandel, N.S.; Hay, N. AMPK regulates NADPH homeostasis to promote tumour cell survival during energy stress. *Nature* **2012**, *485*, 661–665. [CrossRef] [PubMed]
65. Jeon, S.M.; Hay, N. The dark face of AMPK as an essential tumor promoter. *Cell Logist.* **2012**, *2*, 197–202. [CrossRef]
66. Saunders, M.P.; Salisbury, A.J.; O'Byrne, K.J.; Long, L.; Whitehouse, R.M.; Talbot, D.C.; Mawer, E.B.; Harris, A.L. A novel cyclic adenosine monophosphate analog induces hypercalcemia via production of 1,25-dihydroxyvitamin D in patients with solid tumors. *J. Clin. Endocrinol. Metab.* **1997**, *82*, 4044–4048. [CrossRef] [PubMed]
67. Propper, D.J.; Saunders, M.P.; Salisbury, A.J.; Long, L.; O'Byrne, K.J.; Braybrooke, J.P.; Dowsett, M.; Taylor, M.; Talbot, D.C.; Ganesan, T.S.; et al. Phase I study of the novel cyclic AMP (cAMP) analogue 8-chloro-cAMP in patients with cancer: Toxicity, hormonal, and immunological effects. *Clin. Cancer Res.* **1999**, *5*, 1682–1689.
68. Huk, D.J.; Ashtekar, A.; Magner, A.; La Perle, K.; Kirschner, L.S. Deletion of Rap1b, but not Rap1a or Epac1, Reduces Protein Kinase A-Mediated Thyroid Cancer. *Thyroid* **2018**, *28*, 1153–1161. [CrossRef]
69. Tsygankova, O.M.; Saavedra, A.; Rebhun, J.F.; Quilliam, L.A.; Meinkoth, J.L. Coordinated regulation of Rap1 and thyroid differentiation by cyclic AMP and protein kinase A. *Mol. Cell. Biol.* **2001**, *21*, 1921–1929. [CrossRef]
70. Ribeiro-Neto, F.; Leon, A.; Urbani-Brocard, J.; Lou, L.; Nyska, A.; Altschuler, D.L. cAMP-dependent oncogenic action of Rap1b in the thyroid gland. *J. Biol. Chem.* **2004**, *279*, 46868–46875. [CrossRef]
71. Gutmann, D.H.; Saporito-Irwin, S.; DeClue, J.E.; Wienecke, R.; Guha, A. Alterations in the rap1 signaling pathway are common in human gliomas. *Oncogene* **1997**, *15*, 1611–1616. [CrossRef]
72. Chevillard, S.; Ugolin, N.; Vielh, P.; Ory, K.; Levalois, C.; Elliott, D.; Clayman, G.L.; El-Naggar, A.K. Gene expression profiling of differentiated thyroid neoplasms: Diagnostic and clinical implications. *Clin. Cancer Res.* **2004**, *10*, 6586–6597. [CrossRef] [PubMed]
73. Hattori, M.; Minato, N. Rap1 GTPase: Functions, regulation, and malignancy. *J. Biochem.* **2003**, *134*, 479–484. [CrossRef]
74. Chen, C.H.; Chuang, H.C.; Huang, C.C.; Fang, F.M.; Huang, H.Y.; Tsai, H.T.; Su, L.J.; Shiu, L.Y.; Leu, S.; Chien, C.Y. Overexpression of Rap-1A indicates a poor prognosis for oral cavity squamous cell carcinoma and promotes tumor cell invasion via Aurora-A modulation. *Am. J. Pathol.* **2013**, *182*, 516–528. [CrossRef]
75. de Rooij, J.; Zwartkruis, F.J.; Verheijen, M.H.; Cool, R.H.; Nijman, S.M.; Wittinghofer, A.; Bos, J.L. Epac is a Rap1 guanine-nucleotide-exchange factor directly activated by cyclic AMP. *Nature* **1998**, *396*, 474–477. [CrossRef] [PubMed]

76. Kawasaki, H.; Springett, G.M.; Mochizuki, N.; Toki, S.; Nakaya, M.; Matsuda, M.; Housman, D.E.; Graybiel, A.M. A family of cAMP-binding proteins that directly activate Rap1. *Science* **1998**, *282*, 2275–2279. [CrossRef] [PubMed]
77. Dremier, S.; Milenkovic, M.; Blancquaert, S.; Dumont, J.E.; Doskeland, S.O.; Maenhaut, C.; Roger, P.P. Cyclic adenosine 3′,5′-monophosphate (cAMP)-dependent protein kinases, but not exchange proteins directly activated by cAMP (Epac), mediate thyrotropin/cAMP-dependent regulation of thyroid cells. *Endocrinology* **2007**, *148*, 4612–4622. [CrossRef]
78. Almahariq, M.; Tsalkova, T.; Mei, F.C.; Chen, H.; Zhou, J.; Sastry, S.K.; Schwede, F.; Cheng, X. A novel EPAC-specific inhibitor suppresses pancreatic cancer cell migration and invasion. *Mol. Pharmacol.* **2013**, *83*, 122–128. [CrossRef]
79. Cheng, X.; Ji, Z.; Tsalkova, T.; Mei, F. Epac and PKA: A tale of two intracellular cAMP receptors. *Acta Biochim. Biophys. Sin.* **2008**, *40*, 651–662. [CrossRef] [PubMed]
80. Wang, X.; Luo, C.; Cheng, X.; Lu, M. Lithium and an EPAC-specific inhibitor ESI-09 synergistically suppress pancreatic cancer cell proliferation and survival. *Acta Biochim. Biophys. Sin.* **2017**, *49*, 573–580. [CrossRef]
81. Takahashi, M.; Li, Y.; Dillon, T.J.; Stork, P.J. Phosphorylation of Rap1 by cAMP-dependent Protein Kinase (PKA) Creates a Binding Site for KSR to Sustain ERK Activation by cAMP. *J. Biol. Chem.* **2017**, *292*, 1449–1461. [CrossRef]
82. Wang, Z.; Dillon, T.J.; Pokala, V.; Mishra, S.; Labudda, K.; Hunter, B.; Stork, P.J. Rap1-mediated activation of extracellular signal-regulated kinases by cyclic AMP is dependent on the mode of Rap1 activation. *Mol. Cell. Biol.* **2006**, *26*, 2130–2145. [CrossRef]
83. Takahashi, M.; Dillon, T.J.; Liu, C.; Kariya, Y.; Wang, Z.; Stork, P.J. Protein kinase A-dependent phosphorylation of Rap1 regulates its membrane localization and cell migration. *J. Biol. Chem.* **2013**, *288*, 27712–27723. [CrossRef]
84. Vogel, K.S.; Klesse, L.J.; Velasco-Miguel, S.; Meyers, K.; Rushing, E.J.; Parada, L.F. Mouse tumor model for neurofibromatosis type 1. *Science* **1999**, *286*, 2176–2179. [CrossRef] [PubMed]
85. Takeda, H.; Miyoshi, H.; Kojima, Y.; Oshima, M.; Taketo, M.M. Accelerated onsets of gastric hamartomas and hepatic adenomas/carcinomas in Lkb1+/-p53-/- compound mutant mice. *Oncogene* **2006**, *25*, 1816–1820. [CrossRef]
86. Cichowski, K.; Shih, T.S.; Schmitt, E.; Santiago, S.; Reilly, K.; McLaughlin, M.E.; Bronson, R.T.; Jacks, T. Mouse models of tumor development in neurofibromatosis type 1. *Science* **1999**, *286*, 2172–2176. [CrossRef]
87. Almeida, M.Q.; Muchow, M.; Boikos, S.; Bauer, A.J.; Griffin, K.J.; Tsang, K.M.; Cheadle, C.; Watkins, T.; Wen, F.; Starost, M.F.; et al. Mouse Prkar1a haploinsufficiency leads to an increase in tumors in the Trp53+/− or Rb1+/− backgrounds and chemically induced skin papillomas by dysregulation of the cell cycle and Wnt signaling. *Hum. Mol. Genet.* **2010**, *19*, 1387–1398. [CrossRef] [PubMed]
88. Carney, J.A.; Gordon, H.; Carpenter, P.C.; Shenoy, B.V.; Go, V.L. The complex of myxomas, spotty pigmentation, and endocrine overactivity. *Medicine* **1985**, *64*, 270–283. [CrossRef]
89. Stratakis, C.A.; Courcoutsakis, N.A.; Abati, A.; Filie, A.; Doppman, J.L.; Carney, J.A.; Shawker, T. Thyroid gland abnormalities in patients with the syndrome of spotty skin pigmentation, myxomas, endocrine overactivity, and schwannomas (Carney complex). *J. Clin. Endocrinol. Metab.* **1997**, *82*, 2037–2043. [CrossRef]
90. Casey, M.; Vaughan, C.J.; He, J.; Hatcher, C.J.; Winter, J.M.; Weremowicz, S.; Montgomery, K.; Kucherlapati, R.; Morton, C.C.; Basson, C.T. Mutations in the protein kinase A R1alpha regulatory subunit cause familial cardiac myxomas and Carney complex. *J. Clin. Investig.* **2000**, *106*, R31–R38. [CrossRef] [PubMed]
91. Dumont, J.E.; Jauniaux, J.C.; Roger, P.P. The cyclic AMP-mediated stimulation of cell proliferation. *Trends Biochem. Sci.* **1989**, *14*, 67–71. [CrossRef]
92. Roger, P.; Taton, M.; Van Sande, J.; Dumont, J.E. Mitogenic effects of thyrotropin and adenosine 3′,5′-monophosphate in differentiated normal human thyroid cells in vitro. *J. Clin. Endocrinol. Metab.* **1988**, *66*, 1158–1165. [CrossRef]
93. Hishinuma, A.; Yamanaka, T.; Kasai, K.; So, S.; Tseng, C.C.; Bamba, N.; Ohtake, H.; Shimoda, S. Different growth control of the two human thyroid cell lines of adenomatous goiter and papillary carcinoma. *Thyroid* **1995**, *5*, 41–46. [CrossRef] [PubMed]
94. Sarlis, N.J. Expression patterns of cellular growth-controlling genes in non-medullary thyroid cancer: Basic aspects. *Rev. Endocr. Metab. Disord.* **2000**, *1*, 183–196. [CrossRef]
95. Eng, C. Familial papillary thyroid cancer–many syndromes, too many genes? *J. Clin. Endocrinol. Metab.* **2000**, *85*, 1755–1757. [CrossRef] [PubMed]
96. van der Laan, B.F.; Freeman, J.L.; Asa, S.L. Expression of growth factors and growth factor receptors in normal and tumorous human thyroid tissues. *Thyroid* **1995**, *5*, 67–73. [CrossRef]
97. Farid, N.R.; Zou, M.; Shi, Y. Genetics of follicular thyroid cancer. *Endocrinol. Metab. Clin. N. Am.* **1995**, *24*, 865–883. [CrossRef]
98. Maenhaut, C.; Roger, P.P.; Reuse, S.; Dumont, J.E. Activation of the cyclic AMP cascade as an oncogenic mechanism: The thyroid example. *Biochimie* **1991**, *73*, 29–36. [CrossRef]
99. Bertherat, J.; Horvath, A.; Groussin, L.; Grabar, S.; Boikos, S.; Cazabat, L.; Libe, R.; Rene-Corail, F.; Stergiopoulos, S.; Bourdeau, I.; et al. Mutations in regulatory subunit type 1A of cyclic adenosine 5′-monophosphate-dependent protein kinase (PRKAR1A): Phenotype analysis in 353 patients and 80 different genotypes. *J. Clin. Endocrinol. Metab.* **2009**, *94*, 2085–2091. [CrossRef]
100. Carney, J.A.; Lyssikatos, C.; Seethala, R.R.; Lakatos, P.; Perez-Atayde, A.; Lahner, H.; Stratakis, C.A. The Spectrum of Thyroid Gland Pathology in Carney Complex: The Importance of Follicular Carcinoma. *Am. J. Surg. Pathol.* **2018**, *42*, 587–594. [CrossRef]
101. Adeniran, A.J.; Zhu, Z.; Gandhi, M.; Steward, D.L.; Fidler, J.P.; Giordano, T.J.; Biddinger, P.W.; Nikiforov, Y.E. Correlation between genetic alterations and microscopic features, clinical manifestations, and prognostic characteristics of thyroid papillary carcinomas. *Am. J. Surg. Pathol.* **2006**, *30*, 216–222. [CrossRef]

102. Kimura, E.T.; Nikiforova, M.N.; Zhu, Z.; Knauf, J.A.; Nikiforov, Y.E.; Fagin, J.A. High prevalence of BRAF mutations in thyroid cancer: Genetic evidence for constitutive activation of the RET/PTC-RAS-BRAF signaling pathway in papillary thyroid carcinoma. *Cancer Res.* **2003**, *63*, 1454–1457. [PubMed]
103. Soares, P.; Trovisco, V.; Rocha, A.S.; Lima, J.; Castro, P.; Preto, A.; Maximo, V.; Botelho, T.; Seruca, R.; Sobrinho-Simoes, M. BRAF mutations and RET/PTC rearrangements are alternative events in the etiopathogenesis of PTC. *Oncogene* **2003**, *22*, 4578–4580. [CrossRef] [PubMed]
104. Frattini, M.; Ferrario, C.; Bressan, P.; Balestra, D.; De Cecco, L.; Mondellini, P.; Bongarzone, I.; Collini, P.; Gariboldi, M.; Pilotti, S.; et al. Alternative mutations of BRAF, RET and NTRK1 are associated with similar but distinct gene expression patterns in papillary thyroid cancer. *Oncogene* **2004**, *23*, 7436–7440. [CrossRef] [PubMed]
105. Nikiforov, Y.E.; Nikiforova, M.N. Molecular genetics and diagnosis of thyroid cancer. *Nat. Rev. Endocrinol.* **2011**, *7*, 569–580. [CrossRef] [PubMed]
106. Marques, A.R.; Espadinha, C.; Catarino, A.L.; Moniz, S.; Pereira, T.; Sobrinho, L.G.; Leite, V. Expression of PAX8-PPAR gamma 1 rearrangements in both follicular thyroid carcinomas and adenomas. *J. Clin. Endocrinol. Metab.* **2002**, *87*, 3947–3952. [CrossRef]
107. Nikiforova, M.N.; Biddinger, P.W.; Caudill, C.M.; Kroll, T.G.; Nikiforov, Y.E. PAX8-PPARgamma rearrangement in thyroid tumors: RT-PCR and immunohistochemical analyses. *Am. J. Surg. Pathol.* **2002**, *26*, 1016–1023. [CrossRef]
108. Dwight, T.; Thoppe, S.R.; Foukakis, T.; Lui, W.O.; Wallin, G.; Hoog, A.; Frisk, T.; Larsson, C.; Zedenius, J. Involvement of the PAX8/peroxisome proliferator-activated receptor gamma rearrangement in follicular thyroid tumors. *J. Clin. Endocrinol. Metab.* **2003**, *88*, 4440–4445. [CrossRef] [PubMed]
109. Nikiforova, M.N.; Lynch, R.A.; Biddinger, P.W.; Alexander, E.K.; Dorn, G.W., 2nd; Tallini, G.; Kroll, T.G.; Nikiforov, Y.E. RAS point mutations and PAX8-PPAR gamma rearrangement in thyroid tumors: Evidence for distinct molecular pathways in thyroid follicular carcinoma. *J. Clin. Endocrinol. Metab.* **2003**, *88*, 2318–2326. [CrossRef]
110. Ezzat, S.; Zheng, L.; Kolenda, J.; Safarian, A.; Freeman, J.L.; Asa, S.L. Prevalence of activating ras mutations in morphologically characterized thyroid nodules. *Thyroid* **1996**, *6*, 409–416. [CrossRef]
111. Karga, H.; Lee, J.K.; Vickery, A.L., Jr.; Thor, A.; Gaz, R.D.; Jameson, J.L. Ras oncogene mutations in benign and malignant thyroid neoplasms. *J. Clin. Endocrinol. Metab.* **1991**, *73*, 832–836. [CrossRef] [PubMed]
112. Namba, H.; Rubin, S.A.; Fagin, J.A. Point mutations of ras oncogenes are an early event in thyroid tumorigenesis. *Mol. Endocrinol.* **1990**, *4*, 1474–1479. [CrossRef]
113. Manenti, G.; Pilotti, S.; Re, F.C.; Della Porta, G.; Pierotti, M.A. Selective activation of ras oncogenes in follicular and undifferentiated thyroid carcinomas. *Eur. J. Cancer* **1994**, *30A*, 987–993. [CrossRef]
114. Motoi, N.; Sakamoto, A.; Yamochi, T.; Horiuchi, H.; Motoi, T.; Machinami, R. Role of ras mutation in the progression of thyroid carcinoma of follicular epithelial origin. *Pathol. Res. Pract.* **2000**, *196*, 1–7. [CrossRef]
115. Esapa, C.T.; Johnson, S.J.; Kendall-Taylor, P.; Lennard, T.W.; Harris, P.E. Prevalence of Ras mutations in thyroid neoplasia. *Clin. Endocrinol.* **1999**, *50*, 529–535. [CrossRef]
116. Suarez, H.G.; du Villard, J.A.; Severino, M.; Caillou, B.; Schlumberger, M.; Tubiana, M.; Parmentier, C.; Monier, R. Presence of mutations in all three ras genes in human thyroid tumors. *Oncogene* **1990**, *5*, 565–570.
117. Zhu, Z.; Gandhi, M.; Nikiforova, M.N.; Fischer, A.H.; Nikiforov, Y.E. Molecular profile and clinical-pathologic features of the follicular variant of papillary thyroid carcinoma. An unusually high prevalence of ras mutations. *Am. J. Clin. Pathol.* **2003**, *120*, 71–77. [CrossRef] [PubMed]
118. Garcia-Rostan, G.; Zhao, H.; Camp, R.L.; Pollan, M.; Herrero, A.; Pardo, J.; Wu, R.; Carcangiu, M.L.; Costa, J.; Tallini, G. *ras* mutations are associated with aggressive tumor phenotypes and poor prognosis in thyroid cancer. *J. Clin. Oncol.* **2003**, *21*, 3226–3235. [CrossRef]
119. Saavedra, H.I.; Knauf, J.A.; Shirokawa, J.M.; Wang, J.; Ouyang, B.; Elisei, R.; Stambrook, P.J.; Fagin, J.A. The RAS oncogene induces genomic instability in thyroid PCCL3 cells via the MAPK pathway. *Oncogene* **2000**, *19*, 3948–3954. [CrossRef]
120. Basolo, F.; Pisaturo, F.; Pollina, L.E.; Fontanini, G.; Elisei, R.; Molinaro, E.; Iacconi, P.; Miccoli, P.; Pacini, F. N-ras mutation in poorly differentiated thyroid carcinomas: Correlation with bone metastases and inverse correlation to thyroglobulin expression. *Thyroid* **2000**, *10*, 19–23. [CrossRef]
121. Fagin, J.A. Minireview: Branded from the start-distinct oncogenic initiating events may determine tumor fate in the thyroid. *Mol. Endocrinol.* **2002**, *16*, 903–911. [CrossRef]
122. Hou, P.; Liu, D.; Xing, M. Functional characterization of the T1799-1801del and A1799-1816ins BRAF mutations in papillary thyroid cancer. *Cell Cycle* **2007**, *6*, 377–379. [CrossRef] [PubMed]
123. Carta, C.; Moretti, S.; Passeri, L.; Barbi, F.; Avenia, N.; Cavaliere, A.; Monacelli, M.; Macchiarulo, A.; Santeusanio, F.; Tartaglia, M.; et al. Genotyping of an Italian papillary thyroid carcinoma cohort revealed high prevalence of BRAF mutations, absence of RAS mutations and allowed the detection of a new mutation of BRAF oncoprotein (BRAF(V599lns)). *Clin. Endocrinol.* **2006**, *64*, 105–109. [CrossRef]
124. Trovisco, V.; Vieira de Castro, I.; Soares, P.; Maximo, V.; Silva, P.; Magalhaes, J.; Abrosimov, A.; Guiu, X.M.; Sobrinho-Simoes, M. BRAF mutations are associated with some histological types of papillary thyroid carcinoma. *J. Pathol.* **2004**, *202*, 247–251. [CrossRef]
125. Begum, S.; Rosenbaum, E.; Henrique, R.; Cohen, Y.; Sidransky, D.; Westra, W.H. BRAF mutations in anaplastic thyroid carcinoma: Implications for tumor origin, diagnosis and treatment. *Mod. Pathol.* **2004**, *17*, 1359–1363. [CrossRef]

126. Nikiforova, M.N.; Kimura, E.T.; Gandhi, M.; Biddinger, P.W.; Knauf, J.A.; Basolo, F.; Zhu, Z.; Giannini, R.; Salvatore, G.; Fusco, A.; et al. BRAF mutations in thyroid tumors are restricted to papillary carcinomas and anaplastic or poorly differentiated carcinomas arising from papillary carcinomas. *J. Clin. Endocrinol. Metab.* **2003**, *88*, 5399–5404. [CrossRef] [PubMed]
127. Namba, H.; Nakashima, M.; Hayashi, T.; Hayashida, N.; Maeda, S.; Rogounovitch, T.I.; Ohtsuru, A.; Saenko, V.A.; Kanematsu, T.; Yamashita, S. Clinical implication of hot spot BRAF mutation, V599E, in papillary thyroid cancers. *J. Clin. Endocrinol. Metab.* **2003**, *88*, 4393–4397. [CrossRef]
128. Xing, M. BRAF mutation in thyroid cancer. *Endocr. Relat. Cancer* **2005**, *12*, 245–262. [CrossRef] [PubMed]
129. Ito, T.; Seyama, T.; Mizuno, T.; Tsuyama, N.; Hayashi, T.; Hayashi, Y.; Dohi, K.; Nakamura, N.; Akiyama, M. Unique association of p53 mutations with undifferentiated but not with differentiated carcinomas of the thyroid gland. *Cancer Res.* **1992**, *52*, 1369–1371.
130. Dobashi, Y.; Sugimura, H.; Sakamoto, A.; Mernyei, M.; Mori, M.; Oyama, T.; Machinami, R. Stepwise participation of p53 gene mutation during dedifferentiation of human thyroid carcinomas. *Diagn. Mol. Pathol.* **1994**, *3*, 9–14. [CrossRef]
131. Garcia-Rostan, G.; Tallini, G.; Herrero, A.; D'Aquila, T.G.; Carcangiu, M.L.; Rimm, D.L. Frequent mutation and nuclear localization of beta-catenin in anaplastic thyroid carcinoma. *Cancer Res.* **1999**, *59*, 1811–1815.
132. Kurihara, T.; Ikeda, S.; Ishizaki, Y.; Fujimori, M.; Tokumoto, N.; Hirata, Y.; Ozaki, S.; Okajima, M.; Sugino, K.; Asahara, T. Immunohistochemical and sequencing analyses of the Wnt signaling components in Japanese anaplastic thyroid cancers. *Thyroid* **2004**, *14*, 1020–1029. [CrossRef]
133. Block, M.A.; Jackson, C.E.; Greenawald, K.A.; Yott, J.B.; Tashjian, A.H., Jr. Clinical characteristics distinguishing hereditary from sporadic medullary thyroid carcinoma. Treatment implications. *Arch. Surg.* **1980**, *115*, 142–148. [CrossRef]
134. Kouvaraki, M.A.; Shapiro, S.E.; Perrier, N.D.; Cote, G.J.; Gagel, R.F.; Hoff, A.O.; Sherman, S.I.; Lee, J.E.; Evans, D.B. RET proto-oncogene: A review and update of genotype-phenotype correlations in hereditary medullary thyroid cancer and associated endocrine tumors. *Thyroid* **2005**, *15*, 531–544. [CrossRef]
135. Brandi, M.L.; Gagel, R.F.; Angeli, A.; Bilezikian, J.P.; Beck-Peccoz, P.; Bordi, C.; Conte-Devolx, B.; Falchetti, A.; Gheri, R.G.; Libroia, A.; et al. Guidelines for diagnosis and therapy of MEN type 1 and type 2. *J. Clin. Endocrinol. Metab.* **2001**, *86*, 5658–5671. [CrossRef] [PubMed]
136. Romei, C.; Pardi, E.; Cetani, F.; Elisei, R. Genetic and clinical features of multiple endocrine neoplasia types 1 and 2. *J. Oncol.* **2012**, *2012*, 705036. [CrossRef] [PubMed]
137. Wohllk, N.; Schweizer, H.; Erlic, Z.; Schmid, K.W.; Walz, M.K.; Raue, F.; Neumann, H.P. Multiple endocrine neoplasia type 2. *Best Pract. Res. Clin. Endocrinol. Metab.* **2010**, *24*, 371–387. [CrossRef] [PubMed]
138. Eng, C.; Clayton, D.; Schuffenecker, I.; Lenoir, G.; Cote, G.; Gagel, R.F.; van Amstel, H.K.; Lips, C.J.; Nishisho, I.; Takai, S.I.; et al. The relationship between specific RET proto-oncogene mutations and disease phenotype in multiple endocrine neoplasia type 2: International RET mutation consortium analysis. *JAMA* **1996**, *276*, 1575–1579. [CrossRef]
139. Lodish, M.B.; Stratakis, C.A. RET oncogene in MEN2, MEN2B, MTC and other forms of thyroid cancer. *Expert Rev. Anticancer Ther.* **2008**, *8*, 625–632. [CrossRef]
140. Wells, S.A., Jr. Advances in the management of MEN2: From improved surgical and medical treatment to novel kinase inhibitors. *Endocr. Relat. Cancer* **2018**, *25*, T1–T13. [CrossRef]
141. Romei, C.; Ciampi, R.; Elisei, R. A comprehensive overview of the role of the RET proto-oncogene in thyroid carcinoma. *Nat. Rev. Endocrinol.* **2016**, *12*, 192–202. [CrossRef]
142. Mulligan, L.M. RET revisited: Expanding the oncogenic portfolio. *Nat. Rev. Cancer* **2014**, *14*, 173–186. [CrossRef] [PubMed]
143. Elisei, R.; Tacito, A.; Ramone, T.; Ciampi, R.; Bottici, V.; Cappagli, V.; Viola, D.; Matrone, A.; Lorusso, L.; Valerio, L.; et al. Twenty-Five Years Experience on RET Genetic Screening on Hereditary MTC: An Update on The Prevalence of Germline RET Mutations. *Genes* **2019**, *10*, 698. [CrossRef] [PubMed]
144. Romei, C.; Ugolini, C.; Cosci, B.; Torregrossa, L.; Vivaldi, A.; Ciampi, R.; Tacito, A.; Basolo, F.; Materazzi, G.; Miccoli, P.; et al. Low prevalence of the somatic M918T RET mutation in micro-medullary thyroid cancer. *Thyroid* **2012**, *22*, 476–481. [CrossRef] [PubMed]
145. Romei, C.; Casella, F.; Tacito, A.; Bottici, V.; Valerio, L.; Viola, D.; Cappagli, V.; Matrone, A.; Ciampi, R.; Piaggi, P.; et al. New insights in the molecular signature of advanced medullary thyroid cancer: Evidence of a bad outcome of cases with double RET mutations. *J. Med. Genet.* **2016**, *53*, 729–734. [CrossRef] [PubMed]
146. Molinaro, E.; Romei, C.; Biagini, A.; Sabini, E.; Agate, L.; Mazzeo, S.; Materazzi, G.; Sellari-Franceschini, S.; Ribechini, A.; Torregrossa, L.; et al. Anaplastic thyroid carcinoma: From clinicopathology to genetics and advanced therapies. *Nat. Rev. Endocrinol.* **2017**, *13*, 644–660. [CrossRef]
147. Deeken-Draisey, A.; Yang, G.Y.; Gao, J.; Alexiev, B.A. Anaplastic thyroid carcinoma: An epidemiologic, histologic, immunohistochemical, and molecular single-institution study. *Hum. Pathol.* **2018**, *82*, 140–148. [CrossRef] [PubMed]
148. Wreesmann, V.B.; Ghossein, R.A.; Patel, S.G.; Harris, C.P.; Schnaser, E.A.; Shaha, A.R.; Tuttle, R.M.; Shah, J.P.; Rao, P.H.; Singh, B. Genome-wide appraisal of thyroid cancer progression. *Am. J. Pathol.* **2002**, *161*, 1549–1556. [CrossRef]
149. Charles, R.P.; Silva, J.; Iezza, G.; Phillips, W.A.; McMahon, M. Activating BRAF and PIK3CA mutations cooperate to promote anaplastic thyroid carcinogenesis. *Mol. Cancer Res.* **2014**, *12*, 979–986. [CrossRef]
150. Garcia-Rostan, G.; Costa, A.M.; Pereira-Castro, I.; Salvatore, G.; Hernandez, R.; Hermsem, M.J.; Herrero, A.; Fusco, A.; Cameselle-Teijeiro, J.; Santoro, M. Mutation of the PIK3CA gene in anaplastic thyroid cancer. *Cancer Res.* **2005**, *65*, 10199–10207. [CrossRef]

151. Gauchotte, G.; Philippe, C.; Lacomme, S.; Leotard, B.; Wissler, M.P.; Allou, L.; Toussaint, B.; Klein, M.; Vignaud, J.M.; Bressenot, A. BRAF, p53 and SOX2 in anaplastic thyroid carcinoma: Evidence for multistep carcinogenesis. *Pathology* **2011**, *43*, 447–452. [CrossRef]
152. Landa, I.; Ibrahimpasic, T.; Boucai, L.; Sinha, R.; Knauf, J.A.; Shah, R.H.; Dogan, S.; Ricarte-Filho, J.C.; Krishnamoorthy, G.P.; Xu, B.; et al. Genomic and transcriptomic hallmarks of poorly differentiated and anaplastic thyroid cancers. *J. Clin. Investig.* **2016**, *126*, 1052–1066. [CrossRef]
153. Tiedje, V.; Ting, S.; Herold, T.; Synoracki, S.; Latteyer, S.; Moeller, L.C.; Zwanziger, D.; Stuschke, M.; Fuehrer, D.; Schmid, K.W. NGS based identification of mutational hotspots for targeted therapy in anaplastic thyroid carcinoma. *Oncotarget* **2017**, *8*, 42613–42620. [CrossRef]
154. Baloch, Z.W.; LiVolsi, V.A. Special types of thyroid carcinoma. *Histopathology* **2018**, *72*, 40–52. [CrossRef]
155. Aschebrook-Kilfoy, B.; Ward, M.H.; Sabra, M.M.; Devesa, S.S. Thyroid cancer incidence patterns in the United States by histologic type, 1992–2006. *Thyroid* **2011**, *21*, 125–134. [CrossRef]
156. Brose, M.S.; Nutting, C.M.; Jarzab, B.; Elisei, R.; Siena, S.; Bastholt, L.; de la Fouchardiere, C.; Pacini, F.; Paschke, R.; Shong, Y.K.; et al. Sorafenib in radioactive iodine-refractory, locally advanced or metastatic differentiated thyroid cancer: A randomised, double-blind, phase 3 trial. *Lancet* **2014**, *384*, 319–328. [CrossRef]
157. Schlumberger, M.; Tahara, M.; Wirth, L.J.; Robinson, B.; Brose, M.S.; Elisei, R.; Habra, M.A.; Newbold, K.; Shah, M.H.; Hoff, A.O.; et al. Lenvatinib versus placebo in radioiodine-refractory thyroid cancer. *N. Engl. J. Med.* **2015**, *372*, 621–630. [CrossRef] [PubMed]
158. Cabanillas, M.E.; Schlumberger, M.; Jarzab, B.; Martins, R.G.; Pacini, F.; Robinson, B.; McCaffrey, J.C.; Shah, M.H.; Bodenner, D.L.; Topliss, D.; et al. A phase 2 trial of lenvatinib (E7080) in advanced, progressive, radioiodine-refractory, differentiated thyroid cancer: A clinical outcomes and biomarker assessment. *Cancer* **2015**, *121*, 2749–2756. [CrossRef] [PubMed]
159. Wells, S.A., Jr.; Robinson, B.G.; Gagel, R.F.; Dralle, H.; Fagin, J.A.; Santoro, M.; Baudin, E.; Elisei, R.; Jarzab, B.; Vasselli, J.R.; et al. Vandetanib in patients with locally advanced or metastatic medullary thyroid cancer: A randomized, double-blind phase III trial. *J. Clin. Oncol.* **2012**, *30*, 134–141. [CrossRef] [PubMed]
160. Elisei, R.; Schlumberger, M.J.; Muller, S.P.; Schoffski, P.; Brose, M.S.; Shah, M.H.; Licitra, L.; Jarzab, B.; Medvedev, V.; Kreissl, M.C.; et al. Cabozantinib in progressive medullary thyroid cancer. *J. Clin. Oncol.* **2013**, *31*, 3639–3646. [CrossRef]
161. Capdevila, J.; Wirth, L.J.; Ernst, T.; Ponce Aix, S.; Lin, C.C.; Ramlau, R.; Butler, M.O.; Delord, J.P.; Gelderblom, H.; Ascierto, P.A.; et al. PD-1 Blockade in Anaplastic Thyroid Carcinoma. *J. Clin. Oncol.* **2020**, *38*, 2620–2627. [CrossRef] [PubMed]
162. Dierks, C.; Seufert, J.; Aumann, K.; Ruf, J.; Klein, C.; Kiefer, S.; Rassner, M.; Boerries, M.; Zielke, A.; la Rosee, P.; et al. Combination of Lenvatinib and Pembrolizumab Is an Effective Treatment Option for Anaplastic and Poorly Differentiated Thyroid Carcinoma. *Thyroid* **2021**, *31*, 1076–1085. [CrossRef] [PubMed]
163. Bouys, L.; Bertherat, J. Management of Endocrine Disease: Carney complex: Clinical and genetic update 20 years after the identification of the CNC1 (PRKAR1A) gene. *Eur. J. Endocrinol.* **2021**, *184*, R99–R109. [CrossRef] [PubMed]
164. Stratakis, C.A.; Raygada, M. Carney Complex. In *GeneReviews(R)*; Adam, M.P., Ardinger, H.H., Pagon, R.A., Wallace, S.E., Bean, L.J.H., Mirzaa, G., Amemiya, A., Eds.; University of Washington: Seattle, WA, USA, 1993.

cancers

MDPI

Article

Head-to-Head Comparison of Neck ^{18}F-FDG PET/MR and PET/CT in the Diagnosis of Differentiated Thyroid Carcinoma Patients after Comprehensive Treatment

Yangmeihui Song [1,2,†], Fang Liu [1,2,†], Weiwei Ruan [1,2], Fan Hu [1,2], Muhsin H. Younis [3,4], Zairong Gao [1,2], Jie Ming [5], Tao Huang [5], Weibo Cai [3,4] and Xiaoli Lan [1,2,*]

1 Department of Nuclear Medicine, Union Hospital, Tongji Medical College, Huazhong University of Science and Technology, Wuhan 430022, China; songymh@hust.edu.cn (Y.S.); fangliu72@hust.edu.cn (F.L.); 2017xh0388@hust.edu.cn (W.R.); hufan1201@163.com (F.H.); gaobonn@hust.edu.cn (Z.G.)
2 Hubei Province Key Laboratory of Molecular Imaging, Wuhan 430030, China
3 Department of Radiology, University of Wisconsin-Madison, Madison, WI 53705, USA; myounis@wisc.edu (M.H.Y.); wcai@uwhealth.org (W.C.)
4 Department of Medical Physics, University of Wisconsin-Madison, Madison, WI 53705, USA
5 Department of Breast and Thyroid Surgery, Union Hospital, Tongji Medical College, Huazhong University of Science and Technology, Wuhan 430022, China; mingjiewh@hust.edu.cn (J.M.); huangtaowh@163.com (T.H.)
* Correspondence: xiaoli_lan@hust.edu.cn
† Yangmeihui Song and Fang Liu contributed equally to this work.

Citation: Song, Y.; Liu, F.; Ruan, W.; Hu, F.; Younis, M.H.; Gao, Z.; Ming, J.; Huang, T.; Cai, W.; Lan, X. Head-to-Head Comparison of Neck ^{18}F-FDG PET/MR and PET/CT in the Diagnosis of Differentiated Thyroid Carcinoma Patients after Comprehensive Treatment. *Cancers* **2021**, *13*, 3436. https://doi.org/10.3390/cancers13143436

Academic Editors: Fabio Medas and Pier Francesco Alesina

Received: 17 May 2021
Accepted: 28 June 2021
Published: 9 July 2021

Simple Summary: The most advanced positron emission tomography–magnetic resonance (PET/MR) combines the high soft tissue contrast of MRI with the high functional/metabolic sensitivity of PET and has the potential to achieve the highest level of diagnostic performance for refractory malignancies in differentiated thyroid cancer (DTC) patients. The utility of PET/MR in the postoperative follow-up of DTC patients has been relatively ambiguous. This retrospective study compared ^{18}F-fluorodeoxyglucose neck PET/MR with PET/CT head-to-head, in order to evaluate the diagnostic efficacy of PET/MR in assessment malignancy in DTC patients after comprehensive treatment. We determined that PET/MR presented better detection rates, image conspicuity, and sensitivity than PET/CT in recurrent DTC lesions and cervical lymph node metastases. The addition of neck PET/MR scan after whole-body PET/CT may provide more favorable diagnostic information.

Abstract: We explored the clinical value of ^{18}F-FDG PET/MR in a head-to-head comparison with PET/CT in loco-regional recurrent and metastatic cervical lymph nodes of differentiated thyroid carcinoma (DTC) patients after comprehensive treatment. ^{18}F-FDG PET/CT and neck PET/MR scans that were performed in DTC patients with suspected recurrence or cervical lymph node metastasis after comprehensive treatment were retrospectively analyzed. Detection rates, diagnostic efficacy, image conspicuity, and measured parameters were compared between ^{18}F-FDG PET/CT and PET/MR. The gold standard was histopathological diagnosis or clinical and imaging follow-up results for more than 6 months. Among the 37 patients enrolled, no suspicious signs of tumor were found in 10 patients, 24 patients had lymph node metastasis, and 3 patients had both recurrence and lymph node metastases. A total of 130 lesions were analyzed, including 3 malignant and 6 benign thyroid nodules, as well as 74 malignant and 47 benign cervical lymph nodes. Compared with PET/CT, PET/MR presented better detection rates (91.5% vs. 80.8%), image conspicuity (2.74 ± 0.60 vs. 1.9 ± 0.50, $p < 0.001$, especially in complex level II), and sensitivity (80.5% vs. 61.0%). SUVmax differed in benign and malignant lymph nodes in both imaging modalities ($p < 0.05$). For the same lesion, the SUVmax, SUVmean, and diameters measured by PET/MR and PET/CT were consistent and had significant correlation. In conclusion, compared with ^{18}F-FDG PET/CT, PET/MR was more accurate in determining recurrent and metastatic lesions, both from a patient-based and from a lesion-based perspective. Adding local PET/MR after whole-body PET/CT may be recommended to provide more precise diagnostic information and scope of surgical resection without additional ionizing radiation. Further scaling-up prospective studies and economic benefit analysis are expected.

Keywords: thyroid neoplasms; fluorodeoxyglucose F18 (^{18}F-FDG); positron emission tomography (PET); magnetic resonance imaging (MRI); recurrence; neoplasm metastasis

1. Introduction

Thyroid carcinoma is the most common endocrine malignant tumor worldwide, accounting for 2% of all cancers, after a two-fold increase over the last 25 years [1–3]. More than 90% of thyroid carcinomas are differentiated thyroid carcinoma (DTC), which includes papillary carcinoma (PTC) (85%) and follicular carcinoma (FTC) (12%). The prognosis of DTC is generally favorable after comprehensive treatment including surgery, radioactive iodine, and thyroid-stimulating hormone (TSH) suppression [4]. Nevertheless, up to 30% of patients may experience local recurrence and/or metastasis within several decades, which indicates a poor prognosis and a drop of the five-year survival rate from higher than 90% to 35–85% [5,6]. Postoperative recurrence appears most frequently (60–75%) in cervical lymph nodes (LNs) [7]. As a result, strict postoperative follow-up and advances in early detection are essential for a timely intervention in case of relapse and metastatic disease. Conventional ^{131}I whole-body scan (^{131}I-WBS), in association with periodic evaluation of serum thyroglobulin (Tg) and neck ultrasound, have been employed as the routine diagnostic procedure in the protocol of patients thyroidectomized for DTC [8,9]. However, 10–15% of follow-up DTC patients appear with abnormal thyroglobulin levels and negative findings on ^{131}I-WBS [10–12]. In guidelines of different countries, the clinical indication of ^{18}F-fluorodeoxyglucose positron emission tomography–computed tomography (^{18}F-FDG PET/CT) has been widely accepted for postoperative DTC patients who present with the aforementioned discordant findings, as well as for the systemic assessment of patients with suspected metastases [8–10,13–15]. Nevertheless, according to previous reports, the sensitivity and specificity of ^{18}F-FDG PET/CT in detecting DTC recurrence or metastasis are 46–100% and 66–100% respectively, which is considered inadequate [16,17].

Magnetic resonance imaging (MRI) is a useful technique for the diagnosis of thyroid nodules and metastatic cervical lymph nodes, which benefits from excellent soft-tissue contrast, superior spatial resolution, and the ability to functionally characterize tissues by utilizing non-contrast- or contrast-enhanced techniques such as diffusion-weighted imaging (DWI) and apparent diffusion coefficient (ADC) [18–20]. The hybrid PET/MR is a promising imaging modality that combines the high soft tissue contrast of MRI with the high functional/metabolic sensitivity of PET without additional ionizing radiation. For head and neck oncologic imaging, it has the potential to achieve the highest level of diagnostic performance. However, to date, the usefulness of PET/MR in head and neck malignancy has not been fully elucidated [21–23]. It is questionable whether simultaneous PET/MR can provide better diagnostic ability than CT, MRI, and PET/CT in loco-regional recurrent and metastatic cervical lymph nodes [16,24–26].

The purpose of the present study was therefore to evaluate the diagnostic ability of simultaneous neck PET/MRI in a head-to-head comparison with PET/CT for the assessment of malignancy in postoperative differentiated thyroid carcinoma (DTC) patients.

2. Materials and Methods

2.1. Patients and Lesions

We retrospectively reviewed the images of DTC patients who underwent ^{18}F-FDG PET in our center from 23 October 2017 to 29 July 2020. The inclusion criteria were as follows: (1) diagnosis of DTC was confirmed by histopathological analysis; (2) patients had received comprehensive treatment (including total or subtotal thyroidectomy, ^{131}I ablation therapy, or/and thyroid hormone replacement/suppression therapy); (3) patients had one or more of the following high-risk features of recurrence or cervical lymph node metastasis: (1) positive serum Tg and negative ^{131}I-WBS, (2) rising anti-thyroglobulin antibodies (TgAb) after radioactive iodine ablation, (3) suspected widespread metastases throughout the body, eligible for ^{18}F-FDG PET examination according to the available guidelines at that time; (4) patients accepted ^{18}F-FDG PET/CT and subsequent PET/MR examination; (5) patients were available for follow-up including postoperative pathology/fine-needle aspiration biopsy (FNAB) or regular ultrasonography and Tg/TgAb level monitor every 3–6 months. This retrospective study was approved by the Ethics Committee of Union Hospital, Tongji Medical College, Huazhong University of Science and Technology. All patients signed an informed consent before undergoing ^{18}F-FDG PET/MR imaging.

The local thyroid region lesions and cervical lymph nodes included in the present study were involved according to the following criteria: (1) the lesion was diagnosed by pathology after reoperation or FNAB; (2) the lesion was monitored regularly by imaging including neck ultrasonography, ^{131}I-WBS, CT, and/or MRI, for at least 6 months.

2.2. ^{18}F-FDG PET/CT Scan

^{18}F-FDG was produced by a GE Medical Cyclotron (Mini trace, GE Healthcare, Milwaukee, WI, USA) and synthesized by the Tracelab MX FDG (GE Healthcare, Milwaukee, WI, USA) automatic synthesis system. The radiochemical purity was more than 95%. All patients were fasting for more than 6 h, with fasting blood glucose $\leq$ 200 mg/dL before injection. The patients were given an intravenous injection of ^{18}F-FDG 3.70–5.55 MBq/kg according to their body weight. After resting for about 60 min, drinking 200–500 mL of water, and urination, whole-body PET/CT (discovery VCT®, GE Healthcare, Milwaukee, WI, USA) examination was performed. First, 64 slice spiral CT (Discovery VCT®, GE Healthcare, Milwaukee, WI, USA) scanning was performed, operating with tube voltage 110 kV, tube current 110 mA, and layer thickness 3.3 mm. Then, PET imaging was acquired in the three-dimensional acquisition mode, scanning the range from the upper to the middle thigh with 2 min per bed, for a total of 6–7 beds. PET data were reconstructed with the ordered subsets expectation maximization (OSEM) method. The standard reconstruction was performed with a 512 $\times$ 512 matrix and 3.3 mm slice thickness. CT data were used for attenuation correction. Finally, cross-sectional, sagittal, coronal CT, PET, and PET/CT fusion images were obtained by the GE AW4.6 workstation software (GE Healthcare, Milwaukee, WI, USA).

2.3. ^{18}F-FDG PET/MR Scan

After PET/CT acquisition, all patients underwent a neck PET/MR (3.0 T, signa TOF-PET/MR, GE Healthcare, Milwaukee, WI, USA) scan around 120 min after ^{18}F-FDG injection. Head and neck coil and field of view (FOV) were used for PET/MR scanning. The scanning sequence included axial fast spin echo T1 weighted imaging (FSE T1WI), axial, sagittal, and coronal FSE T2WI, and finally axial DWI. PET scanning used 3D acquisition, with about 15 min per bed. The scanning parameters were T1WI (turn angle = 142°, echo time [TE]/repeat time [TR] = 13.2/640 ms, bandwidth = 41.67 KHz, FOV = 24 cm $\times$ 24 cm, matrix = 256 $\times$ 192), T2WI (turn angle = 142°, echo time [TE]/repeat time [TR] = 161/3054 ms, bandwidth = 50 KHz, FOV = 22 cm $\times$ 22 cm, matrix = 288 $\times$ 288), DWI (echo time [TE]/repeat time [TR] = 191/2500 ms, bandwidth = 250 KHz, FOV = 24 cm $\times$ 24 cm, matrix = 96 $\times$ 96, b = 600). The time of flight (TOF) technique and OSEM algorithm were used to reconstruct the PET data with the following parameters: FOV = 30 cm $\times$ 30 cm, matrix = 192 $\times$ 192, filter cutoff = 3.0 mm, subset = 28, iteration = 3. PET attenuation correction was based on atlas MR attenuation correction combined with the Dixon water–fat separation method.

2.4. Image Interpretation and Analysis

All acquired images were analyzed by the AW workstation. Two nuclear medicine physicians (X.L., with 24 years of experience and F.L. with 20 years of experience in radiology and 5 years of experience in nuclear oncology) visually interpreted PET/CT and PET/MR images and collected the following information:

(1) lesion counts detected on PET/CT and PET/MR, respectively;

(2) lesion conspicuity scoring according to [26] (assessed independently): 1 point for no detection; 2 points for detected suspicious morphological correlation; 3 points for clear morphological correlation;
(3) lesion diagnosis (any difference of opinion resolved by consensus): benign or malignant.

Two nuclear medicine physicians (Y.S. and F.L.) delineated the region of interest (ROI) along the edge of the focus segmented on T1WI/T2WI and CT according to the aforementioned detected lesions and collected the following dataset respectively:

(1) lesion diameters: long and short diameters as referred in RECIST 1.1 [27];
(2) standardized uptake value (SUV) for lesions calculated automatically by the workstation: SUVmax and SUVmean.

2.5. Local Recurrence and Metastatic Lymph Nodes

The gold standard for locally recurrent DTC or nodal metastases was determined according to one of the following criteria: (1) histopathological diagnosis of recurrence or metastasis; (2) clinical serum Tg and/or TgAb levels increased continuously during the follow-up of more than 6 months and imaging (neck ultrasound, CT, and/or MR) revealing following malignant features simultaneously.

Ultrasound criteria: nodules or lymph nodes were considered malignant if the short axis diameter was $\geq$10 mm in levels I–II or $\geq$7 mm in levels III–VI, the volume increased more than 50%, or the diameter increased more than 20% or 2 mm. In addition, other signs of malignancy, including spherical or long-to-short axis ratio < 2, absence of an echogenic hilum, microcalcification and cystic changes, could classify the node as malignant, regardless of the size of the lymph node [28–31].

CT or MR criteria: recurrence was determined by size and abnormal density/signal with irregular edges or blurred boundaries on CT/MR; for nodules or lymph nodes, they were perceived as malignant if the maximum axial diameter was $\geq$8 mm in the retropharyngeal space, $\geq$15 mm in levels I–II or $\geq$10 mm in levels III–VII, or the volume increased more than 50%, or the diameter increased more than 20% or 2 mm [32,33]. In addition, other signs of malignancy, including central necrosis, contrast enhancement, intralesional calcifications and cystic changes, could classify the nodule as malignant, irrespective of nodal size [34].

2.6. Statistical Analyses

SPSS 26.0 (IBM, Armonk, New York, NY, USA) and GraphPad Prism 9.0 (GraphPad Software Inc., San Diego, CA, USA) were used for statistical analysis and figure production, respectively. For all variables, the Kolmogorov–Smirnov normal distribution test was performed first. Continuous variables with a normal distribution were expressed as mean $\pm$ SD. Continuous variables that were not normally distributed were expressed as median and interquartile intervals. Categorical variables were expressed as numbers and percentages. The Kappa consistency analysis was used to assess the two physicians' subjective score, and the Wilcoxon signed-ranks test was used to evaluate the image conspicuity difference. The sensitivities, specificities, positive predictive values (PPVs), negative predictive values (NPVs), and accuracies of PET/MR, MR, and PET/CT for diagnosis were determined in accordance with the gold standard. According to the R $\times$ C chi-square test and the fisher exact probability method, the difference in diagnostic performance of PET/MR, MR, PET/CT was tested. The Wilcoxon signed-rank test was used to test the difference of PET/MR and PET/CT parameters (SUVmax, SUVmean, and lymph node diameter) for the same lymph nodes subgroup. The independent-samples Mann–Whitney U test was used to analyze the differences of these parameters between malignant and benign lymph nodes. Spearman's correlation method was used to analyze the correlation between PET/MR and PET/CT parameters and calculate the coefficient of determination (r^2). Bland–Altman analysis was used to compare the two techniques.

3. Results

A total of 37 patients were retrospectively reviewed. Figure 1 shows the case screening. The patients (12 males and 25 females) had a mean age of 38.95 ± 12.03 years (range, 12–68 years). The time interval between PET examination and the first surgery ranged from 4 months to >5 years. In total, 25 patients had elevated non-stimulated Tg levels along with negative ^{131}I-WBS, their median serum Tg was 11.01 ng/mL (range, 3.04– > 500 ng/mL), with thyrotropin levels all < 0 μIU/mL. The TgAb level of five patients rose to 2302.48 ± 1470.59 IU/mL (range 649.4– > 4000 IU/mL). One patient had an increase in both Tg and TgAb. After the PET/MR and PET/CT examinations, seven patients completed reoperation and histopathological examinations, and two patients underwent FNAB. The period of follow-up was between 8 and 24 months. Table 1 presents the general characteristics of the enrolled patients.

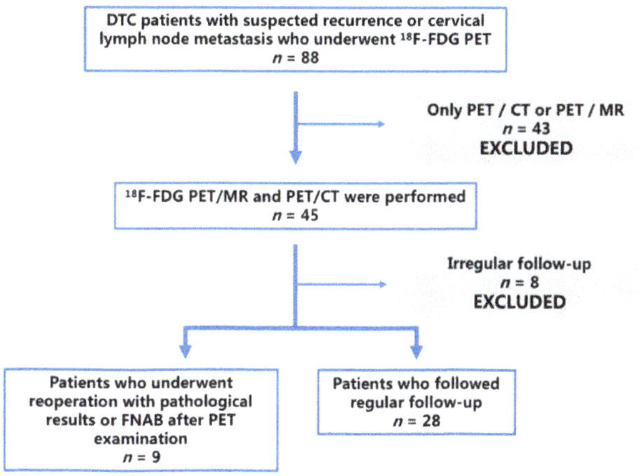

Figure 1. Flow chart of patients who were referred for assessment.

Table 1. Patients' characteristics.

Characteristics		Number
Age	38.95 ± 12.03 years (range, 12–68 years)	
	<55 years	33 (89.2%)
	>55 years	4 (10.8%)
Sex	Male	12 (32.4%)
	Female	25 (67.6%)
Histologic type	PTC [1]	29 (78.4%)
	PTMC [2]	4 (10.8%)
	PTC [1] + PTMC [2]	3 (8.1%)
	FTC [3]	1 (2.7%)
Stage of disease	I	32 (86.5%)
	II	2 (5.4%)
	IV	3 (8.1%)
Clinical indication for PET Imaging	Positive Tg [4] and negative ^{131}I-WBS [5]	25 (67.6%)
	Rising TgAb [6] after radioactive iodine ablation	4 (10.8%)
	Suspected metastasis detection	8 (21.6%)
Gold standard source	Pathology after reoperation	7 (18.9%)
	Fine-needle aspiration	2 (5.4%)
	Regular follow-up	28 (75.7%)

[1] PTC papillary thyroid carcinoma, [2] PTMC papillary thyroid microcarcinoma, [3] FTC follicular thyroid carcinoma, [4] Tg thyroglobulin, [5] ^{131}I-WBS ^{131}Iodine whole body scan, [6] TgAb anti-thyroglobulin antibodies.

3.1. Patient-Based Analysis

Among the 37 patients, no malignant signs were found in 10 patients, while 24 patients had lymph node metastasis, and 3 patients presented coexisted recurrence with lymph node metastases. PET/MR correctly determined the disease status of 36 patients (97.3%), while PET/CT identified 31 cases (83.8%). Of the three coexisting cases, two were correctly identified by PET/MR and one was correctly identified by PET/CT. A recurrent focus was missed by both modalities. Of 10 negative patients, 3 presented pulmonary metastases on whole-body PET/CT, 4 were pathologically confirmed as negative, and the remaining 3 patients were found to have decreased Tg during follow-up. Figure 2 displays a patient with recurrence and lymph node metastasis, where PET/MR successfully identified the recurrent lesion in the thyroid region, but PET/CT missed it. Lymph node metastases in these patients were all successfully identified by both modalities. In the 24 patients with lymph node metastases detected, all were correctly diagnosed by PET/MR, and only 20 patients were recognized by PET/CT. Figure 3 shows a DTC patient with lymph node metastases, which were identified by PET/MR but missed by PET/CT.

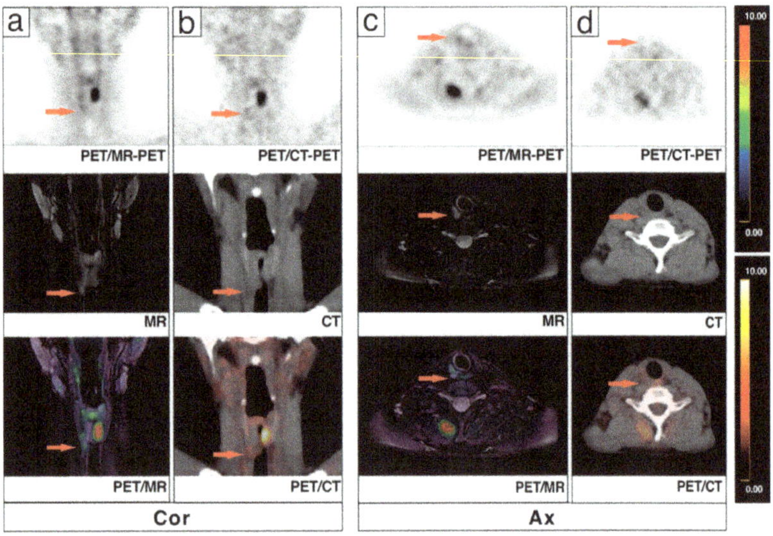

Figure 2. A 17-year-old post-operative DTC patient underwent ^{131}I treatment three times with persistently elevated Tg up to 371.0 ug/L. ^{131}I-WBS showed scattered iodine uptake foci in the right paratracheal area and lung lobes. ^{18}F-FDG PET/CT was performed for whole-body systemic evaluation. ^{18}F-FDG PET/CT showed no significant abnormalities in the thyroid region ((**b**,**d**), red arrows); additional PET/MR of the neck showed a long T2 signal nodule in the right thyroid region with a mild metabolic increase SUVmax 1.7 ((**a**,**c**), red arrows). In combination with medical history and ^{131}I examination, a residual/recurrent thyroid cancer was diagnosed. The patient was subsequently reoperated, and residual/recurrent thyroid cancer was confirmed by histological pathology.

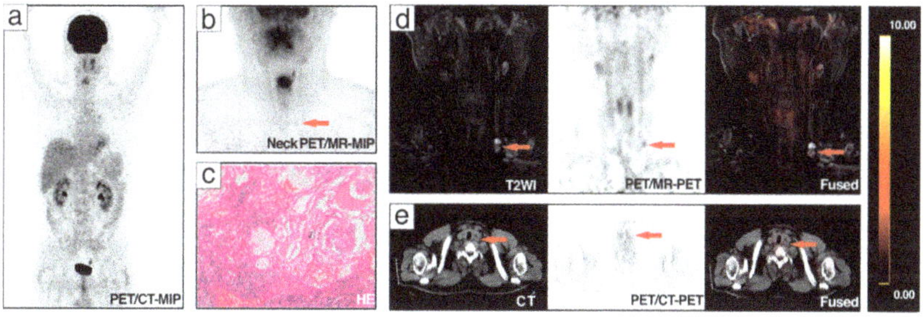

Figure 3. A 36-year-old patient with Tg 39.1 μg/L and negative ^{131}I-WBS after comprehensive treatment was admitted to ^{18}F-FDG PET/CT and underwent additional neck PET/MR. PET/MR clearly presented the morphological and metabolic changes of lymph nodes in the VB region ((**b**,**d**), red arrows). PET/CT showed no significant changes in the corresponding lesions ((**a**,**e**), red arrows). After reoperation, 1 lymph node in the left VB, 8 lymph nodes in the left level IIA, 7 lymph nodes in the left level III, and 10 lymph nodes in the left level IV were taken for pathomorphological examination, and only the lymph node in the VB was pathologically diagnosed to be a metastatic lymph node (**c**).

3.2. Lesion-Based Analysis

Finally, a total of 130 lesions (9 in the original thyroid area, 121 in the cervical lymph node) were examined, including 3 malignant and 6 benign thyroid nodules, as well as 74 malignant and 47 benign cervical lymph nodes. Of all lesions, 44 (33.8%) were analyzed by histopathology, including 32 malignant lesions (1 local recurrence and 31 metastatic lymph nodes) and 12 benign lesions (2 benign thyroid nodules and 10 benign lymph nodes). Other lesions were confirmed by strict follow-up in the aforementioned manner. Among 130 lesions, PET/MR detected 119 (91.5%), but missed 1 recurrent thyroid cancer and 10 metastatic lymph nodes; PET/CT detected 105 (80.8%), but missed 2 recurrent thyroid cancers, 21 metastatic lymph nodes, 1 benign thyroid nodule, and 1 benign lymph node. For 74 lymph node metastases, the detection numbers of PET/MR and PET/CT were, respectively, 64 (86.5%) and 53 (71.6%). Table 2 shows the number of thyroid nodules and lymph nodes detected by ^{18}F-FDG PET/MR and PET/CT.

Table 2. Number of thyroid nodules and lymph nodes detected by ^{18}F-FDG PET/MR and PET/CT.

		Golden Standard	PET/MR	PET/CT
Malignant	Thyroid nodules	3	2	1
	Lymph nodes	74	64	53
Benign	Thyroid nodules	6	6	5
	Lymph nodes	47	47	46
Total		130	119	105

The diagnostic performance of two PET modalities (PET/MR and PET/CT) and MR (alone) is displayed in the Table 3 and Figure 4. The diagnostic sensitivities of PET/MR, MR, and PET/CT were significantly different (80.5%, 77.9%, and 61.0%, p = 0.012). The paired comparison of PET/MR, MR, and PET/CT showed significant differences of sensitivity between PET/CT and the other two techniques (p < 0.001 and p = 0.007 respectively). The specificities of the three modalities (84.9%, 83.0%, and 81.1%, p = 0.875) showed no significant difference, also in paired comparisons. For metastatic lymph nodes, the sensitivities of PET/MR, MR, and PET/CT were 81.1%, 78.4%, and 62.2% (p = 0.018). Paired comparisons also showed significant differences between PET/CT and the other two techniques (p = 0.001 and p < 0.001 respectively). PPVs, NPVs, and accuracies in diagnosing all lesions (recurrent and malignant cervical lymph nodes) were generally consistent in tendencies among the three imaging modalities, among which PET/MR yielded the optimal diagnostic performance. Both imaging modalities yielded false-positive results, either for suspicious thyroid nodules or lymph nodes. Based on the available pathological results, misdiagnosed lesions were mainly fibrofatty tissue.

Table 3. Diagnostic performance of two modalities.

	All Lesions			Malignant Thyroid Nodules			Metastatic Nodes		
	PET/MR	MR	PET/CT	PET/MR	MR	PET/CT	PET/MR	MR	PET/CT
True-positive	62	60	47	2	2	1	60	58	46
True-negative	45	44	43	4	4	4	41	40	39
False-positive	8	9	10	2	2	2	6	7	8
False-negative	15	17	30	1	1	2	14	16	28
Sensitivity (%)	80.5%	77.9%	61.0%	66.7%	66.7%	33.3%	81.1%	78.4%	62.2%
Specificity (%)	84.9%	83.0%	81.1%	66.7%	66.7%	66.7%	87.2%	85.1%	83.0%
PPV (%)	88.6%	87.0%	82.5%	50.0%	50.0%	33.3%	90.9%	89.2%	85.2%
NPV (%)	75.0%	72.1%	58.9%	80.0%	80.0%	66.7%	74.5%	71.4%	58.2%
Accuracy (%)	82.3%	80.0%	69.2%	66.7%	66.7%	55.6%	83.5%	81.0%	70.2%

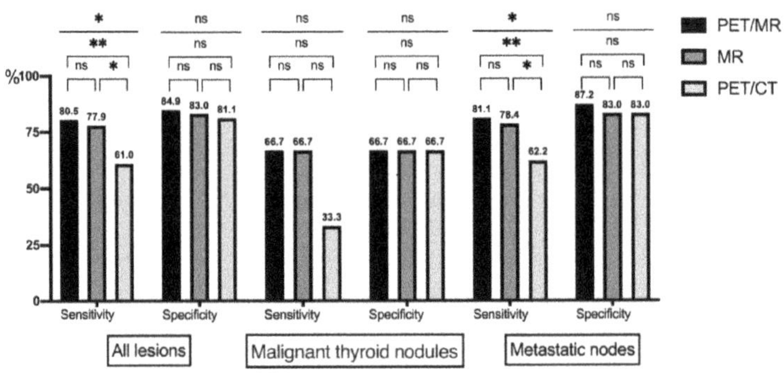

Figure 4. Diagnostic performance of two modalities (ns represents no significance; * represents the p-value < 0.05; ** represents the p-value < 0.01).

The image clarity scores for each region of the lesion are shown in Table 4. For all included lesions, the PET/MR scores were significantly higher than those of PET/CT (2.74 ± 0.60 vs. 1.9 ± 0.50, $p < 0.001$). The largest score was in level II (2.92 ± 0.33), which almost exceeded PET/CT (1.91 ± 0.45) by 1 point. For malignant lesions, there was no difference between PET/MR and PET/CT in the assessment of suspected thyroid nodules, while there were significant differences in the assessment of metastatic lymph nodes of all levels. The largest differences between PET/MR and PET/CT occurred in level II (2.83 ± 0.48 vs. 1.79 ± 0.58) and level V (2.73 ± 0.67 vs. 1.85 ± 0.46), as presented in Figure 3. For benign lesions, PET/MR had better presentation of thyroid nodules and lymph nodes in other regions, especially in levels II (3.00 ± 0.00 versus 2.02 ± 0.25) and IV (3.00 ± 0.00 versus 2.14 ± 0.36). Image conspicuity agreement was excellent (κ = 1 in thyroid nodules, κ = 0.981 in lymph nodes, $p < 0.001$) between the two physicians.

Table 4. Conspicuity score of recurrent or metastatic lesions in relation to location (scoring criteria referring to [26]).

		All Lesions				Malignant				Benign			
		No.	PET/MR	^{18}F-PET/CT	*p*	No.	PET/MR	PET/CT	*p*	No.	PET/MR	^{1}PET/CT	*p*
Thyroid area		9	2.56 ± 0.73	2.00 ± 0.707	0.027	3	2.00 ± 0.894	2.00 ± 0.894	1	6	2.83 ± 0.39	2.00 ± 0.60	0.008
Lymph nodes	II	53 (43.8%)	2.92 ± 0.33	1.91 ± 0.45	<0.001	24 (45.3%)	2.83 ± 0.48	1.79 ± 0.58	<0.001	29 (54.7%)	3.00 ± 0.00	2.02 ± 0.25	<0.001
	III	16 (13.2%)	2.38 ± 0.79	1.84 ± 0.52	<0.001	13 (81.3%)	2.31 ± 0.84	1.81 ± 0.57	0.003	3 (18.8%)	2.67 ± 0.52	2.00 ± 0.00	0.46
	IV	18 (14.9%)	2.67 ± 0.68	1.97 ± 0.56	<0.001	11 (61.1%)	2.45 ± 0.82	1.82 ± 0.60	0.035	7 (38.9%)	3.00 ± 0.00	2.14 ± 0.36	0.001
	V	19 (15.7%)	2.74 ± 0.64	1.92 ± 0.54	<0.001	13 (68.4%)	2.73 ± 0.67	1.85 ± 0.46	<0.001	6 (31.6%)	2.75 ± 0.62	2.08 ± 0.67	0.11
	VI	15 (12.4%)	2.50 ± 0.76	1.73 ± 0.45	0.002	13 (86.7%)	2.54 ± 0.74	1.82 ± 0.55	0.002	2 (13.3%)	3.00 ± 0.00	2.50 ± 0.71	<0.001
	Total	121	2.74 ± 0.60 Kappa = 0.981, $p < 0.001$	1.9 ± 0.50	<0.001	74	2.61 ± 0.72	1.8 ± 0.57	<0.001	47	2.96 ± 0.20	2.04 ± 0.29	<0.001

Table 5 lists the SUVmax, SUVmean, and lymph node diameters in the maximum cross-sectional area of lymph nodes measured by PET/MR and PET/CT. The SUVmax of malignant lymph nodes was significantly higher than that of benign lymph nodes on PET/MR (median 2.6 vs. 2.2, $p = 0.004$) and PET/CT (median 2.0 vs. 1.8, $p = 0.006$). However, SUVmax showed an overlap in benign and malignant lymph nodes (Figure S1). Figure 5 presents an isolated malignant lymph node with intense ^{18}F-FDG uptake on PET/MR. The SUVmean, long diameter, and short diameter indicated no significant differences between benign and malignant nodes on both modalities (Figure S1). For all included lymph nodes, SUVmax, SUVmean, and lymph node diameters of PET/MR were higher than those measured on PET/CT by 17.4%, 22.2%, 11%, and 18% (all $p \leq 0.001$), respectively. The Bland–Altman analysis showed great consistency among modalities between the SUVmax, SUVmean, and diameters (Figure S2). Additionally, there were correlations between the parameters detected on PET/MR and PET/CT (all $p < 0.001$, Figure S3). The correlation coefficient of SUVmax for all lymph nodes was 0.661 (Figure S3).

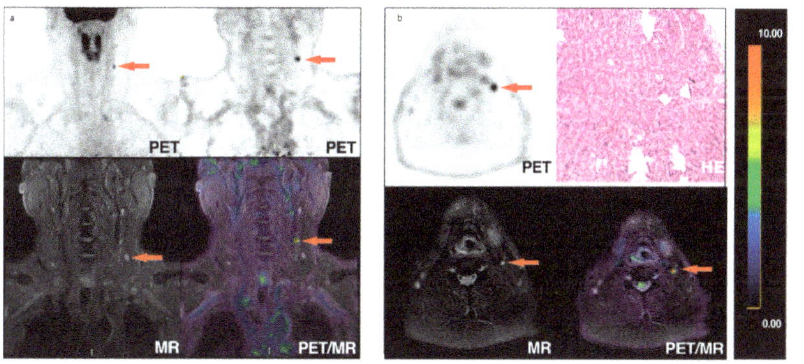

Figure 5. A 51-year-old DTC patient after comprehensive treatment presented with an unexplained increase in Tg (2.88 μg/L). PET/MR depicted an increased uptake of a small lymph node (long diameter, 0.7 cm) in the left level III, with SUVmax 5.1, without other apparently abnormal lymph nodes ((**a**,**b**), red arrows). 30 suspicious lymph nodes were removed by re-operation, and notably, only the lymph node identified on PET/MR was malignant.

Table 5. SUVs, diameters of lymph nodes detected by both PET/MR and PET/CT.

		PET/MR	PET/CT
All detected lymph nodes $n = 99$	SUVmax	2.3 (2.0–2.8) [1]	1.9 (1.5–2.2)
	SUVmean	1.8 (1.5–2.2)	1.4 (1.1–1.8)
	Long axis	9.4 (7.2–11.7)	7.3 (5.3–9.5)
	Short axis	5.0 (4.0–6.2)	4.1 (3.0–5.3)
Malignant $n = 54$	SUVmax	2.6 (2.0–3.5)	2.0 (1.6–2.3)
	SUVmean	1.9 (1.5–2.5)	1.4 (1.2–1.9)
	Long axis	9.7 (7.3–11.4)	7.3 (5.0–9.4)
	Short axis	4.7 (3.8–6.9)	3.7 (3.0–5.0)
Benign $n = 45$	SUVmax	2.2 (1.9–2.6)	1.8 (1.5–2.0)
	SUVmean	1.7 (1.5–2.0)	1.4 (1.0–1.8)
	Long axis	8.9 (7.0–12.7)	7.3 (5.5–9.6)
	Short axis	5.3 (4.5–6.1)	4.4 (3.3–5.4)

[1] The data are uniformly expressed as median (25th–75th %).

4. Discussion

In this study, the head-to-head comparison of PET/MR with PET/CT in DTC patients after comprehensive treatment revealed that PET/MR was more accurate in determining recurrent/residual and metastatic lesions, both from a patient-based and a lesion-based perspective. PET/MR provided superior conspicuity, as shown in clarity score evaluation, making it more useful for the identification of lesions. Both malignant and benign lesions had a significantly higher SUVmax, making it essential to incorporate the morphological content provided by MR to strengthen diagnosis efficacy. Therefore, additional neck PET/MR may be recommended for the detection of recurrence/lymph nodes metastases in DTC patients after comprehensive treatment, as it provides clearer images, more accurate identification, and more precise resection scope to avoid over-resection.

PET/MR can identify recurrent lesions and metastatic lymph nodes more accurately. According to patient analysis, PET/MR detected 26 of 27 patients with tumor burden, while PET/CT only detected 21. Based on lesion analysis, PET/MR combined with the advantages of MR had higher detection rates (91.5% vs. 80.8%), image conspicuity (especially in level II), and diagnostic efficacy than PET/CT. It was found that PET/MR showed higher diagnostic efficacy, and the MR part of PET/MR showed different positive results compared to ^{18}F-FDG PET/CT, which suggested that the combination of the two modalities had a synergistic effect. This is consistent with published research [16,35]. However, there are still false positives for both imaging modalities, which are mainly caused by local postoperative hyperplasia. Based on the available pathological diagnosis in this study, suspicious areas depicted on PET/MR or PET/CT were fibrofatty tissue closely associated with postoperative local hyperplasia. In addition, high physiological ^{18}F-FDG uptake can be observed in Waldeyer's ring, active muscles (vocal cord movement, swallowing), salivary glands, and brown fat [36].

MR plays an important role in the detection of complex thyroid lesions and metastatic lymph nodes [18–20] not only because MR has superior soft tissue contrast and additional imaging techniques, but also because multi-position, multi-parameter, and multi-sequence images can provide several benefits. These benefits include clear lesion contour and location, signal alteration and enhancement, diffusion restriction, and accurate assessment of lesion invasion of surrounding tissue structures (e.g., envelope, cartilage) [37]. On conventional MR, malignant thyroid nodules exhibit irregular margins and blurred boundaries with cystic changes, diffuse enlargement of the thyroid gland, and peripheral and distant invasion. They usually reveal low to intermediate T1- and high T2-weighted signal intensities, or occasionally high T1- and T2-weighted signal intensities with heterogeneous enhancement on enhanced T1WI [38]. On DWI, recurrence or metastases present strong contrast with the dark background signal from fat deposited around, based on metabolic or physiological changes [39,40]. Additionally, one should note that the clear volumetric information provided by MRI may be meaningful for determining the treatment dose [41]. In regard to image conspicuity, PET/MR had obvious advantages over PET/CT in detecting and displaying thyroid nodules as well as suspicious lymph nodes regardless of the region of interest. Compared with PET/CT, high resolution and multiple sequences such as DWI and ADC of MR have made contributions to the imaging of lesions, especially in level II with complex anatomy and high incidence of nonspecific lymph nodes [42]. Of note, the updated NCCN Guidelines of Thyroid Carcinoma (Version 3.2020) recommend that if iodine-131 imaging is negative and stimulated Tg > 2–5 ng/mL, additional non-radioiodine imaging modalities should be considered, including central and lateral neck compartments ultrasound, neck CT with contrast, chest CT with contrast, and PET/CT. However, enhanced CT is not routinely performed in patients with highly suspected recurrence or metastases in our department, in order to avoid the influence of the iodine contrast agent on the subsequent ^{131}I treatment.

^{18}F-FDG PET/CT is mainly used for postoperative surveillance of poorly differentiated thyroid cancer [43]. The uptake ability of ^{18}F-FDG by thyroid cancer depends on the tumor differentiation degree [44,45]. The lower the differentiation of the lesion, the less it takes up ^{131}I, but the more it takes up ^{18}F-FDG, so positive Tg and negative ^{131}I-WBS lesions are prone to be identified. This study also verified that SUVmax associated with ^{18}F-FDG uptake was meaningful for the characterization of cervical lymph nodes. For PET alone, modern PET/MR can provide a superior SUVs than PET/CT, with time-of-flight (TOF) technology based on a new generation of crystals and the latest photovoltaic conversion technology.

There are contradictory results on the value of PET/CT and additional MR according to previous research. On the one hand, Hempel et al. concluded that the combination of PET/CT with MR was not suitable for routine clinical application [16,46]. Loeffelbein et al. reported that there was no significant difference between PET, MRI, and PET + MR in identifying recurrences in the neck [47]. On the other hand, earlier research argued that PET/CT and additional MR can provide additional diagnostic information [48,49]. PET/MR allows accurate, temporally and spatially unified multiparametric imaging of PET and MR. It can provide additional information and further improve the diagnostic efficacy than non-simultaneous PET and MR [50]. Previous studies have reported that PET/MR did not outperform PET/CT or even slightly underperform PET/CT in the detection of lung metastases and bone metastases [26,41]. Our results reveal that PET/MR is comparable to PET/CT in terms of diagnostic specificity. In addition, for the same lesion, SUVmax, SUVmean, and diameters measured on PET/MR and PET/CT were consistent and had significant correlation. Although there were significant differences between the measured parameters of PET/MR and PET/CT, this may be related to different tracer elimination, attenuation correction, and associated scatter correction.

There are several limitations in this study. First, the number of patients and lesions involved was limited. Most lesions were determined by a follow-up combination of Tg levels and imaging (ultrasound, CT, and/or MR) instead of surgical biopsy or FNAB; therefore, the absence of histopathological confirmation of most lesions may potentially affect the final diagnostic accuracy. Second, quantitative comparisons of parameters were limited by different imaging techniques, different attenuation correction and associated scatter correction methods, as well as different tracer elimination caused by the single-injection double-examination protocol. In addition, the study was retrospective and only included patients with DTC who underwent both PET/CT and PET/MR. Multicenter clinical trials that prospectively include patients are necessary to assess the validity of our results. Furthermore, cervical lymph nodes are often inflammatory, which may lead to nonspecific ^{18}F-FDG uptake. Therefore, the exploitation of specific imaging agents should be the orientation of future research. In this study, although ^{18}F-FDG uptake differed between malignant and benign disease, there was also overlap in both SUV values, which may have an impact on the accuracy of the results. Third and lastly, PET/MR examinations are expensive, and the clinical application of this study should also consider the overall benefit to patients in relation to financial expenditures. Further analysis of the economic benefits is expected.

5. Conclusions

This study compared ^{18}F-FDG PET/CT and additional neck PET/MR scans head to head to analyze the detection ability and diagnostic efficacy of recurrent/residual DTC lesions and cervical lymph node metastases, as well as the characteristics of each parameter. The results showed that ^{18}F-FDG PET/MR was more accurate in diagnosing recurrent and metastatic lesions, both from a patient-based and a lesion-based perspective. PET/MR detected more lesions and presented better image conspicuity and diagnostic performance due to the high soft tissue resolution and multi-sequence imaging available with MRI. The addition of neck PET/MR after whole-body PET/CT may be recommended to provide more precise diagnostic information and scope of surgical resection without additional ionizing radiation. Further prospective studies with expanded samples and economic benefit analysis are needed to support the conclusions.

Supplementary Materials: The following are available online at https://www.mdpi.com/article/10.3390/cancers13143436/s1, Figure S1: SUVs, diameters of malignant and benign lymph nodes detected by both PET/MR and PET/CT, Figure S2: Bland–Altman analysis of SUVmax, SUVmean, and diameter measurements provided in two modalities, Figure S3: Correlation of SUVs and lymph node diameters measured on PET/MR and PET/CT.

Author Contributions: X.L., W.C. and F.L. designed the study; Y.S., F.L. and X.L. reviewed all the images, obtained the data, designed the statistical analysis, and finished the interpretation of the patient cohort; T.H., Z.G. and J.M. recruited the patients and provided the clinical data; W.R. and F.H. performed PET/CT and PET/MR examination; Y.S. wrote the manuscript; X.L., M.H.Y. and W.C. revised the manuscript. All authors have read and agreed to the published version of the manuscript.

Funding: This research was funded by the Key Project of National Nature Science Foundation of China (No. 82030052 and 81630049), Key Project of Hubei Province Technical Innovation (No. 2017ACA182), and University of Wisconsin–Madison.

Institutional Review Board Statement: The study was conducted according to the guidelines of the Declaration of Helsinki, and approved by the Institutional Review Board (or Ethics Committee) of Union Hospital, Tongji Medical College, Huazhong University of Science and Technology (2018-48).

Informed Consent Statement: Informed consent was obtained from all subjects involved in the study.

Data Availability Statement: The data presented in this study are available in this article (and supplementary material).

Conflicts of Interest: Weibo Cai is a scientific advisor, stockholder, and grantee of Focus-X Therapeutics, Inc. All other authors declare no conflict of interest.

References

1. Siegel, R.L.; Miller, K.D.; Jemal, A. Cancer statistics, 2020. *CA Cancer J. Clin.* **2020**, *70*, 7–30. [CrossRef] [PubMed]
2. Deng, Y.; Li, H.; Wang, M.; Li, N.; Tian, T.; Wu, Y.; Xu, P.; Yang, S.; Zhai, Z.; Zhou, L.; et al. Global Burden of Thyroid Cancer From 1990 to 2017. *JAMA Netw. Open* **2020**, *3*, e208759. [CrossRef] [PubMed]
3. Goodarzi, E.; Moslem, A.; Feizhadad, H.; Jarrahi, A.; Adineh, H.; Sohrabivafa, M.; Khazaei, Z. Epidemiology, incidence and mortality of thyroid cancer and their relationship with the human development index in the world: An ecology study in 2018. *Adv. Hum. Biol.* **2019**, *9*, 162–167.
4. Sherman, S.I. Thyroid carcinoma. *Lancet* **2003**, *361*, 501–511. [CrossRef]
5. Gao, L.; Jiang, Y.; Liang, Z.; Zhang, L.; Mao, X.; Yang, X.; Wang, Y.; Xu, J.; Liu, R.; Zhu, S.; et al. Cervical soft tissue recurrence of differentiated thyroid carcinoma after thyroidectomy indicates a poor prognosis. *Int. J. Surg.* **2017**, *48*, 254–259. [CrossRef]
6. Han, J.M.; Bae, J.C.; Kim, H.I.; Kwon, S.; Jeon, M.J.; Kim, W.G.; Kim, T.Y.; Shong, Y.K.; Kim, W.B. Clinical Outcomes of Differentiated Thyroid Cancer Patients with Local Recurrence or Distant Metastasis Detected in Old Age. *Endocrinol. Metab.* **2018**, *33*, 459–465. [CrossRef]
7. Liu, F.H.; Kuo, S.F.; Hsueh, C.; Chao, T.C.; Lin, J.D. Postoperative recurrence of papillary thyroid carcinoma with lymph node metastasis. *J. Surg. Oncol.* **2015**, *112*, 149–154. [CrossRef] [PubMed]

8. Thyroid Carcinoma. Available online: https://www.nccn.org/professionals/physician_gls/pdf/thyroid.pdf (accessed on 9 April 2021).
9. Haugen, B.R.; Alexander, E.K.; Bible, K.C.; Doherty, G.M.; Mandel, S.J.; Nikiforov, Y.E.; Pacini, F.; Randolph, G.W.; Sawka, A.M.; Schlumberger, M.; et al. 2015 American Thyroid Association Management Guidelines for Adult Patients with Thyroid Nodules and Differentiated Thyroid Cancer: The American Thyroid Association Guidelines Task Force on Thyroid Nodules and Differentiated Thyroid Cancer. *Thyroid* **2016**, *26*, 1–133. [CrossRef] [PubMed]
10. Bertagna, F.; Bosio, G.; Biasiotto, G.; Rodella, C.; Puta, E.; Gabanelli, S.; Lucchini, S.; Merli, G.; Savelli, G.; Giubbini, R.; et al. F-18 FDG-PET/CT evaluation of patients with differentiated thyroid cancer with negative I-131 total body scan and high thyroglobulin level. *Clin. Nucl. Med.* **2009**, *34*, 756–761. [CrossRef]
11. Lu, C.Z.; Cao, S.S.; Wang, W.; Liu, J.; Fu, N.; Lu, F. Usefulness of PET/CT in the diagnosis of recurrent or metastasized differentiated thyroid carcinoma. *Oncol. Lett.* **2016**, *11*, 2420–2423. [CrossRef] [PubMed]
12. Chao, M. Management of Differentiated Thyroid Cancer with Rising Thyroglobulin and Negative Diagnostic Radioiodine Whole Body Scan. *Clin. Oncol.* **2010**, *22*, 438–447. [CrossRef] [PubMed]
13. Linee Guida SIE-AIMN-AIFM per il Trattamento e Follow-Up del Carcinoma Differenziato della Tiroide. Available online: https://www.aimn.it/pubblicazioni/LG/LG_ca_tiroide.pdf (accessed on 1 February 2019).
14. Filetti, S.; Durante, C.; Hartl, D.; Leboulleux, S.; Locati, L.D.; Newbold, K.; Papotti, M.G.; Berruti, A. Thyroid cancer: ESMO Clinical Practice Guidelines for diagnosis, treatment and follow-up. *Ann. Oncol.* **2019**, *30*, 1856–1883. [CrossRef] [PubMed]
15. Expert Panel on Thyroid Cancer, Guidelines Working Committee of Chinese Society of Clinical Oncology. Guidelines of Chinese So-ciety of Clinical Oncology (CSCO): Persistent/Recurrent and Metastatic Differentiated Thyroid Cancer-2019. *J. Cancer Control. Treat.* **2019**, *32*, 1051–1080.
16. Hempel, J.M.; Kloeckner, R.; Krick, S.; Pinto Dos Santos, D.; Schadmand-Fischer, S.; Boeßert, P.; Bisdas, S.; Weber, M.M.; Fottner, C.; Musholt, T.J.; et al. Impact of combined FDG-PET/CT and MRI on the detection of local recurrence and nodal metastases in thyroid cancer. *Cancer Imaging* **2016**, *16*, 37. [CrossRef] [PubMed]
17. Haslerud, T.; Brauckhoff, K.; Reisæter, L.; Küfner Lein, R.; Heinecke, A.; Varhaug, J.E.; Biermann, M. F18-FDG-PET for recurrent differentiated thyroid cancer: A systematic meta-analysis. *Acta Radiol.* **2016**, *57*, 1193–1200. [CrossRef] [PubMed]
18. Wang, J.C.; Takashima, S.; Takayama, F.; Kawakami, S.; Saito, A.; Matsushita, T.; Matsuba, H.; Kobayashi, S. Tracheal invasion by thyroid carcinoma: Prediction using MR imaging. *AJR Am. J. Roentgenol.* **2001**, *177*, 929–936. [CrossRef] [PubMed]
19. Khizer, A.T.; Raza, S.; Slehria, A.U. Diffusion-weighted MR Imaging and ADC Mapping in Differentiating Benign from Malignant Thyroid Nodules. *J. Coll. Physicians Surg. Pak.* **2015**, *25*, 785–788.
20. Shi, R.; Yao, Q.; Wu, L.; Zhou, Q.; Lu, Q.; Gao, R.; Hu, J.; Kao, L.; Bains, A.; Yan, Z.; et al. T2* mapping at 3.0T MRI for differentiation of papillary thyroid carcinoma from benign thyroid nodules. *J. Magn. Reson. Imaging* **2016**, *43*, 956–961. [CrossRef]
21. Park, J.; Pak, K.; Yun, T.J.; Lee, E.K.; Ryoo, I.; Lee, J.Y.; Hwang, I.; Yoo, R.E.; Kang, K.M.; Choi, S.H.; et al. Diagnostic Accuracy and Confidence of [18F] FDG PET/MRI in comparison with PET or MRI alone in Head and Neck Cancer. *Sci. Rep.* **2020**, *10*, 9490. [CrossRef]
22. Kim, S.G.; Friedman, K.; Patel, S.; Hagiwara, M. Potential Role of PET/MRI for Imaging Metastatic Lymph Nodes in Head and Neck Cancer. *AJR Am. J. Roentgenol.* **2016**, *207*, 248–256. [CrossRef]
23. Byeon, Y.H.; Choi, J.E.; Park, J.Y.; Song, J.H.; Yeo, K.J.; Kong, E.J.; Kang, S.H.; Lee, S.J. Diagnostic Accuracy of PET/MR for Evaluating Central Lymph Node Status in Patients with Papillary Thyroid Carcinoma. *J. Endocr. Surg.* **2017**, *17*, 122–130. [CrossRef]
24. Platzek, I.; Beuthien-Baumann, B.; Schneider, M.; Gudziol, V.; Kitzler, H.H.; Maus, J.; Schramm, G.; Popp, M.; Laniado, M.; Kotzerke, J.; et al. FDG PET/MR for lymph node staging in head and neck cancer. *Eur. J. Radiol.* **2014**, *83*, 1163–1168. [CrossRef] [PubMed]
25. Schlittenbauer, T.; Zeilinger, M.; Nkenke, E.; Kreißel, S.; Wurm, M.C.; Lell, M.; Kuwert, T.; Beck, M. Positron emission tomography-computed tomography versus positron emission tomography-magnetic resonance imaging for diagnosis of oral squamous cell carcinoma: A pilot study. *J. Craniomaxillofac. Surg.* **2015**, *43*, 2129–2135. [CrossRef] [PubMed]
26. Vrachimis, A.; Burg, M.C.; Wenning, C.; Allkemper, T.; Weckesser, M.; Schäfers, M.; Stegger, L. [(18)F]FDG PET/CT outperforms [(18)F]FDG PET/MRI in differentiated thyroid cancer. *Eur. J. Nucl. Med. Mol. Imaging* **2016**, *43*, 212–220. [CrossRef] [PubMed]
27. Eisenhauer, E.A.; Therasse, P.; Bogaerts, J.; Schwartz, L.H.; Sargent, D.; Ford, R.; Dancey, J.; Arbuck, S.; Gwyther, S.; Mooney, M.; et al. New response evaluation criteria in solid tumours: Revised RECIST guideline (version 1.1). *Eur. J. Cancer* **2009**, *45*, 228–247. [CrossRef] [PubMed]
28. Vassallo, P.; Wernecke, K.; Roos, N.; Peters, P.E. Differentiation of benign from malignant superficial lymphadenopathy: The role of high-resolution US. *Radiology* **1992**, *183*, 215–220. [CrossRef] [PubMed]
29. Rosário, P.W.; de Faria, S.; Bicalho, L.; Alves, M.F.; Borges, M.A.; Purisch, S.; Padrão, E.L.; Rezende, L.L.; Barroso, A.L. Ultrasonographic differentiation between metastatic and benign lymph nodes in patients with papillary thyroid carcinoma. *J. Ultrasound Med.* **2005**, *24*, 1385–1389. [CrossRef]
30. Kuna, S.K.; Bracic, I.; Tesic, V.; Kuna, K.; Herceg, G.H.; Dodig, D. Ultrasonographic differentiation of benign from malignant neck lymphadenopathy in thyroid cancer. *J. Ultrasound Med.* **2006**, *25*, 1531–1537; quiz 1538–1540. [CrossRef] [PubMed]
31. Sadigh, G.; Carlos, R.C.; Neal, C.H.; Dwamena, B.A. Ultrasonographic differentiation of malignant from benign breast lesions: A meta-analytic comparison of elasticity and BIRADS scoring. *Breast Cancer Res. Treat.* **2012**, *133*, 23–35. [CrossRef]

32. Sakai, O.; Curtin, H.D.; Romo, L.V.; Som, P.M. Lymph node pathology. Benign proliferative, lymphoma, and metastatic disease. Radiol. *Clin. North. Am.* **2000**, *38*, 979–998.
33. Kim, E.; Park, J.S.; Son, K.R.; Kim, J.H.; Jeon, S.J.; Na, D.G. Preoperative diagnosis of cervical metastatic lymph nodes in papillary thyroid carcinoma: Comparison of ultrasound, computed tomography, and combined ultrasound with computed tomography. *Thyroid* **2008**, *18*, 411–418. [CrossRef] [PubMed]
34. Seo, Y.L.; Yoon, D.Y.; Baek, S.; Ku, Y.J.; Rho, Y.S.; Chung, E.J.; Koh, S.H. Detection of neck recurrence in patients with differentiated thyroid cancer: Comparison of ultrasound, contrast-enhanced CT and (18)F-FDG PET/CT using surgical pathology as a reference standard: (ultrasound vs. CT vs. (18)F-FDG PET/CT in recurrent thyroid cancer). *Eur. Radiol.* **2012**, *22*, 2246–2254.
35. Becker, M.; Zaidi, H. Imaging in head and neck squamous cell carcinoma: The potential role of PET/MRI. *Br. J. Radiol.* **2014**, *87*, 20130677. [CrossRef]
36. Abouzied, M.M.; Crawford, E.S.; Nabi, H.A. 18F-FDG imaging: Pitfalls and artifacts. *J. Nucl. Med. Technol.* **2005**, *33*, 145–155, quiz 162–143. [PubMed]
37. Owrangi, A.M.; Greer, P.B.; Glide-Hurst, C.K. MRI-only treatment planning: Benefits and challenges. *Phys. Med. Biol.* **2018**, *63*, 05tr01. [CrossRef]
38. Som, P.M.; Brandwein, M.; Lidov, M.; Lawson, W.; Biller, H.F. The varied presentations of papillary thyroid carcinoma cervical nodal disease: CT and MR findings. *AJNR Am. J. Neuroradiol.* **1994**, *15*, 1123.
39. Park, S.-H.; Hahm, M.H.; Bae, B.K.; Chong, G.O.; Jeong, S.Y.; Na, S.; Jeong, S.; Kim, J.-C. Magnetic resonance imaging features of tumor and lymph node to predict clinical outcome in node-positive cervical cancer: A retrospective analysis. *Radiat. Oncol.* **2020**, *15*, 86. [CrossRef] [PubMed]
40. Mao, Y.; Hedgire, S.; Harisinghani, M. Radiologic Assessment of Lymph Nodes in Oncologic Patients. *Curr. Radiol. Rep.* **2014**, *2*, 36. [CrossRef]
41. Binse, I.; Poeppel, T.D.; Ruhlmann, M.; Gomez, B.; Umutlu, L.; Bockisch, A.; Rosenbaum-Krumme, S.J. Imaging with (124)I in differentiated thyroid carcinoma: Is PET/MRI superior to PET/CT? *Eur. J. Nucl. Med. Mol. Imaging* **2016**, *43*, 1011–1017. [CrossRef]
42. Chong, V. Cervical lymphadenopathy: What radiologists need to know. *Cancer Imaging* **2004**, *4*, 116–120. [CrossRef]
43. Yang, J.H.; Maciel, R.M.B.; Nakabashi, C.C.D.; Janovsky, C.; Padovani, R.P.; Macellaro, D.; Camacho, C.P.; Osawa, A.; Wagner, J.; Biscolla, R.P.M. Clinical utility of 18F-FDG PET/CT in the follow-up of a large cohort of patients with high-risk differentiated thyroid carcinoma. *Arch. Endocrinol. Metab.* **2017**, *61*, 416–425. [CrossRef]
44. von Falck, C.; Boerner, A.R.; Galanski, M.; Knapp, W.H. Neuroendocrine tumour of the mediastinum: Fusion of 18F-FDG and 68Ga-DOTATOC PET/CT datasets demonstrates different degrees of differentiation. *Eur. J. Nucl. Med. Mol. Imaging* **2007**, *34*, 812. [CrossRef]
45. Kurokawa, T.; Yoshida, Y.; Kawahara, K.; Tsuchida, T.; Okazawa, H.; Fujibayashi, Y.; Yonekura, Y.; Kotsuji, F. Expression of GLUT-1 glucose transfer, cellular proliferation activity and grade of tumor correlate with [F-18]-fluorodeoxyglucose uptake by positron emission tomography in epithelial tumors of the ovary. *Int. J. Cancer* **2004**, *109*, 926–932. [CrossRef] [PubMed]
46. Subesinghe, M.; Scarsbrook, A.F.; Sourbron, S.; Wilson, D.J.; McDermott, G.; Speight, R.; Roberts, N.; Carey, B.; Forrester, R.; Gopal, S.V.; et al. Alterations in anatomic and functional imaging parameters with repeated FDG PET-CT and MRI during radiotherapy for head and neck cancer: A pilot study. *BMC Cancer* **2015**, *15*, 137. [CrossRef] [PubMed]
47. Loeffelbein, D.J.; Souvatzoglou, M.; Wankerl, V.; Dinges, J.; Ritschl, L.M.; Mücke, T.; Pickhard, A.; Eiber, M.; Schwaiger, M.; Beer, A.J. Diagnostic value of retrospective PET-MRI fusion in head-and-neck cancer. *BMC Cancer* **2014**, *14*, 846. [CrossRef] [PubMed]
48. Nakamoto, Y.; Tamai, K.; Saga, T.; Higashi, T.; Hara, T.; Suga, T.; Koyama, T.; Togashi, K. Clinical value of image fusion from MR and PET in patients with head and neck cancer. *Mol. Imaging Biol.* **2009**, *11*, 46–53. [CrossRef] [PubMed]
49. Seiboth, L.; Van Nostrand, D.; Wartofsky, L.; Ousman, Y.; Jonklaas, J.; Butler, C.; Atkins, F.; Burman, K. Utility of PET/neck MRI digital fusion images in the management of recurrent or persistent thyroid cancer. *Thyroid* **2008**, *18*, 103–111. [CrossRef] [PubMed]
50. Rosenkrantz, A.B.; Friedman, K.; Chandarana, H.; Melsaether, A.; Moy, L.; Ding, Y.S.; Jhaveri, K.; Beltran, L.; Jain, R. Current Status of Hybrid PET/MRI in Oncologic Imaging. *AJR Am. J. Roentgenol.* **2016**, *206*, 162–172. [CrossRef]

cancers

Review

Poorly Differentiated and Anaplastic Thyroid Cancer: Insights into Genomics, Microenvironment and New Drugs

Alessandro Prete [1], Antonio Matrone [1], Carla Gambale [1], Liborio Torregrossa [2], Elisa Minaldi [1], Cristina Romei [1], Raffaele Ciampi [1], Eleonora Molinaro [1] and Rossella Elisei [1,*]

1 Endocrine Unit, Department of Clinical and Experimental Medicine, University Hospital of Pisa, Via Paradisa 2, 56124 Pisa, Italy; a.prete1@studenti.unipi.it or alessandro.prete22@gmail.com (A.P.); antonio.matrone@med.unipi.it (A.M.); gambalecarla@libero.it (C.G.); elisa.minaldi@med.unipi.it (E.M.); cristina.romei@unipi.it (C.R.); raffaele.ciampi@unipi.it (R.C.); e.molinaro@ao-pisa.toscana.it (E.M.)

2 Department of Surgical, Medical, Molecular Pathology and Critical Area, University Hospital of Pisa, 56124 Pisa, Italy; l.torregrossa@ao-pisa.toscana.it

* Correspondence: rossella.elisei@med.unipi.it; Tel.: +39-050-544-723; Fax: +39-050-578-772

Simple Summary: In the last decades, many researchers produced promising data concerning genetics and tumor microenvironment of poorly differentiated thyroid cancer (PDTC) and anaplastic thyroid cancer (ATC). They are trying to tear the veil covering these orphan cancers, suggesting new therapeutic weapons as single or combined therapies.

Abstract: PDTC and ATC present median overall survival of 6 years and 6 months, respectively. In spite of their rarity, patients with PDTC and ATC represent a significant clinical problem, because of their poor survival and the substantial inefficacy of classical therapies. We reviewed the newest findings about genetic features of PDTC and ATC, from mutations occurring in DNA to alterations in RNA. Therefore, we describe their tumor microenvironments (both immune and not-immune) and the interactions between tumor and neighboring cells. Finally, we recapitulate how this upcoming evidence are changing the treatment of PDTC and ATC.

Keywords: anaplastic thyroid cancer; poorly thyroid cancer; genetic landscape; tumor microenvironment; genetically guided therapy

Citation: Prete, A.; Matrone, A.; Gambale, C.; Torregrossa, L.; Minaldi, E.; Romei, C.; Ciampi, R.; Molinaro, E.; Elisei, R. Poorly Differentiated and Anaplastic Thyroid Cancer: Insights into Genomics, Microenvironment and New Drugs. *Cancers* **2021**, *13*, 3200. https://doi.org/10.3390/cancers13133200

Academic Editors: Fabio Medas and Pier Francesco Alesina

Received: 30 May 2021
Accepted: 24 June 2021
Published: 26 June 2021

1. Introduction

Thyroid cancer is the most common endocrine tumor and its incidence has been raising up over the last 20 years, mostly due to the flowering diagnosis of micro thyroid carcinomas [1]. Thyroid cancer is subcategorized into follicular and non-follicular derived carcinoma (e.g., medullary thyroid carcinoma). Among the first, World Health Organization (WHO) identifies papillary thyroid carcinoma (PTC), follicular thyroid carcinoma (FTC), poorly differentiated thyroid carcinoma (PDTC), and anaplastic thyroid carcinoma (ATC) [2].

Thyroid cancer 5 year-survival is variable among the different hystotypes. According to a recent epidemiological study performed in Denmark by using a national cancer registry, the 5 year-survival rates were 91.1% and 79.9% in PTC and FTC, respectively, 63.6% in PDTC and 12.2% in ATC [3]. Unfortunately, PDTC and ATC median overall survival is 6 years and 6 months, respectively [4,5]. Although PDTC and ATC are rare, therapy for patients affected by PDTC and ATC represents an unmet clinical need that should be addressed, considering their poor survival. In addition, PDTC and ATC harbor diagnostic pitfalls that make difficult their clinical management. Although PDTC was added in WHO classification in 2004, its diagnostic criteria are not widely shared and many pathologists are following criteria of Turin consensus conference [6] and others Memorial Sloan Kettering Cancer Center ones [7]. Likewise, the wide spectrum of ATC hystotypes could challenge the differential diagnosis with other cancers (e.g., angiomatoid variant ATC with thyroid angiosarcoma) [8] or even with benign lesions (e.g., acute thyroiditis) [9] (Figure 1).

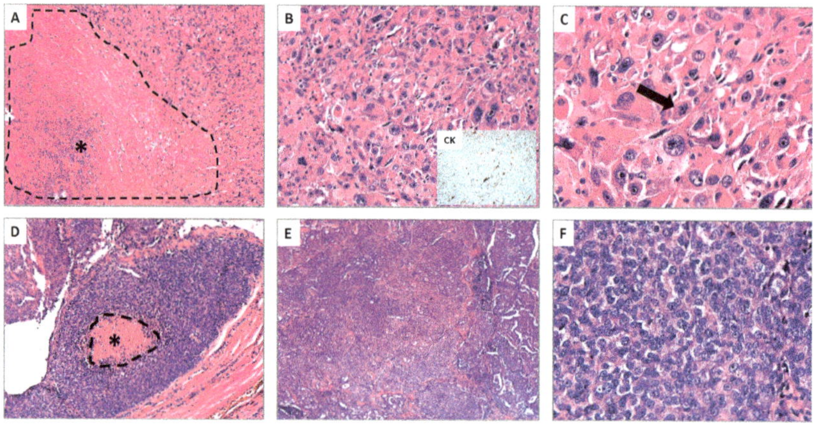

Figure 1. (**A–C**) Anaplastic thyroid carcinoma (ATC) (hematoxylin and eosin stain); (**A**) The presence of extensive tumor necrosis is a typical aspect of ATC (see asterisk *) (original magnification ×10); (**B**) The neoplastic cells show marked nuclear atypia with spindled and pleomorphic morphology, associated to elevated mitotic rate, simulating high-grade pleomorphic sarcoma. In the insert, focal immunostaining for cytokeratins supports the epithelial nature of ATC (original magnification ×20); (**C**) At higher magnification, the pronounced nuclear atypia and an atypical mitosis (see arrow) are shown (original magnification ×40). (**D–F**) Poorly differentiated thyroid carcinoma (PDTC) (hematoxylin and eosin stain); (**D**) The typical example of PDTC is the so-called "insular carcinoma". In this field, the tumor shows a small focus of tumor necrosis (see asterisk *) (original magnification ×10); (**E**) The neoplasm exhibits a prevalent solid growth pattern (original magnification ×20); (**F**) At higher magnification, the tumor cells appear small and uniform, the nuclei are generally rounded and hyperchromatic, in absence of the typical aspects of papillary thyroid carcinoma (original magnification ×40).

In the past, many treatments were proposed to answer this aforementioned need, but with disappointing results [10]. Nowadays many clinicians are proposing genetically guided treatments for PDTC and ATC, according to the new discoveries about their genetic landscape [11,12].

In the current review, as first, we summarize the upcoming findings about genetic features of PDTC and ATC, from mutations occurring in DNA to alterations in RNA; therefore, we describe their tumor microenvironments and the interactions between tumor and other neighboring cells; finally, we recapitulate how this upcoming evidence are changing the treatment of PDTC and ATC.

2. Genetics Features

Genomic instability is universally considered as a driver of carcinogenesis, supporting the generation of all hallmarks of cancer (i.e., resistance to cell death, promotion of proliferative signaling, escape from growth suppressors, invasion and metastasis capacity, activation of replicative immortality, evasion of immune destruction, deregulation cellular energetics and neo-angiogenesis) [13,14]. Across several neoplasia, thyroid cancer presents lower genomic instability, expressed as the number of mutations per tumor, compared to other adult neoplasia (e.g., endometrial and colorectal cancers) [15]; this evidence has also been confirmed in metastatic cases [16]. However, thyroid cancer shows a heterogenous mutational burden across its histotypes: ATC presents an increased number of genetic alterations per tumor (median 4, range 0–29) compared to PTC and FTC [17]; likewise, according to data from Tissue Cancer Genome Atlas (TCGA), PDTC mutational burden is higher than PTC, even if lower than ATC [18,19]. Genomic instability in PDTC and ATC embraces both somatic driver mutations and gene fusions.

2.1. Somatic Driver Mutations

Vogelstein et al. considered a driver mutation as a genomic variant that directly or indirectly induces a selective growth advantage [20]. As shown in Table 1, ATC and PDTC harbor many driver mutations, occurring mainly in both MAPK and PI3K-AKT pathways.

BRAF and RAS genes (HRAS, KRAS, and NRAS) are main members of MAPK pathway. Both of them occur in more than 25% of ATCs, according to catalogue of somatic mutations in cancer (COSMIC) database [21], while 15.38–33.33% and 6.8–41.2% of PDTCs harbor BRAF and RAS mutations, respectively (Table 1) [18,22–24]. Interestingly, although BRAF and RAS mutations are present in a relevant percentage of both ATC and PDTC cases, they seem to play different roles. In ATC, neither BRAF or RAS mutations seem to be sufficient to induce neoplastic cell anaplasia. McFadden et al. produced a thyroid-specific CreER transgenic mouse in order to specifically induce $BRAF^{V600E}$ mutation in thyroid cells; although this mutation induces PTC foci, it was capable to promote ATC tumorigenesis only in the presence of p53 mutation [25]. Likewise, $KRAS^{G12D}$ mutation developed anaplastic foci with complete deregulation of normal thyroid follicular morphology in mice model only in association with a homozygous mutation of TSH receptor [26]. However, BRAF-RAS signaling retains a crucial role in ATC cells and its inhibition by siRNA anti-BRAF produces growth arrest in ATC cell lines [27], even stronger in combination with MEK inhibition [25]. Otherwise, the mechanisms seem to be different in PDTC: Vitagliano et al. were able to promote progression of FTC foci into PDTC in mouse model by $NRAS^{G61K}$ mutation [28].

Table 1. ATC and PDTC genetic landscape: somatic mutations.

Cellular Function		Gene	Mutation Rate (%)	
			ATC [21,29]	PDTC [18,22–24]
Intracellular signaling	MAPK pathway	*BRAF*	27.63	15.38–33.33
		NRAS	19.25	4.35–30.77
		NF1	5.56	0
		KRAS	4.92	0–5.31
		HRAS	4.51	2.45–4.88
	PI3K-AKT pathway	*PIK3CA*	11.24	2.38–19.51
		PTEN	9.27	0–4.35
		NF2	5.10	0
		IRS1	3.64	-
		AKT1	-	0-8.70
	WNT pathway	*AXIN1*	4.51	-
		CTNNB1	3.88	0–2.44
		APC	3.05	17.39
Cell cycle regulation		*TERT promoter*	75	21.95–40.48
		TP53	45.67	8.33–43.48
		ATM	4.91	7.14–13.04
		RB1	4.36	1.19–4.35
		CDKN2A	4.01	-
Chromatin remolding		*KMT2D*	4.42	-
		CREBBP	4.17	-
		ARID2	3.93	-
		ARID1A	3.69	-
		DNMT3A	3.38	-
		KMT2A	3.36	-
DNA damage response		*MDC1*	3.18	-
		MSH2	3.05	-
Protein metabolism		*EIF1AX*	9.24	4.88–10.71
		CALR	4.85	-
		RBM10	3.38	-

In addition to mutations of MAPK pathway, next generation analysis showed that ATC harbors higher prevalence of mutations in PI3K-AKT pathway compared to other histotypes [30]: according to COSMIC database, PI3KCA and PTEN were found mutated in 11.24% and 9.27%, respectively (Table 1) [21]. Likewise, also PDTC harbors frequently PIK3CA or AKT1 mutations (2.38–19.51% and 0–8.70%, respectively) (Table 1) [18,22–24].

Interestingly, in ATC series provided by Liu et al., the 81.3% of samples presented genetic alterations affecting both MAPK and PI3K-AKT pathways [31]. Accordingly, in mouse model, the presence of mutations occurring in both pathways induced ATC foci, confirming the synergistic interactions between these pathways [32]. On one hand, MAPK pathway has a crucial role in cell proliferation and survival, and, on the other hand, upregulated PI3K-AKT pathway has been related to tumor aggressiveness [33].

Beyond mutations occurring at members of MAPK and PI3K-AKT pathways, many variants have been reported in cell cycle regulators. Many reports showed that mutations occurring in p53 and TERT promoter (pTERT) are highly prevalent in ATC, occurring even simultaneously [17,18,21] (Table 1). Likewise, PDTC presents both mutations, even if less frequently than ATC [18,34]. Intriguingly, in the presence of an impaired cell-cycle checkpoint pathway (e.g., p53), the occurrence of a concomitant mutation in telomerase activity (e.g., pTERT) could induce an indefinite cell proliferation [35]. In addition, the interplays between the duet BRAF-pTERT have recently been described by Tan and colleagues [36]. In particular, in case of mutation of both of them, cancer cells suppress apoptosis mainly thank to pTERT activity, while in case of mutation occurring only on BRAF gene, apoptosis activity seems to be not significantly affected [36]. Accordingly, the inhibition of TERT activity could represent an Achilles heel, as recently shown in-vitro and in-vivo model by Bu et al. In these models, BIBR1532 (a TERT inhibitor) significantly inhibited tumor growth as well as cell invasion, migration and angiogenesis [37].

If regulation of cell cycle has a crucial role in oncogenesis, also protein metabolism control has been deeply involved in tumorigenesis [14,38]. Not surprisingly, both PDTC and ATC harbor EIF1AX mutations in about 10% of cases (Table 1) [18,22–24]. EIF1AX is a member of 43S preinitiation complexes, responsible of translation initiation, and its mutation has recently been involved in preinitiation complex stabilization and, further, in deregulating protein synthesis [39,40]. Interestingly, EIF1AX mutations are mutually exclusive with other drivers in PTC [19], while they co-occur with RAS mutations in ATC and PDTC [18]. Recently, Krishnamoorthy et al. showed a positive feedback relationship between RAS and EIF1AX proteins, which reinforces c-MYC gene expression [40].

2.2. Gene Fusions

Fusion genes are common driver mutations described in both hematopoietic and solid tumors [41]. They usually involve a driver gene, which expresses a receptor tyrosine kinase (e.g., RET) or its downstream kinase (e.g., BRAF), and a partner gene (e.g., NCOA4). If in physiologic state most of these kinases require the ligand to induce their dimerization, these rearrangements are capable to induce a ligand-independent dimerization and a deregulated kinase activity [42]. In the past, all the tumorigenic effects were considered as consequence of a non-controlled expression of the driver gene; however, new evidence suggests that also the partner gene may play a crucial oncogenic role [43].

Although fusion genes have been extensively described in thyroid cancer, their prevalence is lower compared to other solid tumors [41]. PDTC harbors gene fusions in 10–14% of cases while ATC in 3–5% [44] (Table 2). Interestingly, when present, fusions usually involve the same few oncogenes. RET fusions are the most common, mainly CCDC6-RET (RET/PTC1) and NCOA4-RET (RET/PTC3), while NTRK, ALK and BRAF fusions are quite rare (Table 2) [44]. Recently, Nikitski et al. developed a mouse model of STRN-ALK fusion gene that was capable of inducing PTC, PDTC and ATC foci [45]. This model revealed the presence of two clusters of PDTC with specific cell morphology, immunohistochemical characteristics and different levels of expression of thyroid differentiation markers [45].

Table 2. ATC and PDTC genetic landscape: gene fusions.

Gene Fusions		Mutation Rate [16,18,29,44,46]	
		ATC	PDTC
PAX8-PPARγ Fusions		0	3/84
NTRK fusions	*NTRK1-IRF2BP2*	1/126	0
	NTRK2-CRNDE	1/126	0
	ETV6-NTRK3	0	1/60
RET fusions	*CCDC6-RET*	2/126	3/84, 2/60
	NCOA4-RET	Case report	2/84, 1/23
	PDCD10-RET	0	1/60
	TFG-RET	0	1/60
ALK fusions	*STRN-ALK*	Case report	1/23
	EML4-ALK	0	2/84
BRAF fusions	*KIAA1549-BRAF*	Case report	0
	SCRIB-BRAF	0	1/60
Other fusions	NUT-BRD4	1/33	0

Although rare, gene fusions could represent precious targets for targeted therapies. Moreover, any histotype of thyroid cancers with gene fusions has recently been proposed as a discrete group with specific histologic characteristics such as multinodular growth and extensive fibrotic features. For this reason, they have been named "kinase fusion-related thyroid carcinomas" [46].

2.3. Copy Number Variations

In oncology, copy number variations (CNVs) are well characterized as prognostic factors for recurrence and death [47]. This evidence has been confirmed also in advanced thyroid cancer [18]. If they are quite rare in differentiated thyroid cancer (less than 10%) [19], in PDTC and ATC they are widespread, especially in cancers without known driver mutation (losses of 1p, 8p, 13q, 15q, 17p, 22q, and gains of 1q and 20q) [18]. Interestingly, they seem to be hystotipes-specific: 8p and 17p losses and 20q gains are more frequent in ATC while loss of 1p was substantially more recurring in PDTCs [18]. Moreover, CNVs correlate with gene context where occur: 1p, 13q, and 15q losses were enriched in PDTCs without known driver mutation while loss of 22q was associated with RAS-mutated PDTCs [18]. In ATC, beyond large chromosomal variations, Pozdeyev et al. reported more restricted CNVs such as losses of CDKN2A and CDKN2B or amplification of KIT, PDGFRA and KDR, further confirmed by other authors [17,24].

Finally, since CNVs have recently been related to resistance to target therapies in thyroid cancer [48], it would be very interesting to ascertain if some of them (e.g., PDGFRA amplification) could induce resistance to target therapy (e.g., multikinase inhibitors, MKIs) in ATC and PDTC.

2.4. RNA Alterations

It is universally recognized that messenger RNA (mRNA) synthesis and translation are deeply modified in cancer; however, new evidence shows that all kinds of RNA are universally impaired [49]. In normal condition, cells produce different types of RNAs: mRNA, ribosomal RNA (rRNA), transfer RNA (tRNA), microRNA (miRNA), long non-coding (lncRNA) and circular RNA (circRNA). Accordingly, neoplastic cells could deregulate all kinds of RNAs that could promote the cells growth and invasiveness [49].

In particular, miRNA are usually 20–23 nucleotides in length that can bind multiple mRNA, regulating their catabolism and further their translation [50]. 127 and 18 different miRNAs have been characterized in ATC and PDTC, respectively. Among them, 69 miRNAs resulted decreased and 54 increased in ATC, while 10 resulted decreased and

8 increased in PDTC. If their role in PDTC is not fully elucidated and they might be used as an ancillary diagnostic tool and prognostic marker [51], they have been fully characterized in ATC. According to literature data, we grouped them into 3 main roles: regulation of growth tumor, invasiveness and resistance to therapy (Figure 2). We found that 9 miRNA were related to tumor growth [52–61], 14 to tumor growth and invasiveness [62–69], 28 to invasiveness [67,70–76], and 66 to therapies resistance (62 to anti-BRAF treatment, 3 to chemotherapy and 1 to radiotherapy) [77–81]. Additionally, 10 miRNAs were considered as an ancillary diagnostic tool [82,83] (Figure 2).

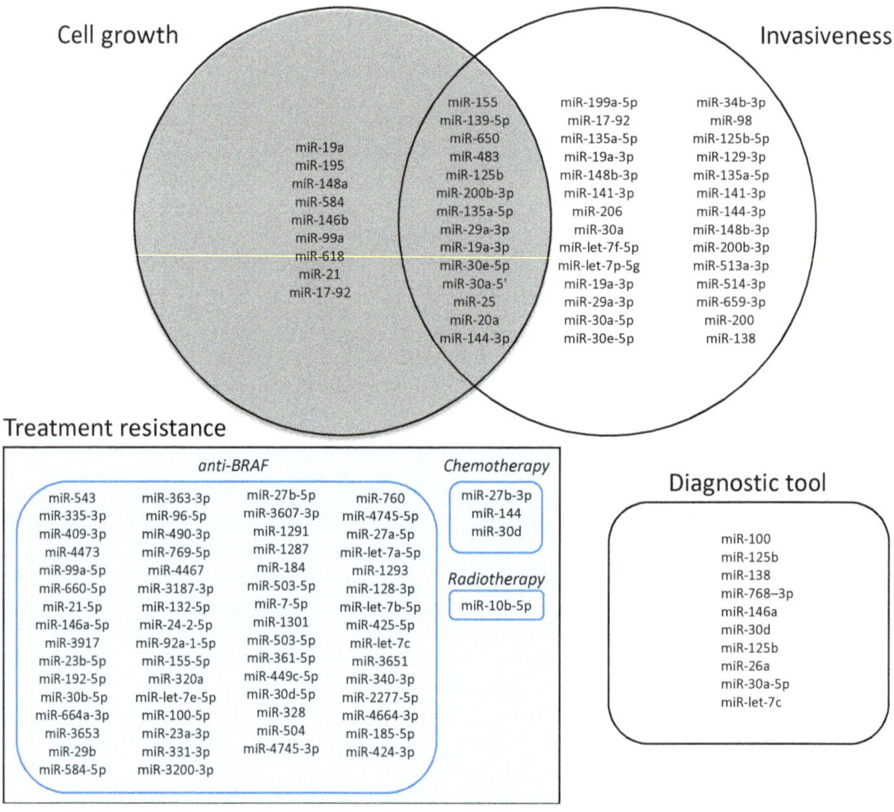

Figure 2. miRNA that were discovered in ATC according to their function.

Beyond miRNA, growing evidence is showing the role of lncRNAs in cancer. lncRNA are RNAs longer than 200 nucleotides that do not encode proteins but regulate gene expression, splicing and nucleation of subnuclear domains [49]; moreover, lncRNAs may have cytoplasmic functions, such as miRNA sponging, interaction with signaling proteins, and further modulation of mRNA translation [49]. In ATC, lncRNAs may regulate tumor growth [84,85], invasiveness [86], and both tumor growth and invasiveness [87–91]; they can also regulate cancer sensitivity to treatments [92]. In particular, lncRNA PTCSC3 was described at low levels both in ATC tissue and cell lines and it was demonstrated that its upregulation inhibited the resistance to doxorubicin by suppressing stem cell proprieties [92].

Finally, circRNAs are usually consequence of back-splicing events, producing in a covalently closed circRNA molecule instead of linear ones. Although circRNAs have usually been detected at low levels in normal and in cancer cells, some of them are at higher concentration and have functional roles: miRNA sponging and proteins stabilization [49]. In ATC, a recent study showed that circRNA may produce resistance to chemotherapy. In particular, Liu et al. showed that circRNA EIF6 could sponge miR-144-3p to promote autophagy and cisplatin-resistance [93].

3. Tumor Microenvironment

Tumor microenvironment (TME) is the dynamic milieu that harbors tumor cells [94]. It comprises blood vessels, extracellular matrix (ECM), non-neoplastic cells, and signaling molecules [95]. Neoplastic cells interact with other TME members in order to regulate self-growth, invasiveness and resistance to therapy [94]. In thyroid, many reports showed that TME may promote tumor growth, metastatic power, and resistance to therapy, both in differentiated and anaplastic thyroid cancer [96–98].

In TME we should distinguish not immune and immune related cells. Among the former, cancer associated fibroblasts play a relevant role in both ATC and PDTC [99,100]. In ATC, tumor cells present paracrine communication with fibroblast: ATC cells activate fibroblasts by reprogramming their metabolism, phenotype and secretome, and then activated fibroblasts reinforce thyroid cancer progression, by enhancing tumor invasion and proliferation [100]. Likewise, interactions between PDTC cells and cancer associated fibroblasts may potentiate tumor progression, by collagen remodeling [99]. Analog interplays have been recently demonstrated between ATC and endothelial cells, partially rescued by sorafenib [94].

Giannini et al. provided significant evidence about immune TME in ATC and PDTC [101]. ATC TME was enriched of tumor infiltrating leukocytes (both macrophage and lymphocytes) and characterized by hot or altered–immunosuppressed phenotype, since a relevant part of CD8+ lymphocytes presented exhausted features. Accordingly, Caillou et al. showed that tumor-associated macrophages build up a dense network in whom cancer cells reside [102,103] and their presence is associated with a worse prognosis in ATC [104]. Cameselle-García and colleagues elucidated that ATC tumors are enriched of tumor infiltrating lymphocytes (mainly CD8+ cytotoxic T cells), which mainly reside in the interface between tumor ant thyroid tissue [105]. Otherwise, PDTC harbored less tumor infiltrating leukocytes compared to ATC, and presented a cold immune contexture in 65% of cases [101]. In these immune contexts, PD/PD-L1 pathway (programmed cell death protein-1/programmed cell death ligand-1) plays a crucial role in ATC and less frequently also in PDTC [97,105,106]. If in physiologic conditions, PD/PD-L1 pathway regulates T cell immune suppression, in neoplastic milieu it is exploited by cancer cells in order to avoid immune attack, by inducing T-cell exhaustion [107]. In ATC, PD/PD-L1 proteins expression was shown to be regulated by BRAF mutation and is was associated to a worst prognosis [106,108]. Accordingly, Brauner et al. demonstrated that dual inhibition of BRAF and PD/PD-L1 pathways induced a powerful shrinkage of ATC tumor in orthotopic immune-competent mouse model [108].

4. Contemporary Treatment in ATC and PDTC

Traditionally, treatments against ATC and PDTC globally provided disappointing results [12,109]. ATC presents very low median overall survival [109,110]. Although PDTC presents higher 5-year survival (62%) compared to ATC [111], disease control in patients with metastatic PDTC is still poor (59%) and 85% of their disease specific deaths is related to the presence of distant metastasis [12]. In both of them, surgery represents a cornerstone of multimodal treatment; nonetheless, systemic treatment is necessary in case of diffuse disease. Systemic treatment comprises chemotherapy (in case of ATC, elsewhere reviewed [112]), anti-angiogenic therapy, immunotherapy and genetically guided therapy (Figure 3). Since their individual use provided encouraging but insufficient results, they have recently been proposed in multimodal approach.

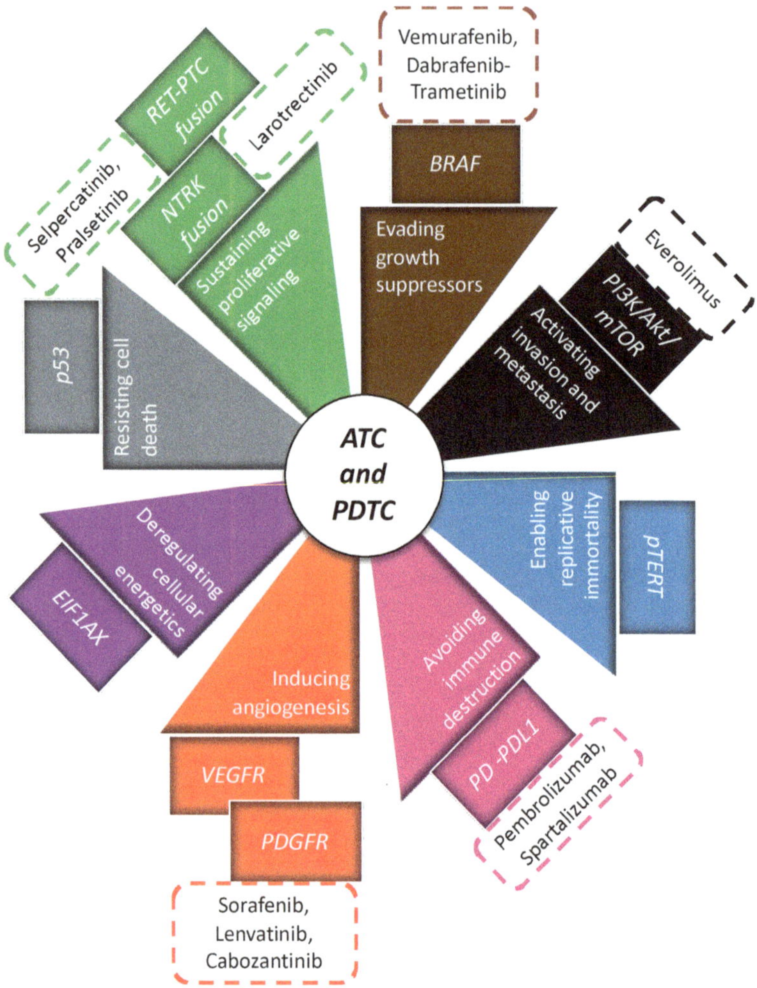

Figure 3. All innovative therapies that have been suggested in ATC and PDTC (rectangular box with dotted lines); each of them has been related to a specific inhibition of hallmark of cancer (triangle box) and cellular pathway (rectangular box).

4.1. Antiangiogenic Therapy

As previously shown, neo-angiogenesis is a main hallmark of cancer, sustaining its limitless growth [113]. Accordingly, neoplastic cells regulate neo-angiogenesis in order to guarantee their progression in ATC as well as in PDTC [114,115]. Many anti-angiogenic drugs have been employed to inhibit ATC and PDTC growth. Year by year, sorafenib, lenvatinib, cabozantinib, pazopanib, gefitinib and imatinib have been used with fluctuating results.

Sorafenib was the first anti-angiogenic drug proposed for ATC treatment. It was employed in two different phase-2 trials [116,117]; in both of them, disease control (partial response and stable disease) was reached in about 40% of patients but the median overall survival was still lower than 5 months [116,117]. Similarly, sorafenib seemed not to produce exciting results in PDTC [118]. From 2009 to 2011, 40 patients with PDTC were randomly allocated to sorafenib and placebo arms in a randomized, double-blind, multicentric, phase-3 trial (DECISION trial). Although not statistically significant, the sub analysis on PDTC showed a consistent improvement of PFS in patients treated with sorafenib as in all the other histotypes [119]. As reported in DECISION trial, sorafenib toxicity is mainly characterized by grade 1 and grade 2 adverse events such as hand–foot skin reaction, diarrhoea, alopecia, rash/desquamation, fatigue, weight loss, and hypertension [119].

Lenvatinib had very promising results in in-vitro and in-vivo models of ATC that were partially confirmed in clinical settings [120]. Takahashi et al. performed a phase II clinical trial, showing an overall survival of 10.6 months (95% CI: 3.8–19.8) and disease control in 16 out of 17 patients [121]. However, different results were given by a recent post-marketing observational study which reviewed 124 patients affected by ATC and treated with lenvatinib [122]. It showed a disease control in 76.2% (66.89–83.96%) of patients; however, this response seemed to be only transient, because the time-to-treatment failure was 74.5 (57.0–108.0) days, and the median overall survival was still poor (3.4, 95% CI 2.66–4.33 months) [122]. At the same time, baseline clinical conditions of enrolled patients were poor (ECOG > 1) in more than 70% and this could partially explain these disappointing findings. Further studies should be employed in order to verify lenvatinib efficacy in ATC patients with better clinical conditions. Otherwise, lenvatinib produced interesting results for PDTC patients. In SELECT trial, which explored lenvatinib efficacy in patients with radioiodine-refractory thyroid cancer, 28 patients harboring PDTC were enrolled. In this selected population, lenvatinib confirmed its efficacy compared to placebo (HR 0.21, 0.08–0.56) [123]. Accordingly, a retrospective multicentric analysis of real-world data confirmed these encouraging results [124]. In this analysis of clinical practice in Austria enrolling 43 patients, the overall survival seemed to be not modified by tumor subtype (differentiated vs. poorly differentiated/anaplastic TC), whereas a maintenance dosage higher than 14 mg was associated with better prognosis [124]. About toxicity, in spite of high proportion of adverse events with grade $\geq$ III in SELECT trial (75.9%), Austrian, Italian, and French real-world data reported lower rates of adverse events of grade $\geq$ III (44%, 22.3% and 48%, respectively) [123–126]. Fatigue, hypertension, diarrhea, decreased weight, stomatitis, and anorexia are the most common reported adverse events [125,126].

More recently, cabozantinib has been explored as a salvage therapy for patients with radioiodine-refractory thyroid cancer already treated with MKIs. In this trial, 7 patients with PDTC were enrolled to receive cabozantinib and all of them presented clinical benefit (3 PR and 4 SD) [127]. Other antiangiogenic agents (pazopanib, gefitinib and imatinib) were employed for ATC therapy but they did not produce encouraging results [128–130].

4.2. Genetically Guided Therapy

Many reports showed that ATC has a singular genomic and transcriptomic landscape (ATC-like) [131]. In this singular genomic landscape, BRAF-MEK pathway was proposed as a potential target.

After the exciting results of BRAF inhibition in BRAF-mutated melanoma [132], a multicenter prospective "basket" trial, encompassing tumors with BRAF mutation, enrolled 7 patients affected by ATC for treatment with vemurafenib: 2 of them experienced a durable partial response (more than 11 months) [133]. In order to produce a stronger inhibition of BRAF-MEK pathway, dual inhibition of BRAF and MEK with dabrafenib and trametinib was proposed. Accordingly, in in-vitro ATC model, combined therapy induced greater growth inhibition than single agents [134]. Likewise, dabrafenib-trametinib therapy produced about 80% of 12-months progression free survival and overall survival in phase II clinical trial enrolling 16 patients [135]. Moreover, 1 patient experienced a complete response, 10 partial response, 3 stable disease and only 1 disease progression. In this trial, fatigue (44%), pyrexia (31%), and nausea (31%), were the most common adverse events, although the 50% of enrolled patients reported an adverse event with grade $\geq$ III [135]. This trial permitted the approval of this combination by FDA for treatment of $BRAF^{V600E}$ mutated ATC.

As previously reported, PI3K/Akt/mTOR has a crucial role in ATC cells and also anti-mTOR inhibitors have been proposed with conflicting results. Everolimus was used to treat one patient with ATC harboring a mutation of Tuberous Sclerosis 2 protein (TSC2), member of PI3K/AKT/mTOR pathway, obtaining an extraordinary 18-month response [136]. However, these promising results were not confirmed in other studies [137,138].

New perspectives have recently been opened for patients with ATC or PDTC harboring RET fusion genes, since highly selective RET inhibitors, such as selpercatinib and pralsetinib, are currently under investigation [139,140]. In 2020, a phase 1–2 clinical trial enrolled patients with thyroid cancer harboring an activating RET alteration for treatment with selpercatinib (LIBRETTO-001). In this trial, one patient with ATC and 3 with PDTC were enrolled. Interestingly, the patient with ATC reached PR as best response as well as 2 out of 3 patients with PDTC, while the other one with PDTC obtained SD [139]. Furthermore, selpercatinib presents a more tolerable toxicity profile with a rate of adverse events $\geq$ III of only 30% compared to other targeted therapies and the most common reported adverse events were hypertension, increased alanine or aspartate aminotransferase level, hyponatremia and diarrhea. Likewise, Cabanillas et al. have recently presented data about the use of larotrectinib, a NTRK fusion gene inhibitor, in 7 patients with ATC. Intriguingly, 3 out of 7 reached PR and SD, while 3 patients experienced PD [141]. Grade $\geq$ III adverse events occurred in 46% of patients, although only 7% of patients presented ones that were considered related to larotrectinib [141]. Recently, an excellent response was documented with crizotinib in one patient with ATC, harboring ALK-RET fusion gene [142].

Other agents such as HDAC inhibitors have been used but with disappointing results (NCT03002623 trial).

4.3. Immunotherapy

Immunotherapy is inducing a deep change in anticancer therapy, regulating immune cells attack against neoplastic cells. Interestingly, many reports showed that ATC presents higher PD-L1^{+} cells compared to DTC, proposing PD/PD-L1 pathway as targetable [101,143], and, as shown above, preclinical data produced interesting result in mouse model [108]. Accordingly, PD-1 antibodies (e.g., pembrolizumab and spartalizumab), after promising data about their use in BRAF-mutated melanoma [144], have been used as single agents in patients affected by ATC [145].

Pembrolizumab induced a durable response (16 months) in one patient with unresectable ATC: after its second cycle the patient referred a significant improvement of dysphagia and after 3 cycle a complete response was almost reached [146]. However, after a severe toxicity related to pembrolizumab (grade 4 colitis), it was suspended and the patient died 8 months later, after the appearance of cerebral metastasis [146]. On the other hand, it seemed to do not produce the same result when co-administrated with chemoradiotherapy. Chintakuntlawar et al. treated 3 patients with pembrolizumab and chemoradiotherapy, but, in spite of a prompt an early tumor response, all patients passed away <6 months [147].

Spartalizumab toxicity and efficacy were evaluated in a phase I/II trial enrolling 42 patients with locally advanced and/or metastatic anaplastic thyroid carcinoma [148]. The overall response rate was 19% in the whole cohort, while it was higher in patients defined as PD-L1–positive (29%), and even better in the subset of patients with PD-L1 expression > 50% (35%). In this last subset of patients, the 1-year survival rate reached 52.1% [148]. About toxicity profile, the most frequent adverse events were diarrhea, pruritus, fatigue, and pyrexia and grade $\geq$ III adverse events related to treatment were observed in 10% of patients [148].

4.4. Multimodal Therapy

Considering the promising data about single regimens, many clinicians proposed a multimodal therapy against ATC in order to reduce therapy resistance. Moreover, driver mutations such as BRAF were proposed as master regulators of immune TME in thyroid cancer [114,149].

Multimodal therapy against immune TME and main mutated pathways could induce a deep inhibition of ATC growth and progression, evading resistance mechanisms.

In 2018, Cabanillas et al. showed one case of locally aggressive unresectable ATC treated with neo-adjuvant therapy composed by dabrafenib, trametinib and pembrolizumab (DTP) [150]. Interestingly, the patient had a relevant response, allowing a complete surgical resection followed by postoperative chemoradiation. Likewise, other 4 clinical cases have recently been reported about DTP use as neoadjuvant therapy in ATC, with unexpected high PFS (19.5, 95% CI: 13.75–24.5, months) [151].

Immunotherapy has been proposed also in adjuvant therapy with dabrafenib and trametinib or lenvatinib. Iyer et al. [152] used pembrolizumab as salvage therapy in 5 patients treated with dabrafenib and trametinib, 1 with trametinib, and 6 with lenvatinib. Although 2 patients experienced PD, 5 patients had PR and 5 had SD and, from the start of targeted therapies, the median OS was 10.4 months (95% CI = 6.02, 14.83, range 5.4–40 months) [152]. In this series, fatigue, anemia and hypertension were the most common AEs associated with this combination and drug-induced rash and altered mental status (likely related to PD) induced drug interruption [152]. Similarly, Dierks et al. showed interesting results about lenvatinib and pembrolizumab combined treatment both in ATC and PDTC: 5/6 patients with ATC reached CR/PR and 2/2 with PDTC obtained PR [153]. Similarly, nivolumab (anti-PD1 antibody) was added to vemurafenib in patients affected by metastatic ATC, obtaining a prolonged response (more than 20 months) [154]. According to these results, new clinical trials are ongoing (e.g., NCT03181100).

In 2017, 6 patients with PDTC and 2 with ATC were enrolled to receive sorafenib and temsirolimus (mTOR inhibitor) in a non-randomized clinical trial. In one hand, results in patients with PDTC were encouraging and 4 patients reached PR and 2 SD; on the other hand, one patient with ATC had PR and the other one had PD [155]. Furthermore, 14% of enrolled patients discontinued the treatment for toxicity and most common adverse events grade ≥ 3 were hyperglycemia, fatigue, anemia, and oral mucositis [155].

5. Conclusions

PDTC and ATC are rare but, unfortunately, they are lethal although a relevant different 5-year survival rate (5 years vs. 6 months). Nowadays, we know many elements of their genetic landscape and tumor microenvironment. This knowledge helped the scientific community to identify therapies which specifically target these cancers. Some of them (e.g., DTP) has recently reached the clinical practice and could be prescribed for BRAF^{V600E} mutated ATC. However, their therapeutic benefit is still scarce and many other studies are necessary to answer these unmet clinical needs.

Funding: This research received no external funding.

Conflicts of Interest: The authors declare no conflict of interest.

References

1. Kitahara, C.M.; Sosa, J.A. The Changing Incidence of Thyroid Cancer. *Nat. Rev. Endocrinol.* **2016**, *12*, 646–653. [CrossRef] [PubMed]
2. Borda, A.; Zahan, A.-E.; Piciu, D.; Barbuș, E.; Berger, N.; Nechifor-Boilă, A. A 15 Year Institutional Experience of Well-Differentiated Follicular Cell-Derived Thyroid Carcinomas; Impact of the New 2017 TNM and WHO Classifications of Tumors of Endocrine Organs on the Epidemiological Trends and Pathological Characteristics. *Endocrine* **2020**, *67*, 630–642. [CrossRef]
3. Mirian, C.; Grønhøj, C.; Jensen, D.H.; Jakobsen, K.K.; Karnov, K.; Jensen, J.S.; Hahn, C.H.; Klitmøller, T.A.; Bentzen, J.; von Buchwald, C. Trends in Thyroid Cancer: Retrospective Analysis of Incidence and Survival in Denmark 1980–2014. *Cancer Epidemiol.* **2018**, *55*, 81–87. [CrossRef] [PubMed]
4. de la Fouchardière, C.; Decaussin-Petrucci, M.; Berthiller, J.; Descotes, F.; Lopez, J.; Lifante, J.C.; Peix, J.L.; Giraudet, A.L.; Delahaye, A.; Masson, S.; et al. Predictive Factors of Outcome in Poorly Differentiated Thyroid Carcinomas. *Eur. J. Cancer* **2018**. [CrossRef]
5. Smallridge, R.C.; Copland, J.A. Anaplastic Thyroid Carcinoma: Pathogenesis and Emerging Therapies. *Clin. Oncol.* **2010**. [CrossRef] [PubMed]

6. Volante, M.; Collini, P.; Nikiforov, Y.E.; Sakamoto, A.; Kakudo, K.; Katoh, R.; Lloyd, R.V.; LiVolsi, V.A.; Papotti, M.; Sobrinho-Simoes, M.; et al. Poorly Differentiated Thyroid Carcinoma: The Turin Proposal for the Use of Uniform Diagnostic Criteria and an Algorithmic Diagnostic Approach. *Am. J. Surg. Pathol.* **2007**, *31*, 1256–1264. [CrossRef] [PubMed]
7. Hiltzik, D.; Carlson, D.L.; Tuttle, R.M.; Chuai, S.; Ishill, N.; Shaha, A.; Shah, J.P.; Singh, B.; Ghossein, R.A. Poorly Differentiated Thyroid Carcinomas Defined on the Basis of Mitosis and Necrosis: A Clinicopathologic Study of 58 Patients. *Cancer* **2006**, *106*, 1286–1295. [CrossRef] [PubMed]
8. Njim, L.; Moussa, A.; Hadhri, R.; Gassab, I.; Ben Yahia, N.; Mahmoudi, H.; Zakhama, A. Angiomatoid tumor of the thyroid gland: Primitive angiosarcoma or variant of anaplastic carcinoma? *Ann. Pathol.* **2008**, *28*, 221–224. [CrossRef] [PubMed]
9. Prete, A.; Cosentino, G.; Manetti, L.; Ambrosini, C.E.; Papini, P.; Marinò, M.; Torregrossa, L.; Marcocci, C.; Elisei, R.; Lupi, I. Firm Mass in Thyroid of an Elderly Patient: Not Always Cancer. *Endocrinol. Diabetes Metab. Case Rep.* **2020**, *2020*. [CrossRef]
10. Ain, K.B. Anaplastic Thyroid Carcinoma: Behavior, Biology, and Therapeutic Approaches. *Thyroid* **1998**, *8*, 715–726. [CrossRef]
11. Molinaro, E.; Romei, C.; Biagini, A.; Sabini, E.; Agate, L.; Mazzeo, S.; Materazzi, G.; Sellari-Franceschini, S.; Ribechini, A.; Torregrossa, L.; et al. Anaplastic Thyroid Carcinoma: From Clinicopathology to Genetics and Advanced Therapies. *Nat. Rev. Endocrinol.* **2017**, *13*, 644–660. [CrossRef]
12. Ibrahimpasic, T.; Ghossein, R.; Shah, J.P.; Ganly, I. Poorly Differentiated Carcinoma of the Thyroid Gland: Current Status and Future Prospects. *Thyroid* **2019**, *29*, 311–321. [CrossRef] [PubMed]
13. Andor, N.; Maley, C.C.; Ji, H.P. Genomic Instability in Cancer: Teetering on the Limit of Tolerance. *Cancer Res.* **2017**, *77*, 2179–2185. [CrossRef]
14. Hanahan, D.; Weinberg, R.A. Hallmarks of Cancer: The Next Generation. *Cell* **2011**, *144*, 646–674. [CrossRef]
15. Martincorena, I.; Raine, K.M.; Gerstung, M.; Dawson, K.J.; Haase, K.; Van Loo, P.; Davies, H.; Stratton, M.R.; Campbell, P.J. Universal Patterns of Selection in Cancer and Somatic Tissues. *Cell* **2017**, *171*, 1029–1041.e21. [CrossRef] [PubMed]
16. Zehir, A.; Benayed, R.; Shah, R.H.; Syed, A.; Middha, S.; Kim, H.R.; Srinivasan, P.; Gao, J.; Chakravarty, D.; Devlin, S.M.; et al. Mutational Landscape of Metastatic Cancer Revealed from Prospective Clinical Sequencing of 10,000 Patients. *Nat. Med.* **2017**, *23*, 15.
17. Pozdeyev, N.; Gay, L.M.; Sokol, E.S.; Hartmaier, R.; Deaver, K.E.; Davis, S.; French, J.D.; Borre, P.V.; LaBarbera, D.V.; Tan, A.-C.; et al. Genetic Analysis of 779 Advanced Differentiated and Anaplastic Thyroid Cancers. *Clin. Cancer Res.* **2018**, *24*, 3059–3068. [CrossRef]
18. Landa, I.; Ibrahimpasic, T.; Boucai, L.; Sinha, R.; Knauf, J.A.; Shah, R.H.; Dogan, S.; Ricarte-Filho, J.C.; Krishnamoorthy, G.P.; Xu, B.; et al. Genomic and Transcriptomic Hallmarks of Poorly Differentiated and Anaplastic Thyroid Cancers. *J. Clin. Investig.* **2016**, *126*, 1052–1066. [CrossRef] [PubMed]
19. Cancer Genome Atlas Research Network Integrated Genomic Characterization of Papillary Thyroid Carcinoma. *Cell* **2014**, *159*, 676–690. [CrossRef] [PubMed]
20. Vogelstein, B.; Papadopoulos, N.; Velculescu, V.E.; Zhou, S.; Diaz, L.A.; Kinzler, K.W. Cancer Genome Landscapes. *Science* **2013**, *339*, 1546–1558. [CrossRef]
21. Tate, J.G.; Bamford, S.; Jubb, H.C.; Sondka, Z.; Beare, D.M.; Bindal, N.; Boutselakis, H.; Cole, C.G.; Creatore, C.; Dawson, E.; et al. COSMIC: The Catalogue Of Somatic Mutations In Cancer. *Nucleic Acids Res.* **2019**, *47*, D941–D947. [CrossRef]
22. Gerber, T.S.; Schad, A.; Hartmann, N.; Springer, E.; Zechner, U.; Musholt, T.J. Targeted Next-Generation Sequencing of Cancer Genes in Poorly Differentiated Thyroid Cancer. *Endocr. Connect.* **2018**, *7*, 47–55. [CrossRef] [PubMed]
23. Duan, H.; Li, Y.; Hu, P.; Gao, J.; Ying, J.; Xu, W.; Zhao, D.; Wang, Z.; Ye, J.; Lizaso, A.; et al. Mutational Profiling of Poorly Differentiated and Anaplastic Thyroid Carcinoma by the Use of Targeted Next-Generation Sequencing. *Histopathology* **2019**, *75*, 890–899. [CrossRef] [PubMed]
24. Chen, H.; Luthra, R.; Routbort, M.J.; Patel, K.P.; Cabanillas, M.E.; Broaddus, R.R.; Williams, M.D. Molecular Profile of Advanced Thyroid Carcinomas by Next-Generation Sequencing: Characterizing Tumors Beyond Diagnosis for Targeted Therapy. *Mol. Cancer Ther.* **2018**, *17*, 1575–1584. [CrossRef] [PubMed]
25. McFadden, D.G.; Vernon, A.; Santiago, P.M.; Martinez-McFaline, R.; Bhutkar, A.; Crowley, D.M.; McMahon, M.; Sadow, P.M.; Jacks, T. P53 Constrains Progression to Anaplastic Thyroid Carcinoma in a Braf-Mutant Mouse Model of Papillary Thyroid Cancer. *Proc. Natl. Acad. Sci. USA* **2014**, *111*, E1600–E1609. [CrossRef] [PubMed]
26. Zhu, X.; Zhao, L.; Park, J.W.; Willingham, M.C.; Cheng, S.-Y. Synergistic Signaling of KRAS and Thyroid Hormone Receptor β Mutants Promotes Undifferentiated Thyroid Cancer through MYC Up-Regulation. *Neoplasia* **2014**, *16*, 757–769. [CrossRef]
27. Salvatore, G.; De Falco, V.; Salerno, P.; Nappi, T.C.; Pepe, S.; Troncone, G.; Carlomagno, F.; Melillo, R.M.; Wilhelm, S.M.; Santoro, M. BRAF Is a Therapeutic Target in Aggressive Thyroid Carcinoma. *Clin. Cancer Res.* **2006**, *12*, 1623–1629. [CrossRef]
28. Vitagliano, D.; Portella, G.; Troncone, G.; Francione, A.; Rossi, C.; Bruno, A.; Giorgini, A.; Coluzzi, S.; Nappi, T.C.; Rothstein, J.L.; et al. Thyroid Targeting of the N-Ras(Gln61Lys) Oncogene in Transgenic Mice Results in Follicular Tumors That Progress to Poorly Differentiated Carcinomas. *Oncogene* **2006**, *25*, 5467–5474. [CrossRef]
29. Xu, B.; Ghossein, R. Genomic Landscape of Poorly Differentiated and Anaplastic Thyroid Carcinoma. *Endocr. Pathol.* **2016**, *27*, 205–212. [CrossRef] [PubMed]
30. Li, Z.; Zhang, Y.; Wang, R.; Zou, K.; Zou, L. Genetic Alterations in Anaplastic Thyroid Carcinoma and Targeted Therapies. *Exp. Ther. Med.* **2019**, *18*, 2369–2377. [CrossRef]

31. Liu, Z.; Hou, P.; Ji, M.; Guan, H.; Studeman, K.; Jensen, K.; Vasko, V.; El-Naggar, A.K.; Xing, M. Highly Prevalent Genetic Alterations in Receptor Tyrosine Kinases and Phosphatidylinositol 3-Kinase/Akt and Mitogen-Activated Protein Kinase Pathways in Anaplastic and Follicular Thyroid Cancers. *J. Clin. Endocrinol. Metab.* **2008**, *93*, 3106–3116. [CrossRef] [PubMed]
32. Charles, R.-P.; Silva, J.; Iezza, G.; Phillips, W.A.; McMahon, M. Activating BRAF and PIK3CA Mutations Cooperate to Promote Anaplastic Thyroid Carcinogenesis. *Mol. Cancer Res.* **2014**, *12*, 979–986. [CrossRef] [PubMed]
33. Xing, M. Molecular Pathogenesis and Mechanisms of Thyroid Cancer. *Nat. Rev. Cancer* **2013**, *13*, 184–199. [CrossRef]
34. Romei, C.; Tacito, A.; Molinaro, E.; Piaggi, P.; Cappagli, V.; Pieruzzi, L.; Matrone, A.; Viola, D.; Agate, L.; Torregrossa, L.; et al. Clinical, Pathological and Genetic Features of Anaplastic and Poorly Differentiated Thyroid Cancer: A Single Institute Experience. *Oncol. Lett.* **2018**, *15*, 9174–9182. [CrossRef] [PubMed]
35. Shay, J.W.; Wright, W.E. Senescence and Immortalization: Role of Telomeres and Telomerase. *Carcinogenesis* **2005**, *26*, 867–874. [CrossRef]
36. Tan, J.; Liu, R.; Zhu, G.; Umbricht, C.B.; Xing, M. TERT Promoter Mutation Determines Apoptotic and Therapeutic Responses of BRAF-Mutant Cancers to BRAF and MEK Inhibitors: Achilles Heel. *Proc. Natl. Acad. Sci USA* **2020**, *117*, 15846–15851. [CrossRef]
37. Bu, R.; Siraj, A.K.; Divya, S.P.; Kong, Y.; Parvathareddy, S.K.; Al-Rasheed, M.; Al-Obaisi, K.A.S.; Victoria, I.G.; Al-Sobhi, S.S.; Al-Dawish, M.; et al. Telomerase Reverse Transcriptase Mutations Are Independent Predictor of Disease-Free Survival in Middle Eastern Papillary Thyroid Cancer. *Int. J. Cancer* **2018**, *142*, 2028–2039. [CrossRef]
38. Vander Heiden, M.G.; DeBerardinis, R.J. Understanding the Intersections between Metabolism and Cancer Biology. *Cell* **2017**, *168*, 657–669. [CrossRef]
39. Pestova, T.V.; Borukhov, S.I.; Hellen, C.U. Eukaryotic Ribosomes Require Initiation Factors 1 and 1A to Locate Initiation Codons. *Nature* **1998**, *394*, 854–859. [CrossRef] [PubMed]
40. Krishnamoorthy, G.P.; Davidson, N.R.; Leach, S.D.; Zhao, Z.; Lowe, S.W.; Lee, G.; Landa, I.; Nagarajah, J.; Saqcena, M.; Singh, K.; et al. EIF1AX and RAS Mutations Cooperate to Drive Thyroid Tumorigenesis through ATF4 and C-MYC. *Cancer Discov.* **2019**, *9*, 264–281. [CrossRef] [PubMed]
41. Stransky, N.; Cerami, E.; Schalm, S.; Kim, J.L.; Lengauer, C. The Landscape of Kinase Fusions in Cancer. *Nat. Commun.* **2014**, *5*, 4846. [CrossRef] [PubMed]
42. Gao, Q.; Liang, W.-W.; Foltz, S.M.; Mutharasu, G.; Jayasinghe, R.G.; Cao, S.; Liao, W.-W.; Reynolds, S.M.; Wyczalkowski, M.A.; Yao, L.; et al. Driver Fusions and Their Implications in the Development and Treatment of Human Cancers. *Cell Rep.* **2018**, *23*, 227–238. [CrossRef] [PubMed]
43. Santoro, M.; Carlomagno, F. Central Role of RET in Thyroid Cancer. *Cold Spring Harb. Perspect. Biol.* **2013**, *5*, a009233. [CrossRef]
44. Yakushina, V.D.; Lerner, L.V.; Lavrov, A.V. Gene Fusions in Thyroid Cancer. *Thyroid* **2018**, *28*, 158–167. [CrossRef] [PubMed]
45. Nikitski, A.V.; Rominski, S.L.; Condello, V.; Kaya, C.; Wankhede, M.; Panebianco, F.; Yang, H.; Altschuler, D.L.; Nikiforov, Y.E. Mouse Model of Thyroid Cancer Progression and Dedifferentiation Driven by STRN-ALK Expression and Loss of P53: Evidence for the Existence of Two Types of Poorly Differentiated Carcinoma. *Thyroid* **2019**, *29*, 1425–1437. [CrossRef] [PubMed]
46. Chu, Y.-H.; Wirth, L.J.; Farahani, A.A.; Nosé, V.; Faquin, W.C.; Dias-Santagata, D.; Sadow, P.M. Clinicopathologic Features of Kinase Fusion-Related Thyroid Carcinomas: An Integrative Analysis with Molecular Characterization. *Mod. Pathol.* **2020**, *33*, 2458–2472. [CrossRef]
47. Hieronymus, H.; Murali, R.; Tin, A.; Yadav, K.; Abida, W.; Moller, H.; Berney, D.; Scher, H.; Carver, B.; Scardino, P.; et al. Tumor Copy Number Alteration Burden Is a Pan-Cancer Prognostic Factor Associated with Recurrence and Death. *Elife* **2018**, *7*. [CrossRef] [PubMed]
48. Antonello, Z.A.; Hsu, N.; Bhasin, M.; Roti, G.; Joshi, M.; Van Hummelen, P.; Ye, E.; Lo, A.S.; Karumanchi, S.A.; Bryke, C.R.; et al. Vemurafenib-Resistance via de Novo RBM Genes Mutations and Chromosome 5 Aberrations Is Overcome by Combined Therapy with Palbociclib in Thyroid Carcinoma with BRAFV600E. *Oncotarget* **2017**, *8*, 84743–84760. [CrossRef] [PubMed]
49. Goodall, G.J.; Wickramasinghe, V.O. RNA in Cancer. *Nat. Rev. Cancer* **2021**, *21*, 22–36. [CrossRef]
50. Lin, S.; Gregory, R.I. MicroRNA Biogenesis Pathways in Cancer. *Nat. Rev. Cancer* **2015**, *15*, 321–333. [CrossRef]
51. Dettmer, M.S.; Perren, A.; Moch, H.; Komminoth, P.; Nikiforov, Y.E.; Nikiforova, M.N. MicroRNA Profile of Poorly Differentiated Thyroid Carcinomas: New Diagnostic and Prognostic Insights. *J. Mol. Endocrinol.* **2014**, *52*, 181–189. [CrossRef]
52. Calabrese, G.; Dolcimascolo, A.; Caruso, G.; Forte, S. MiR-19a Is Involved In Progression And Malignancy Of Anaplastic Thyroid Cancer Cells. *Onco Targets Ther.* **2019**, *12*, 9571–9583. [CrossRef] [PubMed]
53. Maroof, H.; Irani, S.; Arianna, A.; Vider, J.; Gopalan, V.; Lam, A.K.-Y. Interactions of Vascular Endothelial Growth Factor and P53 with MiR-195 in Thyroid Carcinoma: Possible Therapeutic Targets in Aggressive Thyroid Cancers. *Curr. Cancer Drug Targets* **2019**, *19*, 561–570. [CrossRef] [PubMed]
54. Sheng, W.; Chen, Y.; Gong, Y.; Dong, T.; Zhang, B.; Gao, W. MiR-148a Inhibits Self-Renewal of Thyroid Cancer Stem Cells via Repressing INO80 Expression. *Oncol. Rep.* **2016**, *36*, 3387–3396. [CrossRef]
55. Orlandella, F.M.; Di Maro, G.; Ugolini, C.; Basolo, F.; Salvatore, G. TWIST1/MiR-584/TUSC2 Pathway Induces Resistance to Apoptosis in Thyroid Cancer Cells. *Oncotarget* **2016**, *7*, 70575–70588. [CrossRef] [PubMed]
56. Wang, S.; Chen, Y.; Bai, Y. P21 Participates in the Regulation of Anaplastic Thyroid Cancer Cell Proliferation by MiR-146b. *Oncol. Lett.* **2016**, *12*, 2018–2022. [CrossRef]

57. Haghpanah, V.; Fallah, P.; Tavakoli, R.; Naderi, M.; Samimi, H.; Soleimani, M.; Larijani, B. Antisense-MiR-21 Enhances Differentiation/Apoptosis and Reduces Cancer Stemness State on Anaplastic Thyroid Cancer. *Tumour Biol.* **2016**, *37*, 1299–1308. [CrossRef]
58. Huang, H.-G.; Luo, X.; Wu, S.; Jian, B. MiR-99a Inhibits Cell Proliferation and Tumorigenesis through Targeting MTOR in Human Anaplastic Thyroid Cancer. *Asian Pac. J. Cancer Prev.* **2015**, *16*, 4937–4944. [CrossRef] [PubMed]
59. Cheng, Q.; Zhang, X.; Xu, X.; Lu, X. MiR-618 Inhibits Anaplastic Thyroid Cancer by Repressing XIAP in One ATC Cell Line. *Ann. Endocrinol. (Paris)* **2014**, *75*, 187–193. [CrossRef]
60. Frezzetti, D.; De Menna, M.; Zoppoli, P.; Guerra, C.; Ferraro, A.; Bello, A.M.; De Luca, P.; Calabrese, C.; Fusco, A.; Ceccarelli, M.; et al. Upregulation of MiR-21 by Ras in Vivo and Its Role in Tumor Growth. *Oncogene* **2011**, *30*, 275–286. [CrossRef]
61. Takakura, S.; Mitsutake, N.; Nakashima, M.; Namba, H.; Saenko, V.A.; Rogounovitch, T.I.; Nakazawa, Y.; Hayashi, T.; Ohtsuru, A.; Yamashita, S. Oncogenic Role of MiR-17-92 Cluster in Anaplastic Thyroid Cancer Cells. *Cancer Sci.* **2008**, *99*, 1147–1154. [CrossRef]
62. Zhang, W.; Ji, W.; Zhao, X. MiR-155 Promotes Anaplastic Thyroid Cancer Progression by Directly Targeting SOCS1. *BMC Cancer* **2019**, *19*, 1093. [CrossRef]
63. Montero-Conde, C.; Graña-Castro, O.; Martín-Serrano, G.; Martínez-Montes, Á.M.; Zarzuela, E.; Muñoz, J.; Torres-Perez, R.; Pita, G.; Cordero-Barreal, A.; Leandro-García, L.J.; et al. Hsa-MiR-139-5p Is a Prognostic Thyroid Cancer Marker Involved in HNRNPF-Mediated Alternative Splicing. *Int. J. Cancer* **2020**, *146*, 521–530. [CrossRef] [PubMed]
64. Orlandella, F.M.; Mariniello, R.M.; Iervolino, P.L.C.; Imperlini, E.; Mandola, A.; Verde, A.; De Stefano, A.E.; Pane, K.; Franzese, M.; Esposito, S.; et al. MiR-650 Promotes Motility of Anaplastic Thyroid Cancer Cells by Targeting PPP2CA. *Endocrine* **2019**, *65*, 582–594. [CrossRef] [PubMed]
65. Zhang, X.; Liu, L.; Deng, X.; Li, D.; Cai, H.; Ma, Y.; Jia, C.; Wu, B.; Fan, Y.; Lv, Z. MicroRNA 483-3p Targets Pard3 to Potentiate TGF-B1-Induced Cell Migration, Invasion, and Epithelial-Mesenchymal Transition in Anaplastic Thyroid Cancer Cells. *Oncogene* **2019**, *38*, 699–715. [CrossRef] [PubMed]
66. Bu, Q.; You, F.; Pan, G.; Yuan, Q.; Cui, T.; Hao, L.; Zhang, J. MiR-125b Inhibits Anaplastic Thyroid Cancer Cell Migration and Invasion by Targeting PIK3CD. *Biomed. Pharmacother.* **2017**, *88*, 443–448. [CrossRef] [PubMed]
67. Liu, G.; Wu, K.; Sheng, Y. Elucidation of the Molecular Mechanisms of Anaplastic Thyroid Carcinoma by Integrated MiRNA and MRNA Analysis. *Oncol. Rep.* **2016**, *36*, 3005–3013. [CrossRef] [PubMed]
68. Aherne, S.T.; Smyth, P.; Freeley, M.; Smith, L.; Spillane, C.; O'Leary, J.; Sheils, O. Altered Expression of Mir-222 and Mir-25 Influences Diverse Gene Expression Changes in Transformed Normal and Anaplastic Thyroid Cells, and Impacts on MEK and TRAIL Protein Expression. *Int. J. Mol. Med.* **2016**, *38*, 433–445. [CrossRef]
69. Xiong, Y.; Zhang, L.; Kebebew, E. MiR-20a Is Upregulated in Anaplastic Thyroid Cancer and Targets LIMK1. *PLoS ONE* **2014**, *9*, e96103. [CrossRef] [PubMed]
70. Hao, F.; Bi, Y.-N.; Wang, L.; Wang, Y.; Ma, J.; Cui, P.; Li, X.; Sun, S.; Ning, L.; Huang, Y.; et al. MiR-199a-5p Suppresses Epithelial-Mesenchymal-Transition in Anaplastic Thyroid Carcinoma Cells via Targeting Snail Signals. *Cancer Biomark.* **2020**, *29*, 317–326. [CrossRef] [PubMed]
71. Fuziwara, C.S.; Saito, K.C.; Kimura, E.T. Thyroid Follicular Cell Loss of Differentiation Induced by MicroRNA MiR-17-92 Cluster Is Attenuated by CRISPR/Cas9n Gene Silencing in Anaplastic Thyroid Cancer. *Thyroid* **2020**, *30*, 81–94. [CrossRef]
72. Zhang, W.-L.; Lv, W.; Sun, S.-Z.; Wu, X.-Z.; Zhang, J.-H. MiR-206 Inhibits Metastasis-Relevant Traits by Degrading MRTF-A in Anaplastic Thyroid Cancer. *Int. J. Oncol.* **2015**, *47*, 133–142. [CrossRef] [PubMed]
73. Boufraqech, M.; Nilubol, N.; Zhang, L.; Gara, S.K.; Sadowski, S.M.; Mehta, A.; He, M.; Davis, S.; Dreiling, J.; Copland, J.A.; et al. MiR30a Inhibits LOX Expression and Anaplastic Thyroid Cancer Progression. *Cancer Res.* **2015**, *75*, 367–377. [CrossRef]
74. Hébrant, A.; Floor, S.; Saiselet, M.; Antoniou, A.; Desbuleux, A.; Snyers, B.; La, C.; de Saint Aubain, N.; Leteurtre, E.; Andry, G.; et al. MiRNA Expression in Anaplastic Thyroid Carcinomas. *PLoS ONE* **2014**, *9*, e103871. [CrossRef] [PubMed]
75. Braun, J.; Hoang-Vu, C.; Dralle, H.; Hüttelmaier, S. Downregulation of MicroRNAs Directs the EMT and Invasive Potential of Anaplastic Thyroid Carcinomas. *Oncogene* **2010**, *29*, 4237–4244. [CrossRef] [PubMed]
76. Mitomo, S.; Maesawa, C.; Ogasawara, S.; Iwaya, T.; Shibazaki, M.; Yashima-Abo, A.; Kotani, K.; Oikawa, H.; Sakurai, E.; Izutsu, N.; et al. Downregulation of MiR-138 Is Associated with Overexpression of Human Telomerase Reverse Transcriptase Protein in Human Anaplastic Thyroid Carcinoma Cell Lines. *Cancer Sci.* **2008**, *99*, 280–286. [CrossRef] [PubMed]
77. Xu, Y.; Han, Y.-F.; Ye, B.; Zhang, Y.-L.; Dong, J.-D.; Zhu, S.-J.; Chen, J. MiR-27b-3p Is Involved in Doxorubicin Resistance of Human Anaplastic Thyroid Cancer Cells via Targeting Peroxisome Proliferator-Activated Receptor Gamma. *Basic Clin. Pharmacol. Toxicol.* **2018**, *123*, 670–677. [CrossRef]
78. Liu, J.; Feng, L.; Zhang, H.; Zhang, J.; Zhang, Y.; Li, S.; Qin, L.; Yang, Z.; Xiong, J. Effects of MiR-144 on the Sensitivity of Human Anaplastic Thyroid Carcinoma Cells to Cisplatin by Autophagy Regulation. *Cancer Biol. Ther.* **2018**, *19*, 484–496. [CrossRef] [PubMed]
79. Penha, R.C.C.; Pellecchia, S.; Pacelli, R.; Pinto, L.F.R.; Fusco, A. Ionizing Radiation Deregulates the MicroRNA Expression Profile in Differentiated Thyroid Cells. *Thyroid* **2018**, *28*, 407–421. [CrossRef] [PubMed]
80. Varmeh, S.; Borre, P.V.; Gunda, V.; Brauner, E.; Holm, T.; Wang, Y.; Sadreyev, R.I.; Parangi, S. Genome-Wide Analysis of Differentially Expressed MiRNA in PLX4720-Resistant and Parental Human Thyroid Cancer Cell Lines. *Surgery* **2016**, *159*, 152–162. [CrossRef]

81. Zhang, Y.; Yang, W.Q.; Zhu, H.; Qian, Y.Y.; Zhou, L.; Ren, Y.J.; Ren, X.C.; Zhang, L.; Liu, X.P.; Liu, C.G.; et al. Regulation of Autophagy by MiR-30d Impacts Sensitivity of Anaplastic Thyroid Carcinoma to Cisplatin. *Biochem. Pharmacol.* **2014**, *87*, 562–570. [CrossRef]
82. Vriens, M.R.; Weng, J.; Suh, I.; Huynh, N.; Guerrero, M.A.; Shen, W.T.; Duh, Q.-Y.; Clark, O.H.; Kebebew, E. MicroRNA Expression Profiling Is a Potential Diagnostic Tool for Thyroid Cancer. *Cancer* **2012**, *118*, 3426–3432. [CrossRef]
83. Schwertheim, S.; Sheu, S.-Y.; Worm, K.; Grabellus, F.; Schmid, K.W. Analysis of Deregulated MiRNAs Is Helpful to Distinguish Poorly Differentiated Thyroid Carcinoma from Papillary Thyroid Carcinoma. *Horm. Metab. Res.* **2009**, *41*, 475–481. [CrossRef] [PubMed]
84. Xu, B.; Qin, T.; Yu, J.; Giordano, T.J.; Sartor, M.A.; Koenig, R.J. Novel Role of ASH1L Histone Methyltransferase in Anaplastic Thyroid Carcinoma. *J. Biol. Chem.* **2020**, *295*, 8834–8845. [CrossRef] [PubMed]
85. Zhou, Q.; Chen, J.; Feng, J.; Wang, J. Long Noncoding RNA PVT1 Modulates Thyroid Cancer Cell Proliferation by Recruiting EZH2 and Regulating Thyroid-Stimulating Hormone Receptor (TSHR). *Tumour Biol.* **2016**, *37*, 3105–3113. [CrossRef] [PubMed]
86. Zhang, R.; Hardin, H.; Huang, W.; Chen, J.; Asioli, S.; Righi, A.; Maletta, F.; Sapino, A.; Lloyd, R.V. MALAT1 Long Non-Coding RNA Expression in Thyroid Tissues: Analysis by In Situ Hybridization and Real-Time PCR. *Endocr. Pathol.* **2017**, *28*, 7–12. [CrossRef] [PubMed]
87. Kim, D.; Lee, W.K.; Jeong, S.; Seol, M.-Y.; Kim, H.; Kim, K.-S.; Lee, E.J.; Lee, J.; Jo, Y.S. Upregulation of Long Noncoding RNA LOC100507661 Promotes Tumor Aggressiveness in Thyroid Cancer. *Mol. Cell Endocrinol.* **2016**, *431*, 36–45. [CrossRef] [PubMed]
88. Wang, Y.; Hou, Z.; Li, D. Long Noncoding RNA UCA1 Promotes Anaplastic Thyroid Cancer Cell Proliferation via MiR-135a-mediated C-myc Activation. *Mol. Med. Rep.* **2018**, *18*, 3068–3076. [CrossRef]
89. Pellecchia, S.; Sepe, R.; Decaussin-Petrucci, M.; Ivan, C.; Shimizu, M.; Coppola, C.; Testa, D.; Calin, G.A.; Fusco, A.; Pallante, P. The Long Non-Coding RNA Prader Willi/Angelman Region RNA5 (PAR5) Is Downregulated in Anaplastic Thyroid Carcinomas Where It Acts as a Tumor Suppressor by Reducing EZH2 Activity. *Cancers* **2020**, *12*, 235. [CrossRef] [PubMed]
90. Tan, X.; Wang, P.; Lou, J.; Zhao, J. Knockdown of LncRNA NEAT1 Suppresses Hypoxia-Induced Migration, Invasion and Glycolysis in Anaplastic Thyroid Carcinoma Cells through Regulation of MiR-206 and MiR-599. *Cancer Cell Int.* **2020**, *20*, 132. [CrossRef] [PubMed]
91. Zhang, L.; Zhang, J.; Li, S.; Zhang, Y.; Liu, Y.; Dong, J.; Zhao, W.; Yu, B.; Wang, H.; Liu, J. Genomic Amplification of Long Noncoding RNA HOTAIRM1 Drives Anaplastic Thyroid Cancer Progression via Repressing MiR-144 Biogenesis. *RNA Biol.* **2021**, *18*, 547–562. [CrossRef]
92. Wang, X.-M.; Liu, Y.; Fan, Y.-X.; Liu, Z.; Yuan, Q.-L.; Jia, M.; Geng, Z.-S.; Gu, L.; Lu, X.-B. LncRNA PTCSC3 Affects Drug Resistance of Anaplastic Thyroid Cancer through STAT3/INO80 Pathway. *Cancer Biol. Ther.* **2018**, *19*, 590–597. [CrossRef] [PubMed]
93. Liu, F.; Zhang, J.; Qin, L.; Yang, Z.; Xiong, J.; Zhang, Y.; Li, R.; Li, S.; Wang, H.; Yu, B.; et al. Circular RNA EIF6 (Hsa_circ_0060060) Sponges MiR-144-3p to Promote the Cisplatin-Resistance of Human Thyroid Carcinoma Cells by Autophagy Regulation. *Aging (Albany N.Y.)* **2018**, *10*, 3806–3820. [CrossRef]
94. Hui, L.; Chen, Y. Tumor Microenvironment: Sanctuary of the Devil. *Cancer Lett.* **2015**, *368*, 7–13. [CrossRef]
95. Junttila, M.R.; de Sauvage, F.J. Influence of Tumour Micro-Environment Heterogeneity on Therapeutic Response. *Nature* **2013**, *501*, 346–354. [CrossRef] [PubMed]
96. Bergdorf, K.; Ferguson, D.C.; Mehrad, M.; Ely, K.; Stricker, T.; Weiss, V.L. Papillary Thyroid Carcinoma Behavior: Clues in the Tumor Microenvironment. *Endocr. Relat. Cancer* **2019**, *26*, 601–614. [CrossRef] [PubMed]
97. Bastman, J.J.; Serracino, H.S.; Zhu, Y.; Koenig, M.R.; Mateescu, V.; Sams, S.B.; Davies, K.D.; Raeburn, C.D.; McIntyre, R.C.; Haugen, B.R.; et al. Tumor-Infiltrating T Cells and the PD-1 Checkpoint Pathway in Advanced Differentiated and Anaplastic Thyroid Cancer. *J. Clin. Endocrinol. Metab.* **2016**, *101*, 2863–2873. [CrossRef]
98. Prete, A.; Lo, A.S.; Sadow, P.M.; Bhasin, S.S.; Antonello, Z.A.; Vodopivec, D.M.; Ullas, S.; Sims, J.N.; Clohessy, J.; Dvorak, A.M.; et al. Pericytes Elicit Resistance to Vemurafenib and Sorafenib Therapy in Thyroid Carcinoma via the TSP-1/TGFβ1 Axis. *Clin. Cancer Res.* **2018**, *24*, 6078–6097. [CrossRef]
99. Jolly, L.A.; Novitskiy, S.; Owens, P.; Massoll, N.; Cheng, N.; Fang, W.; Moses, H.L.; Franco, A.T. Fibroblast-Mediated Collagen Remodeling Within the Tumor Microenvironment Facilitates Progression of Thyroid Cancers Driven by BrafV600E and Pten Loss. *Cancer Res.* **2016**, *76*, 1804–1813. [CrossRef]
100. Fozzatti, L.; Alamino, V.A.; Park, S.; Giusiano, L.; Volpini, X.; Zhao, L.; Stempin, C.C.; Donadio, A.C.; Cheng, S.-Y.; Pellizas, C.G. Interplay of Fibroblasts with Anaplastic Tumor Cells Promotes Follicular Thyroid Cancer Progression. *Sci. Rep.* **2019**, *9*, 8028. [CrossRef]
101. Giannini, R.; Moretti, S.; Ugolini, C.; Macerola, E.; Menicali, E.; Nucci, N.; Morelli, S.; Colella, R.; Mandarano, M.; Sidoni, A.; et al. Immune Profiling of Thyroid Carcinomas Suggests the Existence of Two Major Phenotypes: An ATC-Like and a PDTC-Like. *J. Clin. Endocrinol. Metab.* **2019**, *104*, 3557–3575. [CrossRef]
102. Varricchi, G.; Loffredo, S.; Marone, G.; Modestino, L.; Fallahi, P.; Ferrari, S.M.; de Paulis, A.; Antonelli, A.; Galdiero, M.R. The Immune Landscape of Thyroid Cancer in the Context of Immune Checkpoint Inhibition. *Int. J. Mol. Sci.* **2019**, *20*, 3934. [CrossRef]
103. Caillou, B.; Talbot, M.; Weyemi, U.; Pioche-Durieu, C.; Al Ghuzlan, A.; Bidart, J.M.; Chouaib, S.; Schlumberger, M.; Dupuy, C. Tumor-Associated Macrophages (TAMs) Form an Interconnected Cellular Supportive Network in Anaplastic Thyroid Carcinoma. *PLoS ONE* **2011**, *6*, e22567. [CrossRef] [PubMed]

104. Ryder, M.; Ghossein, R.A.; Ricarte-Filho, J.C.; Knauf, J.A.; Fagin, J.A. Increased Density of Tumor Associated Macrophages Is Associated with Decreased Survival in Advanced Thyroid Cancer. *Endocr. Relat. Cancer* **2008**, *15*, 1069–1074. [CrossRef] [PubMed]
105. Cameselle-García, S.; Abdulkader-Sande, S.; Sánchez-Ares, M.; Rodríguez-Carnero, G.; Garcia-Gómez, J.; Gude-Sampedro, F.; Abdulkader-Nallib, I.; Cameselle-Teijeiro, J.M. PD-L1 Expression and Immune Cells in Anaplastic Carcinoma and Poorly Differentiated Carcinoma of the Human Thyroid Gland: A Retrospective Study. *Oncol. Lett.* **2021**, *22*, 553. [CrossRef] [PubMed]
106. Chintakuntlawar, A.V.; Rumilla, K.M.; Smith, C.Y.; Jenkins, S.M.; Foote, R.L.; Kasperbauer, J.L.; Morris, J.C.; Ryder, M.; Alsidawi, S.; Hilger, C.; et al. Expression of PD-1 and PD-L1 in Anaplastic Thyroid Cancer Patients Treated With Multimodal Therapy: Results From a Retrospective Study. *J. Clin. Endocrinol. Metab.* **2017**, *102*, 1943–1950. [CrossRef] [PubMed]
107. Hirsch, L.; Zitvogel, L.; Eggermont, A.; Marabelle, A. PD-Loma: A Cancer Entity with a Shared Sensitivity to the PD-1/PD-L1 Pathway Blockade. *Br. J. Cancer* **2019**, *120*, 3–5. [CrossRef]
108. Brauner, E.; Gunda, V.; Vanden Borre, P.; Zurakowski, D.; Kim, Y.S.; Dennett, K.V.; Amin, S.; Freeman, G.J.; Parangi, S. Combining BRAF Inhibitor and Anti PD-L1 Antibody Dramatically Improves Tumor Regression and Anti Tumor Immunity in an Immunocompetent Murine Model of Anaplastic Thyroid Cancer. *Oncotarget* **2016**, *7*, 17194–17211. [CrossRef] [PubMed]
109. Alobuia, W.; Gillis, A.; Kebebew, E. Contemporary Management of Anaplastic Thyroid Cancer. *Curr. Treat. Opt. Oncol.* **2020**, *21*, 78. [CrossRef]
110. Xu, B.; Fuchs, T.; Dogan, S.; Landa, I.; Katabi, N.; Fagin, J.A.; Tuttle, R.M.; Sherman, E.; Gill, A.J.; Ghossein, R. Dissecting Anaplastic Thyroid Carcinoma: A Comprehensive Clinical, Histologic, Immunophenotypic, and Molecular Study of 360 Cases. *Thyroid* **2020**, *30*, 1505–1517. [CrossRef]
111. Ibrahimpasic, T.; Ghossein, R.; Carlson, D.L.; Nixon, I.; Palmer, F.L.; Shaha, A.R.; Patel, S.G.; Tuttle, R.M.; Shah, J.P.; Ganly, I. Outcomes in Patients with Poorly Differentiated Thyroid Carcinoma. *J. Clin. Endocrinol. Metab.* **2014**, *99*, 1245–1252. [CrossRef] [PubMed]
112. Tiedje, V.; Stuschke, M.; Weber, F.; Dralle, H.; Moss, L.; Führer, D. Anaplastic Thyroid Carcinoma: Review of Treatment Protocols. *Endocr. Relat. Cancer* **2018**, *25*, R153–R161. [CrossRef] [PubMed]
113. Bergers, G.; Hanahan, D. Modes of Resistance to Anti-Angiogenic Therapy. *Nat. Rev. Cancer* **2008**, *8*, 592–603. [CrossRef] [PubMed]
114. Husain, A.; Hu, N.; Sadow, P.M.; Nucera, C. Expression of Angiogenic Switch, Cachexia and Inflammation Factors at the Crossroad in Undifferentiated Thyroid Carcinoma with BRAF(V600E). *Cancer Lett.* **2016**, *380*, 577–585. [CrossRef]
115. Song, Y.S.; Kim, M.J.; Sun, H.J.; Kim, H.H.; Shin, H.S.; Kim, Y.A.; Oh, B.-C.; Cho, S.W.; Park, Y.J. Aberrant Thyroid-Stimulating Hormone Receptor Signaling Increases VEGF-A and CXCL8 Secretion of Thyroid Cancer Cells, Contributing to Angiogenesis and Tumor Growth. *Clin. Cancer Res.* **2019**, *25*, 414–425. [CrossRef]
116. Savvides, P.; Nagaiah, G.; Lavertu, P.; Fu, P.; Wright, J.J.; Chapman, R.; Wasman, J.; Dowlati, A.; Remick, S.C. Phase II Trial of Sorafenib in Patients with Advanced Anaplastic Carcinoma of the Thyroid. *Thyroid* **2013**, *23*, 600–604. [CrossRef] [PubMed]
117. Ito, Y.; Onoda, N.; Ito, K.-I.; Sugitani, I.; Takahashi, S.; Yamaguchi, I.; Kabu, K.; Tsukada, K. Sorafenib in Japanese Patients with Locally Advanced or Metastatic Medullary Thyroid Carcinoma and Anaplastic Thyroid Carcinoma. *Thyroid* **2017**, *27*, 1142–1148. [CrossRef] [PubMed]
118. Gupta-Abramson, V.; Troxel, A.B.; Nellore, A.; Puttaswamy, K.; Redlinger, M.; Ransone, K.; Mandel, S.J.; Flaherty, K.T.; Loevner, L.A.; O'Dwyer, P.J.; et al. Phase II Trial of Sorafenib in Advanced Thyroid Cancer. *J. Clin. Oncol.* **2008**, *26*, 4714–4719. [CrossRef]
119. Brose, M.S.; Nutting, C.M.; Jarzab, B.; Elisei, R.; Siena, S.; Bastholt, L.; de la Fouchardiere, C.; Pacini, F.; Paschke, R.; Shong, Y.K.; et al. Sorafenib in Radioactive Iodine-Refractory, Locally Advanced or Metastatic Differentiated Thyroid Cancer: A Randomised, Double-Blind, Phase 3 Trial. *Lancet* **2014**, *384*, 319–328. [CrossRef]
120. Tohyama, O.; Matsui, J.; Kodama, K.; Hata-Sugi, N.; Kimura, T.; Okamoto, K.; Minoshima, Y.; Iwata, M.; Funahashi, Y. Antitumor Activity of Lenvatinib (E7080): An Angiogenesis Inhibitor That Targets Multiple Receptor Tyrosine Kinases in Preclinical Human Thyroid Cancer Models. *J. Thyroid Res.* **2014**, *2014*, 638747. [CrossRef]
121. Takahashi, S.; Kiyota, N.; Yamazaki, T.; Chayahara, N.; Nakano, K.; Inagaki, L.; Toda, K.; Enokida, T.; Minami, H.; Imamura, Y.; et al. A Phase II Study of the Safety and Efficacy of Lenvatinib in Patients with Advanced Thyroid Cancer. *Future Oncol.* **2019**, *15*, 717–726. [CrossRef]
122. Takahashi, S.; Tahara, M.; Ito, K.; Tori, M.; Kiyota, N.; Yoshida, K.; Sakata, Y.; Yoshida, A. Safety and Effectiveness of Lenvatinib in 594 Patients with Unresectable Thyroid Cancer in an All-Case Post-Marketing Observational Study in Japan. *Adv. Ther.* **2020**, *37*, 3850–3862. [CrossRef]
123. Schlumberger, M.; Tahara, M.; Wirth, L.J.; Robinson, B.; Brose, M.S.; Elisei, R.; Habra, M.A.; Newbold, K.; Shah, M.H.; Hoff, A.O.; et al. Lenvatinib versus Placebo in Radioiodine-Refractory Thyroid Cancer. *N. Engl. J. Med.* **2015**, *372*, 621–630. [CrossRef] [PubMed]
124. Rendl, G.; Sipos, B.; Becherer, A.; Sorko, S.; Trummer, C.; Raderer, M.; Hitzl, W.; Ardelt, M.; Gallowitsch, H.J.; Pirich, C. Real-World Data for Lenvatinib in Radioiodine-Refractory Differentiated Thyroid Cancer (RELEVANT): A Retrospective Multicentric Analysis of Clinical Practice in Austria. *Int. J. Endocrinol.* **2020**, *2020*, 1–8. [CrossRef]
125. Locati, L.D.; Piovesan, A.; Durante, C.; Bregni, M.; Castagna, M.G.; Zovato, S.; Giusti, M.; Ibrahim, T.; Puxeddu, E.; Fedele, G.; et al. Real-World Efficacy and Safety of Lenvatinib: Data from a Compassionate Use in the Treatment of Radioactive Iodine-Refractory Differentiated Thyroid Cancer Patients in Italy. *Eur. J. Cancer* **2019**, *118*, 35–40. [CrossRef]

126. Berdelou, A.; Borget, I.; Godbert, Y.; Nguyen, T.; Garcia, M.-E.; Chougnet, C.N.; Ferru, A.; Buffet, C.; Chabre, O.; Huillard, O.; et al. Lenvatinib for the Treatment of Radioiodine-Refractory Thyroid Cancer in Real-Life Practice. *Thyroid* **2018**, *28*, 72–78. [CrossRef] [PubMed]
127. Cabanillas, M.E.; de Souza, J.A.; Geyer, S.; Wirth, L.J.; Menefee, M.E.; Liu, S.V.; Shah, K.; Wright, J.; Shah, M.H. Cabozantinib As Salvage Therapy for Patients With Tyrosine Kinase Inhibitor-Refractory Differentiated Thyroid Cancer: Results of a Multicenter Phase II International Thyroid Oncology Group Trial. *J. Clin. Oncol.* **2017**, *35*, 3315–3321. [CrossRef] [PubMed]
128. Ha, H.T.; Lee, J.S.; Urba, S.; Koenig, R.J.; Sisson, J.; Giordano, T.; Worden, F.P. A Phase II Study of Imatinib in Patients with Advanced Anaplastic Thyroid Cancer. *Thyroid* **2010**, *20*, 975–980. [CrossRef] [PubMed]
129. Pennell, N.A.; Daniels, G.H.; Haddad, R.I.; Ross, D.S.; Evans, T.; Wirth, L.J.; Fidias, P.H.; Temel, J.S.; Gurubhagavatula, S.; Heist, R.S.; et al. A Phase II Study of Gefitinib in Patients with Advanced Thyroid Cancer. *Thyroid* **2008**, *18*, 317–323. [CrossRef] [PubMed]
130. Bible, K.C.; Suman, V.J.; Menefee, M.E.; Smallridge, R.C.; Molina, J.R.; Maples, W.J.; Karlin, N.J.; Traynor, A.M.; Kumar, P.; Goh, B.C.; et al. A Multiinstitutional Phase 2 Trial of Pazopanib Monotherapy in Advanced Anaplastic Thyroid Cancer. *J. Clin. Endocrinol. Metab.* **2012**, *97*, 3179–3184. [CrossRef] [PubMed]
131. Yoo, S.-K.; Song, Y.S.; Lee, E.K.; Hwang, J.; Kim, H.H.; Jung, G.; Kim, Y.A.; Kim, S.; Cho, S.W.; Won, J.-K.; et al. Integrative Analysis of Genomic and Transcriptomic Characteristics Associated with Progression of Aggressive Thyroid Cancer. *Nat. Commun.* **2019**, *10*, 2764. [CrossRef] [PubMed]
132. Flaherty, K.T.; Puzanov, I.; Kim, K.B.; Ribas, A.; McArthur, G.A.; Sosman, J.A.; O'Dwyer, P.J.; Lee, R.J.; Grippo, J.F.; Nolop, K.; et al. Inhibition of Mutated, Activated BRAF in Metastatic Melanoma. *N. Engl. J. Med.* **2010**, *363*, 809–819. [CrossRef] [PubMed]
133. Hyman, D.M.; Puzanov, I.; Subbiah, V.; Faris, J.E.; Chau, I.; Blay, J.-Y.; Wolf, J.; Raje, N.S.; Diamond, E.L.; Hollebecque, A.; et al. Vemurafenib in Multiple Nonmelanoma Cancers with BRAF V600 Mutations. *N. Engl. J. Med.* **2015**, *373*, 726–736. [CrossRef] [PubMed]
134. Kurata, K.; Onoda, N.; Noda, S.; Kashiwagi, S.; Asano, Y.; Hirakawa, K.; Ohira, M. Growth Arrest by Activated BRAF and MEK Inhibition in Human Anaplastic Thyroid Cancer Cells. *Int. J. Oncol.* **2016**, *49*, 2303–2308. [CrossRef]
135. Subbiah, V.; Kreitman, R.J.; Wainberg, Z.A.; Cho, J.Y.; Schellens, J.H.M.; Soria, J.C.; Wen, P.Y.; Zielinski, C.; Cabanillas, M.E.; Urbanowitz, G.; et al. Dabrafenib and Trametinib Treatment in Patients With Locally Advanced or Metastatic BRAF V600-Mutant Anaplastic Thyroid Cancer. *J. Clin. Oncol.* **2018**, *36*, 7–13. [CrossRef] [PubMed]
136. Wagle, N.; Grabiner, B.C.; Van Allen, E.M.; Amin-Mansour, A.; Taylor-Weiner, A.; Rosenberg, M.; Gray, N.; Barletta, J.A.; Guo, Y.; Swanson, S.J.; et al. Response and Acquired Resistance to Everolimus in Anaplastic Thyroid Cancer. *N. Engl. J. Med.* **2014**, *371*, 1426–1433. [CrossRef]
137. Harris, E.J.; Hanna, G.J.; Chau, N.; Rabinowits, G.; Haddad, R.; Margalit, D.N.; Schoenfeld, J.; Tishler, R.B.; Barletta, J.A.; Nehs, M.; et al. Everolimus in Anaplastic Thyroid Cancer: A Case Series. *Front. Oncol.* **2019**, *9*, 106. [CrossRef] [PubMed]
138. Schneider, T.C.; de Wit, D.; Links, T.P.; van Erp, N.P.; van der Hoeven, J.J.M.; Gelderblom, H.; Roozen, I.C.F.M.; Bos, M.; Corver, W.E.; van Wezel, T.; et al. Everolimus in Patients With Advanced Follicular-Derived Thyroid Cancer: Results of a Phase II Clinical Trial. *J. Clin. Endocrinol. Metab.* **2017**, *102*, 698–707. [CrossRef] [PubMed]
139. Wirth, L.J.; Sherman, E.; Robinson, B.; Solomon, B.; Kang, H.; Lorch, J.; Worden, F.; Brose, M.; Patel, J.; Leboulleux, S.; et al. Efficacy of Selpercatinib in RET-Altered Thyroid Cancers. *N. Engl. J. Med.* **2020**, *383*, 825–835. [CrossRef]
140. Subbiah, V.; Yang, D.; Velcheti, V.; Drilon, A.; Meric-Bernstam, F. State-of-the-Art Strategies for Targeting RET-Dependent Cancers. *J. Clin. Oncol.* **2020**, *38*, 1209–1221. [CrossRef] [PubMed]
141. Cabanillas, M.E.; Drilon, A.; Farago, A.F.; Brose, M.S.; McDermott, R.; Sohal, D.; Oh, D.-Y.; Almubarak, M.; Bauman, J.; Chu, E.; et al. 1916P Larotrectinib Treatment of Advanced TRK Fusion Thyroid Cancer. *Ann. Oncol.* **2020**, *31*, S1086. [CrossRef]
142. Godbert, Y.; Henriques de Figueiredo, B.; Bonichon, F.; Chibon, F.; Hostein, I.; Pérot, G.; Dupin, C.; Daubech, A.; Belleannée, G.; Gros, A.; et al. Remarkable Response to Crizotinib in Woman With Anaplastic Lymphoma Kinase–Rearranged Anaplastic Thyroid Carcinoma. *JCO* **2014**, *33*, e84–e87. [CrossRef] [PubMed]
143. Ahn, J.; Jin, M.; Song, E.; Ryu, Y.-M.; Song, D.E.; Kim, S.-Y.; Kim, T.Y.; Kim, W.B.; Shong, Y.K.; Jeon, M.J.; et al. Immune Profiling of Advanced Thyroid Cancers Using Fluorescent Multiplex Immunohistochemistry. *Thyroid* **2021**, *31*, 61–67. [CrossRef]
144. Robert, C.; Schachter, J.; Long, G.V.; Arance, A.; Grob, J.J.; Mortier, L.; Daud, A.; Carlino, M.S.; McNeil, C.; Lotem, M.; et al. Pembrolizumab versus Ipilimumab in Advanced Melanoma. *N. Engl. J. Med.* **2015**, *372*, 2521–2532. [CrossRef] [PubMed]
145. De Leo, S.; Trevisan, M.; Fugazzola, L. Recent Advances in the Management of Anaplastic Thyroid Cancer. *Thyroid Res.* **2020**, *13*, 17. [CrossRef] [PubMed]
146. Spalart, V.; Legius, B.; Segers, K.; Coolen, J.; Maes, B.; Decoster, L. Dramatic Response to First Line Single Agent Pembrolizumab in Anaplastic Thyroid Carcinoma. *Case Rep. Endocrinol.* **2019**, *2019*, 9095753. [CrossRef]
147. Chintakuntlawar, A.V.; Yin, J.; Foote, R.L.; Kasperbauer, J.L.; Rivera, M.; Asmus, E.; Garces, N.I.; Janus, J.R.; Liu, M.; Ma, D.J.; et al. A Phase 2 Study of Pembrolizumab Combined with Chemoradiotherapy as Initial Treatment for Anaplastic Thyroid Cancer. *Thyroid* **2019**, *29*, 1615–1622. [CrossRef]
148. Capdevila, J.; Wirth, L.J.; Ernst, T.; Ponce Aix, S.; Lin, C.-C.; Ramlau, R.; Butler, M.O.; Delord, J.-P.; Gelderblom, H.; Ascierto, P.A.; et al. PD-1 Blockade in Anaplastic Thyroid Carcinoma. *J. Clin. Oncol.* **2020**, *38*, 2620–2627. [CrossRef] [PubMed]

149. Vanden Borre, P.; McFadden, D.G.; Gunda, V.; Sadow, P.M.; Varmeh, S.; Bernasconi, M.; Jacks, T.; Parangi, S. The next Generation of Orthotopic Thyroid Cancer Models: Immunocompetent Orthotopic Mouse Models of BRAF V600E-Positive Papillary and Anaplastic Thyroid Carcinoma. *Thyroid* **2014**, *24*, 705–714. [CrossRef] [PubMed]
150. Cabanillas, M.E.; Ferrarotto, R.; Garden, A.S.; Ahmed, S.; Busaidy, N.L.; Dadu, R.; Williams, M.D.; Skinner, H.; Gunn, G.B.; Grosu, H.; et al. Neoadjuvant BRAF- and Immune-Directed Therapy for Anaplastic Thyroid Carcinoma. *Thyroid* **2018**, *28*, 945–951. [CrossRef]
151. Wang, J.R.; Zafereo, M.E.; Dadu, R.; Ferrarotto, R.; Busaidy, N.L.; Lu, C.; Ahmed, S.; Gule-Monroe, M.K.; Williams, M.D.; Sturgis, E.M.; et al. Complete Surgical Resection Following Neoadjuvant Dabrafenib Plus Trametinib in BRAFV600E-Mutated Anaplastic Thyroid Carcinoma. *Thyroid* **2019**, *29*, 1036–1043. [CrossRef] [PubMed]
152. Iyer, P.C.; Dadu, R.; Gule-Monroe, M.; Busaidy, N.L.; Ferrarotto, R.; Habra, M.A.; Zafereo, M.; Williams, M.D.; Gunn, G.B.; Grosu, H.; et al. Salvage Pembrolizumab Added to Kinase Inhibitor Therapy for the Treatment of Anaplastic Thyroid Carcinoma. *J. Immunother. Cancer* **2018**, *6*, 68. [CrossRef] [PubMed]
153. Dierks, C.; Seufert, J.; Aumann, K.; Ruf, J.; Klein, C.; Kiefer, S.; Rassner, M.; Boerries, M.; Zielke, A.; La Rosée, P.; et al. The Lenvatinib/Pembrolizumab Combination Is an Effective Treatment Option for Anaplastic and Poorly Differentiated Thyroid Carcinoma. *Thyroid* **2021**. [CrossRef] [PubMed]
154. Kollipara, R.; Schneider, B.; Radovich, M.; Babu, S.; Kiel, P.J. Exceptional Response with Immunotherapy in a Patient with Anaplastic Thyroid Cancer. *Oncologist* **2017**, *22*, 1149–1151. [CrossRef] [PubMed]
155. Sherman, E.J.; Dunn, L.A.; Ho, A.L.; Baxi, S.S.; Ghossein, R.A.; Fury, M.G.; Haque, S.; Sima, C.S.; Cullen, G.; Fagin, J.A.; et al. Phase 2 Study Evaluating the Combination of Sorafenib and Temsirolimus in the Treatment of Radioactive Iodine-Refractory Thyroid Cancer. *Cancer* **2017**, *123*, 4114–4121. [CrossRef] [PubMed]

cancers

Review

Next-Generation Molecular Imaging of Thyroid Cancer

Yuchen Jin [1,2,3,†], Beibei Liu [4,†], Muhsin H. Younis [5], Gang Huang [1], Jianjun Liu [1], Weibo Cai [5,6,*] and Weijun Wei [1,*]

1 Department of Nuclear Medicine, Renji Hospital, School of Medicine, Shanghai Jiao Tong University, 1630 Dongfang Rd., Shanghai 200127, China; yuchenjin@sjtu.edu.cn (Y.J.); huang2802@163.com (G.H.); nuclearj@163.com (J.L.)
2 Department of Nuclear Medicine, Shanghai Sixth People's Hospital Affiliated to Shanghai Jiao Tong University, Shanghai 200233, China
3 Human Oncology and Pathogenesis Program, Memorial Sloan-Kettering Cancer Center, New York, NY 10065, USA
4 Institute of Diagnostic and Interventional Radiology, Shanghai Sixth People's Hospital Affiliatede to Shanghai Jiao Tong University, Shanghai 200233, China; beibei4906@163.com
5 Departments of Radiology and Medical Physics, University of Wisconsin–Madison, Madison, WI 53705-2275, USA; muhsinhy@gmail.com
6 Carbone Cancer Center, University of Wisconsin, Madison, WI 53705, USA
* Correspondence: wcai@uwhealth.org (W.C.); weijun.wei@outlook.com (W.W.); Tel.: +86-160-8262-1749 (W.C.)
† Yuchen Jin and Beibei Liu contributed equally to this work.

Simple Summary: Molecular imaging utilizes radionuclides or artificially modified molecules to image particular targets or pathways which are important in the pathogenesis of a certain disease. Transporter-based probes like radioiodine and [^{18}F]fluoro-D-glucose ([^{18}F]FDG) are widely used for diagnosing thyroid cancer (TC) and predicting the prognosis thereafter. However, newly developed probes (peptide, antibody, nanoparticle probes, and aptamer) image the fine molecular changes involved in the pathogenesis of TC and enable target-specific diagnosis and treatment of TC. Furthermore, novel molecular probes have high specificity and sensitivity, imparting a high level of objectivity to the research areas of TC.

Abstract: An essential aspect of thyroid cancer (TC) management is personalized and precision medicine. Functional imaging of TC with radioiodine and [^{18}F]FDG has been frequently used in disease evaluation for several decades now. Recently, advances in molecular imaging have led to the development of novel tracers based on aptamer, peptide, antibody, nanobody, antibody fragment, and nanoparticle platforms. The emerging targets—including HER2, CD54, SHP2, CD33, and more—are promising targets for clinical translation soon. The significance of these tracers may be realized by outlining the way they support the management of TC. The provided examples focus on where preclinical investigations can be translated. Furthermore, advances in the molecular imaging of TC may inspire the development of novel therapeutic or theranostic tracers. In this review, we summarize TC-targeting probes which include transporter-based and immuno-based imaging moieties. We summarize the most recent evidence in this field and outline how these emerging strategies may potentially optimize clinical practice.

Keywords: thyroid cancer; molecular imaging; theranostics; companion diagnostics; immunoPET

Citation: Jin, Y.; Liu, B.; Younis, M.H.; Huang, G.; Liu, J.; Cai, W.; Wei, W. Next-Generation Molecular Imaging of Thyroid Cancer. *Cancers* **2021**, *13*, 3188. https://doi.org/10.3390/cancers13133188

Academic Editors: Fabio Medas and Pier Francesco Alesina

Received: 4 May 2021
Accepted: 22 June 2021
Published: 25 June 2021

1. Introduction

Thyroid cancer (TC) is one of the most common cancer types and its occurrence has been rapidly increasing over the last several years [1]. TC represents around 2–2.3% of new cancer cases and 0.2–0.4% of deaths from all cancer types [2,3]. In 2021, the USA may have approximately 44,280 new cases of TC and about 2200 deaths [2]. Around 90,000 new cases along with 6800 deaths were estimated in 2015 in China [2]. By 2030, TC is anticipated to become the second-most common type of cancer in females and the ninth in males [3]. 90–95% of cases present either papillary TC (PTC) or follicular TC (FTC), both of which originate from follicular cells in the thyroid and can be referred to as differentiated TC (DTC) [1].

In DTC, the thyroid retains the ability to absorb and store nearly all of the iodine in the whole body, providing the rationale for combined therapeutics with thyroidectomy and ^{131}I (a beta-emitting radioisotope of iodine) therapy [4]. A total or near-total thyroidectomy removes all or most of the thyroid and DTC tissue, facilitating DTC control and the subsequent ^{131}I ablation, adjuvant therapy, or therapy for DTCs [5]. The ^{131}I tends to concentrate in remnant thyroid tissue, latent DTC foci, and metastatic DTC lesions. The radiation can damage the remnant thyroid tissue and DTC cells, helping DTC re-staging and improving DTC prognosis [5,6]. Unfortunately, within 10 years of an initial thyroidectomy, local recurrence and distant metastases take place in approximately 10–20% of DTCs. Notwithstanding ^{131}I management, only one-third of DTCs could be regarded as having shown "complete response" with the remaining DTCs refractory to ^{131}I (i.e., radioiodine refractory DTC, RR-DTC) having a poor prognosis [7].

Two less common types of TC are medullary TC (MTC) and anaplastic TC (ATC), accounting for <5% of all TC cases. Notably, however, 50–80% of MTCs show widespread metastasis at the initial diagnosis, with a five-year survival rate of 38% [8]. Furthermore, ATC is tremendously aggressive with its median overall survival of less than one year [8,9]. Thus, it is necessary to find latent lesions, precisely evaluate the grade of malignancy, adopt the most effective therapeutics, and take precautions against local recurrence or distant metastasis on time.

Traditional diagnosis methods include thyroid physical exams, blood tests (for testing biomarkers such as thyroglobulin and calcitonin), ultrasound imaging (for helping determine whether a thyroid nodule or lymph node is likely to be benign or cancerous), and other imaging tests such as CT and MRI (for TC staging and determining TC spread) [5]. In recent decades, molecular imaging (MI) has become an increasingly popular approach, applying radionuclides or artificially modified molecules to assist clinicians in locating biomarkers, potential therapeutic targets, or describing signaling pathways [10,11]. These targets play a vital role in the diagnosis and management of TC, allowing for characterization and quantification of the molecular composition of tumor tissues [12]. MI has been shown to improve diagnosis of TC, personalized management, and long-term predictive prognosis index [13]. Moreover, MI is crucial to actualizing multimodality-based theranostic strategies for TCs [14].

Over the past decade, significant progress has been made in the application of MI to TC. For instance, nanobodies and aptamers have been used to elucidate the bio-features of TC. These tracers show an antigen-binding ability resembling that of traditional antibodies [15–18]. Furthermore, immuno-single photon emission computerized tomography (immunoSPECT) and immuno-positron emission tomography (immunoPET) have encouraged the development of new theranostic methods intended for complex clinical settings, particularly for the RR-DTCs or ATCs [19]. These methods provide opportunities for obtaining deep insights into the pathogenesis of TC and as well as novel therapeutic targets for TC. Indeed, the discovery and translation of new probes enabling precise theranostics of TC are urgently needed, especially for RR-DTCs and ATCs.

Primary references are mainly derived from PubMed (available before 7 June 2021), comprehensively including the pivotal evidence in the field. In this review, transporter-based platforms are updated, and newer tracers like aptamer-, peptide-, antibody-, nanobody-, and nanoparticle-based platforms for TC are summarized. We highlight some of the potentially translatable probes in the current review. We also outline how these emerging strategies may potentially improve clinical practice.

2. Transporter-Targeting Probes

Most transporter-targeting probes are small-size molecules, carried into the intracellular space by transporters on the cell surface. Some transporter-associated probes may take part in cell metabolism [20,21]. Many transporter-based isotopes, including radioiodine, are routinely to image the recurrence and metastases of TC. Several alternatives to radioiodine can identify RR-DTC metastases lacking radioiodine uptake. Other transporter-based radiotracers like [^{201}Tl]TlCl, [^{99m}Tc]Tc-sestamibi ([^{99m}Tc]Tc-MIBI), [^{99}mTc]Tc-tetrofosmin, [^{99m}Tc]Tc-depreotide, [^{111}In]In-diethylenetriaminepentaacetic acid-octreotide ([^{111}In]In-DTPA-octreotide), and [^{18}F]fluoro-D-glucose ([^{18}F]FDG) have been synthesized, tested, and validated as beneficial for diagnosing TC [5,22]. In particular, [^{18}F]FDG has been widely applied in the management of TC [5].

2.1. *Sodium Iodine Symporter (NIS)-Targeting Probes*

NIS is the protein mainly locating at the cell plasma membrane, which carries Na^+/I^- ions from the extracellular matrix into the intracellular fluid [23]. The transported iodine, as an element, helps produce thyroid hormone (iodide organification) [24]. Unlike the expression pattern of other tumor targets (low expression in normal tissues and high expression in tumor tissues), NIS is usually present at high levels in normal thyroid tissues and DTC cells, enabling radioiodine collection in normal thyroid and TC cells [25]. Nevertheless, NIS downregulation happens in RR-DTCs, poorly differentiated TCs (PDTCs), and ATCs, causing these TC cells hard to benefit much from radioiodine treatment [26].

2.1.1. Radioiodine

Radioiodine, a widely used radioisotope, has a crucial role in the diagnosis and treatment of DTC. There are several medically useful radioisotopes of iodine (^{125}I, ^{131}I, and ^{124}I, etc.). However, only ^{131}I and ^{124}I are commonly applied in clinical settings due to their clinically acceptable radiation half-life, diagnostic or therapeutic performance, economic cost, and safety [27]. [^{131}I]NaI can track thyroid and TC cells with γ radiation on SPECT, and damage those cells by emitting β^- radiation [28]. [^{131}I]NaI allows ablation of thyroid remnant, adjuvant therapy of TC, and therapy of TC, which vastly improves the prognosis of patients with TC [5]. ^{124}I is another isotope of iodine emitting positron, which can be exploited for PET imaging. [^{124}I]NaI-PET/CT has superior spatial resolution and quantification ability over [^{131}I]NaI SPECT [29].

Recently, numerous reports have focused on radioiodine for improving the diagnosis performance, and efficacy of treatment [30–32]. Tg tests coupled with iodine uptake assay [32], or [^{124}I]NaI PET/CT only [30,31], are used for ^{131}I dosimetry. Apart from performing dosimetry before ^{131}I treatment, much attention should be given to increase the membranous expression of NIS, induce the concentration of ^{131}I, and improve the therapeutic efficacy of ^{131}I treatment. For RR-DTC, PDTC, and ATC, it is essential to explore agents that could increase NIS expression and augment the migration of NIS to the cell membrane. These agents mainly include but are not limited to, retinoic acid [33], mechanistic target of rapamycin kinase (mTOR) inhibitors [34], and very recently, V-Raf murine sarcoma viral oncogene homolog B (BRAF) and mitogen-activated protein kinase kinase (MAP2K1/2, MEK1/2) inhibitors, which inhibit the extracellular signal-regulated kinase (ERK) pathway responsible for tumor progression and radioiodine uptake [35,36] (Figure 1). RR-DTCs would be stabilized, or shrinkage after treatment with kinase inhibitors, owing to the suppressed signaling pathway and enhanced ^{131}I treatment efficacy [26,37].

Lately, estrogen-related receptor gamma (ERRγ), one of the estrogen-related receptors, has gained more traction as a potential target to enhance or enable radioiodine uptake. ERRγ, a member of NR3B nuclear receptor superfamily, is a biomarker for multiple cancers, including breast cancer and prostate cancer [38]. Previous reports have shown that the ERRγ inverse agonist GSK5182 increased NIS expression and NIS-mediated iodine uptake in Kirsten rat sarcoma viral oncogene homolog (KRAS) or BRAF mutated ATC cells in vitro [39]. In addition, another ERRγ inverse agonist, DN200434, was recently shown to increase the uptake of radioiodine in ATC tumors, identifying ERRγ as a target to enhance ^{131}I therapy responsiveness [40] (Figure 2). It remains to be determined if DN200434 has a re-differentiative effect in patients with either RR-DTC or ATC.

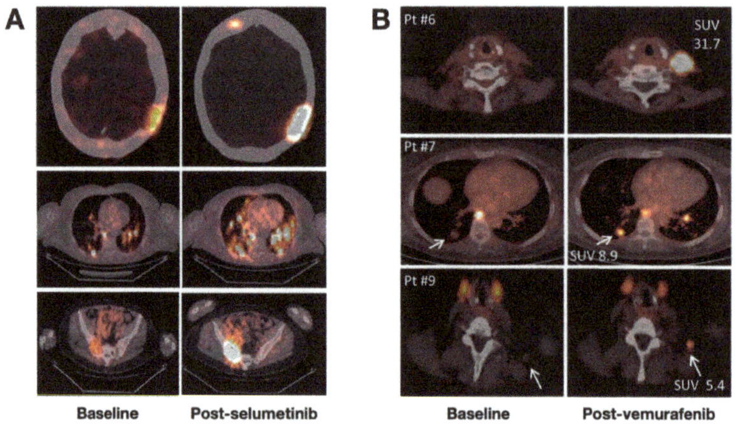

Figure 1. [^{124}I]NaI PET/CT images of patients with RR-DTC or PDTC with or without kinase inhibitors. (**A**) PET/CT images showed enhanced iodine uptake of lesions post-treatment with selumetinib in nearly all previously negative head, lung, and sacroiliac bone metastases. Reproduced with permission from [35], copyright 2013 Massachusetts Medical Society. (**B**) PET/CT images showed enhanced radioiodine uptake of lesions in the neck and lung after treatment with vemurafenib, a specific BRAF^{V600E} inhibitor. Reproduced with permission from [36], copyright 2019 Endocrine Society.

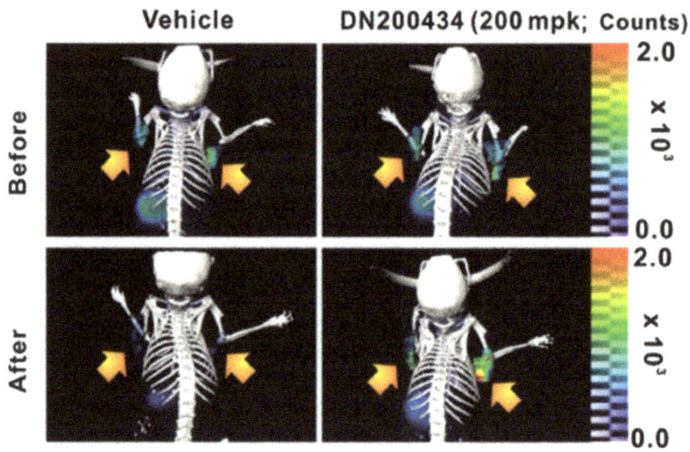

Figure 2. [^{124}I]NaI-PET/CT demonstrates enhanced iodine uptake in CAL62 ATC tumor after treatment with DN200434. The arrows indicate the ATC tumor. Reproduced with permission from [40], copyright 2019 American Association for Cancer Research.

2.1.2. [^{18}F]Tetrafluoroborate ([^{18}F]TFB)

Detecting local recurrence and metastases of DTC in radioiodine imaging is particularly important for the arrangement of local treatments, e.g., surgery or radiotherapy [5]. Whereas negative radioiodine imaging with increased serum thyroglobulin is a barrier for finding malignant lesions, the so-called "Thyroglobulin Elevated and Negative Iodine

Scintigraphy" (TENIS) needs radically diverse diagnostic and therapeutic methods [26]. TENIS could be caused by poor NIS expression, iodide organification defect, or radioiodine stunning [41,42]. A failure to find NIS-expressing DTC lesions might delay the diagnosis and also the timely onset of the treatment [43]. Despite [^{18}F]FDG-PET/CT could be applied for finding TENIS metastases, but its uptake might be partially caused by tumor-infiltrating immune cells [44]. Recently, [^{18}F]TFB, [^{18}F]Fluorosulfate ([^{18}F]FS), and [^{18}F]hexafluorophosphate ([^{18}F]HFP) have been discovered for imaging DTCs [45–48].

[^{18}F]TFB is an analog to radioiodine, having similar NIS affinities, same charge, and similar ionic radius to iodide. Therefore, [^{18}F]TFB can be transported by NIS [46,49] differed from radioiodine, [^{18}F]TFB can be readily synthesized at medical cyclotrons, and it provides a satisfactory half-life, dosing, biodistribution, and PET imaging quality [46,47] (Figure 3). [^{18}F]TFB-PET can exclusively reveal NIS expression in tumor cells, therefore reclassifying TENIS metastases into partial or complete dedifferentiation, and helping metastasis localization and prognosis evaluation [47]. [^{18}F]FS and [^{18}F]HFP are two other newly discovered NIS-targeting tracers having favorable targeting efficiency, image contrasts, and biodistribution features [45,48]. Although it has been reported that FS and HFP had higher NIS affinity than TFB [45], it remains unclear if [^{18}F]HFP and [^{18}F]FS are superior to [^{18}F]TFB. The clinical evaluation of the [^{18}F]HFP and [^{18}F]FS are still needed.

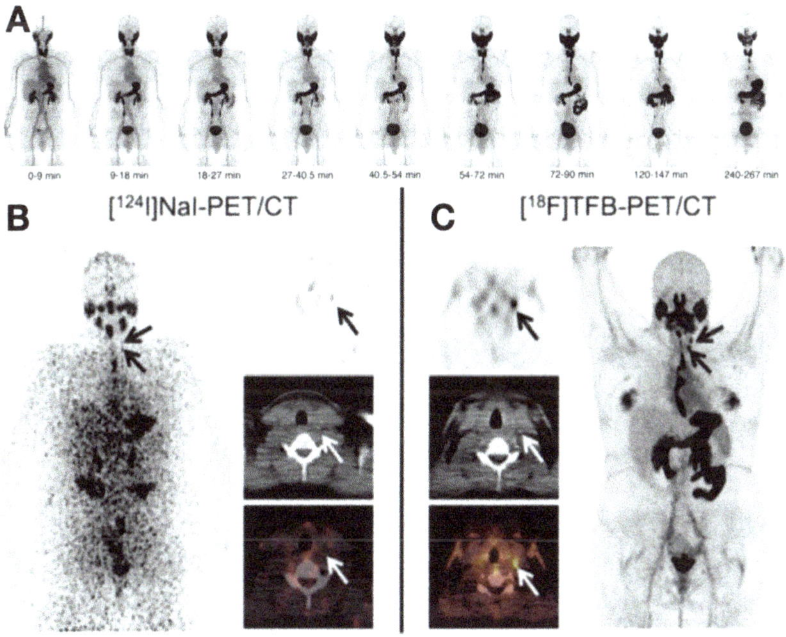

Figure 3. Evaluation of thyroid cancer via [^{18}F]TFB-PET/CT and [^{124}I]NaI-PET/CT. (**A**) Biodistribution of [^{18}F]TFB at various time points on PET images. [^{18}F]TFB accumulated rapidly in the thyroid and other normal tissues like the salivary gland and stomach within 10–30 min. Reproduced with permission from [50], copyright 2017 Society of Nuclear Medicine and Molecular Imaging. (**B**,**C**) A comparison between [^{124}I]NaI-PET/CT and [^{18}F]TFB-PET/CT in a 26-year-old patient post-thyroidectomy. (**B**) [^{124}I]NaI-PET/CT was unremarkable for PTC. (**C**) In contrast, [^{18}F]TFB-PET/CT revealed two foci in the left lateral cervical region. Reproduced with permission from [51], copyright 2018 Wolters Kluwer Health.

2.2. Glucose Transporter-Targeting Probes

[^{18}F]FDG, mainly transported by glucose-transporter family-1 (GLUT1), is a well-known radiopharmaceutical glucose analog used in clinical PET imaging [52]. Aggressive TCs with low radioiodine uptake generally show high levels of [^{18}F]FDG uptake [53].

[^{18}F]FDG-PET/CT has shown great sensitivity in patients who otherwise do not benefit from ^{131}I treatment. This is because metastases without radioiodine uptake tend to have high glycolytic rates, causing enhanced [^{18}F]FDG uptake [54]. Furthermore, [^{18}F]FDG can help detect TC recurrence or metastases and predict radioiodine uptake [54,55]. More specifically, [^{18}F]FDG maximum standard unit value (SUVmax) higher than 4.0 would predict poor radioiodine uptake [54]. Besides, most PDTC, ATC, and MTC cells do not concentrate ^{131}I. Thus, in these entities, [^{18}F]FDG PET/CT imaging is useful in initial diagnosis, subsequent disease grading, treatment, and follow-up after treatment. Even though numerous glucose analog tracers other than [^{18}F]FDG were created [56], their head-to-head comparisons with the widely used [^{18}F]FDG are lacking.

2.3. *Amino Acid Transporter-Targeting Probes*

Alternatives to [^{18}F]FDG are a subject of interest. Occasionally, [^{18}F]FDG may yield inexplicable images. The false-positive [^{18}F]FDG uptake happens in Hashimoto's disease and Graves' disease. In addition, it is hard to find brain metastasis on [^{18}F]FDG PET/CT images because of the intense background signals [57,58]. In recent years, amino acid probes have obtained incremental attraction as alternatives to [^{18}F]FDG. Amino acids probes include [^{18}F]fluoro-α-methyl tyrosine ([^{18}F]FAMT), [^{18}F]fluoro-dihydroxyphenylalanine ([^{18}F]FDOPA), L-[methyl-^{11}C]-methionine ([^{11}C]MET), [^{18}F]fluoroethyl-tyrosine ([^{18}F]FET), [^{18}F]fluoroglutamine ([^{18}F]FGln), and the newly discovered [^{18}F]NKO-035. Of these, [^{18}F]FDOPA, [^{11}C]MET, and [^{18}F]FGln have been investigated in TCs [59–63].

2.3.1. [^{18}F]FDOPA

[^{18}F]FDOPA is a large neutral amino acid that resembles natural L-dopa, which can be transported by L-type amino acid transporter 1 (LAT1, SLC7A5) and L-type amino acid transporter 2 (LAT2, SLC7A8) [64]. [^{18}F]FDOPA is a satisfactory probe for detecting MTC metastasis, persistence, and residual disease [59]. However, if [^{18}F]FDOPA imaging is negative or unavailable, [^{18}F]FDG should be considered, especially for aggressive MTCs displaying signs of dedifferentiation or rising carcinoma embryonic antigen (CEA) concentration in serum [59,65].

2.3.2. [^{11}C]MET

[^{11}C]MET, transported mainly by SLC7A5, is often used to visualize parathyroid adenoma and enable focused parathyroidectomy [66–68]. Published data for [^{11}C]MET in TC is limited. Only one case with hyperparathyroidism has been reported, which showed intense focal [^{11}C]MET uptake in a cold nodule with highly increased sestamibi uptake. The nodule was finally diagnosed as FTC, indicating the incremental value of [^{11}C]MET in imaging DTCs [63]. [^{11}C]MET is currently being studied as a surrogate for [^{18}F]FDG in other tumor types, such as brain tumors [69,70] and laryngeal cancer [71]. To date, there is no evidence showing the superiority of [^{11}C]MET over [^{18}F]FDG. Although complementary uptake of ^{11}C-MET and [^{18}F]FDG has been reported in recurrent or metastatic DTCs [72], further clarification and longitudinal study are still required to illustrate the actual value of the [^{11}C]MET in clinic settings. The downside of [^{11}C]MET is the short half-life of ^{11}C (20.4 min), which limits its broad application [73].

2.3.3. [^{18}F]FGln

[^{18}F]FGln, an analog of natural glutamine regulated by several glutamine (Gln) transporters (solute carrier family 1 member 5, SLC1A5; solute carrier family 38 member 1, SLC38A1; and SLC7A5; etc.), has been tested and subsequently considered as a promising probe for assessing glutamine metabolism in tumors [61]. Its use is justified by the understanding that tumor cells need extra nutrition and energy for rapid growth and proliferation, while glutamine metabolism is occasionally used by the cell as an alternative to glucose [74]. [^{18}F]FGln can further complement the diagnostic capacity of [^{18}F]FDG by detecting Gln metabolic changes in PTCs [62]. In [^{18}F]FGln imaging, excellent contrast images can be made only 10 min after injection, while late-phase imaging (60 min) would cause a high background to some extent [62] (Figure 4).

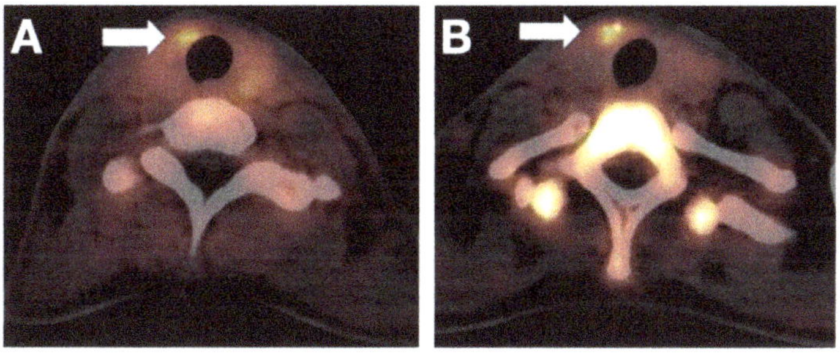

Figure 4. Example of a PTC revealed by [^{18}F]FGln at 10 min (**A**) and 60 min (**B**) post-injection, respectively. The arrows indicate the malignant lesion. Reproduced with permission from [62], copyright 2020 Springer Nature Inc.

[^{18}F]FAMT, [^{18}F]FET, and the newly reported [^{18}F]NKO-035 are all transported by L-type amino acid transporters, which are overexpressed in tumor cells [21,75]. However, data for those probes remain inadequate now. Furthermore, unlike other amino acid tracers transported by multiple unspecific amino acid transporters, [^{18}F]FAMT has an α-methyl moiety that allows it to be exclusively specific to SLC7A5, making it highly tumor-specific [76,77]. Furthermore, [^{18}F]FAMT is more specific for tumors than [^{18}F]FDG, although their sensitivities are similar. However, [^{18}F]FAMT imaging is comparable to [^{18}F]FDG imaging in diagnosing tumors other than TCs [20]. Future studies are warranted to investigate the amino acid metabolism in TCs and the diagnostic value of amino acid tracers in large cohorts.

2.4. Nucleoside Transporter-Targeting Probes

Radiolabeled or fluorescent nucleobase analogs are currently used to diagnose solid tumors, including cancers of the bladder, breast, lung, ovary, and pancreas. Regarding diagnosis of TC specifically, only [^{18}F]fluorothymidine ([^{18}F]FLT) has been tested to date. [^{18}F]FLT, which can be taken up by equilibrative nucleoside transporter 1 (ENT1), is a marker of cell proliferation [78]. In one study, 20 DTCs were assessed with [^{18}F]FLT and [^{18}F]FDG on PET/CT. While 69% of the metastatic lesions were identified by focal increases in [^{18}F]-FLT uptake, a lower result than the 92% identified by [^{18}F]FDG PET/CT. It is also demonstrated that [^{18}F]FDG has the advantage in terms of specificity and accuracy over [^{18}F]FLT in finding local lymph node malignancy and distant metastases [79]. So far, [^{18}F]FLT PET/CT has not progressed very far in diagnosing TCs.

3. Peptide-Based Probes

Peptide tracers have played vital roles in MI due to their unique advantages, notably their low molecular weight and ability to bind tumor biomarkers specifically, with low toxicity to surrounding non-cancer cells. Multiple tracers, like [^{68}Ga]Ga-dodecane tetraacetic acid labeled RGD2 ([^{68}Ga]Ga-DOTA-RGD2; RGD: Arg-Gly-Asp), [^{68}Ga]Ga-prostate specific membrane antigen ligand ([^{68}Ga]Ga-PSMA) with conjugates of N,N′-bis[2 -hydroxy-5-(carboxyethyl)benzyl]ethylene diamine-N,N′-diacetic acid (HBED-CC) or DOTA, [^{68}Ga]Ga-DOTA-DGlu-Ala-Tyr-Gly-Trp-(N-Me)Nle-Asp-1-Nal-NH2 ([^{68}Ga]Ga-DOTA-MGS5), [^{111}In]In-DTPA-octreotide, and other somatostatin analogs have been developed for imaging TCs, particularly MTCs and RR-DTCs [80].

3.1. Somatostatin Receptor (SSTR)-Targeting Probes

Somatostatin receptors have become typical therapeutic targets in neuroendocrine tumors (NETs) because they are often overexpressed on the surface of tumor cells. This has led to the development of several ^{68}Ga-labelled somatostatin analogs as PET imaging probes [81], which could be used for the diagnosis of MTC [80]. ^{68}Ga-labeled somatostatin analogs, including [^{68}Ga]Ga-DOTA-(1-Nal^3)-octreotide ([^{68}Ga]Ga-DOTANOC), [^{68}Ga]Ga-DOTA(0)-Phe(1)-Tyr(3)-octreotide ([^{68}Ga]Ga-DOTATOC), and [^{68}Ga]Ga-DOTA-(Tyr3)-octreotate ([^{68}Ga]Ga-DOTATATE), are valuable diagnostic tools showing excellent performance in the majority of patients with NETs [82]. Nevertheless, studies reporting the diagnostic value of SSTR-targeted PET in recurrent MTC are limited. A meta-analysis involving nine studies reported that the tumor detection rate on SSTR-based PET or PET/CT is only 63.5% in recurrent MTC, which is lower than that in other NETs [83].

3.2. *αvβ3 Integrin-Targeting Probes*

The integrin αvβ3 expression on epithelial cells and mature endothelial cells is relatively low, however, it is commonly and highly expressed in solid tumors. RGD and RGD_2 are peptides that bind integrin αvβ3 [84]. Recently, the dimeric [^{68}Ga]Ga-DOTA-RGD_2 has been successfully applied for PET imaging of RR-DTCs in clinical settings [85], showing sensitivity, specificity, and accuracy of 82.3%, 100%, and 86.4%, respectively, which exceeds the same measurements in [^{18}F]FDG of 82.3%, 50%, and 75%, respectively. For RR-DTCs, the advantage provided by [^{68}Ga]Ga-DOTA-RGD2 is the ability to detect lesions not detected by [^{18}F]FDG [85] (Figure 5). Furthermore, diagnosis of RR-DTCs using [^{68}Ga]Ga-DOTA-RGD_2 is better accompanied by [^{177}Lu]Lu-DOTA-RGD_2, a potential treatment option for RR-DTCs [86]. Considering that [^{68}Ga]Ga-DOTA-RGD_2 and [^{177}Lu]Lu-DOTA-RGD_2 are a useful theranostic pair for RR-DTCs, the potential to improve the theranostic landscape of RR-DTCs by sequentially using these agents is high. Nuclear medicine approaches have revolutionized the theranostic arsenal for DTCs, and we are confident that there is room to optimize the management of RR-DTCs with these novel agents.

3.3. *PSMA-Targeting Probes*

PSMA is overexpressed on the prostate cancer cell membrane. Recently, several studies found unexpected PSMA-targeted radiotracer uptake by TCs, including RR-DTCs [87–91] (Figure 6). In addition, ~50% of TC microvessels showed high expression of PSMA related to tumor size and vascular invasion [89]. Thus, it is reasonable that high-grade TCs can be targeted by PSMA-specific radioligands like [^{177}Lu]Lu-PSMA and [^{225}Ac]Ac-PSMA [92], establishing a novel theranostic platform for TCs that are refractory to radioiodine treatment. Currently, the clinical interest and focus of PSMA-targeted theranostics remain primarily oriented towards prostate cancers. It is worth exploring the performance of PSMA-targeted agents in RR-DTCs. The authors wonder if PSMA-targeted agents will open a new horizon for RR-DTCs in the future.

3.4. *Cholecystokinin-2 Receptor (CCK2R)-Targeting Probes*

CCK2R is highly expressed in 90% of MTC, 50% of small cell lung cancers, 60% of astrocytomas, insulinomas, stromal ovarian cancers, gastrointestinal stromal tumors, and more than 20% of gastroenteropancreatic tumors [93–95]. As a new peptide tracer targeting CCK2R, ^{68}Ga-DOTA-MGS5 is supposed to be superior to [^{18}F]FDOPA in diagnosing MTCs. The comparison between the [^{68}Ga]Ga-DOTA-MGS5 and [^{18}F]FDOPA was performed in a 75-year-old female patient with recurrent MTC (calcitonin: 2726 ng/l), who underwent consecutive [^{68}Ga]Ga-DOTA-MGS5 and [^{18}F]FDOPA-PET/CT. [^{68}Ga]Ga-DOTA-MGS5 found three obvious liver lesions with higher uptake than [^{18}F]FDOPA-PET/CT (SUVmax = 6.4–8.3 vs. 3.7) and showed a good lesion-to-background contrast in the liver, which might yield complementary information to [^{18}F]FDOPA-PET in patients with recurrent MTC [96] (Figure 7). The background of [^{68}Ga]Ga-DOTA-MGS5 seems higher than that of [^{18}F]FDOPA in our opinion.

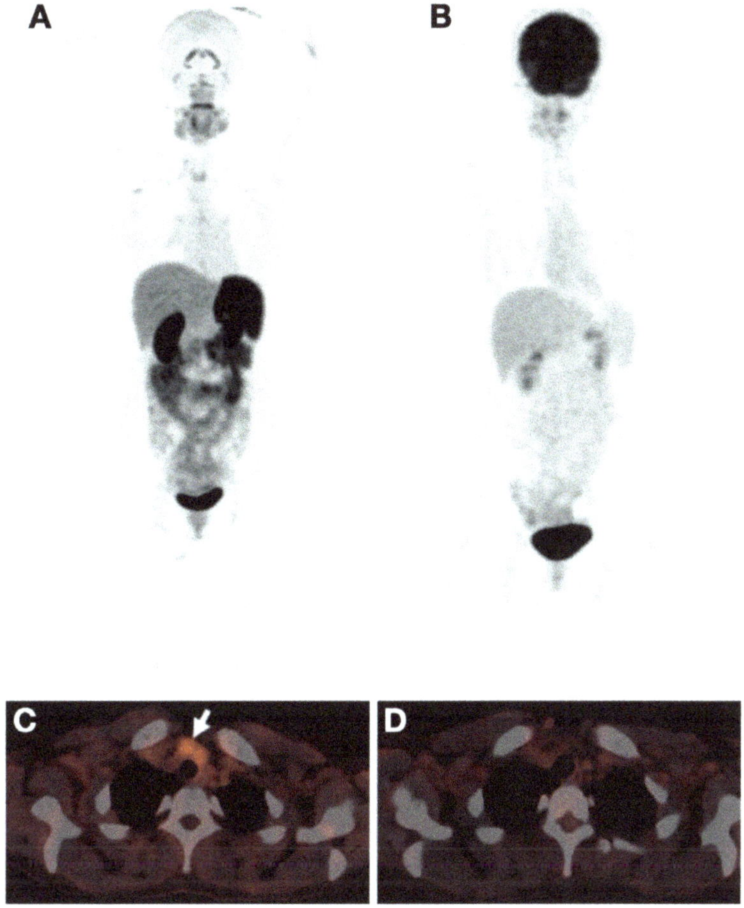

Figure 5. PET/CT imaging comparing [^{68}Ga]Ga-DOTA-RGD2 and [^{18}F]FDG. The RR-DTC case showed a high level of stimulated Tg (85 ng/mL) and negative ^{131}I post-therapy whole-body scan. Histopathology confirmed the metastatic lesions. (**A**) A maximum intensity projection (MIP) image showed [^{68}Ga]Ga-DOTA-RGD2 positive foci in the lower cervical region. (**B**) The corresponding MIP image of [^{18}F]FDG. (**C**) Fused PET/CT showed the metastatic foci was [^{68}Ga]Ga-DOTA-RGD2 positive; (**D**) the corresponding foci is negative on [^{18}F]FDG fused PET/CT. Reproduced with permission from [85], copyright 2020 Mary Ann Liebert Inc.

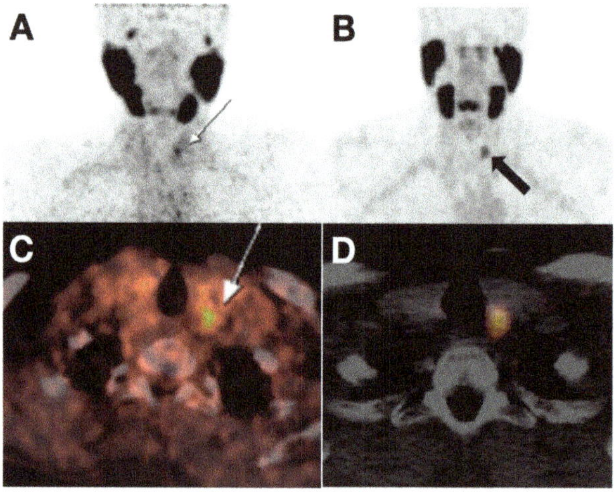

Figure 6. (**A**,**C**) PET and PET/CT fusion images showed slight [^{68}Ga]Ga-PSMA uptake in the thyroid nodule of a 62-year-old patient with prostate cancer. The thyroid nodule was validated as Hürthle cell angioinvasive FTC by post-thyroidectomy pathology. Reproduced with permission from [88] copyright 2016 Society of Nuclear Medicine and Molecular Imaging. (**B**,**D**) PET and PET/CT fusion image marked ^{68}Ga-PSMA uptake in the thyroid nodule of a 65-year-old man with metastatic prostate cancer. The thyroid nodule was regarded as TC proved by post-thyroidectomy pathology. Reproduced with permission from [91], copyright 2017 Wolters Kluwer Health Inc.

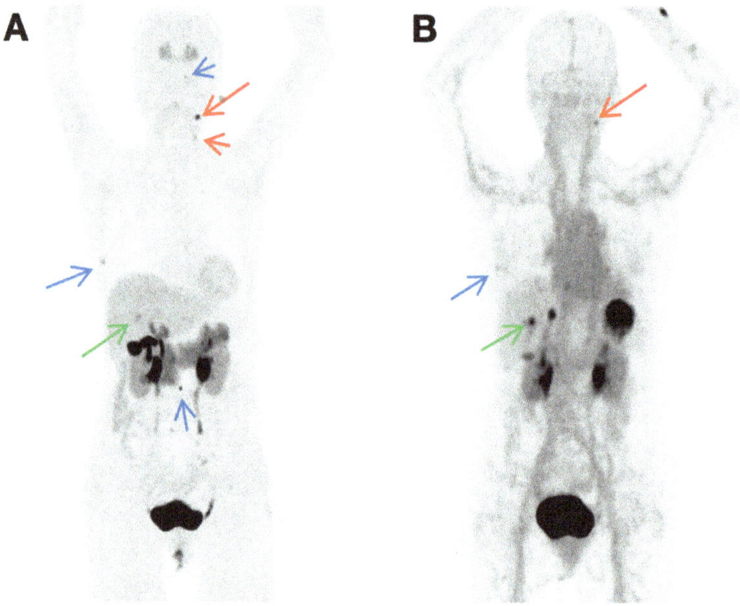

Figure 7. Comparison of [^{18}F]FDOPA and [^{68}Ga]Ga-DOTA-MGS5 in MTC patients. (**A**) [^{18}F]FDOPA PET imaging at one hour post-injection. (**B**) ^{68}Ga-Ga-DOTA-MGS5 PET imaging at one-hour post-injection. [^{68}Ga]Ga-DOTA-MGS5 yields complementary information to [^{18}F]FDOPA-PET. Reproduced with permission from [96], copyright 2021, Springer Nature Inc.

4. Antibody-Based Probes

Antibodies are high-affinity molecules with strict targeting abilities that are used for highly specific binding [97]. The development and translational use of antibody therapeutics have shaped the model of molecular targeted therapy and immunotherapy. The high affinity of monoclonal antibodies for their targets promotes the rational and efficacious use of antibody therapeutics [98]. We have advocated that PET imaging with radiolabeled antibodies or antibody fragments (i.e., immunoPET) provides a powerful platform for visualizing the tumor targets, selecting suitable patients for targeted therapies or immunotherapies, and assessing the therapeutic responses thereafter [19]. The first-generation monoclonal antibodies (mAbs) were of murine origin, making them immunogenic, limited for their clinical use. Consequently, chimeric mAbs, humanized mAbs, and complete human mAbs were produced to solve this issue [98]. One limitation of the full-size antibody probes is their considerable size (~150 kDa), which leads to a long circulatory half-life and reduced tissue penetration [99]. To ameliorate the imaging quality and efficiency and accelerate clinical translation, some smaller molecule substitute probes have been investigated, including antigen-binding fragments (Fabs) and engineered Fab variants, single-chain variable fragments (scFv), diabodies, minibodies (~25–100 kDa), and other types of therapeutic proteins, such as affibodies and nanobodies [19]. Facilitated by these developments, multiple antibodies, and antibody derivatives have been designed as either imaging probes or therapeutic agents to induce cancer cell death and elicit host immune effector responses in TC [19].

4.1. Single Target Immunoglobulin G (IgG) Probes

Full-size IgG antibody probes have been applied to tumor detection, staging, guidance of local treatment, identification or validation of tumor targets, and assessment of therapeutic response or tumor prognosis [100]. Once the first-rank antigen has been selected, the corresponding IgG can be labeled with a radionuclide or fluorescent tag [19]. The radionuclide labeled IgG can be visualized via immunoPET imaging, and the fluorescent tags can be visualized through the fluorescence system during thyroidectomy or metastasectomy [101].

4.1.1. Epidermal Growth Factor Receptor (HER2, ERBB2)-Targeting Probes

The human HER2, which is expressed on the cell plasma membrane [102], is a typical molecular marker for breast cancers and a subset of aggressive thyroid cancers [103,104]. HER2 overexpression was found in 44% of FTCs, 18% of PTCs [105], and certain ATCs [106]. Several HER2-specific agents—such as trastuzumab, lapatinib, and pertuzumab—have primarily ameliorated the prognosis in HER2-positive breast cancers [107,108]. Outside of breast cancers and TCs, HER2 is also widely overexpressed in multiple malignancies, including bladder, pancreatic, ovarian, and stomach cancers [109–111]. CUDC-101 (an inhibitor of epidermal growth factor receptor (EGFR), HER2, and histone deacetylase (HDAC)) inhibited tumor growth and metastases in metastatic ATC models [112], and lapatinib (an inhibitor of HER2 and EGFR) overcame the ERK and v-akt murine thymoma viral oncogene homolog 1 (AKT) rebound in PLX4032 resistant TC cells [113]. These studies indicate that HER2 is a potential target for developing theranostic interventions for advanced TCs.

By labeling the HER2-targeting mAb pertuzumab with ^{89}Zr, we have developed the [^{89}Zr]Zr-DFO-pertuzumab and evaluated its diagnostic efficacy in subcutaneous and orthotopic ATC models [114] (Figure 8). ImmunoPET and fluorescence imaging indicated that radiolabeled or fluorescence-labeled HER2 probes are promising for the management of ATCs, which may become helpful tools for image-guided tumor removal or identifying HER2-positive ATCs for HER2-targeted therapies. However, clinical studies are needed for further translation. To facilitate clinical translation and broad clinical use, we have developed a series of novel nanobody-based tracers to delineate HER2 expression. We will test the performance of the tracers in TC models very soon.

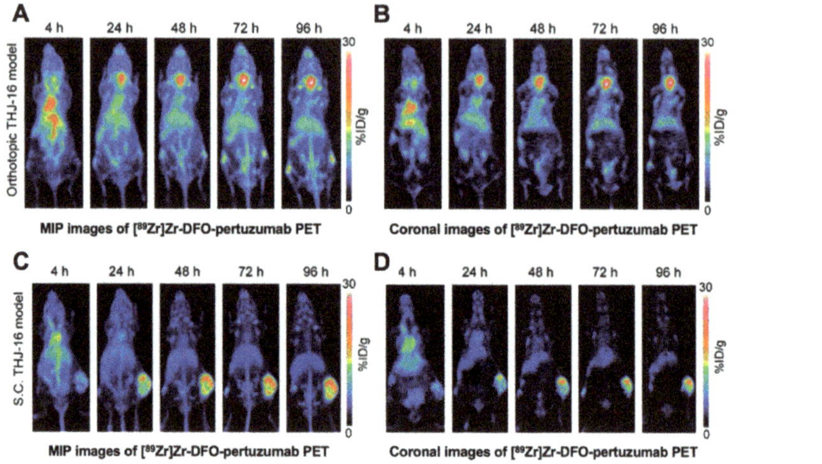

Figure 8. PET imaging with [^{89}Zr]Zr-DFO-pertuzumab in xenografts (cell line: THJ-16T). (**A**) Maximum intensity projection (MIP) showed the ability of [^{89}Zr]Zr-DFO-pertuzumab for visualizing TCs in an orthotopic model. (**B**) Coronal imaging in an orthotopic model. (**C**) MIP in a subcutaneous model. (**D**) Coronal imaging in a subcutaneous model. Reproduced with permission from [114], copyright 2019 e-Century Publishing Corporation.

4.1.2. Intercellular Adhesion Molecule-1 (ICAM-1, CD54)-Targeting Probes

ICAM-1, belonging to the immunoglobulin superfamily of cell adhesion molecules, consists of five extracellular IgG-like domains and one cytoplasmic tail [115]. ICAM-1 is found to be expressed at low levels in normal tissue, but at high levels in multiple types of cancer, including TCs [116,117]. One of its important features is that it can initiate tumor transmigration and invasion [116,118]. Furthermore, ICAM-1-targeted chimeric antigen receptor T (CAR-T) cells can robustly kill TC cells [119,120]. Research thus far has suggested ICAM-1 as an ideal target for TC diagnosis and treatments. For this purpose, Wei et al. created an immunoPET probe [^{64}Cu]Cu-NOTA-ICAM-1, which targets ICAM-1. [^{64}Cu]Cu-NOTA-ICAM-1 immunoPET imaging showed high contrast in diagnosing the subcutaneous and orthotopic ATCs in preclinical settings [101] (Figure 9). With the published data and unpublished data in hand, we believe that ICAM-1 may serve as a viable biomarker for certain types of TCs. However, it remains to see the diagnostic utility of ICAM-1–targeted tracers in patients with TCs.

4.1.3. Lectin Galactoside-Binding Soluble 3 (LGALS3, Galectin-3, or Gal3)-Targeting Probes

Gal-3 is a protein that is undetectable in normal and benign thyroid tissues but highly expressed in DTC cytosol, cell membranes, and intercellular substance [121]. The expression of galectin-3 as a biomarker for TCs has been validated in two multicenter studies [122,123]. The sensitivity and specificity of Gal-3 immunodetection reached 94% and 98% in distinguishing benign from TC lesions, with positive and negative predictive values of 98% and 94%, respectively, and diagnostic accuracy of 96% [122]. [^{89}Zr]Zr-labeled Gal3 mAb ([^{89}Zr]Zr-DFO-Gal3) or Gal-3 mAb with F(ab′)$_2$ conjunction ([^{89}Zr]Zr-Gal3-F(ab′)$_2$) has shown good binding to TC in vivo, allowing it to be potentially used for the detection of recurrence and metastases [124,125] (Figure 10). The particular design of [^{89}Zr]Zr-DFO-Gal3-F(ab′)$_2$, a protein formed of two F(ab′) fragments, results in faster blood clearance and lower liver uptake than traditional mAb-based tracers [125]. The high uptake of [^{89}Zr]Zr-DFO-Gal3-F(ab′)$_2$ in kidneys is due to the urinary excretion [125], which should not be problematic because metastatic TC to the kidney is very rare [126]. For a diagnostic purpose, the dose is usually quite low and so is the nephrotoxicity. Thus [^{89}Zr]Zr-DFO-

Gal3-F(ab′)$_2$ might be an excellent candidate for translation into the preoperative evaluation and postoperative follow-up.

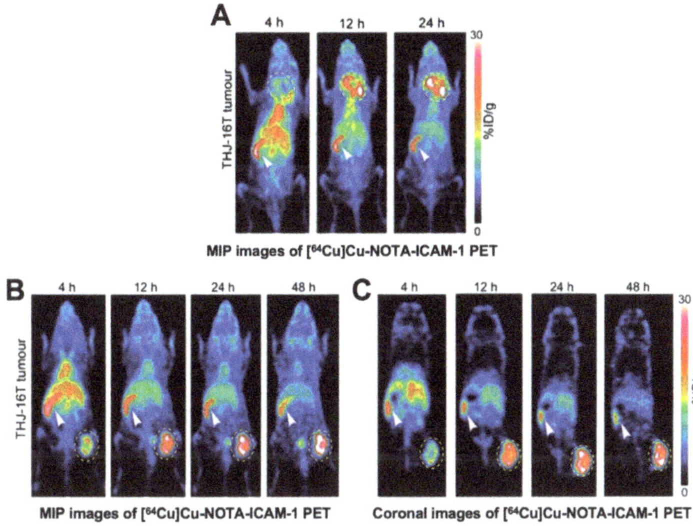

Figure 9. [^{64}Cu]Cu-NOTA-ICAM-1 immunoPET imaging in ATC xenografts (cell line: THJ-16T). (**A**) Maximum intensity projection (MIP) images in an orthotopic model. (**B**) MIP images in a subcutaneous model. (**C**) Coronal images of the same model. Reproduced with permission from [101], copyright 2020 Springer Nature Inc.

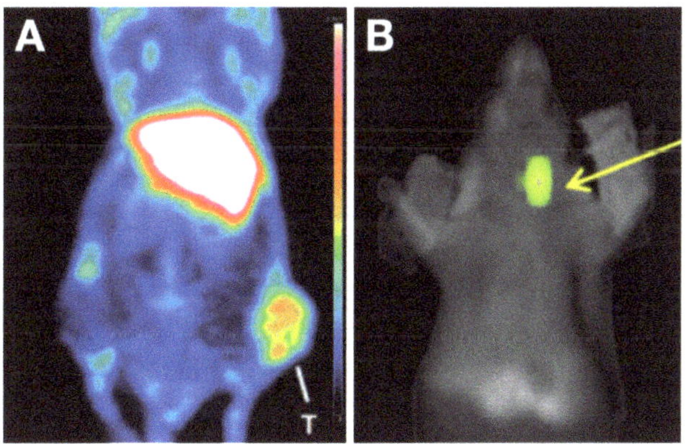

Figure 10. Characterization of [^{89}Zr]Zr-Gal-3 in TC xenografts. (**A**) PET image acquired at 48 h post radiotracer injection in a subcutaneous TC model showed an apparent accumulation of [^{89}Zr]Zr-Gal-3 in a tumor at the right thigh; Reproduced with permission from copyright 2016 American Association for Cancer Research [124]. (**B**) TC in an orthotopic model was visualized after injection of Cy5.5-Gal-3 with fluorescence imaging in the neck. Reproduced with permission from [125] copyright 2019 Society of Nuclear Medicine and Molecular Imaging.

4.2. Bispecific IgG Probes

Bispecific antibody (BsAb) probes have filled the vacancy of single target IgG probes in theranostics by providing higher antigen-binding capacity in tumor tissues than the monomeric counterparts [19]. Additionally, the pharmacokinetics of BsAbs could be improved by protein modification. The ability of BsAbs to bind to two targets allows these bispecific IgG probes to display an enhanced role for targeting two antigens on a tumor cell surface, linking the tumor cells and immune cells, for instance [127,128]. However, until recently, only one BsAb targeting CEA and HSG has been thoroughly investigated in the diagnosis of MTC.

As stated previously, the intense expression of CEA is a biomarker of MTC. Prior clinical studies have shown the high sensitivity of the combination of anti-CEA BsAbs and ^{111}In or ^{131}I labeled haptens-peptides [129–131]. IMP288, an HSG hapten, was reported to have the ability to bind multiple radionuclides [132]. Meanwhile, a trivalent BsAb (called TF2), was engineered composing one HSG glycine Fab fragment and two anti-CEA Fab fragments [133]. The combination of ^{68}Ga labeled IMP288 and TF2 in PET imaging yields high sensitivity and specificity; Nevertheless, the pretargeting conditions may still need to be modified to reduce or avoid IMP288-induced adverse effects (malaise, bronchospasm, tachycardia, and hypertension) [132,134]. The delivery method of the tracer may challenge patients' acceptability because the combination of IMP288 and TF2 requires two injections: the first injection for TF2 BsAb, and a second injection for [^{68}Ga]Ga-IMP288, with a time lag (one or two days) between the two injections [134] (Figure 11). The pretargeting strategy was used for the diagnostic purpose in the study. Replacement of ^{68}Ga with beta-emitter (e.g., ^{177}Lu) or alpha-emitter (e.g., ^{225}Ac) will further develop pretargeting therapeutic strategies, which will hopefully maximize the therapeutic index and minimize the adverse effects.

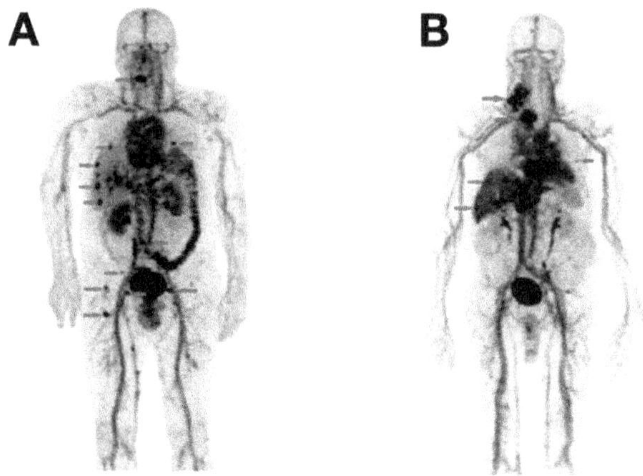

Figure 11. [^{68}Ga]Ga-IMP288 plus TF2 PET revealed a considerable number of MTC foci. (**A**) Patient #1: foci were detected in multiple places, including supradiaphragmatic nodes, lung, liver, and bone, etc. (**B**) Patient #2: foci were detected in supradiaphragmatic nodes and liver, etc. Reproduced with permission from [134], copyright 2016 Society of Nuclear Medicine and Molecular Imaging.

4.3. Fab-Based Probes

Fab is characterized by a light chain and a heavy chain of an immunoglobulin, containing variable regions, constant domain of the light chain (CL), and first constant domain of the heavy chain (CH1) [135]. The Fab, therefore, takes the specificity of the immunoglobulin. Unlike the traditional antibodies (produced from mammalian cells), Fabs could be generally and easily produced from bacteria cells, like *E. coli* [136]. One drawback of Fab is the limited retention on the antigen and rapid clearance [137]. Some Fabs have been discovered for the treatment of TC (targeting cluster of differentiation 276 [CD276] [138], etc.), and some publications reported the potential value of Fab as diagnostic probes targeting Galectin-3 [125,139,140].

[^{89}Zr]Zr-DFO-αGal3-Fab-PAS_{200}, an imunoPET probe fused with 200 Pro, Ala, and Ser residues (PAS_{200}) and conjugated with [^{89}Zr]Zr-deferoxamine ([^{89}Zr]Zr-DFO), is a recently reported Fab-based probe derived from the rat anti-Gal3 mAb. Similar to the full-size [^{89}Zr]Zr-labeled Gal-3 mAb (mentioned in Section 4.1.3) [125], the [^{89}Zr]Zr-DFO-αGal3-Fab-PAS_{200} can bind the Gal-3 well [139] (Figure 12). Unlike the uptake of full-size ^{89}Zr-labeled Gal-3 mAb which lasts over five days after injection, the [^{89}Zr]Zr-DFO-αGal3-Fab-PAS_{200} was supposed to have a shorter lasting time, but the exact time was undetermined [125]. Research concerning a head-to-head comparison between the anti-Gal3 IgG probe and the corresponding fragment probe is lacking.

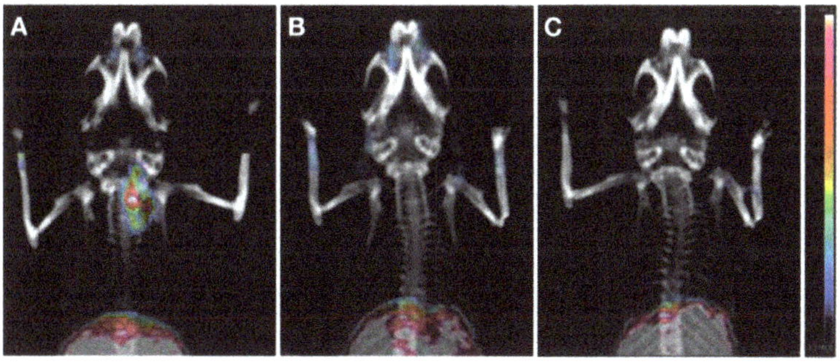

Figure 12. PET/CT images of mice at 24 h after intravenous injections. (**A**) Injection with 3 MBq of [^{89}Zr]Zr-DFO-αGal3-Fab-PAS_{200}. (**B**) Co-injection of 3 MBq of [^{89}Zr]Zr-DFO-αGal3-Fab-PAS_{200} and 1000-fold of nonradioactive aGal3-Fab-PAS_{200} (for blocking). (**C**) Control. Color scale bars: 3.3–7.8%ID/g. Reproduced with permission from [139], copyright 2020 Mary Ann Liebert, Inc.

4.4. Nanobody-Based Probes

A single-domain antibody (sdAb, nanobody) is an engineered antibody fragment containing a single monomeric variable antibody domain. Compared to the large size of full-size antibodies (~150 kDa), nanobodies (~15 kDa) can be delivered to tumors with comparatively less obstruction [141]. Nanobodies can be reconstructed to Fc-domains or conjugated to molecular inhibitors, radioisotopes, fluorescent dye, and nanoparticles, making them suitable for targeting tumors with many applications [142]. For example, Jailkhani et al. established nanobody libraries against extracellular matrix (ECM) proteins, which are hallmarks of many diseases, including cancers. PET/CT imaging showed that ^{64}Cu-labeled NJB2 nanobody probes targeted ECM and detected breast cancer and melanoma *for* primary and metastatic foci (including thyroid) with excellent contrast [143]. Thus, nanobody probes may open up a promising opportunity for application in TCs. So far, nanobody probes remain absent in TC research [144]. Our team has developed a series of nanobodies targeting various targets (e.g., tumor-associated calcium signal transducer 2 [TACSTD2, TROP-2], ICAM-1, integrin associated protein [CD47], and melanoma cell adhesion molecule [MCAM, CD146]) and are fully exploring the theranostic potential of the nanobodies in TCs.

5. Other Probes

5.1. Aptamer-Based Probes

Aptamers are nucleic acids with antigen selectivity rivaling that of antibodies [145]. They bind to their target through electrostatic interactions, hydrophobic interactions, and induced fitting. Aptamers also offer target recognition that is comparable to traditional antibodies. Unlike antibodies, however, aptamers can be produced more feasibly. Its additional advantages include favorable storage properties and limited immunogenicity in vivo [146]. The major drawback of aptamers is the lack of stability in vivo. Regarding their application in TC, only a few aptamer probes have been reported [15].

5.1.1. Prominin 1 (PROM1, CD133)-Targeting Probes

CD133 is a kind of glycoprotein mainly expressed in hematopoietic stem and progenitor cells [147]. As a marker of cancer stem cells of brain tumor, colon cancer, melanoma, and ATCs [148–151], it is known to be responsible for the rapid growth of ATC and PTC cells [152,153]. Ge et al. synthesized and characterized an aptamer AP-1-M targeting CD133 in an ATC xenograft model. The synthesized AP-1-M-doxorubicin conjugates can effectively bind CD133-expressing tumor cells, and an intense signal may reflect the tumor proliferation at a fast pace [15] (Figure 13).

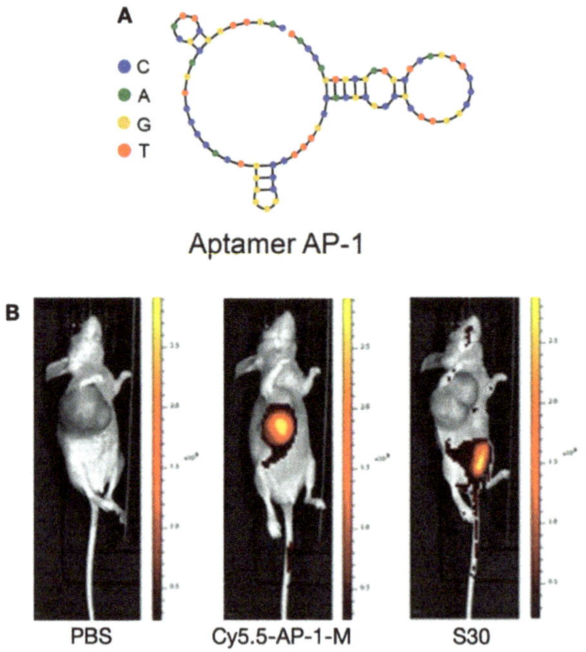

Figure 13. (**A**) Predicated structure of aptamer precursor AP-1. (**B**) Distribution of AP-1-M in a FRO xenograft model on fluorescence imaging at 48 h post-injection of PBS, Cy5.5-labeled AP-1-M, and control aptamer S30. Reproduced with permission from [15], copyright 2013 Royal Society of Chemistry.

5.1.2. PTC Tissue-Targeting Probes

Zhong et al. generated a PTC tissue-specific aptamer (TC-6) via tissue-based systematic evolution of ligands by exponential enrichment (SELEX), with clinical PTC tissues (positive control) and non-tumor thyroid tissues (negative control). The TC-6 can specifically distinguish PTC from other non-tumor tissues (Figure 14), and suppress the migration and invasion of PTC cells [16]. However, the exact molecular target remains unknown.

5.2. Nanoparticles-Based Probes

Nanoparticles have been emerging with widespread attention in MI, drug delivery, and disease treatment. Nanoparticles have brought their potential as MI agents to TC, primarily through their applicability in fluorescence imaging, ultrasound, and MRI [154,155]. These modalities enable nanoparticles to accumulate in cells by activation through US, light, temperature, and pH change, depending on the nanoparticle structures and their surface molecules. The ligand options for targeted nanoparticles are somewhat limited. Antibodies and peptides are the primary ligand choices due to their specific affinity to targets in TC fields. Although applications of targeted nanoparticles in TC have so far been limited, there have been publications investigating nanoparticles conjugated to antibodies targeting epidermal growth factor receptor (EGFR) or Src homology 2 (SH2) domain-containing phosphatase 2 (SHP2) [154,155].

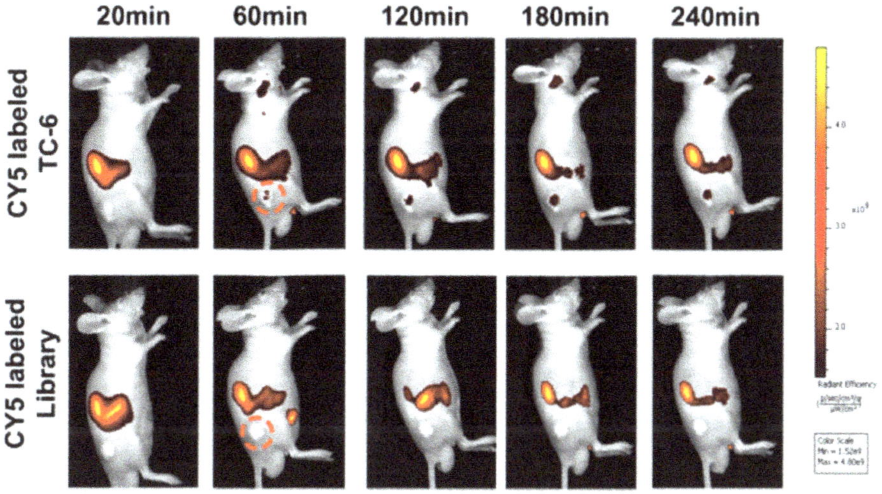

Figure 14. Time-lapse fluorescence imaged post-injection of Cy5-labeled TC-6 (**upper**) or library control (**lower**) in a TPC1 xenograft model. Reproduced with permission from [16], copyright 2016 American Association for Cancer Research.

5.2.1. EGFR-Targeting Probes

EGFR is a receptor binding the extracellular epidermal growth factor family (EGF family) [156]. In many tumor types, including TC, increased EGFR expression or activity initiates the tumor cell progression [112]. Recently, EGFR has been the target of the newly created nanoparticle (called C-HPNs) based on a core-shell system loaded with EGFR-targeted cetuximab and 10-hydroxycamptothecin (10-HCPT, chemotherapy agent). The EGFR antibody ligands enable nanoparticles to attach to cells which overexpress EGFR. With low-intensity focused ultrasound (LIFU) assistance, the liquid perfluoropentane (PFP) core in the nanoparticles would become vaporized and transformed into microbubbles, enhancing ultrasound contrast for tumor diagnosing. The core explosion induced by PFP boiling causes the release of 10-HCPT, providing more targeted delivery of the chemotherapeutic drug [154] (Figure 15)

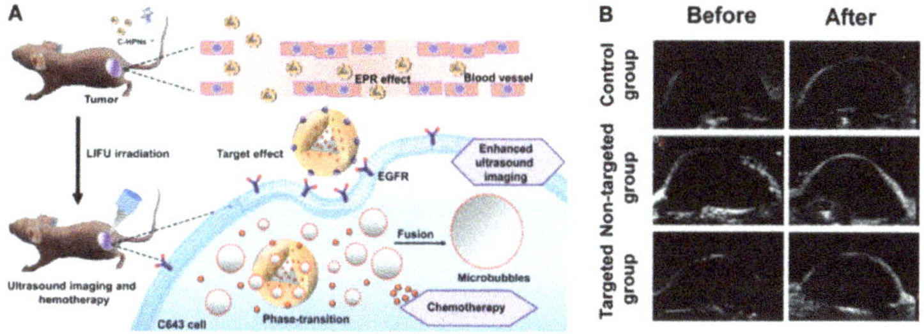

Figure 15. Theranostic applications of nanoparticles targeting EGFR. (**A**) Schematic illustration of the nanoparticles for chemotherapy drug delivery and enhanced diagnosis via LIFU. (**B**) Ultrasound imaging of tumors in B-mode before and after LIFU treatments. Reproduced with permission from [154], copyright 2019 Royal Society of Chemistry.

5.2.2. Protein Tyrosine Phosphatase Non-Receptor Type 11 (PTPN11, SHP2)-Targeting Probes

Another example is the SHP2, which is a tumor biomarker, acting as a signal of cell proliferation and immortality [157]. Hu et al. created an SHP2-targeted core-shell nanoparticle chelated with the contrast agent Gd^{3+} on the surface (NPs-SHP2). Similar to the EGFR-targeted nanoparticles mentioned previously, PFP-based LIFU can facilitate the probe carrying contrast agent been accumulated in the thyroid tumor area for enhanced MRI [155] (Figure 16).

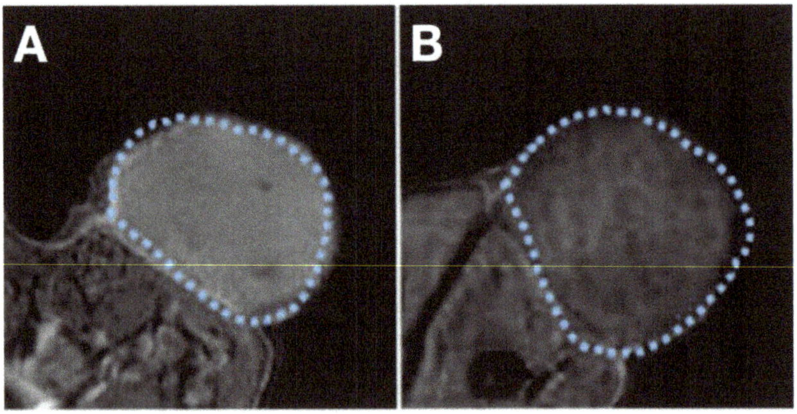

Figure 16. MRI in subcutaneous thyroid squamous cell cancer (TSCC) xenograft (blue dashed line) with NPs-SHP2 nanoparticles after LIFU treatment. (**A**) injection of SHP2-targeted nanoparticles. (**B**) injection of non-targeted nanoparticles (control). Reproduced with permission from [155], copyright Dove Medical Press Inc.

6. Conclusions and Future Perspectives

In summary, MI plays a vital role in evaluating and managing TCs, especially in accurately finding occult foci that are undetected by traditional ultrasound, CT, and MRI, thereby helping TC patients get the precise therapeutics (Table 1). Transporter-based probes tend to have high sensitivity, and immune-based probes generally have high specificity. So far, there is no single probe to reveal all the lesions both specifically and sensitively. Moreover, although TCs can be classified in a single pathological category, the biomarker expression in TC can vary dramatically. The apparent heterogeneity of TC requires the availability of more than one therapeutic method. By fully elucidating the biological characteristics of TCs and thoroughly exploring the biomarkers enriched in TCs [26,158,159], we believe that we can discover helpful targets for developing diagnostic probes and companion therapeutic agents for different molecular types of TC, not limited to pathological typing and phenotyping.

Table 1. A synoptic view of the MI radiotracers and their potential clinical value.

Tracer Types	Target	TC Type	Typical Roles	LoE [Ref.]
Transporter-targeting probes				
[^{124}I]NaI, [^{131}I]NaI	NIS	DTC	LL, TS, PE, TT, RD	Clinical [35,36]
[^{18}F]TFB, [^{18}F]FS, [^{18}F]HFP	NIS	DTC	LL, TS, PE, IUE	Clinical [50,51]
[^{18}F]FDG	GLUT1	TC	LL, TS, PE, PIU	Clinical [5,54,55]
[^{18}F]FDOPA	SLC7A5, SLC7A8	MTC	LL, TS, PE	Clinical [59,65]
[^{11}C]MET	SLC7A5	FTC	LL, TS, PE	Clinical [63]
[^{18}F]FGln	SLC7A5, SLC1A5, SLC38A1	PTC	LL, TS, PE	Clinical [62]
[^{18}F]FLT	ENT1	DTC	LL, TS, PE	Clinical [79,160]

Table 1. *Cont.*

Tracer Types	Target	TC Type	Typical Roles	LoE [Ref.]
Peptide-based probes				
^{68}Ga/^{177}Lu/^{90}Y/^{111}In labelled somatostatin analogue	SSTRs	TC	LL, TS, PE, PRRT	Clinical [161–163]
^{68}Ga/^{177}Lu labelled RGD$_2$	$\alpha v\beta 3$	TC	LL, TS, PE, PRRT	Clinical [85,86]
^{68}Ga/^{177}Lu labelled PSMA-ligand	PSMA	DTC	LL, TS, PE, PRRT	Clinical [88,91,164,165]
^{68}Ga/^{177}Lu labelled MGS5	CCK2R	MTC	LL, TS, PE, PRRT	Clinical [96] and preclinical [95]
Antibody-based probes				
Single target IgG-based probes				
^{89}Zr or RDye 800CW labeled pertuzumab	HER2	ATC	LL, TS	Preclinical [114]
^{64}Cu or RDye 800CW labeled ICAM-1 Ab	ICAM-1	ATC	LL, TS	Preclinical [101]
^{89}Zr labeled Gal3 Ab	Gal3	DTC	LL, TS	Preclinical [124]
Bispecific IgG-based probes				
^{68}Ga/^{177}Lu labelled IMP288 plus TF2 BsAb	CEA × HSG	MTC	LL, TS, PE, PRRT	Clinical [134,166]
Fab-based probes				
^{89}Zr or Cy5.5 labeled αGal3-Fab	Gal3	DTC	LL, TS	Preclinical [125,139,140]
Nanobody-based probes				
Targeting TROP-2 probes	TROP-2	TC (SP [167])	LL, TS, PRRT	Preclinical (OS)
Targeting CD47 probes	CD47	TC (SP [168])	LL, TS, PRRT	Preclinical (OS)
Targeting CD146 probes	CD146	TC (SP [169])	LL, TS, PRRT	Preclinical (OS)
Other probes				
Aptamer-based probes				
Cy5.5-AP-1-M	CD133	ATC	LL, TS	Preclinical [15]
Cy5-TC-6	PTC tissue	PTC	LL, TS	Preclinical [16]
Nanoparticles-based probes				
C-HPNs	EGFR	ATC	LL, TS, TT	Preclinical [154]
NPs-SHP2	SHP2	TC	LL, TS	Preclinical [155]

MI, molecular imaging; SP, speculative; LoE, level of evidence; LL, lesion localization; PE, prognosis evaluation; TT, tumor therapy; RD, radioiodine-131 dosimetry, [^{131}I]NaI dosimetry; TS, tumor staging; IUE, iodine uptake evaluation; PIU, predicting iodine uptake; OS, ongoing study; PRRT, pre-evaluation for receptor radionuclide therapy; TC, thyroid cancer; PTC, papillary thyroid cancer; MTC, medullary thyroid cancer; ATC, anaplastic thyroid cancer; DTC, differentiated thyroid cancer; BsAb, bispecific antibody; Ab, antibody; Fab, antigen-binding fragment.

With the development of biological techniques and imaging tools, more valuable imaging methods are emerging. Integration of multiple imaging modalities and anatomical features would help physicians diagnose and treat TCs in a timely target-specific manner. Nanoparticles may enable anti-TC drug delivery and multimodality imaging, which may further improve the management of TC. However, the authors are cautious because of the limited clinical evidence in the field of TC. Bispecific MI probes have gained more traction in the past decade. The synthesis of bispecific antibody or antibody fragment tracers has been thoroughly elucidated elsewhere [170]. The importance of bispecific probes is that they enable enhanced affinity and high image quality, providing the ability targeting more occult foci than traditional single-target probes, and inducing more comprehensive application across TC patients with complex biological characteristics.

For antibody probe design, the traditional antibody-based radioactive or fluorescent probes for TCs have simply been prepared by non-selective conjugation on lysine/cysteine residues with or without chelators [171,172]. This approach may reduce target binding affinity, especially at a high conjugate/protein ratio, and in any case, leads to a mixture of products with different numbers of tags per protein molecule [173]. The method may also cause undesirable biodistribution (e.g., high kidney uptake and poor tumor targeting due to in vivo cleavage of the S–S linkage) and pharmacokinetics (fast antibody clearance for modification of interchain disulfide cysteine) [174]. Protein engineering techniques are progressing very rapidly. In this setting, the site-specific and homogeneous introduction of the tags into the targeting moieties would be more advantageous. The emerging techniques mainly include chelator conjunction to the antibody glycan region, enzyme-assisted chelator attachment, and incorporating and chelating radioisotope into amino acid sequences [171]. This may help us design molecular imaging agents and companion therapeutic agents with increased possibility for clinical translation.

For the diagnosis of TC, the superiority of MI over conventional anatomical imaging is clear, with advantages of favorable spatial and temporal resolution and functional imaging [175]. The emergence of MI has fundamentally changed the management of TC. For instance, [^{18}F]FDG PET/CT plays its role in optimizing initial therapy, which is mandatory for improving DTC outcome. [^{18}F]FDG PET/CT could be conducted if some foci are radioiodine non-avid before treatment planning. Rosenbaum-Krumme et al. found that the TNM staging and management were changed from standard therapy (surgery plus ^{131}I therapy) to individual therapy (standard therapy plus external beam therapy or targeted therapy etc.) because of the [^{18}F]FDG PET/CT results in 21% of the high-risk DTCs [176]. We suppose that MI in TCs would become a helpful modality for tumor staging, prognosis evaluation, which may lead to immense changes in what treatments the TC patients are given, maximizing the benefits of individual therapy.

For TC therapy, despite the rapid progress in molecular imaging, we firmly believe that the innovation of therapeutic agents should accompany the development of diagnostic agents. For example, radionuclides such as ^{177}Lu, ^{225}Ac ^{188}Re, ^{67}Cu, ^{47}Sc, ^{166}Ho, ^{90}Y, ^{161}Tb, ^{149}Tb, ^{212}Pb, and ^{213}Bi emitting α-particles, β-particles, and Auger electrons can be feasibly chelated with DOTA, NOTA, etc., which is similar to the diagnostic isotopes mentioned in this review, ^{64}Cu or ^{68}Ga chelated with NOTA or DOTA [177]. For theranostic application, diagnostic probes with a chelating agent and a radionuclide suitable for imaging (e.g., NOTA and ^{64}Cu) can be used to map the target and assess the therapeutic potential of the same probe labelled with the same chelating agent and a therapeutic radionuclide (e.g., NOTA and ^{67}Cu) [19]. ^{149}Tb is another theranostic radioisotope that has not been investigated in thyroid cancer research to date. ^{149}Tb can simultaneously emit positrons (β^+ particles), α-particles, and γ-radiation, allowing PET and α particle-based therapy to go on at the same time [177]. The current review focuses on emerging probes for imaging with examples. Further introduction and discussion about the concept of TC therapy or theranostics will be updated and illustrated in an upcoming review. We hope the ever-developing diagnostic and therapeutic probes and theranostic applications can substantially improve the management of TCs, especially the aggressive RR-DTCs, MTCs, and ATCs.

In the last two decades, there has been a general increase in the prevalence of TC. The phenomenon is partially due to environmental factors (e.g., chemical pollution, anthropogenic or natural radiation), but is also due to overdiagnosis by increased screening with more sensitive methods (e.g., high-resolution ultrasound), especially in developed countries (e.g., South Korea and the United States), leading to unnecessary treatment. As mentioned previously, most incident TCs are low-risk DTCs that tend to retain their stability over the years until death due to aging. Therefore, it is unnecessary to treat indolent TCs because of the low cost-effectiveness and the practically unchanged mortality. Something to note is that the ever-developing MI techniques might more sensitively detect TCs, potentially causing overdiagnosis for indolent TC and overtreatment via invasive methods (e.g., thyroidectomy or metastasectomy) or noninvasive therapeutics (e.g., chemotherapy agents or multikinase inhibitors). To avoid these pitfalls, future work could focus on discovering prognosis- or progress-related targets or probes, thereby classifying TCs into indolent and active disease. In other words, future MI research should not be limited to the field of finding latent TC lesions.

Author Contributions: Conceptualization, Y.J., W.W. and W.C.; Methodology, Y.J., B.L. and W.W.; Writing—original draft preparation, Y.J.; Writing—review and editing, B.L., M.H.Y. and W.W.; Visualization, Y.J.; Supervision, W.W. and W.C.; Project administration, W.W. and W.C.; Funding acquisition, W.W., W.C., J.L. and G.H. All authors have read and agreed to the published version of the manuscript.

Funding: This research was funded by the National Key Research and Development Program of China (grant no. 2020YFA0909000), the National Natural Science Foundation of China (grant no. 82001878), the Shanghai Rising-Star Program (Grant No. 20QA1406100), and the University of Wisconsin–Madisons. Y.J. is supported by a postgraduate scholarship from the China Scholarship Council.

Institutional Review Board Statement: Not applicable.

Informed Consent Statement: Not applicable.

Data Availability Statement: No new data were created or analyzed in this study. Data sharing is not applicable to this article.

Conflicts of Interest: Weibo Cai is a scientific advisor, stockholder, and grantee of Focus-X Therapeutics, Inc. All other authors declare no conflict of interest.

References

1. Lim, H.; Devesa, S.S.; Sosa, J.A.; Check, D.; Kitahara, C.M. Trends in Thyroid Cancer Incidence and Mortality in the United States, 1974–2013. *JAMA* **2017**, *317*, 1338. [CrossRef] [PubMed]
2. Chen, W.; Zheng, R.; Baade, P.D.; Zhang, S.; Zeng, H.; Bray, F.; Jemal, A.; Yu, X.Q.; He, J. Cancer Statistics in China, 2015. *CA Cancer J. Clin.* **2016**, *66*, 115–132. [CrossRef] [PubMed]
3. Rahib, L.; Smith, B.D.; Aizenberg, R.; Rosenzweig, A.B.; Fleshman, J.M.; Matrisian, L.M. Projecting Cancer Incidence and Deaths to 2030: The Unexpected Burden of Thyroid, Liver, and Pancreas Cancers in the United States. *Cancer Res.* **2014**, *74*, 2913–2921. [CrossRef] [PubMed]
4. De la Vieja, A.; Riesco-Eizaguirre, G. Radio-Iodide Treatment: From Molecular Aspects to the Clinical View. *Cancers* **2021**, *13*, 995. [CrossRef] [PubMed]
5. Haugen, B.R.; Alexander, E.K.; Bible, K.C.; Doherty, G.M.; Mandel, S.J.; Nikiforov, Y.E.; Pacini, F.; Randolph, G.W.; Sawka, A.M.; Schlumberger, M.; et al. 2015 American Thyroid Association Management Guidelines for Adult Patients with Thyroid Nodules and Differentiated Thyroid Cancer: The American Thyroid Association Guidelines Task Force on Thyroid Nodules and Differentiated Thyroid Cancer. *Thyroid* **2016**, *26*, 1–133. [CrossRef]
6. Schlumberger, M.; Leboulleux, S. Current Practice in Patients with Differentiated Thyroid Cancer. *Nat. Rev. Endocrinol.* **2021**, *17*, 176–188. [CrossRef]
7. Durante, C.; Haddy, N.; Baudin, E.; Leboulleux, S.; Hartl, D.; Travagli, J.P.; Caillou, B.; Ricard, M.; Lumbroso, J.D.; Vathaire, F.D.; et al. Long-Term Outcome of 444 Patients with Distant Metastases from Papillary and Follicular Thyroid Carcinoma: Benefits and Limits of Radioiodine Therapy. *J. Clin Endocrinol Metab.* **2006**, *91*, 2892–2899. [CrossRef]
8. ACS Thyroid Cancer Survival Rates, by Type and Stage. Available online: https://www.cancer.org/cancer/thyroid-cancer/detection-diagnosis-staging/survival-rates.html (accessed on 5 June 2021).
9. Lin, B.; Ma, H.; Ma, M.; Zhang, Z.; Sun, Z.; Hsieh, I.-Y.; Okenwa, O.; Guan, H.; Li, J.; Lv, W. The Incidence and Survival Analysis for Anaplastic Thyroid Cancer: A SEER Database Analysis. *Am. J. Transl. Res.* **2019**, *11*, 5888–5896.
10. James, M.L.; Gambhir, S.S. A Molecular Imaging Primer: Modalities, Imaging Agents, and Applications. *Physiol. Rev.* **2012**, *92*, 897–965. [CrossRef]
11. Wahl, R.L.; Chareonthaitawee, P.; Clarke, B.; Drzezga, A.; Lindenberg, L.; Rahmim, A.; Thackeray, J.; Ulaner, G.A.; Weber, W.; Zukotynski, K.; et al. Mars Shot for Nuclear Medicine, Molecular Imaging, and Molecularly Targeted Radiopharmaceutical Therapy. *J. Nucl. Med. Off. Publ. Soc. Nucl. Med.* **2021**, *62*, 6–14. [CrossRef]
12. Piccardo, A.; Trimboli, P.; Foppiani, L.; Treglia, G.; Ferrarazzo, G.; Massollo, M.; Bottoni, G.; Giovanella, L. PET/CT in Thyroid Nodule and Differentiated Thyroid Cancer Patients. The Evidence-Based State of the Art. *Rev. Endocr. Metab. Disord.* **2019**, *20*, 47–64. [CrossRef]

13. Kendler, D.B.; Araújo, M.L., Jr.; Alencar, R.; Accioly, M.T.D.S.; Bulzico, D.A.; Pessoa, C.C.D.N.; Accioly, F.A.; De Farias, T.P.; Lopes, F.P.P.L.; Corbo, R.; et al. Somatostatin Receptor Subtype 1 Might Be a Predictor of Better Response to Therapy in Medullary Thyroid Carcinoma. *Endocrine* **2017**, *58*, 474–480. [CrossRef]
14. Ambrosini, V.; Kunikowska, J.; Baudin, E.; Bodei, L.; Bouvier, C.; Capdevila, J.; Cremonesi, M.; de Herder, W.W.; Dromain, C.; Falconi, M.; et al. Consensus on Molecular Imaging and Theranostics in Neuroendocrine Neoplasms. *Eur. J. Cancer* **2021**, *146*, 56–73. [CrossRef]
15. Ge, M.H.; Zhu, X.H.; Shao, Y.M.; Wang, C.; Huang, P.; Wang, Y.; Jiang, Y.; Maimaitiyiming, Y.; Chen, E.; Yang, C.; et al. Synthesis and Characterization of CD133 Targeted Aptamer–Drug Conjugates for Precision Therapy of Anaplastic Thyroid Cancer. *Biomater. Sci.* **2020**. [CrossRef]
16. Zhong, W.; Pu, Y.; Tan, W.; Liu, J.; Liao, J.; Liu, B.; Chen, K.; Yu, B.; Hu, Y.; Deng, Y.; et al. Identification and Application of an Aptamer Targeting Papillary Thyroid Carcinoma Using Tissue-SELEX. *Anal. Chem.* **2019**, *91*, 8289–8297. [CrossRef]
17. Zhu, C.; Li, L.; Fang, S.; Zhao, Y.; Zhao, L.; Yang, G.; Qu, F. Selection and Characterization of an SsDNA Aptamer against Thyroglobulin. *Talanta* **2021**, *223*, 121690. [CrossRef]
18. Kumarasamy, J.; Ghorui, S.K.; Gholve, C.; Jain, B.; Dhekale, Y.; Gupta, G.D.; Damle, A.; Banerjee, S.; Rajan, M.G.R.; Kulkarni, S. Production, Characterization and in-Vitro Applications of Single-Domain Antibody against Thyroglobulin Selected from Novel T7 Phage Display Library. *J. Immunol. Methods* **2021**, *492*, 112990. [CrossRef]
19. Wei, W.; Rosenkrans, Z.T.; Liu, J.; Huang, G.; Luo, Q.-Y.; Cai, W. ImmunoPET: Concept, Design, and Applications. *Chem. Rev.* **2020**, *120*, 3787–3851. [CrossRef]
20. Achmad, A.; Bhattarai, A.; Yudistiro, R.; Heryanto, Y.D.; Higuchi, T.; Tsushima, Y. The Diagnostic Performance of 18F-FAMT PET and 18F-FDG PET for Malignancy Detection: A Meta-Analysis. *BMC Med. Imaging* **2017**, *17*, 66. [CrossRef]
21. Enomoto, K.; Hotomi, M. Amino Acid Transporters as Potential Therapeutic Targets in Thyroid Cancer. *Endocrinol. Metab.* **2020**, *35*, 227–236. [CrossRef]
22. Fu, H.; Sa, R.; Cheng, L.; Jin, Y.; Qiu, X.; Liu, M.; Chen, L. An updated review on nuclear molecular imaging of thyroid cancers. *Endocr. Pract.* **2020**, *27*, 494–502. [CrossRef] [PubMed]
23. Portulano, C.; Paroder-Belenitsky, M.; Carrasco, N. The Na+/I− Symporter (NIS): Mechanism and Medical Impact. *Endocr. Rev.* **2013**, *35*, 106–149. [CrossRef] [PubMed]
24. Mariani, G.; Tonacchera, M.; Grosso, M.; Orsolini, F.; Vitti, P.; Strauss, H.W. The Role of Nuclear Medicine in the Clinical Management of Benign Thyroid Disorders, Part 1: Hyperthyroidism. *J. Nucl. Med.* **2021**, *62*, 304–312. [CrossRef] [PubMed]
25. Oh, J.M.; Ahn, B.-C. Molecular Mechanisms of Radioactive Iodine Refractoriness in Differentiated Thyroid Cancer: Impaired Sodium Iodide Symporter (NIS) Expression Owing to Altered Signaling Pathway Activity and Intracellular Localization of NIS. *Theranostics* **2021**, *11*, 6251–6277. [CrossRef] [PubMed]
26. Jin, Y.; Nostrand, D.V.; Cheng, L.; Liu, M.; Chen, L. Radioiodine Refractory Differentiated Thyroid Cancer. *Crit. Rev. Oncol. Hemat.* **2018**, *125*, 111–120. [CrossRef] [PubMed]
27. Nagarajah, J.; Janssen, M.; Hetkamp, P.; Jentzen, W. Iodine Symporter Targeting with 124 I/ 131 I Theranostics. *J. Nucl. Med.* **2017**, *58*, 34S–38S. [CrossRef]
28. Wyszomirska, A. Iodine-131 for Therapy of Thyroid Diseases. Physical and Biological Basis. *Nucl. Med. Rev. Cent. East. Eur.* **2012**, *15*, 120–123.
29. Gulec, S.A.; Kuker, R.A.; Goryawala, M.; Fernandez, C.; Perez, R.; Khan-Ghany, A.; Apaza, A.; Harja, E.; Harrell, M. 124 I PET/CT in Patients with Differentiated Thyroid Cancer: Clinical and Quantitative Image Analysis. *Thyroid* **2016**, *26*, 441–448. [CrossRef]
30. Jentzen, W.; Verschure, F.; van Zon, A.; van de Kolk, R.; Wierts, R.; Schmitz, J.; Bockisch, A.; Binse, I. 124I PET Assessment of Response of Bone Metastases to Initial Radioiodine Treatment of Differentiated Thyroid Cancer. *J. Nucl. Med.* **2016**, *57*, 1499–1504. [CrossRef]
31. Ruhlmann, M.; Jentzen, W.; Ruhlmann, V.; Pettinato, C.; Rossi, G.; Binse, I.; Bockisch, A.; Rosenbaum-Krumme, S. High Level of Agreement Between Pretherapeutic 124I PET and Intratherapeutic 131I Imaging in Detecting Iodine-Positive Thyroid Cancer Metastases. *J. Nucl. Med.* **2016**, *57*, 1339–1342. [CrossRef]
32. Jin, Y.; Ruan, M.; Cheng, L.; Fu, H.; Liu, M.; Sheng, S.; Chen, L. Radioiodine Uptake and Thyroglobulin-Guided Radioiodine Remnant Ablation in Patients with Differentiated Thyroid Cancer: A Prospective, Randomized, Open-Label, Controlled Trial. *Thyroid* **2019**, *29*, 101–110. [CrossRef]
33. Simon, D.; Körber, C.; Krausch, M.; Segering, J.; Groth, P.; Görges, R.; Grünwald, F.; Müller-Gärtner, H.; Schmutzler, C.; Köhrle, J.; et al. Clinical Impact of Retinoids in Redifferentiation Therapy of Advanced Thyroid Cancer: Final Results of a Pilot Study. *Eur. J. Nucl. Med. Mol. Imaging* **2002**, *29*, 775–782. [CrossRef]
34. Plantinga, T.S.; Heinhuis, B.; Gerrits, D.; Netea, M.G.; Joosten, L.A.B.; Hermus, A.R.M.M.; Oyen, W.J.G.; Schweppe, R.E.; Haugen, B.R.; Boerman, O.C.; et al. MTOR Inhibition Promotes TTF1-Dependent Redifferentiation and Restores Iodine Uptake in Thyroid Carcinoma Cell Lines. *J. Clin. Endocrinol. Metab.* **2014**, *99*, E1368–E1375. [CrossRef]
35. Ho, A.L.; Grewal, R.K.; Leboeuf, R.; Sherman, E.J.; Pfister, D.G.; Deandreis, D.; Pentlow, K.S.; Zanzonico, P.B.; Haque, S.; Gavane, S.; et al. Selumetinib-Enhanced Radioiodine Uptake in Advanced Thyroid Cancer. *N. Engl. J. Med.* **2013**, *368*, 623–632. [CrossRef]
36. Dunn, L.A.; Sherman, E.J.; Baxi, S.S.; Tchekmedyian, V.; Grewal, R.K.; Larson, S.M.; Pentlow, K.S.; Haque, S.; Tuttle, R.M.; Sabra, M.M.; et al. Vemurafenib Redifferentiation of BRAF Mutant, RAI-Refractory Thyroid Cancers. *J. Clin. Endocrinol. Metab.* **2018**, *104*, 1417–1428. [CrossRef]

37. Vaisman, F.; Carvalho, D.P.; Vaisman, M. A New Appraisal of Iodine Refractory Thyroid Cancer. *Endocr. Relat. Cancer* **2015**, *22*, R301–R310. [CrossRef]
38. Misawa, A.; Inoue, S. Estrogen-Related Receptors in Breast Cancer and Prostate Cancer. *Front. Endocrinol.* **2015**, *6*, 83. [CrossRef]
39. Singh, T.D.; Jeong, S.Y.; Lee, S.-W.; Ha, J.-H.; Lee, I.-K.; Kim, S.H.; Kim, J.; Cho, S.J.; Ahn, B.-C.; Lee, J.; et al. Inverse Agonist of Estrogen-Related Receptor γ Enhances Sodium Iodide Symporter Function Through Mitogen-Activated Protein Kinase Signaling in Anaplastic Thyroid Cancer Cells. *J. Nucl. Med. Off. Publ. Soc. Nucl. Med.* **2015**, *56*, 1690–1696. [CrossRef]
40. Singh, T.D.; Song, J.; Kim, J.; Chin, J.; Ji, H.D.; Lee, J.-E.; Lee, S.B.; Yoon, H.; Yu, J.H.; Kim, S.K.; et al. A Novel Orally Active Inverse Agonist of Estrogen-Related Receptor Gamma (ERRγ), DN200434, A Booster of NIS in Anaplastic Thyroid Cancer. *Clin. Cancer Res.* **2019**, *25*, 5069–5081. [CrossRef]
41. Hershman, J.M. To Avoid Stunning, Give Treatment Doses of Radioiodine-131 within Three Days after Completing the Diagnostic Scan or Wait Seven Days. *Clin. Thyroid.* **2015**, *27*, 341–343. [CrossRef]
42. Silberstein, E.B.; Alavi, A.; Balon, H.R.; Clarke, S.E.M.; Divgi, C.; Gelfand, M.J.; Goldsmith, S.J.; Jadvar, H.; Marcus, C.S.; Martin, W.H.; et al. The SNMMI Practice Guideline for Therapy of Thyroid Disease with 131I 3.0. *J. Nucl. Med.* **2012**, *53*, 1633–1651. [CrossRef] [PubMed]
43. Silberstein, E.B. The Problem of the Patient with Thyroglobulin Elevation but Negative Iodine Scintigraphy: The TENIS Syndrome. *Semin. Nucl. Med.* **2011**, *41*, 113–120. [CrossRef] [PubMed]
44. Kim, M.J.; Sun, H.J.; Song, Y.S.; Yoo, S.-K.; Kim, Y.A.; Seo, J.-S.; Park, Y.J.; Cho, S.W. CXCL16 Positively Correlated with M2-Macrophage Infiltration, Enhanced Angiogenesis, and Poor Prognosis in Thyroid Cancer. *Sci. Rep.* **2019**, *9*, 13288. [CrossRef] [PubMed]
45. Jiang, H.; Bansal, A.; Goyal, R.; Peng, K.-W.; Russell, S.J.; DeGrado, T.R. Synthesis and Evaluation of 18F-Hexafluorophosphate as a Novel PET Probe for Imaging of Sodium/Iodide Symporter in a Murine C6-Glioma Tumor Model. *Bioorg. Med. Chem.* **2018**, *26*, 225–231. [CrossRef]
46. Jiang, H.; DeGrado, T.R. [18F]Tetrafluoroborate ([18F]TFB) and Its Analogs for PET Imaging of the Sodium/Iodide Symporter. *Theranostics* **2018**, *8*, 3918–3931. [CrossRef]
47. Dittmann, M.; Carvalho, J.M.G.; Rahbar, K.; Schäfers, M.; Claesener, M.; Riemann, B.; Seifert, R. Incremental Diagnostic Value of [18F]Tetrafluoroborate PET-CT Compared to [131I]Iodine Scintigraphy in Recurrent Differentiated Thyroid Cancer. *Eur. J. Nucl. Med. Mol. Imaging* **2020**, *47*, 2639–2646. [CrossRef]
48. Khoshnevisan, A.; Chuamsaamarkkee, K.; Boudjemeline, M.; Jackson, A.; Smith, G.E.; Gee, A.D.; Fruhwirth, G.O.; Blower, P.J. 18F-Fluorosulfate for PET Imaging of the Sodium–Iodide Symporter: Synthesis and Biologic Evaluation In Vitro and In Vivo. *J. Nucl. Med.* **2017**, *58*, 156–161. [CrossRef]
49. Concilio, S.C.; Zhekova, H.R.; Noskov, S.Y.; Russell, S.J. Inter-Species Variation in Monovalent Anion Substrate Selectivity and Inhibitor Sensitivity in the Sodium Iodide Symporter (NIS). *PLoS ONE* **2020**, *15*, e0229085. [CrossRef]
50. O'Doherty, J.; Jauregui-Osoro, M.; Brothwood, T.; Szyszko, T.; Marsden, P.K.; O'Doherty, M.J.; Cook, G.J.R.; Blower, P.J.; Lewington, V. 18 F-Tetrafluoroborate, a PET Probe for Imaging Sodium/Iodide Symporter Expression: Whole-Body Biodistribution, Safety, and Radiation Dosimetry in Thyroid Cancer Patients. *J. Nucl. Med.* **2017**, *58*, 1666–1671. [CrossRef]
51. Samnick, S.; Al-Momani, E.; Schmid, J.-S.; Mottok, A.; Buck, A.K.; Lapa, C. Initial Clinical Investigation of [18F]Tetrafluoroborate PET/CT in Comparison to [124I]Iodine PET/CT for Imaging Thyroid Cancer. *Clin. Nucl. Med.* **2018**, *43*, 162–167. [CrossRef]
52. Zhang, Y.; Wang, J. Targeting Uptake Transporters for Cancer Imaging and Treatment. *Acta Pharm. Sin. B* **2019**, *10*, 79–90. [CrossRef]
53. Nagarajah, J.; Ho, A.L.; Tuttle, R.M.; Weber, W.A.; Grewal, R.K. Correlation of BRAFV600E Mutation and Glucose Metabolism in Thyroid Cancer Patients: An 18F-FDG PET Study. *J. Nucl. Med.* **2015**, *56*, 662–667. [CrossRef]
54. Liu, M.; Cheng, L.; Jin, Y.; Ruan, M.; Sheng, S.; Chen, L. Predicting 131I-Avidity of Metastases from Differentiated Thyroid Cancer Using 18F-FDG PET/CT in Postoperative Patients with Elevated Thyroglobulin. *Sci. Rep.* **2018**, *8*, 4352. [CrossRef]
55. Kang, S.Y.; Bang, J.-I.; Kang, K.W.; Lee, H.; Chung, J.-K. FDG PET/CT for the Early Prediction of RAI Therapy Response in Patients with Metastatic Differentiated Thyroid Carcinoma. *PLoS ONE* **2019**, *14*, e0218416. [CrossRef]
56. Feng, H.; Wang, X.; Chen, J.; Cui, J.; Gao, T.; Gao, Y.; Zeng, W. Nuclear Imaging of Glucose Metabolism: Beyond 18F-FDG. *Contrast Media Mol. Imaging* **2019**, *2019*, 7954854. [CrossRef]
57. Galldiks, N.; Langen, K.-J.; Albert, N.L.; Chamberlain, M.; Soffietti, R.; Kim, M.M.; Law, I.; Rhun, E.L.; Chang, S.; Schwarting, J.; et al. PET Imaging in Patients with Brain Metastasis—Report of the RANO/PET Group. *Neuro-Oncology* **2019**, *21*, 585–595. [CrossRef]
58. Pagano, L.; Samà, M.T.; Morani, F.; Prodam, F.; Rudoni, M.; Boldorini, R.; Valente, G.; Marzullo, P.; Baldelli, R.; Appetecchia, M.; et al. Thyroid Incidentaloma Identified by ^{18}F-Fluorodeoxyglucose Positron Emission Tomography with CT (FDG-PET/CT): Clinical and Pathological Relevance. *Clin. Endocrinol.* **2011**, *75*, 528–534. [CrossRef]
59. Giovanella, L.; Treglia, G.; Iakovou, I.; Mihailovic, J.; Verburg, F.A.; Luster, M. EANM Practice Guideline for PET/CT Imaging in Medullary Thyroid Carcinoma. *Eur. J. Nucl. Med. Mol. Imaging* **2020**, *47*, 61–77. [CrossRef]
60. Beheshti, M.; Pöcher, S.; Vali, R.; Waldenberger, P.; Broinger, G.; Nader, M.; Kohlfürst, S.; Pirich, C.; Dralle, H.; Langsteger, W. The Value of 18F-DOPA PET CT in Patients with Medullary Thyroid Carcinoma. Comparison with 18F-FDG PET-CT. *Eur. Radiol.* **2009**, *19*, 1425–1434. [CrossRef]

61. Liu, F.; Xu, X.; Zhu, H.; Zhang, Y.; Yang, J.; Zhang, L.; Li, N.; Zhu, L.; Kung, H.F.; Yang, Z. PET Imaging of 18 F-(2S,4R)4-Fluoroglutamine Accumulation in Breast Cancer: From Xenografts to Patients. *Mol Pharm.* **2018**, *15*, 3448–3455. [CrossRef]
62. Xu, X.; Zhu, H.; Liu, F.; Zhang, Y.; Yang, J.; Zhang, L.; Xie, Q.; Zhu, L.; Li, N.; Kung, H.F.; et al. Dynamic PET/CT Imaging of 18F-(2S, 4R)4-Fluoroglutamine in Healthy Volunteers and Oncological Patients. *Eur. J. Nucl. Med. Mol. Imaging* **2020**, *47*, 2280–2292. [CrossRef]
63. Jochumsen, M.R.; Iversen, P.; Arveschoug, A.K. Follicular Thyroid Cancer Avid on C-11 Methionine PET/CT. *Endocrinol. Diabetes Metab. Case Rep.* **2018**, *2018*. [CrossRef]
64. Barollo, S.; Bertazza, L.; Watutantrige-Fernando, S.; Censi, S.; Cavedon, E.; Galuppini, F.; Pennelli, G.; Fassina, A.; Citton, M.; Rubin, B.; et al. Overexpression of L-Type Amino Acid Transporter 1 (LAT1) and 2 (LAT2): Novel Markers of Neuroendocrine Tumors. *PLoS ONE* **2016**, *11*, e0156044. [CrossRef]
65. Yang, J.H.; Camacho, C.P.; Lindsey, S.C.; Valente, F.O.F.; Andreoni, D.M.; Yamaga, L.Y.; Wagner, J.; Biscolla, R.P.M.; Maciel, R.M.B. The Combined Use of Calcitonin Doubling Time and 18F-FDG PET/CT Improves Prognostic Values in Medullary Thyroid Carcinoma: The Clinical Utility of 18F-FDG PET/CT. *Endocr. Pract.* **2017**, *23*, 942–948. [CrossRef]
66. Weber, T.; Gottstein, M.; Schwenzer, S.; Beer, A.; Luster, M. Is C-11 Methionine PET/CT Able to Localise Sestamibi-Negative Parathyroid Adenomas? *World J. Surg.* **2017**, *41*, 980–985. [CrossRef]
67. Yuan, L.; Liu, J.; Kan, Y.; Yang, J.; Wang, X. The Diagnostic Value of 11C-Methionine PET in Hyperparathyroidism with Negative 99mTc-MIBI SPECT: A Meta-Analysis. *Acta Radiol.* **2016**, *58*, 558–564. [CrossRef]
68. Lenschow, C.; Gassmann, P.; Wenning, C.; Senninger, N.; Colombo-Benkmann, M. Preoperative ^{11}C-Methionine PET/CT Enables Focused Parathyroidectomy in MIBI-SPECT Negative Parathyroid Adenoma. *World J. Surg.* **2015**, *39*, 1750–1757. [CrossRef]
69. Hotta, M.; Minamimoto, R.; Miwa, K. 11C-Methionine-PET for Differentiating Recurrent Brain Tumor from Radiation Necrosis: Radiomics Approach with Random Forest Classifier. *Sci. Rep.* **2019**, *9*, 15666. [CrossRef]
70. He, Q.; Zhang, L.; Zhang, B.; Shi, X.; Yi, C.; Zhang, X. Diagnostic Accuracy of 13N-Ammonia PET, 11C-Methionine PET and 18F-Fluorodeoxyglucose PET: A Comparative Study in Patients with Suspected Cerebral Glioma. *BMC Cancer* **2019**, *19*, 332. [CrossRef]
71. Wedman, J.; Pruim, J.; Putten, L.; Hoekstra, O.S.; Bree, R.; Dijk, B.A.C.; Laan, B.F.A.M. Is C-11 Methionine PET an Alternative to 18-F FDG-PET for Identifying Recurrent Laryngeal Cancer after Radiotherapy? *Clin. Otolaryngol.* **2019**, *44*, 124–130. [CrossRef]
72. Phan, H.T.T.; Jager, P.L.; Plukker, J.T.M.; Wolffenbuttel, B.H.R.; Dierckx, R.A.; Links, T.P. Comparison of 11C-Methionine PET and 18F-Fluorodeoxyglucose PET in Differentiated Thyroid Cancer. *Nucl. Med. Commun.* **2008**, *29*, 711–716. [CrossRef] [PubMed]
73. Morimoto, M.; Kudomi, N.; Maeda, Y.; Kobata, T.; Oishi, A.; Matsumoto, K.; Monden, T.; Iwasaki, T.; Mitamura, K.; Norikane, T.; et al. Effect of Quantitative Values on Shortened Acquisition Duration in Brain Tumor 11C-Methionine PET/CT. *EJNMMI Phys.* **2021**, *8*, 34. [CrossRef] [PubMed]
74. Nguyen, T.-L.; Durán, R.V. Glutamine Metabolism in Cancer Therapy. *Cancer Drug Resist.* **2018**. [CrossRef]
75. Sohda, M.; Miyazaki, T.; Honjyo, H.; Hara, K.; Ozawa, D.; Sakai, M.; Yokobori, T.; Higuchi, T.; Tsushima, Y.; Kuwano, H. 18F-FAMT PET Is Useful to Distinguish between Specific Uptake and Nonspecific Uptake Compared to 18F-Flourodeoxyglucose Position Emission Tomography in Esophageal Cancer Patients. *Dig. Surg.* **2018**, *35*, 383–388. [CrossRef]
76. Wei, L.; Tominaga, H.; Ohgaki, R.; Wiriyasermkul, P.; Hagiwara, K.; Okuda, S.; Kaira, K.; Oriuchi, N.; Nagamori, S.; Kanai, Y. Specific Transport of 3-fluoro-l-α-methyl-tyrosine by LAT1 Explains Its Specificity to Malignant Tumors in Imaging. *Cancer Sci.* **2016**, *107*, 347–352. [CrossRef]
77. Wiriyasermkul, P.; Nagamori, S.; Tominaga, H.; Oriuchi, N.; Kaira, K.; Nakao, H.; Kitashoji, T.; Ohgaki, R.; Tanaka, H.; Endou, H.; et al. Transport of 3-Fluoro-l-α-Methyl-Tyrosine by Tumor-Upregulated L-Type Amino Acid Transporter 1: A Cause of the Tumor Uptake in PET. *J. Nucl. Med.* **2012**, *53*, 1253–1261. [CrossRef]
78. Saidijam, M.; Afshar, S.; Ahmad, I.; Patching, S. Nucleoside Transporters in PET Imaging of Proliferating Cancer Cells Using 3′-Deoxy-3′-[18F]Fluoro-L-Thymidine. *J. Diagn. Imaging* **2018**, *5*, 1–13. [CrossRef]
79. Nakajo, M.; Nakajo, M.; Jinguji, M.; Tani, A.; Kajiya, Y.; Tanabe, H.; Fukukura, Y.; Nakabeppu, Y.; Koriyama, C. Diagnosis of Metastases from Postoperative Differentiated Thyroid Cancer: Comparison between FDG and FLT PET/CT Studies. *Radiology* **2013**, *267*, 891–901. [CrossRef]
80. Sun, X.; Li, Y.; Liu, T.; Li, Z.; Zhang, X.; Chen, X. Peptide-Based Imaging Agents for Cancer Detection. *Adv. Drug Deliv. Rev.* **2017**, *110*, 38–51. [CrossRef]
81. Pauwels, E.; Cleeren, F.; Bormans, G.; Deroose, C.M. Somatostatin Receptor PET Ligands-the next Generation for Clinical Practice. *Am. J. Nucl. Med. Mol. Imaging* **2018**, *8*, 311–331.
82. Staderini, M.; Megia-Fernandez, A.; Dhaliwal, K.; Bradley, M. Peptides for Optical Medical Imaging and Steps towards Therapy. *Bioorg. Med. Chem.* **2018**, *26*, 2816–2826. [CrossRef]
83. Treglia, G.; Tamburello, A.; Giovanella, L. Detection Rate of Somatostatin Receptor PET in Patients with Recurrent Medullary Thyroid Carcinoma: A Systematic Review and a Meta-Analysis. *Horm. Athens Greece* **2017**, *16*, 262–272. [CrossRef]
84. Agthoven, J.F.V.; Xiong, J.-P.; Alonso, J.L.; Rui, X.; Adair, B.D.; Goodman, S.L.; Arnaout, M.A. Structural Basis for Pure Antagonism of Integrin AVβ3 by a High-Affinity Form of Fibronectin. *Nat. Struct. Mol. Biol.* **2014**, *21*, 383–388. [CrossRef]

85. Parihar, A.S.; Mittal, B.R.; Kumar, R.; Shukla, J.; Bhattacharya, A. 68Ga-DOTA-RGD2 Positron Emission Tomography/Computed Tomography in Radioiodine Refractory Thyroid Cancer: Prospective Comparison of Diagnostic Accuracy with 18F-FDG Positron Emission Tomography/Computed Tomography and Evaluation Toward Potential Theranostics. *Thyroid Off. J. Am. Thyroid Assoc.* **2020**, *30*, 557–567. [CrossRef]
86. Parihar, A.S.; Sood, A.; Kumar, R.; Bhusari, P.; Shukla, J.; Mittal, B.R. Novel Use of 177Lu-DOTA-RGD2 in Treatment of 68Ga-DOTA-RGD2-Avid Lesions in Papillary Thyroid Cancer with TENIS. *Eur. J. Nucl. Med. Mol. Imaging* **2018**, *45*, 1836–1837. [CrossRef]
87. Heitkötter, B.; Steinestel, K.; Trautmann, M.; Grünewald, I.; Barth, P.; Gevensleben, H.; Bögemann, M.; Wardelmann, E.; Hartmann, W.; Rahbar, K.; et al. Neovascular PSMA Expression Is a Common Feature in Malignant Neoplasms of the Thyroid. *Oncotarget* **2018**, *9*, 9867–9874. [CrossRef]
88. Sager, S.; Vatankulu, B.; Uslu, L.; Sönmezoglu, K. Incidental Detection of Follicular Thyroid Carcinoma in 68Ga-PSMA PET/CT Imaging. *J. Nucl. Med. Technol.* **2016**, *44*, 199–200. [CrossRef]
89. Bychkov, A.; Vutrapongwatana, U.; Tepmongkol, S.; Keelawat, S. PSMA Expression by Microvasculature of Thyroid Tumors–Potential Implications for PSMA Theranostics. *Sci. Rep.* **2017**, *7*, 5202. [CrossRef]
90. Taywade, S.K.; Damle, N.A.; Bal, C. PSMA Expression in Papillary Thyroid Carcinoma. *Clin. Nucl. Med.* **2016**, *41*, e263–e265. [CrossRef]
91. Derlin, T.; Kreipe, H.-H.; Schumacher, U.; Soudah, B. PSMA Expression in Tumor Neovasculature Endothelial Cells of Follicular Thyroid Adenoma as Identified by Molecular Imaging Using 68Ga-PSMA Ligand PET/CT. *Clin. Nucl. Med.* **2017**, *42*, e173–e174. [CrossRef]
92. Khreish, F.; Ebert, N.; Ries, M.; Maus, S.; Rosar, F.; Bohnenberger, H.; Stemler, T.; Saar, M.; Bartholom?, M.; Ezziddin, S. 225 Ac-PSMA-617/ 177 Lu-PSMA-617 Tandem Therapy of Metastatic Castration-Resistant Prostate Cancer: Pilot Experience. *Nuklearmed* **2020**, *59*, 93. [CrossRef]
93. Klingler, M.; Rangger, C.; Summer, D.; Kaeopookum, P.; Decristoforo, C.; Guggenberg, E. von Cholecystokinin-2 Receptor Targeting with Novel C-Terminally Stabilized HYNIC-Minigastrin Analogs Radiolabeled with Technetium-99m. *Pharm* **2019**, *12*, 13. [CrossRef]
94. Klingler, M.; Hörmann, A.A.; Guggenberg, E.V. Cholecystokinin-2 Receptor Targeting with Radiolabeled Peptides: Current Status and Future Directions. *Curr. Med. Chem.* **2020**, *27*, 7112–7132. [CrossRef] [PubMed]
95. Klingler, M.; Summer, D.; Rangger, C.; Haubner, R.; Foster, J.; Sosabowski, J.; Decristoforo, C.; Virgolini, I.; Guggenberg, E. von DOTA-MGS5, a New Cholecystokinin-2 Receptor-Targeting Peptide Analog with an Optimized Targeting Profile for Theranostic Use. *J. Nucl. Med.* **2018**, *60*, 1010–1016. [CrossRef] [PubMed]
96. Uprimny, C.; von Guggenberg, E.; Svirydenka, A.; Mikołajczak, R.; Hubalewska-Dydejczyk, A.; Virgolini, I.J. Comparison of PET/CT Imaging with [18F]FDOPA and Cholecystokinin-2 Receptor Targeting [68Ga]Ga-DOTA-MGS5 in a Patient with Advanced Medullary Thyroid Carcinoma. *Eur. J. Nucl. Med. Mol. Imaging* **2020**, 1–2. [CrossRef]
97. Zahavi, D.; Weiner, L. Monoclonal Antibodies in Cancer Therapy. *Antibodies* **2020**, *9*, 34. [CrossRef]
98. Lu, R.-M.; Hwang, Y.-C.; Liu, I.-J.; Lee, C.-C.; Tsai, H.-Z.; Li, H.-J.; Wu, H.-C. Development of Therapeutic Antibodies for the Treatment of Diseases. *J. Biomed. Sci.* **2020**, *27*, 1. [CrossRef]
99. Keizer, R.J.; Huitema, A.D.R.; Schellens, J.H.M.; Beijnen, J.H. Clinical Pharmacokinetics of Therapeutic Monoclonal Antibodies. *Clin. Pharm.* **2010**, *49*, 493–507. [CrossRef]
100. Warram, J.M.; de Boer, E.; Sorace, A.G.; Chung, T.K.; Kim, H.; Pleijhuis, R.G.; van Dam, G.M.; Rosenthal, E.L. Antibody-Based Imaging Strategies for Cancer. *Cancer Metastasis Rev.* **2014**, *33*, 809–822. [CrossRef]
101. Wei, W.; Jiang, D.; Lee, H.J.; Li, M.; Kutyreff, C.J.; Engle, J.W.; Liu, J.; Cai, W. Development and Characterization of CD54-Targeted ImmunoPET Imaging in Solid Tumors. *Eur. J. Nucl. Med. Mol. Imaging* **2020**, *47*, 2765–2775. [CrossRef]
102. Iqbal, N.; Iqbal, N. Human Epidermal Growth Factor Receptor 2 (HER2) in Cancers: Overexpression and Therapeutic Implications. *Mol. Biol. Int.* **2014**, *2014*, 852748. [CrossRef]
103. Jiang, D.; Im, H.-J.; Sun, H.; Valdovinos, H.F.; England, C.G.; Ehlerding, E.B.; Nickles, R.J.; Lee, D.S.; Cho, S.Y.; Huang, P.; et al. Radiolabeled Pertuzumab for Imaging of Human Epidermal Growth Factor Receptor 2 Expression in Ovarian Cancer. *Eur. J. Nucl. Med. Mol. Imaging* **2017**, *44*, 1296–1305. [CrossRef]
104. Hyman, D.M.; Piha-Paul, S.A.; Won, H.; Rodon, J.; Saura, C.; Shapiro, G.I.; Juric, D.; Quinn, D.I.; Moreno, V.; Doger, B.; et al. HER Kinase Inhibition in Patients with HER2- and HER3-Mutant Cancers. *Nature* **2018**, *554*, 189–194. [CrossRef]
105. Ruggeri, R.M.; Campennì, A.; Giuffrè, G.; Giovanella, L.; Siracusa, M.; Simone, A.; Branca, G.; Scarfì, R.; Trimarchi, F.; Ieni, A.; et al. HER2 Analysis in Sporadic Thyroid Cancer of Follicular Cell Origin. *Int. J. Mol. Sci.* **2016**, *17*, 2040. [CrossRef]
106. Kunstman, J.W.; Juhlin, C.C.; Goh, G.; Brown, T.C.; Stenman, A.; Healy, J.M.; Rubinstein, J.C.; Choi, M.; Kiss, N.; Nelson-Williams, C.; et al. Characterization of the Mutational Landscape of Anaplastic Thyroid Cancer via Whole-Exome Sequencing. *Hum. Mol. Genet.* **2015**, *24*, 2318–2329. [CrossRef]
107. Ahmed, S.; Sami, A.; Xiang, J. HER2-Directed Therapy: Current Treatment Options for HER2-Positive Breast Cancer. *Breast Cancer* **2015**, *22*, 101–116. [CrossRef]
108. Pondé, N.F.; Zardavas, D.; Piccart, M. Progress in Adjuvant Systemic Therapy for Breast Cancer. *Nat. Rev. Clin. Oncol.* **2019**, *16*, 27–44. [CrossRef]

109. Bardhan, P.; Bui, M.M.; Minton, S.; Loftus, L.; Carter, W.B.; Laronga, C.; Ismail-Khan, R. HER2-Positive Male Breast Cancer with Thyroid Cancer: An Institutional Report and Review of Literature. *Ann. Clin. Lab. Sci.* **2012**, *42*, 135–139.
110. Handkiewicz-Junak, D.; Swierniak, M.; Rusinek, D.; Oczko-Wojciechowska, M.; Dom, G.; Maenhaut, C.; Unger, K.; Detours, V.; Bogdanova, T.; Thomas, G.; et al. Gene Signature of the Post-Chernobyl Papillary Thyroid Cancer. *Eur. J. Nucl. Med. Mol. Imaging* **2016**, *43*, 1267–1277. [CrossRef]
111. Yan, M.; Schwaederle, M.; Arguello, D.; Millis, S.Z.; Gatalica, Z.; Kurzrock, R. HER2 Expression Status in Diverse Cancers: Review of Results from 37,992 Patients. *Cancer Metastasis Rev.* **2015**, *34*, 157–164. [CrossRef]
112. Zhang, L.; Zhang, Y.; Mehta, A.; Boufraqech, M.; Davis, S.; Wang, J.; Tian, Z.; Yu, Z.; Boxer, M.B.; Kiefer, J.A.; et al. Dual Inhibition of HDAC and EGFR Signaling with CUDC-101 Induces Potent Suppression of Tumor Growth and Metastasis in Anaplastic Thyroid Cancer. *Oncotarget* **2015**, *6*, 9073–9085. [CrossRef]
113. Montero-Conde, C.; Ruiz-Llorente, S.; Dominguez, J.M.; Knauf, J.A.; Viale, A.; Sherman, E.J.; Ryder, M.; Ghossein, R.A.; Rosen, N.; Fagin, J.A. Relief of Feedback Inhibition of HER3 Transcription by RAF and MEK Inhibitors Attenuates Their Antitumor Effects in BRAF-Mutant Thyroid Carcinomas. *Cancer Discov.* **2013**, *3*, 520–533. [CrossRef]
114. Wei, W.; Jiang, D.; Rosenkrans, Z.T.; Barnhart, T.E.; Engle, J.W.; Luo, Q.; Cai, W. HER2-Targeted Multimodal Imaging of Anaplastic Thyroid Cancer. *Am. J. Cancer Res.* **2019**, *9*, 2413–2427.
115. Reina, M.; Espel, E. Role of LFA-1 and ICAM-1 in Cancer. *Cancers* **2017**, *9*, 153. [CrossRef]
116. Zhang, P.; Goodrich, C.; Fu, C.; Dong, C. Melanoma Upregulates ICAM-1 Expression on Endothelial Cells through Engagement of Tumor CD44 with Endothelial E-selectin and Activation of a PKCα–P38-SP-1 Pathway. *FASEB J.* **2014**, *28*, 4591–4609. [CrossRef] [PubMed]
117. Buitrago, D.; Keutgen, X.M.; Crowley, M.; Filicori, F.; Aldailami, H.; Hoda, R.; Liu, Y.-F.; Hoda, R.S.; Scognamiglio, T.; Jin, M.; et al. Intercellular Adhesion Molecule-1 (ICAM-1) Is Upregulated in Aggressive Papillary Thyroid Carcinoma. *Ann. Surg. Oncol.* **2012**, *19*, 973–980. [CrossRef] [PubMed]
118. Galore-Haskel, G.; Baruch, E.N.; Berg, A.L.; Barshack, I.; Zilinsky, I.; Avivi, C.; Besser, M.J.; Schachter, J.; Markel, G. Histopathological Expression Analysis of Intercellular Adhesion Molecule 1 (ICAM-1) along Development and Progression of Human Melanoma. *Oncotarget* **2014**, *5*, 99580–99586. [CrossRef] [PubMed]
119. Min, I.M.; Shevlin, E.; Vedvyas, Y.; Zaman, M.; Wyrwas, B.; Scognamiglio, T.; Moore, M.D.; Wang, W.; Park, S.; Park, S.; et al. CAR T Therapy Targeting ICAM-1 Eliminates Advanced Human Thyroid Tumors. *Clin. Cancer Res. Off. J. Am. Assoc. Cancer Res.* **2017**, *23*, 7569–7583. [CrossRef]
120. Vedvyas, Y.; McCloskey, J.E.; Yang, Y.; Min, I.M.; Fahey, T.J.; Zarnegar, R.; Hsu, Y.-M.S.; Hsu, J.-M.; Besien, K.V.; Gaudet, I.; et al. Manufacturing and Preclinical Validation of CAR T Cells Targeting ICAM-1 for Advanced Thyroid Cancer Therapy. *Sci. Rep.* **2019**, *9*, 10634. [CrossRef]
121. Li, J.; Vasilyeva, E.; Wiseman, S.M. Beyond Immunohistochemistry and Immunocytochemistry: A Current Perspective on Galectin-3 and Thyroid Cancer. *Expert Rev. Anticancer* **2019**, *19*, 1017–1027. [CrossRef]
122. Bartolazzi, A.; Gasbarri, A.; Papotti, M.; Bussolati, G.; Lucante, T.; Khan, A.; Inohara, H.; Marandino, F.; Orlandi, F.; Nardi, F.; et al. Application of an Immunodiagnostic Method for Improving Preoperative Diagnosis of Nodular Thyroid Lesions. *Lancet* **2001**, *357*, 1644–1650. [CrossRef]
123. Bartolazzi, A.; Orlandi, F.; Saggiorato, E.; Volante, M.; Arecco, F.; Rossetto, R.; Palestini, N.; Ghigo, E.; Papotti, M.; Bussolati, G.; et al. Galectin-3-Expression Analysis in the Surgical Selection of Follicular Thyroid Nodules with Indeterminate Fine-Needle Aspiration Cytology: A Prospective Multicentre Study. *Lancet Oncol.* **2008**, *9*, 543–549. [CrossRef]
124. D'Alessandria, C.; Braesch-Andersen, S.; Bejo, K.; Reder, S.; Blechert, B.; Schwaiger, M.; Bartolazzi, A. Noninvasive In Vivo Imaging and Biologic Characterization of Thyroid Tumors by ImmunoPET Targeting of Galectin-3. *Cancer Res.* **2016**, *76*, 3583–3592. [CrossRef]
125. Rose, F.D.; Braeuer, M.; Braesch-Andersen, S.; Otto, A.M.; Steiger, K.; Reder, S.; Mall, S.; Nekolla, S.; Schwaiger, M.; Weber, W.A.; et al. Galectin-3 Targeting in Thyroid Orthotopic Tumors Opens New Ways to Characterize Thyroid Cancer. *J. Nucl. Med.* **2019**, *60*, 770–776. [CrossRef]
126. Nair, L.M.; Anila, K.R.; Sreekumar, A.; Pradeep, V.M. Renal Metastasis from Papillary Carcinoma Thyroid Detected by Whole Body Iodine Scan: A Case Report and Review of the Literature. *Indian J. Nucl. Med. IJNM Off. J. Soc. Nucl. Med. India* **2016**, *31*, 232–234. [CrossRef]
127. Fan, G.; Wang, Z.; Hao, M.; Li, J. Bispecific Antibodies and Their Applications. *J. Hematol. Oncol.* **2015**, *8*, 130. [CrossRef]
128. Krishnamurthy, A.; Jimeno, A. Bispecific Antibodies for Cancer Therapy: A Review. *Pharm. Ther.* **2017**, *185*, 122–134. [CrossRef]
129. Oudoux, A.; Salaun, P.-Y.; Bournaud, C.; Campion, L.; Ansquer, C.; Rousseau, C.; Bardet, S.; Borson-Chazot, F.; Vuillez, J.-P.; Murat, A.; et al. Sensitivity and Prognostic Value of Positron Emission Tomography with F-18-Fluorodeoxyglucose and Sensitivity of Immunoscintigraphy in Patients with Medullary Thyroid Carcinoma Treated with Anticarcinoembryonic Antigen-Targeted Radioimmunotherapy. *J. Clin. Endocrinol. Metab.* **2007**, *92*, 4590–4597. [CrossRef]
130. Peltier, P.; Curtet, C.; Chatal, J.F.; Doussal, J.M.L.; Daniel, G.; Aillet, G.; Gruaz-Guyon, A.; Barbet, J.; Delaage, M. Radioimmunodetection of Medullary Thyroid Cancer Using a Bispecific Anti-CEA/Anti-Indium-DTPA Antibody and an Indium-111-Labeled DTPA Dimer. *J. Nucl. Med. Off. Publ. Soc. Nucl. Med.* **1993**, *34*, 1267–1273.
131. Barbet, J.; Peltier, P.; Bardet, S.; Vuillez, J.P.; Bachelot, I.; Denet, S.; Olivier, P.; Leccia, F.; Corcuff, B.; Huglo, D.; et al. Radiotheranostics: A Roadmap for Future Development. *Lancet Oncol.* **2020**, *21*, e146–e156. [CrossRef]

132. Kraeber-Bodéré, F.; Salaun, P.-Y.; Ansquer, C.; Drui, D.; Mirallié, E.; Faivre-Chauvet, A.; Barbet, J.; Goldenberg, D.M.; Chatal, J.-F. Pretargeted Radioimmunotherapy (PRAIT) in Medullary Thyroid Cancer (MTC). *Tumor Biol.* **2012**, *33*, 601–606. [CrossRef]
133. Schoffelen, R.; Boerman, O.C.; Goldenberg, D.M.; Sharkey, R.M.; van Herpen, C.M.L.; Franssen, G.M.; McBride, W.J.; Chang, C.-H.; Rossi, E.A.; van der Graaf, W.T.A.; et al. Development of an Imaging-Guided CEA-Pretargeted Radionuclide Treatment of Advanced Colorectal Cancer: First Clinical Results. *Brit. J. Cancer* **2013**, *109*, 934–942. [CrossRef]
134. Bodet-Milin, C.; Faivre-Chauvet, A.; Carlier, T.; Rauscher, A.; Bourgeois, M.; Cerato, E.; Rohmer, V.; Couturier, O.; Drui, D.; Goldenberg, D.M.; et al. Immuno-PET Using Anticarcinoembryonic Antigen Bispecific Antibody and 68Ga-Labeled Peptide in Metastatic Medullary Thyroid Carcinoma: Clinical Optimization of the Pretargeting Parameters in a First-in-Human Trial. *J. Nucl. Med.* **2016**, *57*, 1505–1511. [CrossRef]
135. Bates, A.; Power, C.A. David vs. Goliath: The Structure, Function, and Clinical Prospects of Antibody Fragments. *Antibodies* **2019**, *8*, 28. [CrossRef]
136. Kulmala, A.; Huovinen, T.; Lamminmäki, U. Improvement of Fab Expression by Screening Combinatorial Synonymous Signal Sequence Libraries. *Microb. Cell Factories* **2019**, *18*, 157. [CrossRef]
137. Xenaki, K.T.; Oliveira, S.; van Bergen En Henegouwen, P.M.P. Antibody or Antibody Fragments: Implications for Molecular Imaging and Targeted Therapy of Solid Tumors. *Front. Immunol.* **2017**, *8*, 1287. [CrossRef]
138. Duan, H.; Huang, H.; Jing, G. An Antibody Fab Fragment-Based Chimeric Antigen Receptor Could Efficiently Eliminate Human Thyroid Cancer Cells. *J. Cancer* **2019**, *10*, 1890–1895. [CrossRef]
139. Peplau, E.; Rose, F.D.; Reder, S.; Mittelhäuser, M.; Scafetta, G.; Schwaiger, M.; Weber, W.A.; Bartolazzi, A.; Skerra, A.; D'Alessandria, C. Development of a Chimeric Antigen-Binding Fragment Directed Against Human Galectin-3 and Validation as an Immuno-Positron Emission Tomography Tracer for the Sensitive In Vivo Imaging of Thyroid Cancer. *Thyroid* **2020**, *30*, 1314–1326. [CrossRef]
140. Peplau, E.; Rose, F.D.; Eichinger, A.; Reder, S.; Mittelhäuser, M.; Scafetta, G.; Schwaiger, M.; Weber, W.A.; Bartolazzi, A.; D'Alessandria, C.; et al. Effective Rational Humanization of a PASylated Anti-Galectin-3 Fab for the Sensitive PET Imaging of Thyroid Cancer in Vivo. *Sci. Rep.* **2021**, *11*, 7358. [CrossRef]
141. Wu, Y.; Jiang, S.; Ying, T. Single-Domain Antibodies as Therapeutics against Human Viral Diseases. *Front. Immunol.* **2017**, *8*, 1802. [CrossRef] [PubMed]
142. Pleiner, T.; Bates, M.; Trakhanov, S.; Lee, C.-T.; Schliep, J.E.; Chug, H.; Böhning, M.; Stark, H.; Urlaub, H.; Görlich, D. Nanobodies: Site-Specific Labeling for Super-Resolution Imaging, Rapid Epitope-Mapping and Native Protein Complex Isolation. *Elife* **2015**, *4*, e11349. [CrossRef] [PubMed]
143. Jailkhani, N.; Ingram, J.R.; Rashidian, M.; Rickelt, S.; Tian, C.; Mak, H.; Jiang, Z.; Ploegh, H.L.; Hynes, R.O. Noninvasive Imaging of Tumor Progression, Metastasis, and Fibrosis Using a Nanobody Targeting the Extracellular Matrix. *Proc. Natl. Acad. Sci. USA* **2019**, *116*, 14181–14190. [CrossRef] [PubMed]
144. Li, J.; Zhou, C.; Dong, B.; Zhong, H.; Chen, S.; Li, Q.; Wang, Z. Single Domain Antibody-Based Bispecific Antibody Induces Potent Specific Anti-Tumor Activity. *Cancer Biol.* **2016**, *17*, 1231–1239. [CrossRef] [PubMed]
145. Guo, W.; Zhang, C.; Ma, T.; Liu, X.; Chen, Z.; Li, S.; Deng, Y. Advances in Aptamer Screening and Aptasensors' Detection of Heavy Metal Ions. *J. Nanobiotechnol.* **2021**, *19*, 166. [CrossRef]
146. Zhou, J.; Rossi, J. Aptamers as Targeted Therapeutics: Current Potential and Challenges. *Nat. Rev. Drug Discov.* **2016**, *16*, 181–202. [CrossRef]
147. Behrooz, A.B.; Syahir, A.; Ahmad, S. CD133: Beyond a Cancer Stem Cell Biomarker. *J. Drug Target.* **2018**, *27*, 1–31. [CrossRef]
148. Yang, Z.-L.; Zheng, Q.; Yan, J.; Pan, Y.; Wang, Z.-G. Upregulated CD133 Expression in Tumorigenesis of Colon Cancer Cells. *World J. Gastroenterol.* **2011**, *17*, 932–937. [CrossRef]
149. Dhaybi, R.A.; Sartelet, H.; Powell, J.; Kokta, V. Expression of CD133+ Cancer Stem Cells in Childhood Malignant Melanoma and Its Correlation with Metastasis. *Mod. Pathol.* **2010**, *23*, 376–380. [CrossRef]
150. Liu, J.; Brown, R.E. Immunohistochemical Detection of Epithelialmesenchymal Transition Associated with Stemness Phenotype in Anaplastic Thyroid Carcinoma. *Int. J. Clin. Exp. Pathol.* **2010**, *3*, 755–762.
151. Glumac, P.M.; LeBeau, A.M. The Role of CD133 in Cancer: A Concise Review. *Clin. Transl. Med.* **2018**, *7*, 18. [CrossRef]
152. Friedman, S.; Lu, M.; Schultz, A.; Thomas, D.; Lin, R.-Y. CD133+ Anaplastic Thyroid Cancer Cells Initiate Tumors in Immunodeficient Mice and Are Regulated by Thyrotropin. *PLoS ONE* **2009**, *4*, e5395. [CrossRef]
153. Lin, Z.; Lu, X.; Li, W.; Sun, M.; Peng, M.; Yang, H.; Chen, L.; Zhang, C.; Cai, L.; Li, Y. Association of Cancer Stem Cell Markers with Aggressive Tumor Features in Papillary Thyroid Carcinoma. *Cancer Control.* **2015**, *22*, 508–514. [CrossRef]
154. Wang, Y.; Sui, G.; Teng, D.; Wang, Q.; Qu, J.; Zhu, L.; Ran, H.; Wang, Z.; Jin, C.; Wang, H. Low Intensity Focused Ultrasound (LIFU) Triggered Drug Release from Cetuximab-Conjugated Phase-Changeable Nanoparticles for Precision Theranostics against Anaplastic Thyroid Carcinoma. *Biomater. Sci.* **2018**, *7*, 196–210. [CrossRef]
155. Hu, Z.; Qin, J.; Li, T.; Guo, J. Thyroid Cancer MR Molecular Imaging via SHP2-Targeted Nanoparticles. *Int. J. Nanomed.* **2019**, *14*, 7365–7373. [CrossRef]
156. Ayati, A.; Moghimi, S.; Toolabi, M.; Foroumadi, A. Pyrimidine-Based EGFR TK Inhibitors in Targeted Cancer Therapy. *Eur. J. Med. Chem.* **2021**, *221*, 113523. [CrossRef]
157. Hu, Z.-Q.; Ma, R.; Zhang, C.-M.; Li, J.; Li, L.; Hu, Z.-T.; Gao, Q.; Li, W.-M. Expression and Clinical Significance of Tyrosine Phosphatase SHP2 in Thyroid Carcinoma. *Oncol. Lett.* **2015**, *10*, 1507–1512. [CrossRef]

158. Wei, W.-J.; Hardin, H.; Luo, Q.-Y. Targeting Autophagy in Thyroid Cancers. *Endocr. Relat. Cancer* **2019**, *1*, R181–R194. [CrossRef]
159. Jin, Y.; Liu, M.; Sa, R.; Fu, H.; Cheng, L.; Chen, L. Mouse Models of Thyroid Cancer: Bridging Pathogenesis and Novel Therapeutics. *Cancer Lett* **2020**, *469*, 35–53. [CrossRef]
160. Nakajo, M.; Nakajo, M.; Kajiya, Y.; Jinguji, M.; Mori, S.; Aridome, K.; Suenaga, T.; Tanaka, S. High FDG and Low FLT Uptake in a Thyroid Papillary Carcinoma Incidentally Discovered by FDG PET/CT. *Clin. Nucl. Med.* **2012**, *37*, 607. [CrossRef]
161. Souteiro, P.; Gouveia, P.; Ferreira, G.; Belo, S.; Costa, C.; Carvalho, D.; Duarte, H.; Sampaio, I.L. 68Ga-DOTANOC and 18F-FDG PET/CT in Metastatic Medullary Thyroid Carcinoma: Novel Correlations with Tumoral Biomarkers. *Endocrine* **2019**, *64*, 322–329. [CrossRef]
162. Budiawan, H.; Salavati, A.; Kulkarni, H.R.; Baum, R.P. Peptide Receptor Radionuclide Therapy of Treatment-Refractory Metastatic Thyroid Cancer Using (90)Yttrium and (177)Lutetium Labeled Somatostatin Analogs: Toxicity, Response and Survival Analysis. *Am. J. Nucl. Med. Mol. Imaging* **2013**, *4*, 39–52. [CrossRef]
163. Salavati, A.; Puranik, A.; Kulkarni, H.R.; Budiawan, H.; Baum, R.P. Peptide Receptor Radionuclide Therapy (PRRT) of Medullary and Nonmedullary Thyroid Cancer Using Radiolabeled Somatostatin Analogues. *Semin. Nucl. Med.* **2016**, *46*, 215–224. [CrossRef]
164. Assadi, M.; Ahmadzadehfar, H. 177 Lu-DOTATATE and 177 Lu-Prostate-Specific Membrane Antigen Therapy in a Patient with Advanced Metastatic Radioiodine-Refractory Differentiated Thyroid Cancer after Failure of Tyrosine Kinase Inhibitors Treatment. *World J. Nucl. Med.* **2019**, *18*, 406. [CrossRef]
165. De Vries, L.H.; Lodewijk, L.; Braat, A.J.A.T.; Krijger, G.C.; Valk, G.D.; Lam, M.G.E.H.; Rinkes, I.H.M.B.; Vriens, M.R.; Keizer, B. de 68Ga-PSMA PET/CT in Radioactive Iodine-Refractory Differentiated Thyroid Cancer and First Treatment Results with 177Lu-PSMA-617. *EJNMMI Res.* **2020**, *10*, 18. [CrossRef]
166. Bodet-Milin, C.; Bailly, C.; Touchefeu, Y.; Frampas, E.; Bourgeois, M.; Rauscher, A.; Lacoeuille, F.; Drui, D.; Arlicot, N.; Goldenberg, D.M.; et al. Clinical Results in Medullary Thyroid Carcinoma Suggest High Potential of Pretargeted Immuno-PET for Tumor Imaging and Theranostic Approaches. *Front. Med.* **2019**, *6*, 124. [CrossRef]
167. Liu, H.; Shi, J.; Lin, F. The Potential Diagnostic Utility of TROP-2 in Thyroid Neoplasms. *Appl. Immunohistochem. Mol. Morphol.* **2017**, *25*, 525–533. [CrossRef] [PubMed]
168. Schürch, C.M.; Roelli, M.A.; Forster, S.; Wasmer, M.-H.; Brühl, F.; Maire, R.S.; Pancrazio, S.D.; Ruepp, M.-D.; Giger, R.; Perren, A.; et al. Targeting CD47 in Anaplastic Thyroid Carcinoma Enhances Tumor Phagocytosis by Macrophages and Is a Promising Therapeutic Strategy. *Thyroid* **2019**, *29*, 979–992. [CrossRef] [PubMed]
169. Elmageed, Z.Y.A.; Moroz, K.; Kandil, E. Clinical Significance of CD146 and Latexin during Different Stages of Thyroid Cancer. *Mol. Cell Biochem.* **2013**, *381*, 95–103. [CrossRef] [PubMed]
170. Ehlerding, E.B.; Sun, L.; Lan, X.; Zeng, D.; Cai, W. Dual-Targeted Molecular Imaging of Cancer. *J. Nucl. Med.* **2018**, *59*, 390–395. [CrossRef] [PubMed]
171. Morais, M.; Ma, M.T. Site-Specific Chelator-Antibody Conjugation for PET and SPECT Imaging with Radiometals. *Drug Discov. Today Technol.* **2018**, *30*, 91–104. [CrossRef] [PubMed]
172. Li, L.; Crow, D.; Turatti, F.; Bading, J.R.; Anderson, A.-L.; Poku, E.; Yazaki, P.J.; Carmichael, J.; Leong, D.; Wheatcroft, D.; et al. Site-Specific Conjugation of Monodispersed DOTA-PEGn to a Thiolated Diabody Reveals the Effect of Increasing PEG Size on Kidney Clearance and Tumor Uptake with Improved 64-Copper PET Imaging. *Bioconjugate Chem.* **2011**, *22*, 709–716. [CrossRef]
173. Acchione, M.; Kwon, H.; Jochheim, C.M.; Atkins, W.M. Impact of Linker and Conjugation Chemistry on Antigen Binding, Fc Receptor Binding and Thermal Stability of Model Antibody-Drug Conjugates. *mAbs* **2012**, *4*, 362–372. [CrossRef]
174. Adumeau, P.; Sharma, S.K.; Brent, C.; Zeglis, B.M. Site-Specifically Labeled Immunoconjugates for Molecular Imaging—Part 1: Cysteine Residues and Glycans. *Mol. Imaging Biol.* **2016**, *18*, 1–17. [CrossRef]
175. Chen, Z.-Y.; Wang, Y.-X.; Lin, Y.; Zhang, J.-S.; Yang, F.; Zhou, Q.-L.; Liao, Y.-Y. Advance of Molecular Imaging Technology and Targeted Imaging Agent in Imaging and Therapy. *BioMed Res. Int.* **2014**, *2014*, 819324. [CrossRef]
176. Rosenbaum-Krumme, S.J.; Görges, R.; Bockisch, A.; Binse, I. 18F-FDG PET/CT Changes Therapy Management in High-Risk DTC after First Radioiodine Therapy. *Eur. J. Nucl. Med. Mol. Imaging* **2012**, *39*, 1373–1380. [CrossRef]
177. Müller, C.; van der Meulen, N.P.; Benešová, M.; Schibli, R. Therapeutic Radiometals Beyond 177 Lu and 90 Y: Production and Application of Promising α-Particle, β−-Particle, and Auger Electron Emitters. *J. Nucl. Med.* **2017**, *58*, 91S–96S. [CrossRef]

cancers

MDPI

Article

Diagnostic Value of Galectin-3 in Distinguishing Invasive Encapsulated Carcinoma from Noninvasive Follicular Thyroid Neoplasms with Papillary-Like Nuclear Features (NIFTP) †

Guodong Fu [1,*], Olena Polyakova [1,*], Ronald S. Chazen [1], Jeremy L. Freeman [2,3] and Ian J. Witterick [1,2,3,*]

1 Alex and Simona Shnaider Research Laboratory in Molecular Oncology, Lunenfeld-Tanenbaum Research Institute, Sinai Health System, Mount Sinai Hospital, Toronto, ON M5G 1X5, Canada; Ronald.Chazen@sinaihealth.ca

2 Joseph and Mildred Sonshine Family Centre for Head and Neck Diseases, Sinai Health System, Mount Sinai Hospital, Toronto, ON M5G 1X5, Canada; Jeremy.Freeman@sinaihealth.ca

3 Department of Otolaryngology-Head and Neck Surgery, Sinai Health System, Mount Sinai Hospital, University of Toronto, Toronto, ON M5G 1X5, Canada

* Correspondence: David.Fu@sinaihealth.ca (G.F.); polyakoo@mcmaster.ca (O.P.); Ian.Witterick@sinaihealth.ca (I.J.W.)

† This manuscript is a memorial to Dr. Paul G. Walfish (P.G.W.) for the significant contributions he made to thyroid cancer research and the infrastructural support in Mount Sinai Hospital.

Citation: Fu, G.; Polyakova, O.; Chazen, R.S.; Freeman, J.L.; Witterick, I.J. Diagnostic Value of Galectin-3 in Distinguishing Invasive Encapsulated Carcinoma from Noninvasive Follicular Thyroid Neoplasms with Papillary-Like Nuclear Features (NIFTP). *Cancers* **2021**, *13*, 2988. https://doi.org/10.3390/cancers13122988

Academic Editors: Fabio Medas and Pier Francesco Alesina

Received: 28 April 2021
Accepted: 12 June 2021
Published: 15 June 2021

Simple Summary: The reclassification of NIFTP raised the need for rebuilding the clinical, histologic, cytological and molecular parameters, including re-evaluation of the previously examined biomarkers, for assisting in the diagnosis of this subset of indolent noninvasive tumors from invasive encapsulated follicular variant of papillary thyroid carcinoma (EFVPTC). In this retrospective study, Galectin-3 (Gal-3) IHC staining on patient's thyroid tissues showed a statistically significant higher cytoplasmic Gal-3 expression in invasive EFVPTC than in NIFTP and other benign subgroups. Our findings refined the diagnostic value of Gal-3 expression as an ancillary marker in identifying NIFTP among encapsulated follicular variant nodules.

Abstract: *Background*: non-invasive follicular thyroid neoplasms with papillary-like nuclear features (NIFTP), which is considered as low-risk cancer, should be distinguished from the malignant invasive encapsulated follicular variant of papillary thyroid carcinoma (EFVPTC). Improved discrimination of NIFTPs from invasive EFVPTCs using a molecular biomarker test could provide useful insights into pre- and post-surgical management of the indeterminate thyroid nodule. Galectin-3 (Gal-3), a β-galactosyl-binding molecule in the lectin group, is involved in different biological functions in well differentiated thyroid carcinomas. The aim of this study was to determine whether Gal-3 expression as a diagnostic marker could distinguish indolent NIFTP from invasive EFVPTC on tissue specimens from surgical thyroid nodules. *Methods*: immunohistochemical (IHC) analysis of cytoplasmic and nuclear Gal-3 expression was performed in formalin-fixed paraffin-embedded (FFPE) surgical tissues in four specific diagnostic subgroups- benign nodules, NIFTPs, EFVPTCs and lymphocytic/Hashimoto's thyroiditis (LTs). *Results*: cytoplasmic Gal-3 expression (mean ± SD) was significantly increased in invasive EFVPTCs (4.80 ± 1.60) compared to NIFTPs (2.75 ± 1.58, $p < 0.001$) and benign neoplasms (2.09 ± 1.19, $p < 0.001$) with no significant difference between NIFTPs and benign lesions ($p = 0.064$). The presence of LT enhanced cytoplasmic Gal-3 expression (3.80 ± 1.32) compared to NIFTPs ($p = 0.016$) and benign nodules ($p < 0.001$). Nuclear Gal-3 expression in invasive EFVPTCs (1.84 ± 1.30) was significantly higher than in NIFTPs (1.00 ± 0.72, $p = 0.001$), but similar to benign nodules (1.44 ± 1.77, $p = 0.215$), thereby obviating its potential clinical application. *Conclusions*: our observations have indicated that increased cytoplasmic Gal-3 expression shows diagnostic potential in distinguishing NIFTP among encapsulated follicular variant nodules thereby serving as a possible ancillary test to H&E histopathological diagnostic criteria when LT interference is absent, to assist in the detection of the invasive EFVPTC among such nodules.

Keywords: thyroid cancer; Gal-3 expression; NIFTP; EFVPTC; lymphocytic thyroiditis (LT); immunohistochemical (IHC) analysis

1. Introduction

Thyroid cancer has the most rapidly increasing incidence rate among all major cancers, with a triple increase from 4.5 to 14.4 per 100,000 population during 1974–2013 [1]. It was estimated 52,890 new cases in the United States in 2020 and contributed to 0.36% of all cancer deaths [2,3]. Most primary thyroid cancers are follicular cell-derived epithelial tumors, making up four main pathological carcinoma types: papillary thyroid carcinoma (PTC), follicular thyroid carcinoma (FTC), poorly differentiated thyroid carcinoma (PDTC) and anaplastic thyroid carcinoma (ATC). Medullary thyroid carcinomas (MTC) originate from thyroid parafollicular (C) cells. PTC and FTC are differentiated thyroid cancers, whereas ATC is undifferentiated. PTC constitutes up to 90% of all thyroid malignancies [4], followed by FTC (5–10%), ATC (<2%, typically occurring in the elder patients) and MTC (2%) [5]. As the most common type of well-differentiated thyroid cancer [6], PTC comprises numerous histopathologic variants that are well validated clinically and biologically, including classic variant, follicular variant (encapsulated/well demarcated, with tumor capsular invasion), follicular variant (encapsulated/well demarcated, noninvasive), follicular variant (infiltrative), tall cell variant, hobnail variant, cribriform-morular variant, columnar cell variant and diffuse sclerosing variant [7]. Among all variants, the follicular variant of papillary thyroid carcinoma (FVPTC) is one of the most common diagnoses, representing up to 30% of all thyroid carcinoma cases [8]. FVPTC is subdivided into two subtypes: the infiltrating/diffuse variant (infiltrative FVPTC), which has the metastatic tendency of the classic papillary thyroid carcinoma, and the encapsulated variant (EFVPTC), which may present with no capsular or angiolymphatic invasion or metastases [9,10]. The microscopic diagnostic criteria for EFVPTC are mainly encapsulation or clear demarcation, follicular growth patterns, and nuclear features of papillary carcinoma (enlargement, crowding/overlapping, elongation, irregular contours, grooves, pseudoinclusions and chromatin clearing) [11–14]. Controversies have existed for a long time about whether all EFVPTC cases should be classified as malignancy [15–17]. Evidence suggests that a subset of non-invasive EFVPTC, earlier considered as conventional thyroid cancer, has been demonstrated to be a highly indolent tumor showing an overall risk of recurrence (local, regional and distant) of less than 1% [15,16,18–20]. In 2016, a new terminology Non-invasive follicular thyroid neoplasm with papillary-like nuclear features (NIFTP) has been proposed to name the subset of non-invasive EFVPTC [11] to address the indolent behavior of this tumor and avoid the term "carcinoma" and potential over-treatment.

NIFTP presents the following characteristics: (1) main morphological features, including encapsulation or clear demarcation, follicular growth pattern, no well-formed papillae, no psammoma bodies, <30% solid/trabecular/insular growth pattern, nuclear score 2–3, no tumor necrosis, no high mitotic activity; (2) lack of invasion, which separates this tumor from invasive EFVPTC; (3) a very low risk of the adverse outcome when the tumor is non-invasive [11,21,22]. Histopathological examination of the entire tumor remains the gold standard for NIFTP diagnosis. Of note, the initial exclusionary papillae less than 1% that was subjective to apply has been updated to a 0% cut-off to ensure indolent outcome [22,23]. NIFTP is still an evolving diagnosis, and more data need to be established to substantiate this new entity [24]. As neoplasm develops specific alterations at the proteomic and/or genomic level, molecular marker-based ancillary tests at histological or cytological level may be a great asset in improving the accuracy of the diagnosis of NIFTP [4,11,25,26]. Recently, immunohistochemical test of Programmed Death-Ligand 1 expression has been shown to distinguish invasive EFVPTC from the indolent NIFTP and benign nodules [25], and recommended as an auxiliary aid to pathologists [27].

Galectin-3 (Gal-3), a member of the beta-galactoside-binding protein family that is predominantly localized in the cytoplasm, may translocate to the perinuclear membrane, nucleus and/or secreted from the cytoplasm [28,29]. This protein is involved in various physiological and pathological processes, such as cell proliferation, apoptosis, inflammation, cell adhesion, cellular transformation, tumor progression and metastasis of cancer cells [28,30]. Overexpression of *galectin-3* cDNA in vitro generates a transformed phenotype [31]; conversely, inhibition of Gal-3 expression has suppressed tumor growth in mice tumor models [32]. Gal-3 is a p53 physiological target mediating p53-induced apoptosis at the molecular level; therefore, the aberrant expression of Gal-3 blocks the apoptotic program, promoting the development of cancer [33]. Gal-3 is overexpressed in a high proportion of carcinomas, especially of the papillary histotype, but weak or absent from normal or benign thyroid tissue [29,30,34], suggesting its potential biological role in the malignant transformation of thyroid cells. Gal-3 immunohistochemistry has been reported to assist the diagnosis of FVPTC [29,35]; however, the role of Gal-3 expression as an ancillary marker in reclassification to NIFTP has not yet been determined.

The aim of the current study was to determine whether Gal-3 subcellular expression in histological surgical tissues could serve as a useful biomarker to distinguish indolent NIFTP from invasive EFVPTC.

2. Materials and Methods

2.1. Patient Specimen

This retrospective cohort study was performed at Sinai Health System, Mount Sinai Hospital (MSH), a University of Toronto-affiliated hospital and a prime referral center for patients with thyroid disorders in Toronto, Canada. A total of 1859 patients who previously underwent thyroidectomy in MSH between 2010 and 2015 were identified following the approved guidelines of the Sinai Health System Research Ethics Board (REB #07-0212-E). The pathologist (OP) reviewed the patient clinical charts, surgical pathology reports and H&E stained sections [25]. The final diagnosis was made in accordance with the WHO's Classification of Tumors of Endocrine Organs [36], CAP protocol [7,37] and Endocrine Pathology Society Working Group [11]. After the histopathological evaluations based on strictly defined inclusion and exclusion criteria [11,23], a total of 165 archived formalin-fixed paraffin-embedded (FFPE) tissue blocks of thyroid tumors ($\geq$1.0 cm) retrieved from the MSH Tumor Bank were classified into four specific diagnostic subgroups: 42 cases of benign nodules, 41 NIFTPs, 45 invasive EFVPTCs and 37 cases of noninvasive encapsulated FVPTC lesions with co-existing significant lymphocytic/Hashimoto's thyroiditis (LT) [25,37].

2.2. Histological Inclusion/Exclusion Criteria

The detailed inclusion/exclusion criteria were described in recent studies [23,25]. Briefly, for the NIFTP subgroup, the inclusion criteria included major features (encapsulation/clear demarcation, follicular growth pattern, nuclear features of PTC (2–3 points of the 3-point nuclear scoring scheme): enlargement, crowding/overlapping, elongation, irregular contours, grooves, pseudoinclusions, chromatin clearing) [37] and minor features (dark colloid, irregularly shaped follicles, intratumoral fibrosis, "sprinkling" sign, follicles cleft from stroma, multinucleated giant cells within follicles) [11]. The exclusion criteria used for NIFTP were the presence of "true" papillae, psammoma bodies, infiltrative border, tumor necrosis, high mitotic activity, cell/morphologic characteristics of other variants of PTC. EFVPTC with different degrees of capsular transgression exhibited features within an encapsulated or well circumscribed nodule, follicular architecture, PTC nuclear features and papillae [37]. Noninvasive FVPTC with lymphocytic/Hashimoto's thyroiditis (LT) histologically presented with extensive lymphocytic infiltrate with germinal center formation, lymphocytes predominantly and plasma cells, atrophic follicles with abundant Hürthle cells (large, polygonal cells with abundant granular eosinophilic cytoplasm and large hyperchromatic round to oval regular nucleus). Therefore, LT was placed in a separate category to avoid possible false positive interpretation of a co-existing inflammatory environment as a factor in Gal-3 cytoplasmic expression [37–39].

2.3. Immunohistochemical (IHC) Staining

A representative FFPE section from each tissue block (5 μm thickness) was deparaffinized, hydrated with series of graded alcohol and then antigen retrieval at 115 °C for 3 min was performed in Tris-EDTA buffer (10 mM Tris base, 1 mM EDTA, 0.05% Tween 20, pH 9.0) as described previously [40]. Tissues were treated with 3% H_2O_2 in Tris-buffered saline for 8 min to block the endogenous peroxidase activity. Then slides were incubated with a background punisher to block non-specific staining (Biocare Medical, LLC, Concord, CA, USA) for 20 min, and were followed by 1 hr incubation with rabbit anti-Gal-3 antibody at a 1:500 dilution (ab53082, Abcam, Cambridge, MA, USA). The rinsed sections were then incubated with biotinylated anti-rabbit secondary antibody for 20 min, subsequently detected using The VECTASTAIN ABC System (Vector Labs, Burlington, ON, Canada) and peroxidase substrate diaminobenzidine (DAB) as the chromogen until staining signal developed. Sections of a classical variant of PTC known with Gal-3 positivity were included in each batch of immunostaining for Gal-3 antibody incubation to serve as an external positive control as well as for an irrelevant isotype specific IgG in place of the primary antibody as a negative control to exclude a nonspecific staining. All slides were counterstained with hematoxylin and viewed under a light microscope.

2.4. Evaluation of Immunohistochemistry

IHC sections were scored as positive if epithelial cells showed immunoreactivity in the cytoplasm and/or nucleus using a bright-field microscope (Olympus BX50; Olympus, Center Valley, PA, USA). Sections were scanned at low (×40) and high powers (×200), and Gal-3 stained cells were scored semi-quantitatively by three independent observers (GF, OP, and RSC). Immunostaining scores were determined based on the percentage positivity and staining intensity as described previously [25]. Percentage positive scores were assigned according to the scale: 0 (≤10%), 1 (11–30%), 2 (31–50%), 3 (51–70%) and 4 (>70%). Staining intensity was scored semi-quantitatively as follows: 0 (none), 1 (mild), 2 (moderate) and 3 (intense). A total score for each cytoplasmic or nuclear staining was then obtained (ranging from 0 to 7) by adding the percentage positivity and intensity scores for each section. The IHC scoring was blinded from the histopathology report. Representative photomicrographs showing each IHC score category were included in the supplementary file (Figure S1). The final score was given as an average of scores using following formula: ((percentage score 1 + intensity score 1) + (percentage score 2 + intensity score 2) + (percentage score 3 + intensity score 3))/3.

2.5. Statistical Analysis

Gal-3 IHC score data were analyzed using IBM SPSS Statistics version24 (SPSS, Chicago, IL, USA, http://www.ibm.com/analytics/us/en/technology/spss/ (accessed on 2 March 2020). Descriptive statistic was used to describe the patient population and inferential statistic was used to test the Gal-3 expression differences between the groups (one-way ANOVA). Gal-3 positivity scores served as the predictor variable and invasion served as the primary outcome variable (invasiveness). Diagnostic accuracy was assessed by plotting receiver operator characteristics (ROC) curve. The cut off points for Gal-3 positivity expression and area under the curve (AUC) were calculated. The optimal cut-off value was chosen as the threshold that maximized the AUC. The clinical utility of biomarkers was assessed using AUC, positive predictive value (PPV), negative predictive value (NPV) for invasiveness. The association between cytoplasmic Gal-3 positivity and invasiveness was examined by odds ratio (OR) using cross-tabulation. For the accuracy assessment of positive cytoplasmic Gal-3 expression in distinguishing NIFTP and invasive EFVPTC, we calculated the likelihood ratios (LR): (LR+ = sensitivity/(1-specificity)) and

(LR− = ((1-sensitivity)/specificity). The results were considered statistically significant at $p \leq 0.05$.

3. Results

3.1. Patient Characteristics and Clinical Histopathological Features

The patient characteristics and clinical histopathological features of the retrospective study cohort are summarized in Table 1. The median patient age at initial diagnosis was 50 years. (range 16–89) for the subgroup of benign nodules, 55 years. (range 25–80) for NIFTPs, 49 years. (range 19–78) for the invasive EFVPTCs and 52 years. (range 23–75) for the LT subgroup. The majority of patients were females (131, 79%) compared to male's patients (34, 21%). Clinical, radiologic, or pathologic follow-up data were also reviewed. The median duration of follow-up for the benign subgroup was 6.99 years., NIFTPs 4.10 years., invasive EFVPTC 3.26 years. and LT subgroup 4.13 years. No recurrence for malignant cases was found.

Table 1. Demographics and clinicopathologic features of the patient cohort.

Characteristics	Benign	Neoplasm		LT *	Total Cases
Pathological Diagnosis	Hyperplasia & Adenoma *n* = 42	NIFTP *n* = 41	Invasive EFVPTC *n* = 45	Lymphocytic Thyroiditis *n* = 37	All Patients *n* = 165
Age, Mean (range), years	49.0 (15.8–88.9)	52.1 (22.7–79.5)	48.6 (19.0–77.5)	51.0 (22.8–74.8)	50.1 (15.8–88.9)
Sex, No. (%)					
Female	34	34	35	28	131
<45 years	13	12	13	9	47 (28)
≥45 years	21	22	22	19	84 (51)
Male	8	7	10	9	34
<45 years	1	2	5	2	10 (6)
≥45 years	7	5	5	7	24 (15)
Tumor size, mean(range), cm	3.6 ** (1.2–7.4)	2.6 (1.1–5.9)	2.9 (1.0–8.8)	3.0 (1.0–6.4)	3.0 (1.0–8.8)
Surgery	42	41	45	37	165
Lobectomy	3	1	1	1	6
Total thyroidectomy	29	40	44	36	149
Follow-up					
Mean (years)	6.99	4.10	3.26	4.13	4.65

* Advanced thyroiditis was separated from other noninvasive categories due to co-existing significant lymphocytes/Hashimoto's thyroiditis. ** Average of tumor size was calculated from 27 cases out of 42 benign patients because the information of the remaining 13 cases was not available.

According to the clinical histopathological features, all patients were allocated into four study subgroups- 42 benign nodules (25%), 41 NIFTPs (25%), 45 invasive EFVPTCs (27%) and 37 cases (22%) of encapsulated FVPTC lesions with coexisting significant lymphocytic thyroiditis and no capsular or vascular invasion (LT).

3.2. Cytoplasmic Gal-3 Expression Is Increased in Invasive EFVPTC

Gal-3 IHC analysis was carried out to determine its expression at the subcellular level in thyroid benign nodules, NIFTPs, invasive EFVPTCs and LT subgroup (Figure 1A–D and Figure 2A,B). Gal-3 positive control and the negative control with an isotype specific IgG were stained respectively using thyroid cancer tissue in each batch of immunostaining (Figure 1E,F). Gal-3 expression was mainly observed in tumor cells, whereas the stromal component of tumor did not show positive Gal-3 staining. Cytoplasmic Gal-3 expression (mean ± SD) was significantly increased in invasive EFVPTCs subgroup (4.80 ± 1.60) as compared to NIFTPs (2.75 ± 1.58, $p < 0.001$) and benign nodules (2.09 ± 1.19, $p < 0.001$, Tables 2 and 3); and there was no significant difference between NIFTPs and benign lesions ($p = 0.064$). The presence of LT also enhanced cytoplasmic Gal-3 expression (3.80 ± 1.32) compared to NIFTPs ($p = 0.016$) and benign nodules ($p < 0.001$). Nuclear Gal-3 expression in EFVPTC (1.84 ± 1.30) was significantly higher than in NIFTPs (1.04 ± 0.72, $p = 0.001$).

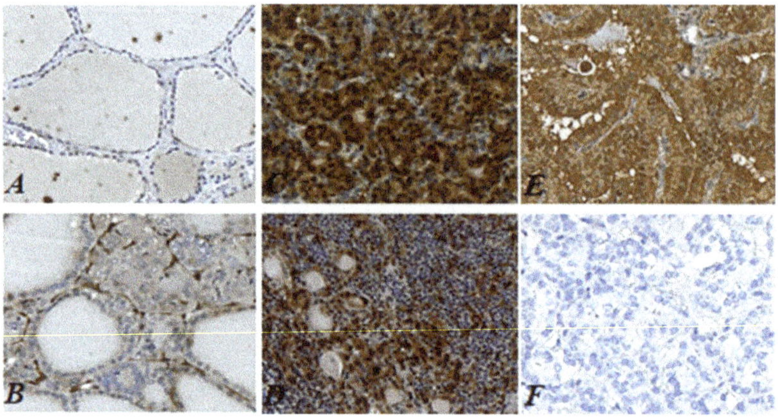

Figure 1. Histological IHC of Gal-3 expression in the tissue sections of Benign Nodules, NIFTP, invasive EFVPTC and LT tissues. (**A**). Lower detectable cytoplasmic Gal-3 expression was observed in the Benign Nodules tissue section. (**B**). Faint cytoplasmic Gal-3 immunostaining was detected in the NIFTP tissue section. (**C**). Moderate to strong cytoplasmic Gal-3 expression was observed in EFVPTC with capsular invasion. (**D**). Mild to moderate cytoplasmic Gal-3 expression was observed in the stained tissue section of LT. (**E**). Positive control, a classic aggressive PTC stained with anti-Gal-3 antibody showed moderate to strong immunostaining. (**F**). Negative control, a classic PTC incubated with isotype specific IgG in place of the anti-Gal-3 antibody did not show detectable immunostaining. All images were shown at original magnification ×200. All images were shown at original magnification ×200.

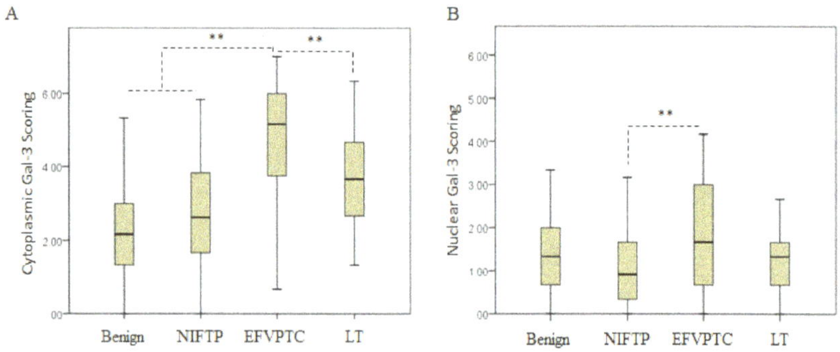

Figure 2. Distribution of Gal-3 expressions in Benign Nodules, NIFTP, EFVPTC and LT tissues. (**A**). Cytoplasmic Gal-3 expression; (**B**). Nuclear Gal-3 expression. The box-and-whisker plot showed the minimum, first quartile, median, third quartile and maximum of each group of data. Double stars (**) denoted a highly significant difference in means between groups at $p < 0.01$ (one-way ANOVA).

Table 2. Gal-3 expression level in cytoplasm and nucleus in tissues from Benign, NIFTP, EFVPTC and Lymphocytic thyroiditis (LT).

Groups	N	Cytoplasmic Gal-3			Nuclear Gal-3		
		Mean ± SD	95% CI		Mean ± SD	95% CI	
			Lower Bound	Upper Bound		Lower Bound	Upper Bound
Benign	42	2.09 ± 1.19	1.72	2.46	1.44 ± 1.07	1.10	1.77
NIFTP	41	2.75 ± 1.58	2.25	3.25	1.04 ± 0.72	0.79	1.23
EFVPTC	45	4.80 ± 1.60	4.32	5.28	1.84 ± 1.30	1.45	2.23
LT	37	3.80 ± 1.32	3.32	4.21	1.23 ± 0.85	0.95	1.51

Table 3. Comparison of cytoplasmic Gal-3 expression among groups of Benign, NIFTP, EFVPTC and Lymphocytic thyroiditis (LT).

(I) Groups	(J) Groups	Mean Difference (I–J)	Std. Error	*p* Value	95% CI	
					Lower Bound	Upper Bound
Benign	NIFTP	−0.659	0.316	0.162	−1.479	0.161
	EFVPTC	−2.737 *	0.312	<0.001	−3.547	−1.927
	LT	−1.703 *	0.328	<0.001	−2.553	−0.852
NIFTP	EFVPTC	−2.05 *	0.311	<0.001	−2.858	−1.479
	LT	−1.017 *	0.326	0.011	−1.864	−0.170
EFVPTC	LT	1.035 *	0.321	0.008	0.202	1.867

* The mean difference is significant at $p < 0.05$ level (F(3162) = 29.395, $p < 0.001$ one-way ANOVA).

However, no significant difference was observed between invasive EFVPTC and benign nodules (1.44 ± 1.07, $p = 0.215$, Tables 2 and 4), which negated the utility of nuclear Gal-3 expression as a reliable diagnostic aid in detecting invasive EFVPTC.

Table 4. Comparison of nuclear Gal-3 expression among Benign, NIFTP, EFVPTC and Lymphocytic thyroiditis (LT).

(I) Groups	(J) Groups	Mean Difference (I–J)	Std. Error	*p* Value	95% CI	
					Lower Bound	Upper Bound
Benign	NIFTP	0.433	0.224	0.219	−0.149	1.014
	EFVPTC	−0.422	0.218	0.215	−0.987	0.142
	LT	0.183	0.229	0.855	−0.411	0.776
NIFTP	EFVPTC	−0.833 *	0.220	0.001	−1.405	−0.262
	LT	−0.228	0.231	0.758	−0.828	0.372
EFVPTC	LT	0.605 *	0.224	0.038	0.024	1.186

* The mean difference is significant at $p < 0.05$ level (F(3162) = 5.166, $p = 0.002$ one-way ANOVA).

3.3. Cytoplasmic Gal-3 Predictive Value for NIFTP versus Invasive EFVPTC

The accuracy of cytoplasmic Gal-3 expression in distinguishing invasive EFVPTC from NIFTP and benign thyroid nodules was determined by the ROC curve analysis. Cytoplasmic Gal-3 emerged as the strongest predictor of invasive EFVPTC in comparison with nonmalignant tissues (AUC = 0.90, (CI 0.83–0.97), $p < 0.001$) thereby underscoring its potential clinical applicability (Table 5 and Figure S2). With a positive cut off value 3.71 (Table S1), cytoplasmic Gal-3 expression in EFVPTC versus in NIFTP showed a sensitivity of 75.6% (95% CI: 63.9–87.2%), specificity 80.5% (95% CI: 68.6–92.4%), positive predictive value (PPV) 81.0% (95% CI: 69.6–92.3%) and negative predictive value (NPV) 75.0% (95% CI: 62.8–87.2%) (Table 5).

Table 5. The clinical utility of biomarkers was assessed using sensitivity, specificity, positive predictive value (PPV), negative predictive value (NPV) and area under the curve (AUC) between benign or NIFTP vs. invasive EFVPTC group.

Gal-3 Staining	Sensitivity (%)	Specificity (%)	PPV (%)	NPV (%)	AUC		
					Area	*p* Value	95% CI
			Benign vs. Invasive EFVPTC				
Cytoplasmic Gal-3	80.0	81.0	81.8	79.1	0.90	<0.001	0.83–0.97
Nuclear Gal-3	48.9	71.4	64.7	56.6	0.58	0.194	0.46–0.70
			NIFTP vs. Invasive EFVPTC				
Cytoplasmic Gal-3	75.6	80.5	81.0	75.0	0.83	<0.001	0.75–0.92
Nuclear Gal-3	46.7	90.2	84.0	60.7	0.66	0.012	0.54–0.77

The cross tabulation analysis of diagnostic odds ratio (OR) showed the positive cytoplasmic Gal-3 expression in invasive EFVPTC was 13 times higher risk of having adverse outcome compared to indolent NIFTP (OR = 12.75, 95% CI: 5.88–49.14). The positive likelihood ratio (LR+ = 3.87, 95% CI: 2.21–7.97) indicated the probability in diagnosing as malignant tumors was increased 2.1 times more in specimens with the positive cytoplasmic Gal-3 expression. However, the negative likelihood ratio (LR- = 0.30, 95% CI: 0.14–0.45) showed the probability of malignancy was decreased by 30% in specimens with the low cytoplasmic Gal-3 expression.

4. Discussion

Indeterminate thyroid nodules are highly prevalent in daily clinical practice and represent up to 30% of all clinically assessed thyroid nodules [41], whereas only less than 20% of this group are malignant. Invasive EFVPTC, noninvasive EFVPTC (not meeting criteria for NIFTP diagnosis) and infiltrative FVPTC were designated as malignant lesions, making the diagnosis of thyroid cancer very difficult in cases where histological hallmarks of invasion are not evident [15–17,37]. A subset of encapsulated follicular tumors, formerly considered to be noninvasive encapsulated/well demarcated follicular variant of PTC, has been reclassified under a new histological nomenclature, NIFTP [11]. The incidence of NIFTP was as high as 13.3% of all PTC cases in North American and European populations [42] and 16.8% of all well-differentiated thyroid cancers in Ontario, Canada [24]. Histopathological examination of the entire capsulated tumor after its resection according to the rigid diagnostic criteria remains the gold standard for NIFTP diagnosis. Malignant behavior (lymph node and/or distant metastasis) has been reported in NIFTP patients [21,43,44]. NIFTP is not entirely considered as a benign thyroid neoplasm, but correct classification of noninvasive EFVPTC that would qualify NITFP is required to ensure an extremely low rate of adverse oncologic outcomes. Molecular marker testing has risen as an auxiliary tool to distinguish malignant invasive EFVPTCs from more indolent NIFTPs and benign nodules [11,25], potentially assisting pathologists in the management of indeterminate thyroid nodules [27]. Scores on the base of the levels of protein marker expression in thyroid nodules may objectively distinguish malignant lesions from indeterminate thyroid nodules, thereby aiding the correct diagnosis and consequent avoidance of over-treatment of NIFTP lesions when the score is low. Our previous study has shown that the degree of cytoplasmic PD-L1 expression could serve as a useful adjunct to traditional H&E histopathology assessment of such nodules, among which with a low expression of cytoplasmic PD-L1 can be considered as benign nodules or NIFTP [25].

Gal-3 expression has been recognized as a promising diagnostic molecular marker of thyroid malignancy due to its differential expression between thyroid carcinomas and normal or benign thyroid tissues [29,45–47]. However, the reclassification of EFVPTC without capsular or vascular invasion to NIFTP not only affects how pathologists evaluate and report this subset of thyroid neoplasms but also raises the need for rebuilding the clinical, histologic, cytologic and molecular parameters for this new entity and accordingly establishing new molecular tests [22]. Therefore, the use of ancillary testing with protein markers previously developed, such as Gal-3 and HBME1, requires to be re-evaluated in the era of NIFTP. In the present study, our data have shown that cytoplasmic Gal-3 expression is significantly increased in invasive EFVPTCs as compared to NIFTPs or benign thyroid nodules in thyroid resection specimens. Concurrently, though there was no significant difference between NIFTPs and benign nodules, cytoplasmic Gal-3 expression in the former was higher than that in the latter, supporting NIFTP cannot be simply considered as a benign lesion. Chronic inflammation can be associated with 30–58% of PTC [48,49]. We also noted that the presence of LT enhances cytoplasmic Gal-3 expression and henceforward the LT increased expression needs to be interpreted with caution. This observation is consistent with the result from another report which showed the increased expression of Gal-3 in an inflammatory environment [50]. Patients with LT were usually under prolonged stimuli from chronic inflammation. The mechanism underlying modulation of Gal-3 expression in thyroid with chronic inflammatory process remains to be determined. Localization of Gal-3 in papillary carcinomas has been reported in both the cytoplasm and nucleus [40,51,52], however, our findings and other's [29] showed predominant expression of Gal-3 in the cytoplasm in PTC rather than the nucleus. Nuclear expression has been observed in some benign thyroid conditions in our study and reports of others [51,52]. The increased cytoplasmic Gal-3 in invasive EFVPTC might contribute to thyroid cancer development through the induction of the capsular, vascular and/or extrathyroidal invasive activity. The detailed correlation between Gal-3 expression and the degree of invasion was not able to be analyzed since most EFVPTC cases were presented with minimal capsular invasion in the current study. Recently, genetic alterations were intensively studied, such as *BRAF*, *RAS* and *TERT* promoter mutations and *RET/PTC* and *PAX8/PPAR*γ rearrangements [53,54]. NIFTPs are commonly detected with the frequent occurrence of RAS mutations and lack of BRAF^{V600E} and TERT promoter mutations [23]. Whether the level of Gal-3 expression can be associated with such mutational status for better identifying NIFTP requires further investigation. Our observations have suggested that cytoplasmic Gal-3 expression can be considered as an ancillary aid to H&E diagnostic criteria in distinguishing invasive EFVPTC from NIFTP and benign nodules.

After four decades of steady increase, thyroid cancer incidence rate reached a plateau and possibly started to decline between 2013 and 2020 in the United States [55]. This reverse trend in the incidence of thyroid cancers has been correlating with the increasing understanding of over-diagnosis and the indolent nature of many thyroid nodules that were more likely classified as cancers previously. NIFTP has emerged as a low risk tumor with an indolent clinical course. The present study was focused on evaluating the diagnostic value of the Gal-3 cytoplasmic expression in the histological tissue samples between NIFTP and EFVPTC. To our knowledge, this is the first report showing the diagnostic value of increased cytoplasmic Gal-3 expression in ruling out the indolent NIFTP from invasive EFVPTC. The Gal-3 test proposed here does not replace conventional surgical histopathological examination but represents an auxiliary diagnostic method, especially for cases where morphologic features of invasion are equivocal, that may affect clinical decision-making with regard to completion thyroidectomy, central lymph node dissection, and adjunctive radioiodine therapy. In practice, Gal-3 staining alone add little to histology evaluation when the diagnosis of NIFTP could be achieved via complete resection of the nodules for histological examination of the entire capsule to rule out invasion. However, in pre-surgical fine needle aspiration (FNA) biopsies, NIFTP can belong to any of four categories of the Bethesda System for Reporting Thyroid Cytopathology (TBSRTC), including benign, atypia of undetermined significance or follicular lesion of undetermined significance (AUS/FLUS), follicular neoplasm or suspicious for a follicular neoplasm (FN/SFN) and suspicious for malignancy (SFM) [56]. The definitive diagnosis of NIFTP cannot be made based on the observation of the preoperative cytology specimens, while molecular tests would be highly useful to improve the accuracy in the diagnostics of NIFTP in FNA biopsies. Gal-3 test could have clinically significant utility in assisting in preoperative diagnosis if it were successfully applied to cytology specimens [57]. We are aware of the limitation of our study which is based upon a single patient cohort from a single tertiary care center. Future studies in a larger patient cohort from multiple centers are needed to validate our observations and conclusions. Furthermore, the NIFTP cases were re-classified based on a thorough review of pathology reports and assessment of H&E slides in this study. NIFTP diagnosis is challenging for pathologist and a potential misclassification error might exist particularly when specimens were managed in a way the entire tumor capsule could not be fully assessed for invasion based on pathology review of slides. We are also cognizant that the clinical outcome analysis for each subtype was limited due to incomplete follow-up information, hence the possible association of cytoplasmic Gal-3 expression with the long-term prognoses of NIFTP verses invasive EFVPTC remains further investigation.

5. Conclusions

In conclusion, our data have demonstrated that increased cytoplasmic Gal-3 expression can (i) significantly distinguish indolent NIFTP from invasive EFVPTC; (ii) assist in the early detection of thyroid tumors with aggressiveness and potential metastatic spread which can be suspected by the increased cytoplasmic Gal-3 expression; (iii) support its clinical application as a useful ancillary test to H&E histopathological diagnostic assessment in distinguishing invasive EFVPTC from NIFTP when there is no significant interference from LT.

Supplementary Materials: The following are available online at https://www.mdpi.com/article/10.3390/cancers13122988/s1, Figure S1: Photomicrographs of IHC scoring of Gal-3 expression in thyroid tissue sections. Figure S2: ROC curve analysis showed each cut-off value of IHC scores. Table S1: The cut-off values for immunopositivity of cytoplasmic Gal-3 expression were compared to Sensitivity and Specificity via ROC analysis.

Author Contributions: Conceptualization and design, G.F., O.P.; methodology and validation, G.F.; cohort classification, O.P.; investigation, G.F. and O.P.; analysis, G.F., O.P. and R.S.C.; resources, J.L.F. and I.J.W.; writing—draft preparation, G.F.; review and editing, G.F., O.P.; R.S.C., J.L.F. and I.J.W.; project administration, G.F.; funding acquisition, I.J.W. All authors have read and agreed to the published version of the manuscript.

Funding: This research was funded by The Mount Sinai Hospital Foundation of Toronto Da Vinci Gala Fundraiser and a donation from The Joyce Wolfish Estate, Mount Sinai Hospital Department of Medicine Research Fund (P.G.W.), Alex and Simona Shnaider Chair in Thyroid Cancer (I.J.W.).

Institutional Review Board Statement: The study was conducted according to the guidelines of the Declaration of Helsinki and approved by the Sinai Health System Research Ethics Board (REB #07-0212-E).

Informed Consent Statement: Informed consent was obtained from all subjects involved in the study.

Acknowledgments: This work was supported by Paul G. Walfish (P.G.W.), who passed away on 28 July 2018.

Conflicts of Interest: The authors declare no conflict of interest. The funders had no role in the design of the study, in the collection, analyses or interpretation of data, and in the writing of the manuscript or in the decision to publish the results.

References

1. Lim, H.; Devesa, S.S.; Sosa, J.A.; Check, D.; Kitahara, C.M. Trends in Thyroid Cancer Incidence and Mortality in the United States, 1974–2013. *JAMA* **2017**, *317*, 1338–1348. [CrossRef] [PubMed]
2. The Surveillance E, and End Results (SEER) Program. Cancer Stat Facts: Thyroid Cancer. 2018. Available online: http://seer.cancer.gov/statfacts/html/thyro.html (accessed on 2 June 2020).
3. Siegel, R.L.; Miller, K.D.; Jemal, A. Cancer statistics, 2020. *CA A Cancer J. Clin.* **2020**, *70*, 7–30. [CrossRef] [PubMed]

4. Xing, M.; Haugen, B.R.; Schlumberger, M. Progress in molecular-based management of differentiated thyroid cancer. *Lancet* **2013**, *381*, 1058–1069. [CrossRef]
5. Katoh, H.; Yamashita, K.; Enomoto, T.; Watanabe, M. Classification and General Considerations of Thyroid Cancer. *Ann. Clin. Pathol.* **2015**, *3*, 1045.
6. Ceresini, G.; Corcione, L.; Michiara, M.; Sgargi, P.; Teresi, G.; Gilli, A.; Usberti, E.; Silini, E.; Ceda, G.P. Thyroid cancer incidence by histological type and related variants in a mildly iodine-deficient area of Northern Italy, 1998 to 2009. *Cancer* **2012**, *118*, 5473–5480. [CrossRef]
7. Mete, O.; Seethala, R.R.; Asa, S.L.; Bullock, M.J.; Carty, S.E.; Hodak, S.P.; McHugh, J.B.; Nikiforov, Y.E.; Pettus, J.; Richardson, M.S.; et al. Protocol for the Examination of Specimens From Patients With Carcinomas of the Thyroid Gland (Version: Thyroid 4.2.0.0); College of American Pathologists (CAP). Protocol Posting Date: August 2019. Available online: https://www.cap.org/protocols-and-guidelines/cancer-reporting-tools/cancer-protocol-templates (accessed on 3 June 2020).
8. Burningham, A.R.; Krishnan, J.; Davidson, B.J.; Ringel, M.D.; Burman, K.D. Papillary and follicular variant of papillary carcinoma of the thyroid: Initial presentation and response to therapy. *Otolaryngol. Head and NeckSurg. Off. J. Am. Acad. Otolaryngol. -Head and Neck Surg.* **2005**, *132*, 840–844. [CrossRef]
9. Gupta, S.; Ajise, O.; Dultz, L.; Wang, B.; Nonaka, D.; Ogilvie, J.; Heller, K.S.; Patel, K.N. Follicular variant of papillary thyroid cancer: Encapsulated, nonencapsulated, and diffuse: Distinct biologic and clinical entities. *Arch. Otolaryngol. Head Neck Surg.* **2012**, *138*, 227–233. [CrossRef]
10. LiVolsi, V.A.; Baloch, Z.W. Follicular-patterned tumors of the thyroid: The battle of benign vs. malignant vs. so-called uncertain. *Endocr. Pathol.* **2011**, *22*, 184–189. [CrossRef]
11. Nikiforov, Y.E.; Seethala, R.R.; Tallini, G.; Baloch, Z.W.; Basolo, F.; Thompson, L.D.; Barletta, J.A.; Wenig, B.M.; Al Ghuzlan, A.; Kakudo, K.; et al. Nomenclature Revision for Encapsulated Follicular Variant of Papillary Thyroid Carcinoma: A Paradigm Shift to Reduce Overtreatment of Indolent Tumors. *JAMA Oncol.* **2016**, *2*, 1023–1029. [CrossRef]
12. Kakudo, K.; Bai, Y.; Liu, Z.; Ozaki, T. Encapsulated papillary thyroid carcinoma, follicular variant: A misnomer. *Pathol. Int.* **2012**, *62*, 155–160. [CrossRef]
13. Liu, J.; Singh, B.; Tallini, G.; Carlson, D.L.; Katabi, N.; Shaha, A.; Tuttle, R.M.; Ghossein, R.A. Follicular variant of papillary thyroid carcinoma: A clinicopathologic study of a problematic entity. *Cancer* **2006**, *107*, 1255–1264. [CrossRef]
14. Yang, G.C.; Liebeskind, D.; Messina, A.V. Diagnostic accuracy of follicular variant of papillary thyroid carcinoma in fine-needle aspirates processed by ultrafast Papanicolaou stain: Histologic follow-up of 125 cases. *Cancer* **2006**, *108*, 174–179. [CrossRef]
15. Baloch, Z.W.; LiVolsi, V.A. Encapsulated follicular variant of papillary thyroid carcinoma with bone metastases. *Modern Pathol.* **2000**, *13*, 861–865. [CrossRef] [PubMed]
16. Daniels, G.H. What if many follicular variant papillary thyroid carcinomas are not malignant? A review of follicular variant papillary thyroid carcinoma and a proposal for a new classification. *Endocr. Pract. Off. J. Am. Coll. Endocrinol. Am. Assoc. Clin. Endocrinol.* **2011**, *17*, 768–787. [CrossRef] [PubMed]
17. Lloyd, R.V.; Erickson, L.A.; Casey, M.B.; Lam, K.Y.; Lohse, C.M.; Asa, S.L.; Chan, J.K.; DeLellis, R.A.; Harach, H.R.; Kakudo, K.; et al. Observer variation in the diagnosis of follicular variant of papillary thyroid carcinoma. *Am. J. Surg. Pathol.* **2004**, *28*, 1336–1340. [CrossRef] [PubMed]
18. Piana, S.; Frasoldati, A.; Di Felice, E.; Gardini, G.; Tallini, G.; Rosai, J. Encapsulated well-differentiated follicular-patterned thyroid carcinomas do not play a significant role in the fatality rates from thyroid carcinoma. *Am. J. Surg. Pathol.* **2010**, *34*, 868–872. [CrossRef]
19. Ganly, I.; Wang, L.; Tuttle, R.M.; Katabi, N.; Ceballos, G.A.; Harach, H.R.; Ghossein, R. Invasion rather than nuclear features correlates with outcome in encapsulated follicular tumors: Further evidence for the reclassification of the encapsulated papillary thyroid carcinoma follicular variant. *Hum. Pathol.* **2015**, *46*, 657–664. [CrossRef]
20. Rosario, P.W.; Penna, G.C.; Calsolari, M.R. Noninvasive encapsulated follicular variant of papillary thyroid carcinoma: Is lobectomy sufficient for tumours >/=1 cm? *Clin. Endocrinol.* **2014**, *81*, 630–632. [CrossRef] [PubMed]
21. Cho, U.; Mete, O.; Kim, M.H.; Bae, J.S.; Jung, C.K. Molecular correlates and rate of lymph node metastasis of non-invasive follicular thyroid neoplasm with papillary-like nuclear features and invasive follicular variant papillary thyroid carcinoma: The impact of rigid criteria to distinguish non-invasive follicular thyroid neoplasm with papillary-like nuclear features. *Mod. Pathol.* **2017**. [CrossRef]
22. Seethala, R.R.; Baloch, Z.W.; Barletta, J.A.; Khanafshar, E.; Mete, O.; Sadow, P.M.; LiVolsi, V.A.; Nikiforov, Y.E.; Tallini, G.; Thompson, L.D. Noninvasive follicular thyroid neoplasm with papillary-like nuclear features: A review for pathologists. *Mod. Pathol.* **2018**, *31*, 39–55. [CrossRef]
23. Nikiforov, Y.E.; Baloch, Z.W.; Hodak, S.P.; Giordano, T.J.; Lloyd, R.V.; Seethala, R.R.; Wenig, B.M. Change in Diagnostic Criteria for Noninvasive Follicular Thyroid Neoplasm With Papillarylike Nuclear Features. *JAMA Oncol.* **2018**, *4*, 1125–1126. [CrossRef] [PubMed]
24. Eskander, A.; Hall, S.F.; Manduch, M.; Griffiths, R.; Irish, J.C. A Population-Based Study on NIFTP Incidence and Survival: Is NIFTP Really a "Benign" Disease? *Ann. Surg. Oncol.* **2019**, *26*, 1376–1384. [CrossRef] [PubMed]
25. Fu, G.; Polyakova, O.; MacMillan, C.; Ralhan, R.; Walfish, P.G. Programmed Death—Ligand 1 Expression Distinguishes Invasive Encapsulated Follicular Variant of Papillary Thyroid Carcinoma from Noninvasive Follicular Thyroid Neoplasm with Papillary-like Nuclear Features. *EBioMedicine* **2017**, *18*, 50–55. [CrossRef]

26. Rivera, M.; Ricarte-Filho, J.; Knauf, J.; Shaha, A.; Tuttle, M.; Fagin, J.A.; Ghossein, R.A. Molecular genotyping of papillary thyroid carcinoma follicular variant according to its histological subtypes (encapsulated vs infiltrative) reveals distinct BRAF and RAS mutation patterns. *Mod. Pathol.* **2010**, *23*, 1191–1200. [CrossRef] [PubMed]
27. Rossi, E.D.; Martini, M. New Insight in a New Entity: NIFTPS and Valuable Role of Ancillary Techniques. The Role of PD-L1. *EBioMedicine* **2017**, *18*, 11–12. [CrossRef] [PubMed]
28. Nangia-Makker, P.; Nakahara, S.; Hogan, V.; Raz, A. Galectin-3 in apoptosis, a novel therapeutic target. *J. Bioenerg. Biomembr.* **2007**, *39*, 79–84. [CrossRef] [PubMed]
29. Chiu, C.G.; Strugnell, S.S.; Griffith, O.L.; Jones, S.J.; Gown, A.M.; Walker, B.; Nabi, I.R.; Wiseman, S.M. Diagnostic utility of galectin-3 in thyroid cancer. *Am. J. Pathol.* **2010**, *176*, 2067–2081. [CrossRef] [PubMed]
30. Cvejic, D.; Savin, S.; Petrovic, I.; Selemetjev, S.; Paunovic, I.; Tatic, S.; Havelka, M. Galectin-3 and proliferating cell nuclear antigen (PCNA) expression in papillary thyroid carcinoma. *Exp. Oncol.* **2005**, *27*, 210–214.
31. Yoshii, T.; Inohara, H.; Takenaka, Y.; Honjo, Y.; Akahani, S.; Nomura, T.; Raz, A.; Kubo, T. Galectin-3 maintains the transformed phenotype of thyroid papillary carcinoma cells. *Int. J. Oncol.* **2001**, *18*, 787–792. [CrossRef]
32. Honjo, Y.; Nangia-Makker, P.; Inohara, H.; Raz, A. Down-regulation of galectin-3 suppresses tumorigenicity of human breast carcinoma cells. *Clin. Cancer Res.* **2001**, *7*, 661–668.
33. Cecchinelli, B.; Lavra, L.; Rinaldo, C.; Iacovelli, S.; Gurtner, A.; Gasbarri, A.; Ulivieri, A.; Del Prete, F.; Trovato, M.; Piaggio, G.; et al. Repression of the antiapoptotic molecule galectin-3 by homeodomain-interacting protein kinase 2-activated p53 is required for p53-induced apoptosis. *Mol. Cell. Biol.* **2006**, *26*, 4746–4757. [CrossRef] [PubMed]
34. Kawachi, K.; Matsushita, Y.; Yonezawa, S.; Nakano, S.; Shirao, K.; Natsugoe, S.; Sueyoshi, K.; Aikou, T.; Sato, E. Galectin-3 expression in various thyroid neoplasms and its possible role in metastasis formation. *Hum. Pathol.* **2000**, *31*, 428–433. [CrossRef] [PubMed]
35. Saggiorato, E.; Aversa, S.; Deandreis, D.; Arecco, F.; Mussa, A.; Puligheddu, B.; Cappia, S.; Conticello, S.; Papotti, M.; Orlandi, F. Galectin-3: Presurgical marker of thyroid follicular epithelial cell-derived carcinomas. *J. Endocrinol. Investig.* **2004**, *27*, 311–317. [CrossRef] [PubMed]
36. Lloyd, R.V.; Osamura, R.Y.; Klèoppel, G.; Rosai, J.; WHO; IARC. *WHO Classification of Tumours of Endocrine Organs*, 4th ed.; International Agency for Research on Cancer (IARC): Lyon, France, 2017; Volume 10.
37. Seethala, R.R.; Asa, S.L.; Bullock, M.J.; Carty, S.E.; Hodak, S.P.; McHugh, J.B.; Nikiforov, Y.E.; Pettus, J.; Richardson, M.S.; Shah, J.; et al. *Protocol for the Examination of Specimens from Patients with Carcinomas of the Thyroid Gland*; Version: Thyroid 4.0.0.0; College of American Pathologists (CAP): Northfield, IL, USA, 2017.
38. van Heerden, J.A.; Hay, I.D.; Goellner, J.R.; Salomao, D.; Ebersold, J.R.; Bergstralh, E.J.; Grant, C.S. Follicular thyroid carcinoma with capsular invasion alone: A nonthreatening malignancy. *Surgery* **1992**, *112*, 1130–1136.
39. Nikiforov, Y.E.; Biddinger, P.W.; Thompson, L.D.R. *Diagnostic Pathology and Molecular Genetics of the Thyroid: A Comprehensive Guide for Practicing Thyroid Pathology*, 2nd ed.; Lippincott Williams & Wilkins: Philadelphia, PA, USA, 2012; pp. 152–182.
40. Ralhan, R.; Veyhl, J.; Chaker, S.; Assi, J.; Alyass, A.; Jeganathan, A.; Somasundaram, R.T.; MacMillan, C.; Freeman, J.; Vescan, A.D.; et al. Immunohistochemical Subcellular Localization of Protein Biomarkers Distinguishes Benign from Malignant Thyroid Nodules: Potential for Fine-Needle Aspiration Biopsy Clinical Application. *Thyroid Off. J. Am. Thyroid Assoc.* **2015**, *25*, 1224–1234. [CrossRef]
41. Haugen, B.R.; Alexander, E.K.; Bible, K.C.; Doherty, G.M.; Mandel, S.J.; Nikiforov, Y.E.; Pacini, F.; Randolph, G.W.; Sawka, A.M.; Schlumberger, M.; et al. 2015 American Thyroid Association Management Guidelines for Adult Patients with Thyroid Nodules and Differentiated Thyroid Cancer: The American Thyroid Association Guidelines Task Force on Thyroid Nodules and Differentiated Thyroid Cancer. *Thyroid Off. J. Am. Thyroid Assoc.* **2016**, *26*, 1–133. [CrossRef]
42. Bychkov, A.; Jung, C.K.; Liu, Z.; Kakudo, K. Noninvasive Follicular Thyroid Neoplasm with Papillary-Like Nuclear Features in Asian Practice: Perspectives for Surgical Pathology and Cytopathology. *Endocr. Pathol.* **2018**, *29*, 276–288. [CrossRef] [PubMed]
43. Parente, D.N.; Kluijfhout, W.P.; Bongers, P.J.; Verzijl, R.; Devon, K.M.; Rotstein, L.E.; Goldstein, D.P.; Asa, S.L.; Mete, O.; Pasternak, J.D. Clinical Safety of Renaming Encapsulated Follicular Variant of Papillary Thyroid Carcinoma: Is NIFTP Truly Benign? *World J. Surg.* **2018**, *42*, 321–326. [CrossRef]
44. Hahn, S.Y.; Shin, J.H.; Lim, H.K.; Jung, S.L.; Oh, Y.L.; Choi, I.H.; Jung, C.K. Preoperative differentiation between noninvasive follicular thyroid neoplasm with papillary-like nuclear features (NIFTP) and non-NIFTP. *Clin. Endocrinol.* **2017**, *86*, 444–450. [CrossRef]
45. Tang, W.; Huang, C.; Tang, C.; Xu, J.; Wang, H. Galectin-3 may serve as a potential marker for diagnosis and prognosis in papillary thyroid carcinoma: A meta-analysis. *OncoTargets Ther.* **2016**, *9*, 455–460. [CrossRef]
46. Bartolazzi, A.; Orlandi, F.; Saggiorato, E.; Volante, M.; Arecco, F.; Rossetto, R.; Palestini, N.; Ghigo, E.; Papotti, M.; Bussolati, G.; et al. Galectin-3-expression analysis in the surgical selection of follicular thyroid nodules with indeterminate fine-needle aspiration cytology: A prospective multicentre study. *Lancet. Oncol.* **2008**, *9*, 543–549. [CrossRef]
47. Li, J.; Vasilyeva, E.; Wiseman, S.M. Beyond immunohistochemistry and immunocytochemistry: A current perspective on galectin-3 and thyroid cancer. *Expert Rev. Anticancer. Ther.* **2019**, *19*, 1017–1027. [CrossRef] [PubMed]
48. Kebebew, E.; Treseler, P.A.; Ituarte, P.H.; Clark, O.H. Coexisting chronic lymphocytic thyroiditis and papillary thyroid cancer revisited. *World J. Surg.* **2001**, *25*, 632–637. [CrossRef] [PubMed]

49. Tamimi, D.M. The association between chronic lymphocytic thyroiditis and thyroid tumors. *Int. J. Surg. Pathol.* **2002**, *10*, 141–146. [CrossRef]
50. Ma, H.; Yan, J.; Zhang, C.; Qin, S.; Qin, L.; Liu, L.; Wang, X.; Li, N. Expression of papillary thyroid carcinoma-associated molecular markers and their significance in follicular epithelial dysplasia with papillary thyroid carcinoma-like nuclear alterations in Hashimoto's thyroiditis. *Int. J. Clin. Exp. Pathol.* **2014**, *7*, 7999–8007. [PubMed]
51. Orlandi, F.; Saggiorato, E.; Pivano, G.; Puligheddu, B.; Termine, A.; Cappia, S.; De Giuli, P.; Angeli, A. Galectin-3 is a presurgical marker of human thyroid carcinoma. *Cancer Res.* **1998**, *58*, 3015–3020.
52. Saggiorato, E.; Cappia, S.; De Giuli, P.; Mussa, A.; Pancani, G.; Caraci, P.; Angeli, A.; Orlandi, F. Galectin-3 as a presurgical immunocytodiagnostic marker of minimally invasive follicular thyroid carcinoma. *J. Clin. Endocrinol. Metab.* **2001**, *86*, 5152–5158. [CrossRef]
53. Nikiforov, Y.E.; Ohori, N.P.; Hodak, S.P.; Carty, S.E.; LeBeau, S.O.; Ferris, R.L.; Yip, L.; Seethala, R.R.; Tublin, M.E.; Stang, M.T.; et al. Impact of mutational testing on the diagnosis and management of patients with cytologically indeterminate thyroid nodules: A prospective analysis of 1056 FNA samples. *J. Clin. Endocrinol. Metab.* **2011**, *96*, 3390–3397. [CrossRef]
54. Decaussin-Petrucci, M.; Descotes, F.; Depaepe, L.; Lapras, V.; Denier, M.L.; Borson-Chazot, F.; Lifante, J.C.; Lopez, J. Molecular testing of BRAF, RAS and TERT on thyroid FNAs with indeterminate cytology improves diagnostic accuracy. *Cytopathol. Off. J. Br. Soc. Clin. Cytol.* **2017**, *28*, 482–487. [CrossRef] [PubMed]
55. Powers, A.E.; Marcadis, A.R.; Lee, M.; Morris, L.G.T.; Marti, J.L. Changes in Trends in Thyroid Cancer Incidence in the United States, 1992 to 2016. *JAMA* **2019**, *322*, 2440–2441. [CrossRef]
56. Brandler, T.C.; Zhou, F.; Liu, C.Z.; Cho, M.; Lau, R.P.; Simsir, A.; Patel, K.N.; Sun, W. Can noninvasive follicular thyroid neoplasm with papillary-like nuclear features be distinguished from classic papillary thyroid carcinoma and follicular adenomas by fine-needle aspiration? *Cancer Cytopathol.* **2017**, *125*, 378–388. [CrossRef] [PubMed]
57. Trimboli, P.; Guidobaldi, L.; Amendola, S.; Nasrollah, N.; Romanelli, F.; Attanasio, D.; Ramacciato, G.; Saggiorato, E.; Valabrega, S.; Crescenzi, A. Galectin-3 and HBME-1 improve the accuracy of core biopsy in indeterminate thyroid nodules. *Endocrine* **2016**, *52*, 39–45. [CrossRef] [PubMed]

cancers

Review

Prognostic and Therapeutic Role of Angiogenic Microenvironment in Thyroid Cancer

Assunta Melaccio [1,†], Lucia Ilaria Sgaramella [2,†], Alessandro Pasculli [2,†], Giovanna Di Meo [2], Angela Gurrado [2], Francesco Paolo Prete [2], Angelo Vacca [1], Roberto Ria [1] and Mario Testini [2,*]

1 Operative Unit of Internal Medicine "G. Baccelli", Department of Biomedical Sciences and Human Oncology, University of Bari "Aldo Moro" Medical School, 70124 Bari, Italy; assunta.melaccio@uniba.it (A.M.); angelo.vacca@uniba.it (A.V.); roberto.ria@uniba.it (R.R.)

2 Academic General Surgery Unit "V. Bonomo", Department of Biomedical Sciences and Human Oncology, University of Bari "Aldo Moro" Medical School, 70124 Bari, Italy; ilaria.sgaramella@policlinico.ba.it (L.I.S.); alessandro.pasculli@uniba.it (A.P.); giovanna.dimeo@policlinico.ba.it (G.D.M.); angela.gurrado@uniba.it (A.G.); francesco.prete@policlinico.ba.it (F.P.P.)

* Correspondence: mario.testini@uniba.it; Tel.: +39-3355370914

† These authors contributed equally to the work.

Simple Summary: Angiogenesis is an essential event for the progression of solid tumors and is promoted by angiogenic cytokines released in the tumor microenvironment by neoplastic and stromal cells. Over the last 20 years, the role of the microenvironment and the implication of several angiogenic factors in tumorigenesis of solid and hematological neoplasms have been widely studied. The tumor microenvironment has also been well-defined for thyroid cancer, clarifying the importance of angiogenesis in cancer progression, spread, and metastasis. Furthermore, recent studies have evaluated the association of circulating angiogenic factors with the clinical outcomes of differentiated thyroid cancer, potentially providing noninvasive, low-cost, and safe tests that can be used in screening, diagnosis, and follow-up. In this review, we highlight the mechanisms of action of these proangiogenic factors and their different molecular pathways, as well as their applications in the treatment and prognosis of thyroid cancer.

Abstract: Thyroid cancer is the most common endocrine malignancy, with a typically favorable prognosis following standard treatments, such as surgical resection and radioiodine therapy. A subset of thyroid cancers progress to refractory/metastatic disease. Understanding how the tumor microenvironment is transformed into an angiogenic microenvironment has a role of primary importance in the aggressive behavior of these neoplasms. During tumor growth and progression, angiogenesis represents a deregulated biological process, and the angiogenic switch, characterized by the formation of new vessels, induces tumor cell proliferation, local invasion, and hematogenous metastases. This evidence has propelled the scientific community's effort to study a number of molecular pathways (proliferation, cell cycle control, and angiogenic processes), identifying mediators that may represent viable targets for new anticancer treatments. Herein, we sought to review angiogenesis in thyroid cancer and the potential role of proangiogenic cytokines for risk stratification of patients. We also present the current status of treatment of advanced differentiated, medullary, and poorly differentiated thyroid cancers with multiple tyrosine kinase inhibitors, based on the rationale of angiogenesis as a potential therapeutic target.

Keywords: thyroid carcinoma; angiogenic microenvironment; prognostic factors; antiangiogenic therapy; therapeutic target; tumor microenvironment; tumor behavior; proliferation pathways; cell cycle control pathways; angiogenesis process

Citation: Melaccio, A.; Sgaramella, L.I.; Pasculli, A.; Di Meo, G.; Gurrado, A.; Prete, F.P.; Vacca, A.; Ria, R.; Testini, M. Prognostic and Therapeutic Role of Angiogenic Microenvironment in Thyroid Cancer. *Cancers* **2021**, *13*, 2775. https://doi.org/10.3390/cancers13112775

Academic Editors: Fabio Medas and Pier Francesco Alesina

Received: 28 April 2021
Accepted: 31 May 2021
Published: 3 June 2021

1. Introduction

Thyroid cancers are the most common endocrine malignancies and have been shown to be one of the fastest-growing malignancies worldwide over the past two decades [1–3]. More than 95% of thyroid carcinomas derive from follicular epithelial cells, and up to 90% of all cases are papillary thyroid cancer (PTC) [4,5]. PTCs usually grow slowly and in an indolent fashion, and their association with lymph node metastasis varies from 30% to 90% of cases [6,7]. Most thyroid carcinomas can be successfully treated with surgical resection and radiometabolic therapy, but a subset of them will progress to refractory/metastatic disease. A role of primary importance in the aggressive behavior of solid and hematological neoplasms has long been identified in the transformation of the tumor microenvironment into an angiogenic microenvironment [8–10]. In fact, during tumor growth and progression, angiogenesis represents a biological process uncontrolled and unlimited in time; the angiogenic switch, characterized by the formation of new vessels (i.e., the transition from the avascular to the vascular phase), induces tumor cell proliferation, local invasion, and hematogenous metastasis [8,9,11]. Identification of tumor biomarkers that might predict disease progression is a medical need. Biomarkers based on genes that appear up- or down-regulated in thyroid cancers have shown poor predictive value and cannot distinguish benign from neoplastic nodules [12]. Moreover, traditional tissue biopsies are somewhat invasive, create discomfort to the patients, and are burdened by contamination from normal tissue and sampling errors [13].

Another area where biomarkers are lacking is the identification of disease persistence after surgery/medical therapy and the ability to distinguish between complete response after treatment or recurrence of disease [13].

Angiogenesis is an essential event for the progression of solid tumors and is promoted by angiogenic cytokines released in the tumor microenvironment by tumor and stromal cells, and can also be found and measured out with a serum assay in terms of circulating angiogenic factors [14]. This is a noninvasive, inexpensive, and safe test that can be potentially used in screening, diagnosis, and follow-up of thyroid cancer patients. Here, we will review the role of angiogenesis in thyroid cancer progression, spread, and metastasis. Moreover, the potential role of proangiogenic cytokines for risk stratification of patients with thyroid cancer will be addressed, as well as the individuation of angiogenesis as a potential therapeutic target.

2. The Thyroid Cancer Microenvironment

Over the last 20 years, the role of the microenvironment in tumorigenesis of thyroid cancer has been well-defined [15]. The components of the thyroid cancer microenvironment (stromal cells, ST, and extracellular matrix components (ECM)) surround and support cancer cells, interacting with them by direct cell-cell and cell-extracellular matrix components interaction. Moreover, a plethora of cytokines and growth factors are produced and released in the cancer microenvironment by cancer cells as well as by ST [16]. It has been demonstrated that cancer-associated fibroblasts (CAFs) surround the tumor cells and play a role in tumor initiation and promotion, tumor cell growth, spreading, and metastasization [17]. Moreover, CAFs are involved in inflammation, metabolism, drug response, and immune surveillance [17]. There is evidence that the expression of CAF-related proteins in stromal and cancer cells varies on the basis of histologic subtype of thyroid carcinomas, $BRAF^{V600E}$ mutation, and subtype of stroma, and an association has been reported between CAF-related proteins and poor survival [18]. It has also been demonstrated that CAFs are involved in the lymphatic spread of thyroid cancers [19], and that, in poorly differentiated thyroid cancer driven by $BRAF^{V600E}$ mutations and loss of Pten, there is a close association between CAF infiltration and collagen I deposition in the tumor microenvironment [20]. Moreover, CAFs produce and release many angiogenic cytokines that contribute to the angiogenic process in the tumor microenvironment [21].

Tumor-associated macrophages (TAMs) are another pivotal component of the thyroid tumor microenvironment associated with tumor cell growth, spread, and poor prognosis [22,23]. In the tumor microenvironment, TAMs contribute to the anti-inflammatory status because of their high expression of interleukin-10 (IL-10) and mannose receptor (MR, CD206), and low expression of IL-12 [24,25]. It has been shown that TAMs present an M2-like activated status, differently from the M1-like circulating macrophages [26,27]. TAMs contribute to angiogenesis of tumors with an increased production of proangiogenic factors, such as vascular endothelial growth factor (VEGF), platelet derived growth factor (PDGF), and basic fibroblast growth factor (bFGF), and produce a high amount of matrix metalloproteases (MMPs), which are responsible for ECM remodeling and facilitate tumor cells spread and invasion [28,29]. The relationship between positive tryptase mast cell (MCs) infiltration and thyroid cancer invasiveness or extrathyroidal extension has been demonstrated. A significantly more abundant presence and distribution of MCs in the intratumoral and peritumoral areas of thyroid cancer has also been shown with respect to adenoma [30,31]. MCs also produce a broad spectrum of chemokines (CXCL8/IL-8, CCL25/TECK, CXCL10/IP-10, CXCL1/GRO-α), interleukins (IL-6), and other molecules (TNF-α) that are involved in the epithelial-to-mesenchymal transition (EMT) activation of thyroid cancer cells [32,33]. Moreover, MCs recruited by several tumor-derived chemotactic factors, such as stem cell factor, VEGF, chemokines, and cytokines, histologically are localized close to epithelia, fibroblasts, and blood and lymphatic vessels and are involved in wound healing, angiogenesis, and lymphangiogenesis [32–34]. Neutrophils are recruited by thyroid cancer cells by releasing CXCL8/IL-8 and granulocyte colony-stimulating factor [35]. In the tumor microenvironment, neutrophils produce and release angiogenic cytokines (onconstatin-M, VEGF-A) and their granule proteins (elastase), which induce cancer cell proliferation, invasiveness, and angiogenesis [36–38]. Our group's complete gene expression profile study demonstrated that the microenvironment components surrounding the thyroid cancer cells express a genomic profile different from that of normal ST [39]. The results of this study indicate that interactions between tumor cells and ST induce in the ST the modulation of genes involved in the control of apoptosis, metabolism, cell movement, cell response to hypoxia, and cell proliferation [39].

2.1. Angiogenesis in Thyroid Cancer

Neovascularization in the cancer microenvironment is a multistep process that is necessary during the progression of solid and hematologic tumors [8,9]. It is a complex and heterogeneous process that includes three different mechanisms: (i) angiogenesis, the sprouting of newly formed vessels from mature preexisting ones; (ii) vasculogenesis, the formation of neovessels starting from endothelial precursor cells, namely hemangioblasts; and (iii) vasculogenic mimicry, the ability of tumor cells or other non-endothelial cells to complete the neovessel wall or to form a complete capillary network without vascular endothelial cells [40,41]. Moreover, tumor-related neovessel formation occurs mainly through sprouting of new capillary vessels out of preexisting ones (angiogenesis), the longitudinal splitting of existing vasculature into two functional vessels (intussusceptive angiogenesis) and the loop-shape expansion of the vessel (looping angiogenesis) involved mainly in wound healing [42–44]. Increased vascularity in the thyroid can occur in hyperplastic goiter, Graves' disease, and cancer [45]. As in other solid and hematologic tumors, the microvessel density (MVD) has been shown to correlate with disease-free survival in thyroid cancers, particularly in PTC and in follicular thyroid carcinoma (FTC) [45–47]. Differences have been demonstrated among tumor types in the patterns of spread and metastasis, probably due to the influence of tumor metastasis route by phenotype, angiogenic or lymphangiogenic, determining a more aggressive behavior [48,49]. Thyroid adenomas, microcarcinomas, PTC, FTC, undifferentiated thyroid carcinomas, and medullary thyroid carcinomas (MTCs) present very different behaviors, clinical outcomes, and metastatic routes (lymphatic or hematic) [48,50]. These differences correlate with different angiogenic regulators released (stimulators or inhibitors), the different expression of receptors, and different extracellular matrix composition in the tumor microenvironment [50].

In thyroid tumors, angiogenesis is activated and maintained by the modulation of the genes involved in angiogenesis and response to hypoxia (HIF1A, TUFT1, BHLHB2), cell survival (RIPK5), proliferation (PTGS2, DUSP5), apoptosis (ZFP36L1, IER3), metabolism (SLCA2A3), cell organization (RAB7B) and protein degradation (SKP1, KLK-4) in the ST surrounding the tumor cells [39]. These alterations are induced and stabilized in the components of the microenvironment through the reciprocal positive and negative interactions between tumor cells and ST (endothelial cells, fibroblasts, macrophages, mast cells) and are mediated by an array of cytokines, receptors, and adhesion molecules [39,51]. Moreover, the communication between cancer cells, ST, and the various stromal cells is mediated by the release of exosomes by the thyroid tumor cells, which contribute to tumor progression, angiogenesis, and metastasis [52].

Evidence indicates that there is a dysregulation of miRNA in thyroid cancer that influences the hallmarks of cancer, including proliferative signaling, evading growth suppressors, resisting cell death, inducing angiogenesis, activating invasion and metastasis, and acquiring the epithelial-mesenchymal transition phenotype [53]. A role in modulating angiogenesis is played by the thyroid hormone (L-thyroxine, T4; 3,5,3′-triiodo-L-thyronine, T3) that represents a valid contributor to this process in thyroid cancers [54]. Thyroid hormone acts by binding the hormone receptor site on $\alpha v\beta 3$ integrin and then modulating angiogenic cytokine (VEGFR and bFGFR) release via integrin activation and signaling in blood vessel cells [47,55]. This modulation is also mediated by hypoxia-inducible factor-alpha (HIF-1α), a transcription factor whose stabilization in cells is regulated by thyroid hormone via $\alpha v\beta 3$ [56,57]. Thyroid-stimulating hormone (TSH), the glycoprotein hormone stimulating the number, size, and activity of thyrocytes as well as the synthesis of thyroid hormone, also contributes to angiogenesis stimulation [40,58,59]. TSH enhances angiogenesis and macrophage recruitment into the thyroid tumor microenvironment and then tumor cell growth through VEGF mRNA and protein induction via the protein kinase C pathway [60,61]. Iodine deprivation causes reactive oxygen species (ROS) production, stabilization of HIF-1α and VEGF release through the activation of signals in the tumor thyrocytes that induce microvascular expansion to facilitate enhanced delivery of iodide [62,63]. Iodine deficiency induces VEGF-A expression by increasing phosphorylation of ribosomal S6 kinase (p70S6K), mediated by mammalian target of rapamycin (mTOR); the latter acts as a positive regulator and AMP-activated protein kinase, in turn stimulating thyroid microvascular activation [64].

2.2. Angiogenic Factors

VEGF is a member of a family of six structurally related proteins, namely, VEGF-A, -B, -C, -D, -E (viral factor), and PDGF; these act by interacting with their relative receptors, which are differentially expressed in various cell types [41,65].The VEGF receptors are differentially implicated in angiogenesis stimulation (VEGF-A, -E/VEGFR-2-neuropilin (NRP)-1, -2), or lymphangiogenesis (VEGF-C, -D/VEGFR-2, -3) [41,66,67]. On the other hand, VEGF also acts on cell types different from vascular cells, modulating various biological activities and primarily tumor cell growth, spread, invasiveness, and drug resistance [68–70].

Our group demonstrated that, as by tumor cells, VEGF is also produced by all the cellular components of the tumor microenvironment and acts via autocrine and paracrine loops to carry out its activity [71,72]. In cancer cells and ST, VEGF expression is modulated by several pathways, including metabolic factor-induced pathways, such as hypoxia and hypoglycemia via ROS production [62,63,73]; lysophosphatidic acid (LPA), via activation of c-Jun N-terminal kinase (JNK) and nuclear factor kappa-light-chain-enhancer of activated B cells (NF-κB) [74]; PI3K/Akt signaling pathway [75]; and transcription factors, such as activator protein-1 (AP-1), NF-κB, and stimulatory protein-1 (SP-1) [76–78]. In thyroid carcinomas, VEGF over-expression has been correlated with increased growth, progression, invasiveness, spread, and metastasis of thyroid cancer cells [79–81]. A consistent increase in VEGF, VEGF-C, and angiopoietin-2 and their tyrosine kinase receptors VEGFR2, VEGFR3, and TEK receptor tyrosine kinase have been demonstrated in thyroid cancer versus normal thyroid tissues, and a strong correlation has been found between this overexpression and tumor size [50]. Moreover, the same authors showed that in the lymph node of metastatic thyroid tumors, there is an increase of VEGF-C expression and, at the same time, a reduced expression of TSP-1 near VEGF and angiopoietin-2 increased production, indicating the hematogenous metastasis capability of thyroid malignancies [50].

bFGF is an angiogenic growth factor that, by interaction with FGF receptor (high-affinity tyrosine kinase (TK) receptor) and with low-affinity heparan sulphate proteoglycans (co-receptors), induces activation, proliferation, chemotaxis, protease production, and vessel formation in endothelial cells [82,83]. In this way, it induces angiogenesis and modulates neovascularization during physiological (wound healing, inflammation) and pathological (atherosclerosis, cancer) conditions [84]. Several studies demonstrated that in thyroid tumors, the expression of bFGF and FGFR are both increased and play a role in tumor progression and angiogenesis [85–88]. As in other solid and hematologic cancers, in thyroid tumors bFGF acts as an angiogenic factor independently in the presence of other factors, such as VEGF, and directly stimulates endothelial and tumor cell growth [45].

MMPs are zinc-endopeptidases of the protease superfamily with specific proteolytic activity against a broad range of substrates located on the ECM [89,90]. MMPs are produced by thyroid tumor and microenvironment stromal cells and promote tumor growth, invasion, migration, and apoptosis inhibition. Moreover, they exert angiogenesis stimulation because the degradation of ECM causes the release of angiogenic factors stored in attachment with heparan sulphate [89,90]. The promotion of tumor growth is primarily related to MMP-2 and MMP-9 through activation of TGF-β [91]. Another growth factor, namely epidermal growth factor (EGF), is involved in promoting cell invasion and angiogenesis in thyroid carcinoma. It acts as a regulator of the production of MMP-9 through focal adhesion kinase (FAK) phosphorylation [92]. Natural inhibitors of MMPs are the tissue inhibitors of metalloproteinases (TIMPs), produced and released in the tumor microenvironment [93]. Published data from our group indicate that the MMPs' proangiogenic and pro-tumoral activities are related to the balance of MMPs and TIMPS in the microenvironment, and that the switch toward an invasive phenotype is mainly due to increased MMP production and release, and not to the reduction of TIMPs (Figure 1) [94,95].

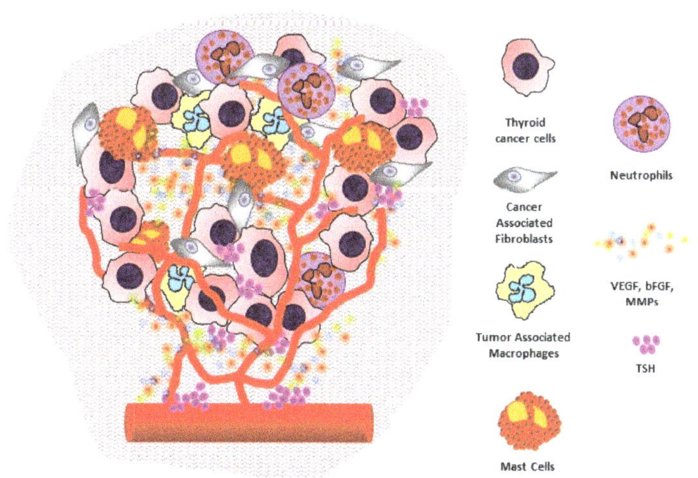

Figure 1. The angiogenic microenvironment of thyroid cancer: interactions between cancer cells, stromal cells, and inflammatory cells to promote angiogenesis and tumor progression.

3. Angiogenesis and Prognosis

Increased MVD, lymphatic vascular density (LVD), and expression of angiogenic and lymphangiogenic factors have been demonstrated in non-neoplastic (multinodular goiter, toxic multinodular goiter, Graves' hyperplasia) and neoplastic conditions (follicular adenoma, papillary thyroid carcinoma, incidental papillary microcarcinoma, follicular carcinoma, and medullary carcinoma) [48,96]. No clear relationship between MVD measurement and thyroid pathology has been demonstrated. In fact, de la Torre et al. showed that MVD is decreased in all thyroid diseases, and LVD is increased in papillary thyroid carcinoma and incidental papillary microcarcinoma [48]. A second study found an increased MVD in PTC compared to normal controls [96]. Other studies demonstrated a high MVD in differentiated thyroid cancers (DTCs) compared to poorly differentiated thyroid cancers and other thyroid tissue samples [97–99]. More consistent results have been obtained with the evaluation of VEGF. Increased distribution and intensity of VEGF-A and VEGF-C have been demonstrated in thyroid cancers compared to normal samples and autoimmune and inflammatory diseases [48,96,98,99]. However, this increased expression was not indicative of multifocal disease, distant metastases at diagnosis, or increased tumor size [48].

Examining angiogenic processes connecting the thyroid cancer cell to its microenvironment could improve many thyroid cancer management steps. The first could be identifying cytologically indeterminate nodules prone to surgical treatment, thus reducing diagnostic thyroidectomies. The second could be the efficient differentiation between aggressive and indolent DTC so that the treatment extension and approach and the follow-up modalities could be correctly adapted. An improvement to correctly identify thyroid cancer in nodules with indeterminate cytology, ruling in or out malignancy, and selecting patients for surveillance, conservative or radical surgery, was the introduction of gene classifiers to be performed on the fine needle aspiration specimen (or even micro-biopsies or surgical specimens) [100–105]. BRAF mutations, and RET-PTC, RAS and PAX8-PPARG, are the most studied factors in this field. The complete genomics of thyroid cancer subtypes will be unveiled, but caution should be exercised in the interpretation and application of the many variants and mutations that are being discovered, because many of them can also be found in benign lesions; there are also thyroid cancers that show none of the known genetic alterations [106]. BRAF mutational status, along with membranous and nuclear galectin-3, HBME-1, CK19, and estrogen receptor beta, had been associated with DTC with aggressive behavior [107]. $BRAF^{V600E}$ mutated microcarcinomas are associated with adverse prognostic factors, whereas BRAF wild-type ones are associated with indolent behavior and a low probability of recurrence [108]. $BRAF^{V600E}$ is associated with tall cell variant PTC, along with mutations of COL5A1, COL1A1, COL10A1, COL11A1, CCL20, and CXCL5 [109]. BRAF is the most prevalent genetic alteration in radioiodine refractory metastatic thyroid cancer patients. BRAF mutation seems to positively influence the median progression-free survival (PFS) in radioiodine refractory patients treated with tyrosine kinase inhibitor, while having a negative prognostic impact in radioiodine-sensitive PTC patients [110]. $BRAF^{V600E}$ mutation is associated with central neck nodal metastases, but concerns were raised for its utility as a stand-alone marker in this field. Indeed, its use along with the analysis of miR-146b-3p, miR-146b-5p, and miR-222 was found to be prognostic of central neck nodal metastases preoperatively [111]. miRNA classifiers are indeed another option to identify and stratify thyroid cancer [53,112,113]. BRAF ^{V600E} appears to identify a subgroup of solitary intraglandular PTC larger than 2 cm and smaller than 4 cm, with a high risk of recurrence, for which a more aggressive treatment should be recommended [114]. There is evidence that $BRAF^{V600E}$ reduces TSP-1 expression in anaplastic thyroid cancer, and this appears to be linked to enhanced proliferation, adherence to collagen, migration, and invasion of the neoplastic thyroid cell. Arguably, this is due to the activation of pericytes in the microenvironment of thyroid cancer, which contributes to stabilizing new vessels through the secretion of PDGRFbeta, VEGF, and other factors [115–117].

VEGF-C and angiopoietin-2, together with their tyrosine kinase receptors KDR, Flt-4, and TEK, were found to be increasingly expressed in thyroid cancers, especially in the transition from a prevascular to vascular phase, and this was also correlated to the tumor size, nodal invasion, and, along with a reduced expression of TSP-1, to distant metastases [50]. It is known that VEGF overexpression correlates with increased microvascular density and, similarly, a reduced expression of TSP-1 is associated with the increased microvascular count [40]. Serum VEGF levels were significantly higher in patients with metastatic thyroid cancer than in healthy subjects and patients in remission [118]. Conversely, VEGF-D serum levels were decreased in patients with metastatic thyroid cancer, and this should be linked to other factors produced by the cancer cell that inhibits the usual production from other tissues of VEGF-D [119]. Moreover, anaplastic tumors show augmented expression of VEGF [45]. The evidence of high VEGF mRNA expression and of high FAL1 expression and cyclin D1 protein levels also shows how angiogenic processes are driven along with enhanced cell proliferation in papillary thyroid cancer [120,121]. In the context of prognostic examinations for patients affected by radioiodine refractory metastatic thyroid cancer, integrin $\alpha v\beta 3$ is essential for tumor angiogenesis, and its expression is high on the surface of activated endothelial cells in newly formed blood vessels. It has been used to trace, using 99mTc-3PRGD2 imaging, metastases that are highly neovascularized. This new angiogenesis imaging modality can provide a new tool to monitor the efficacy of antiangiogenetic therapy [122]. TSH stimulation exerts a regulatory effect on VEGF production from thyroid cancer, probably through the interaction of tissues other than the thyroid itself, and this might have prognostic and therapeutic applications, exploiting the effects of recombinant human TSH administration [60,118,123,124]. The great interest in angiogenesis for prognostic purposes in cancer appears to be tightly connected to the need for circulating markers; this is even true for thyroid cancers, thus avoiding biopsies and other procedures to stratify patients. A possible application for this aim is the assay of miRNA in exosomes, especially miR-21-5p [52,125], which is a decisive proangiogenic factor produced by thyroid cancer cells. VEGF-A and PDGF-BB have been recently indicated as potential circulating biomarkers of PTC treatment [94].

MTC lesions show overexpression of VEGF-A, VEGFR-1, and VEGFR-2 [126], but their prognostic significance is uncertain, although VEGFR-2 and EGFR seem to be related to metastasis [127]. MTC originates from embryologically different tissue, and its management is different from that of DTC. HIF-1α has been associated with an adverse prognosis for MTC [128]. HIF1-1α expression is induced by hypoxia or aberrant signaling and stimulates the expression of VEGF and angiogenesis.

Moreover, MTC shows PSMA expression in the neovasculature, and microvessels showing positivity for PSMA are prognostically favorable. PSMA may become a target for imaging and peptide radioligand therapy [129]. It has been shown that collagen deposition and cross-linking and fibroblast presence in the thyroid cancer microenvironment play a prognostic role, indicating an advanced or aggressive disease, and are driven by PTEN loss BRAF^{V600E} [20,130–133]. The overexpression of MMPs leads to increased VEGF and FGF secretion, related to tumor growth and invasiveness [134,135]. The ratio of MMP-2 to TIMP-2 expression is a prognostic factor for surgically treated MTC, and both of these metalloproteinases play a role in PTC [136–138]. MMP-9 expression is upregulated in PTC and might be a prognostic indicator for more advanced-stage cancer [139–142]. The prognostic role of other components of the extracellular matrix of thyroid cancer tangentially involved in angiogenetic processes, such as macrophages and T lymphocytes, is yet to be clarified [15].

4. Preclinical and Clinical Evidence for Antiangiogenic Therapy

Therapeutic options for thyroid cancers are variable following clinical-pathological staging. Localized and low-risk DTC benefit from surgical treatment (total thyroidectomy) followed by thyroid hormone suppression and adjuvant thyroid ablative therapy with radioactive iodine (RAI) treatment. This management could be applied to 85% of papillary and follicular subtypes [143,144].

In metastatic disease, patients are usually managed with a combination of surgery and RAI treatment. The prognosis depends on metastasis location (if it is suitable for a complete surgical resection) and post-operative radioiodine uptake in the tumor tissue. In the same setting of total thyroidectomy, indeed, patients could be submitted to therapeutic central neck dissection or lateral neck dissection in case of preoperative or intraoperative inspection of lymph nodes that are deemed to be pathologic [145]. However, some tumors are refractory to T4-mediated TSH suppression as well as RAI therapy. Approximately two-thirds of these patients may develop distant metastases resulting in much poorer overall survival rate and a poor prognosis [143,144].

In recent years, the scientific community's effort has been focused on the study of several molecular pathways involved in cancer development. Proliferation pathways, cell cycle control pathways, and angiogenesis processes have been largely evaluated, allowing the identification of mediators that may be useful targets for new anticancer treatments [146]. Multiple tyrosine kinase inhibitors (TKIs) have been identified, and their efficacy on different molecular pathways has been the primary end point of several studies in search of further treatment options for recurrent/metastatic thyroid cancer.

Vandetanib was the first TKI approved by the Food and Drug Administration (FDA) for the treatment of patients with symptomatic, unresectable, locally advanced, or metastatic MTC in the USA (2011) and Europe (2013). This drug acts on EGF, RET, VEGF, and VEGF receptors, leading to a downregulation of proliferative, angiogenic pathways and mediation on apoptosis pathways. The effects have been demonstrated in two phase 2 clinical trials and one phase 3 clinical trial (ZETA trial) in which patients with advanced unresectable MTC were blindly randomized to receive vandetanib at 300 mg daily or placebo [147].

This study demonstrated a significantly longer median PFS duration compared to the placebo group, with a partial response in 44% of cases. A significant difference in the objective response rates and disease control rates as well as in the biochemical response was also discussed. Moreover, vandetanib has also been tested in RAI-refractory DTC patients. A randomized, double-blinded, placebo-controlled phase 2 clinical trial evaluated the effect of this TKI, showing a statistically significant increase in the PFS of patients treated with vandetanib compared to the placebo group [143,148,149].

The second TKI, approved by the FDA in 2012 for the management of advanced and symptomatic MTC, was cabozantinib. This is a TKI with function on the hepatocyte growth factor receptor, RET, and VEGF2 receptors, leading to downregulation or inhibition of angiogenic, proliferative, and apoptotic pathways.

A phase 3 study (EXAM study) evaluated the effect of cabozantinib, showing a statistically significant longer median of PFS in patients treated with the drug (140 mg per day) with respect to those treated with placebo (11.2 versus 4.0 months). In this study, cabozantinib was associated with significant but manageable toxicity [143,149,150].

Sherman et al. published the results of an exploratory analysis of phase 3 trial data evaluating the influence of rearranged during transfection (RET) and RAS (HRAS, KRAS, and NRAS) mutations on cabozantinib clinical activity. They concluded that cabozantinib provides the most significant clinical benefit to patients with MTC who have RET M918T or RAS mutations [151].

Comparing vandetanib with cabozantinib, it seems that vandetanib is more tolerable than cabozantinib, making it the drug of choice for fragile and older patients. This is probably due to differences in patient selection for the two studies in phase 3. In the ZETA study, non-progressive but symptomatic patients were also studied, while the EXAM study enrolled only progressive cases, with adverse events due to cabozantinib higher than the adverse events observed in the ZETA trial. Cabozantinib has stronger antiangiogenic effects than vandetanib; therefore it could be strongly considered in cases of rapid MTC progression.

Cabozantinib and vandetanib have been tested on DTC, without approval [143,149].

In November 2013, sorafenib was the first multiple TKI to be approved by the FDA for the treatment of progressive metastatic DTC refractory to RAI treatment.

It has a documented efficacy in inhibiting all RAF kinases with a specific function on VEGF receptors 1–3, PDGFRB, and RET, which confers to sorafenib proapoptotic propriety and angiogenic effect fitting a molecular rationale for the treatment of all histological subtypes of thyroid cancer. Indeed, some studies have analyzed the use of Sorafenib in patients with metastatic thyroid cancer not suitable for curative surgery, RAI, or radiotherapy with a dose of 400 mg twice a day; these studies report partial response in 32% of cases, stable disease beyond six months, and a toxicity profile similar to that observed in previous studies and managed with dose delay or reduction [152]. Brose et al. investigated sorafenib in a multicenter, randomized, double-blind, placebo-controlled, phase 3 trial (DECISION). Sorafenib was used with the same administration in patients with RAI-refractory, locally advanced, or metastatic DTC that had progressed within the previous 14 months. The results showed how significantly sorafenib improved PFS compared to placebo [153].

Another TKI, lenvatinib, was approved in February 2015 in many countries to treat advanced DTC refractory to RAI. This is a multitargeted TKI of the VEGFRs 1, 2, and 3, FGFRs 1 through 4, PDGFR α, RET, and KIT signaling networks. In a phase 1 study, lenvatinib was associated with a partial response in thyroid cancer as well as melanoma, endometrial, and renal cancers. Subsequently, Sherman et al. performed a phase 2 study involving patients with DTC refractory to RAI, analyzing clinical activity and efficacy of levantinib [154]. Further, a phase 3, randomized, double-blind, multicenter study involving patients with progressive thyroid cancer refractory to iodine-131 was performed (SELECT trial). Schlumberger et al. randomized 261 patients to receive lenvatinib (at a daily dose of 24 mg per day in 28-day cycles) and 131 patients to receive placebo, showing PFS benefit and a high response rate associated with lenvatinib compared to placebo [155]. In an exploratory analysis, Wirth et al. examined treatment-emergent hypertension and its relationship with lenvatinib efficacy and safety in SELECT. They concluded that TE-HTN was significantly correlated with improved outcomes in patients with radioiodine-refractory DTC, indicating that hypertension may be predictive of lenvatinib efficacy in this population [156].

Based on these studies, sorafenib and lenvatinib are now recommended by the National Comprehensive Cancer Network to treat progressive, RAI-refractory DTC [157].

A multicenter phase II study investigated the efficacy and safety of dovitinib in advanced or RAI refractory thyroid cancer. This is another oral TKI with a documented activity on VEGFR, PDGFR, and RET pathways and a unique feature of inhibiting FGFRs. After a phase I study, in which the antitumor activity of dovitinib was evaluated on metastatic renal cell carcinoma [158], Indeed, Lim et al. tested dovitinib orally 500 mg once daily for five consecutive days followed by a 2-day rest every week in patients with PTC, FTC, and MTC with refractory disease. The study showed that dovitinib has modest activity with manageable toxicity with an overall response rate of 20.5% and a disease control rate of 69.1% compared to a relatively short PFS [144].

Another important multitarget tyrosine kinase inhibitor, anlotinib, has been tested for advanced refractory solid tumors. It has a referred action on tumor angiogenesis and growth with a proved effective target on VEGF and their receptors with an inhibition capacity 500 times stronger than sorafenib. Anlotinib also acts on tumor progression and cell proliferation by inhibiting PDGFR alfa/beta, c-Kit, Ret, Aurora-B, c-FMS, and discoidin domain receptor 1 and carrying mutations in PDGFR alfa, c-Kit, Met, and EGFR. In a phase I, open-label study on patients with various types of solid tumor including MTC, Sun et al. showed that at a dose of 12 mg once daily on the 2/1 schedule, anlotinib had a toxicity profile in agreement with that reported for sorafenib and a substantial, broad-spectrum antitumor potential [146]. Subsequently, in a phase II clinical trial, the antitumor activity of anlotinib in patients with advanced or metastatic MTC was confirmed, also demonstrating a manageable adverse event profile [159].

A TKI with selective action on VEGFR1-3, axitinib, has been tested in patients with different types of thyroid cancers. Initially approved for the treatment of renal cell carcinoma, it has been tested in two phase 2 clinical trials for thyroid cancers with a recommended dose of 5 mg twice daily. Both studies described a clinical benefit in refractory and progressive thyroid cancer, tolerability, and a safety profile for axitinib as first-line therapy [160,161].

Pazopanib is another antiangiogenic TKI acting on VEGFR1-3, FGF1/2, PDGF, KIT, and RET receptors. After being approved for renal cancers, it has been tested (at a dose of 800 mg daily) in a phase II clinical trial in patients with metastatic, rapidly progressive, radioiodine-refractory DTC. Another phase II clinical trial tested the antitumor activity on MTC and anaplastic thyroid cancer [162–164].

Recently, another phase II clinical trial of pazopanib in RAI refractory DTC patients with progressive disease confirmed the clinical activity and manageable toxicities of the drug, examining in parallel biomarkers that might precede therapeutic response. However, no predictive biomarkers were found to facilitate a robust early identification of patients likely to respond to pazopanib therapy [165].

Sunitinib is an antiangiogenic TKI able to inhibit the VEGF1–3, PDGF, KIT, and RET receptors. As with other TKIs, it was first approved for other cancers such as renal cell carcinoma and pancreatic neuroendocrine carcinoma and then analyzed for RAI refractory DTC and MTC with FDG-PET-avid disease. Three phase 2 clinical trials reported on sunitinib administered at 37.5 mg daily on a continuous basis. All studies concluded that sunitinib exhibits significant anti-tumor activity in patients with advanced DTC and MTC, with some common adverse events such as fatigue, diarrhea, hand-foot syndrome, neutropenia, and hypertension [166–168].

The knowledge of thyroid tumor behavior, with its ability to produce cytokines and chemokines and consequently promote tumorigenesis, has guided the scientific community for many years in identifying the best TKI. This has led to the testing and approval of different therapeutic options for advanced thyroid tumors that previously had no possibility of treatment (Table 1).

Recently, the development and approval of immunotherapeutics for cancer and the identification of immune checkpoint inhibitors have modified the treatment landscape for many malignancies, taking advantage of the capacity of restoring the state of immunosurveillance on some tumors that were able to evade it [169,170].

Starting from the evidence of increased frequency of aggressive regulatory T cells and the correlation between expression of PD-1 ligand and the worse prognosis for recurrent PTC, the immune system components have been largely studied as therapeutic targets useful in the treatment of thyroid cancer. These are the new fields to be explored in the analysis of target therapy [169].

Table 1. Drugs studied in treatment of thyroid cancer: Tyrosine kinase inhibitors and their multitarget activity.

Drugs	Mechanism of Action: Target(s)	Dose	Study Phase	Tested or Approved for Thyroid Cancer Treatment
Vandetanib	-EGF-R -RET -VEGF-R	300 mg daily	Phase III clinical trial (ZETA trial) [147]	Treatment of patients with symptomatic, unresectable, locally advanced or metastatic MTC
Cabozantinib	-MET -RET -C-Kit -VEGF-R2	140 mg per day	Phase III clinical trial (EXAM trial) [150]	Management of advanced and symptomatic MTC
Sorafenib	-BRAF -VEGF-R1 -VEGF-R3 -PDGF-R -C-Kit -RET	400 mg twice a day	Phase III clinical trial (DECISION trial) [153]	Treatment of progressive metastatic DTC refractory to RAI treatment.
Lenvatinib	-VEGF-R1 -VEGF-R2 -VEGF-R3 -FGF-R1 -FGF-R4 -PDGF-Rα -RET -C-Kit	24 mg once daily	Phase III clinical trial (SELECT trial) [155]	Treatment of advanced DTC refractory to RAI
Dovitinib	-VEGF-R -PDGF-R -RET -FGF-R	500 mg once daily for five consecutive days followed by a 2-day rest every week	Phase II clinical trial [144]	Treatment of advanced or RAI refractory thyroid cancer (PTC, FTC, and MTC)
Anlotinib	-PDGF-R α/β -C-Kit -RET -AURORA-B -C-FMS -DDR1 (DISCOIDIN DOMAIN RECEPTOR 1) -MET -EGF-R	12 mg once daily	Phase II clinical trial [159]	Treatment of advanced refractory solid tumors (including MTC)
Axitinib	-VEGF-R1 -VEGF-R3	5 mg twice daily	Phase II clinical trial [161]	Treatment of different types of thyroid cancers
Pazopanib	-VEGF-R1 -VEGF-R3 -FGF-R1/2 -PDGF-R -C-Kit -RET	800 mg daily	Phase II clinical trials [162–164]	Treatment of different types of thyroid cancers (RAI refractory DTC, MTC, and anaplastic thyroid cancer)
Sunitinib	-VEGF-R1 -VEGF-R3 -PDGF-R -C-Kit -RET	37.5 mg daily	Phase II clinical trials [166–168]	Treatment of RAI refractory DTC and MTC with FDG-PET-avid disease

5. Conclusions

The study of several molecular pathways and the tumor microenvironment involved in cancer development has recently guided the scientific community's effort to clarify tumor behavior. Indeed, proliferation pathways, cell cycle control pathways, and the processes of angiogenesis have been largely evaluated, providing new tools useful in screening, diagnosis, and follow-up of thyroid cancer and allowing the identification of mediators that may be potential targets for new anticancer treatments.

VEGF and its receptors appear to be the major players in the angiogenesis process of thyroid tumors. There have been numerous efforts toward understanding the signaling mechanisms driven by BRAF^{V600E} mutation and loss of Pten as a contribution to the angiogenic process in the thyroid tumor microenvironment. For these reasons, antiangiogenic therapy is used in all histological subtypes of thyroid cancer. In addition, to date, a number of inhibitors of the RAS, RAF and MEK pathways and other types of molecular target therapy have been shown to be effective in vitro and require clinical confirmation.

The tumor microenvironment presents numerous barriers that prevent access to chemotherapies, not only rendering them often ineffective but also potentially increasing the tumor cells' aggressiveness.

Prognostic indicators are based on dynamic interactions between multiple types of cells, especially those with immune functions belonging to the tumor microenvironment.

Further studies are needed to increase knowledge of the tumor microenvironment and to evaluate its changes and remodeling as thyroid cancer progresses.

Additionally, other studies should aim to determine the role of the immune system in thyroid cancer.

Author Contributions: Conceptualization, A.M., L.I.S., A.P., R.R. and M.T.; writing—original draft preparation, A.M., L.I.S. and A.P.; writing—review and editing, A.G., A.V., R.R. and M.T.; methodology, A.M., L.I.S., A.P., A.M., G.D.M., F.P.P., R.R. and M.T.; resources, A.M., G.D.M. and F.P.P.; validation, A.G., A.V., R.R. and M.T.; supervision, A.G., A.V., R.R. and M.T. All authors have read and agreed to the published version of the manuscript.

Funding: This research received no external funding.

Conflicts of Interest: The authors declare no conflict of interest.

References

1. Rahib, L.; Smith, B.D.; Aizenberg, R.; Rosenzweig, A.B.; Fleshman, J.M.; Matrisian, L.M. Projecting cancer incidence and deaths to 2030: The unexpected burden of thyroid, liver, and pancreas cancers in the United States. *Cancer Res.* **2014**, *74*, 2913–2921. [CrossRef]
2. Li, M.; Maso, L.D.; Vaccarella, S. Global trends in thyroid cancer incidence and the impact of overdiagnosis. *Lancet Diabetes Endocrinol.* **2020**, *8*, 468–470. [CrossRef]
3. Howlader, N.; Noone, A.M.; Krapcho, M.; Miller, D.; Brest, A.; Yu, M.; Ruhl, J.; Tatalovich, Z.; Mariotto, A.; Lewis, D.R.; et al. *SEER Cancer Statistics Review, 1975–2016*; National Cancer Institute: Bethesda, MD, USA, April 2019. Available online: https://seer.cancer.gov/csr/1975_2016/ (accessed on 17 March 2021).
4. Ghossein, R. Problems and controversies in the histopathology of thyroid carcinomas of follicular cell origin. *Arch. Pathol. Lab. Med.* **2009**, *133*, 683–691. [CrossRef]
5. Fassnacht, M.; Kreissl, M.C.; Weismann, D.; Allolio, B. New targets and therapeutic approaches for endocrine malignancies. *Pharmacol. Ther.* **2009**, *123*, 117–141. [CrossRef]
6. Kitahara, C.M.; Sosa, J.A. The changing incidence of thyroid cancer. *Nat. Rev. Endocrinol.* **2016**, *12*, 646–653. [CrossRef]
7. Jensen, C.B.; Saucke, M.C.; Francis, D.O.; Voils, C.I.; Pitt, S.C. From Overdiagnosis to Overtreatment of Low-Risk Thyroid Cancer: A Thematic Analysis of Attitudes and Beliefs of Endocrinologists, Surgeons, and Patients. *Thyroid* **2020**, *30*, 696–703. [CrossRef] [PubMed]
8. Folkman, J. Tumor angiogenesis. In *The Molecular Basis of Cancer*; Mendelsohn, J., Howley, P., Liotta, L., Israel, M., Eds.; WB Saunders: Philadelphia, PA, USA, 1995; pp. 206–232.
9. Ribatti, D.; Vacca, A.; Dammacco, F. The Role of the Vascular Phase in Solid Tumor Growth: A Historical Review. *Neoplasia* **1999**, *1*, 293–302. [CrossRef]
10. Martin, T.A.; Ye, L.; Sanders, A.J.; Lane, J.; Jiang, W.G. Cancer invasion and metastasis: Molecular and cellular perspective. In *Metastatic Cancer Clinical and Biological Perspectives*; Landes Bioscienc: Austin, TX, USA, 2013; pp. 135–168.

11. Ribatti, D.; Nico, B.; Crivellato, E.; Roccaro, A.; Vacca, A. The history of the angiogenic switch concept. *Leukemia* **2006**, *21*, 44–52. [CrossRef] [PubMed]
12. Fan, Y.; Shi, L.; Liu, Q.; Dong, R.; Zhang, Q.; Yang, S.; Fan, Y.; Yang, H.; Wu, P.; Yu, J.; et al. Discovery and identification of potential biomarkers of papillary thyroid carcinoma. *Mol. Cancer* **2009**, *8*, 79. [CrossRef] [PubMed]
13. Haugen, B.R.; Alexander, E.K.; Bible, K.C.; Doherty, G.M.; Mandel, S.J.; Nikiforov, Y.E.; Pacini, F.; Randolph, G.W.; Sawka, A.M.; Schlumberger, M.; et al. 2015 American Thyroid Association Management Guidelines for Adult Patients with Thyroid Nodules and Differentiated Thyroid Cancer: The American Thyroid Association Guidelines Task Force on Thyroid Nodules and Differentiated Thyroid Cancer. *Thyroid* **2016**, *26*, 1–133. [CrossRef]
14. Clark, A.G.; Vignjevic, D.M. Modes of cancer cell invasion and the role of the microenvironment. *Curr. Opin. Cell Biol.* **2015**, *36*, 13–22. [CrossRef] [PubMed]
15. Macdonald, L.; Jenkins, J.; Purvis, G.; Lee, J.; Franco, A.T. The Thyroid Tumor Microenvironment: Potential Targets for Therapeutic Intervention and Prognostication. *Horm. Cancer* **2020**, *11*, 1–13. [CrossRef]
16. Turner, H.E.; Harris, A.L.; Melmed, S.; Wass, J.A.H. Angiogenesis in Endocrine Tumors. *Endocr. Rev.* **2003**, *24*, 600–632. [CrossRef]
17. Östman, A. Cancer-associated fibroblasts: Recent developments and emerging challenges. *Semin. Cancer Biol.* **2014**, *25*, 1–2. [CrossRef]
18. Sun, W.Y.; Jung, W.-H.; Koo, J.S. Expression of cancer-associated fibroblast-related proteins in thyroid papillary carcinoma. *Tumor Biol.* **2015**, *37*, 8197–8207. [CrossRef] [PubMed]
19. Cho, J.-G.; Byeon, H.K.; Oh, K.H.; Baek, S.-K.; Kwon, S.-Y.; Jung, K.-Y.; Woo, J.-S. Clinicopathological significance of cancer-associated fibroblasts in papillary thyroid carcinoma: A predictive marker of cervical lymph node metastasis. *Eur. Arch. Oto-Rhino-Laryngol.* **2018**, *275*, 2355–2361. [CrossRef]
20. Jolly, L.A.; Novitskiy, S.; Owens, P.; Massoll, N.; Cheng, N.; Fang, W.; Moses, H.L.; Franco, A. Fibroblast-Mediated Collagen Remodeling Within the Tumor Microenvironment Facilitates Progression of Thyroid Cancers Driven by $BRAF^{V600E}$ and Pten Loss. *Cancer Res.* **2016**, *76*, 1804–1813. [CrossRef]
21. Louault, K.; Li, R.-R.; Declerck, Y.A. Cancer-Associated Fibroblasts: Understanding Their Heterogeneity. *Cancers* **2020**, *12*, 3108. [CrossRef]
22. Crezee, T.; Rabold, K.; De Jong, L.; Jaeger, M.; Netea-Maier, R.T. Metabolic programming of tumor associated macrophages in the context of cancer treatment. *Ann. Transl. Med.* **2020**, *8*, 1028. [CrossRef]
23. Zhang, Q.-W.; Liu, L.; Gong, C.-Y.; Shi, H.-S.; Zeng, Y.-H.; Wang, X.-Z.; Zhao, Y.-W.; Wei, Y.-Q. Prognostic Significance of Tumor-Associated Macrophages in Solid Tumor: A Meta-Analysis of the Literature. *PLoS ONE* **2012**, *7*, e50946. [CrossRef]
24. Mantovani, A.; Marchesi, F.; Malesci, A.; Laghi, L.; Allavena, P. Tumour-associated macrophages as treatment targets in oncology. *Nat. Rev. Clin. Oncol.* **2017**, *14*, 399–416. [CrossRef]
25. Lewis, C.E.; Pollard, J.W. Distinct Role of Macrophages in Different Tumor Microenvironments. *Cancer Res.* **2006**, *66*, 605–612. [CrossRef] [PubMed]
26. Xue, J.; Schmidt, S.V.; Sander, J.; Draffehn, A.; Krebs, W.; Quester, I.; De Nardo, D.; Gohel, T.D.; Emde, M.; Schmidleithner, L.; et al. Transcriptome-based network analysis reveals a spectrum model of human macrophage activation. *Immunity* **2014**, *40*, 274–288. [CrossRef] [PubMed]
27. Murray, P.J.; Allen, J.E.; Biswas, S.K.; Fisher, E.A.; Gilroy, D.W.; Goerdt, S.; Gordon, S.; Hamilton, J.A.; Ivashkiv, L.B.; Lawrence, T.; et al. Macrophage activation and polarization: Nomenclature and experimental guidelines. *Immunity* **2014**, *41*, 14–20. [CrossRef] [PubMed]
28. Cheng, N.; Bai, X.; Shu, Y.; Ahmad, O.; Shen, P. Targeting tumor-associated macrophages as an antitumor strategy. *Biochem. Pharmacol.* **2021**, *183*, 114354. [CrossRef] [PubMed]
29. Ojalvo, L.S.; Whittaker, C.A.; Condeelis, J.S.; Pollard, J.W. Gene Expression Analysis of Macrophages That Facilitate Tumor Invasion Supports a Role for Wnt-Signaling in Mediating Their Activity in Primary Mammary Tumors. *J. Immunol.* **2009**, *184*, 702–712. [CrossRef]
30. Melillo, R.M.; Guarino, V.; Avilla, E.; Galdiero, M.R.; Liotti, F.; Prevete, N.; Rossi, F.W.; Basolo, F.; Ugolini, C.; De Paulis, A.; et al. Mast cells have a protumorigenic role in human thyroid cancer. *Oncogene* **2010**, *29*, 6203–6215. [CrossRef]
31. Proietti, A.; Ugolini, C.; Melillo, R.M.; Crisman, G.; Elisei, R.; Santoro, M.; Minuto, M.; Vitti, P.; Miccoli, P.; Basolo, F. Higher Intratumoral Expression of CD1a, Tryptase, and CD68 in a Follicular Variant of Papillary Thyroid Carcinoma Compared to Adenomas: Correlation with Clinical and Pathological Parameters. *Thyroid* **2011**, *21*, 1209–1215. [CrossRef]
32. Visciano, C.; Prevete, N.; Liotti, F.; Marone, G. Tumor-Associated Mast Cells in Thyroid Cancer. *Int. J. Endocrinol.* **2015**, *2015*, 705169. [CrossRef]
33. Visciano, C.; Liotti, F.; Prevete, N.; Cali', G.; Franco, R.; Collina, F.; De Paulis, A.; Marone, G.; Santoro, M.; Melillo, R.M. Mast cells induce epithelial-to-mesenchymal transition and stem cell features in human thyroid cancer cells through an IL-8–Akt–Slug pathway. *Oncogene* **2015**, *34*, 5175–5186. [CrossRef]
34. Carlini, M.J.; Dalurzo, M.C.L.; Lastiri, J.M.; Smith, D.E.; Vasallo, B.C.; Puricelli, L.I.; De Cidre, L.S.L. Mast cell phenotypes and microvessels in non–small cell lung cancer and its prognostic significance. *Hum. Pathol.* **2010**, *41*, 697–705. [CrossRef] [PubMed]
35. Galdiero, M.R.; Varricchi, G.; Loffredo, S.; Bellevicine, C.; Lansione, T.; Ferrara, A.L.; Iannone, R.; Di Somma, S.; Borriello, F.; Clery, E.; et al. Potential involvement of neutrophils in human thyroid cancer. *PLoS ONE* **2018**, *13*, e0199740. [CrossRef]

36. Jablonska, J.; Leschner, S.; Westphal, K.; Lienenklaus, S.; Weiss, S. Neutrophils responsive to endogenous IFN-β regulate tumor angiogenesis and growth in a mouse tumor model. *J. Clin. Investig.* **2010**, *120*, 1151–1164. [CrossRef]
37. Scapini, P.; Cassatella, M.A. Social networking of human neutrophils within the immune system. *Blood* **2014**, *124*, 710–719. [CrossRef]
38. Scapini, P.; Morini, M.; Tecchio, C.; Minghelli, S.; DI Carlo, E.; Tanghetti, E.; Albini, A.; Lowell, C.; Berton, G.; Noonan, D.M.; et al. CXCL1/Macrophage Inflammatory Protein-2-Induced Angiogenesis In Vivo Is Mediated by Neutrophil-Derived Vascular Endothelial Growth Factor-A. *J. Immunol.* **2004**, *172*, 5034–5040. [CrossRef] [PubMed]
39. Ria, R.; Simeon, V.; Melaccio, A.; Di Meo, G.; Trino, S.; Mazzoccoli, C.; Saltarella, I.; Lamanuzzi, A.; Morano, A.; Gurrado, A.; et al. Gene expression profiling of normal thyroid tissue from patients with thyroid carcinoma. *Oncotarget* **2016**, *7*, 29677–29688. [CrossRef]
40. Rajabi, S.; Dehghan, M.H.; Dastmalchi, R.; Mashayekhi, F.J.; Salami, S.; Hedayati, M. The roles and role-players in thyroid cancer angiogenesis. *Endocr. J.* **2019**, *66*, 277–293. [CrossRef]
41. Ria, R.; Melaccio, A.; Racanelli, V.; Vacca, A. Anti-VEGF Drugs in the Treatment of Multiple Myeloma Patients. *J. Clin. Med.* **2020**, *9*, 1765. [CrossRef] [PubMed]
42. Benest, A.V.; Augustin, H.G. Tension in the vasculature. *Nat. Med.* **2009**, *15*, 608–610. [CrossRef]
43. Dvorak, H.F. Tumor Stroma, Tumor Blood Vessels, and Antiangiogenesis Therapy. *Cancer J.* **2015**, *21*, 237–243. [CrossRef] [PubMed]
44. Bugyik, E.; Renyi-Vamos, F.; Szabo, V.; Dezso, K.; Ecker, N.; Rokusz, A.; Nagy, P.; Dome, B.; Paku, S. Mechanisms of vascularization in murine models of primary and metastatic tumor growth. *Chin. J. Cancer* **2016**, *35*, 1–8. [CrossRef] [PubMed]
45. Ramsden, J.D. Angiogenesis in the thyroid gland. *J. Endocrinol.* **2000**, *166*, 475–480. [CrossRef]
46. Sprindzuk, M.V. Angiogenesis in Malignant Thyroid Tumors. *World J. Oncol.* **2010**, *1*, 221–231. [CrossRef]
47. Mousa, S.A.; Lin, H.-Y.; Tang, H.Y.; Hercbergs, A.; Luidens, M.K.; Davis, P.J. Modulation of angiogenesis by thyroid hormone and hormone analogues: Implications for cancer management. *Angiogenesis* **2014**, *17*, 463–469. [CrossRef]
48. De La Torre, N.G.; Buley, I.; Wass, J.A.H.; Turner, H.E. Angiogenesis and lymphangiogenesis in thyroid proliferative lesions: Relationship to type and tumour behaviour. *Endocr.-Relat. Cancer* **2006**, *13*, 931–944. [CrossRef] [PubMed]
49. Pierotti, M.A.; Bongarzone, I.; Borello, M.G.; Greco, A.; Pilotti, S.; Sozzi, G. Cytogenetics and molecular genetics of carcinomas arising from thyroid epithelial follicular cells. *Genes Chromosomes Cancer* **1996**, *16*, 1–14. [CrossRef]
50. Bunone, G.; Vigneri, P.; Mariani, L.; Butó, S.; Collini, P.; Pilotti, S.; Pierotti, M.A.; Bongarzone, I. Expression of Angiogenesis Stimulators and Inhibitors in Human Thyroid Tumors and Correlation with Clinical Pathological Features. *Am. J. Pathol.* **1999**, *155*, 1967–1976. [CrossRef]
51. Justus, C.R.; Sanderlin, E.J.; Yang, L.V. Molecular Connections between Cancer Cell Metabolism and the Tumor Microenvironment. *Int. J. Mol. Sci.* **2015**, *16*, 11055–11086. [CrossRef] [PubMed]
52. Feng, K.; Ma, R.; Zhang, L.; Li, H.; Tang, Y.; Du, G.; Niu, D.; Yin, D. The Role of Exosomes in Thyroid Cancer and Their Potential Clinical Application. *Front. Oncol.* **2020**, *10*. [CrossRef]
53. Santiago, K.; Wongworawat, Y.C.; Khan, S. Differential MicroRNA-Signatures in Thyroid Cancer Subtypes. *J. Oncol.* **2020**, *2020*, 2052396. [CrossRef]
54. Luidens, M.K.; Mousa, S.; Davis, F.B.; Lin, H.-Y.; Davis, P.J. Thyroid hormone and angiogenesis. *Vasc. Pharmacol.* **2010**, *52*, 142–145. [CrossRef] [PubMed]
55. Davis, P.J.; Davis, F.B.; Mousa, S.; Luidens, M.K.; Lin, H.-Y. Membrane Receptor for Thyroid Hormone: Physiologic and Pharmacologic Implications. *Annu. Rev. Pharmacol. Toxicol.* **2011**, *51*, 99–115. [CrossRef] [PubMed]
56. Wong, V.W.; Crawford, J.D. Vasculogenic Cytokines in Wound Healing. *BioMed Res. Int.* **2013**, *2013*, 190486. [CrossRef]
57. Lin, H.-Y.; Sun, M.; Tang, H.-Y.; Lin, C.; Luidens, M.K.; Mousa, S.A.; Incerpi, S.; Drusano, G.L.; Davis, F.B.; Davis, P.J. l-Thyroxine vs. 3,5,3′-triiodo-l-thyronine and cell proliferation: Activation of mitogen-activated protein kinase and phosphatidylinositol 3-kinase. *Am. J. Physiol. Physiol.* **2009**, *296*, C980–C991. [CrossRef]
58. Sarapura, V.D.; Gordon, D.F.; Samuels, M.H. Chapter 6—Thyroid-stimulating Hormone. In *The Pituitary*, 3rd ed.; Melmed, S., Ed.; Academic Press: San Diego, CA, USA, 2011; pp. 167–203.
59. Freudenthal, B.; Williams, G. Thyroid Stimulating Hormone Suppression in the Long-term Follow-up of Differentiated Thyroid Cancer. *Clin. Oncol.* **2017**, *29*, 325–328. [CrossRef]
60. Soh, E.Y.; Sobhi, S.A.; Wong, M.G.; Meng, Y.G.; Siperstein, A.; Clark, O.H.; Duh, Q.-Y. Thyroid-stimulating hormone promotes the secretion of vascular endothelial growth factor in thyroid cancer cell lines. *Surgery* **1996**, *120*, 944–947. [CrossRef]
61. Hoffmann, S.; Hofbauer, L.C.; Scharrenbach, V.; Wunderlich, A.; Hassan, I.; Lingelbach, S.; Zielke, A. Thyrotropin (TSH)-Induced Production of Vascular Endothelial Growth Factor in Thyroid Cancer Cellsin Vitro: Evaluation of TSH Signal Transduction and of Angiogenesis-Stimulating Growth Factors. *J. Clin. Endocrinol. Metab.* **2004**, *89*, 6139–6145. [CrossRef] [PubMed]
62. Gérard, A.-C.; Poncin, S.; Audinot, J.-N.; Denef, J.-F.; Colin, I.M. Iodide deficiency-induced angiogenic stimulus in the thyroid occurs via HIF- and ROS-dependent VEGF-A secretion from thyrocytes. *Am. J. Physiol. Metab.* **2009**, *296*, E1414–E1422. [CrossRef] [PubMed]
63. Gérard, A.-C.; Humblet, K.; Wilvers, C.; Poncin, S.; Derradji, H.; Goyet, C.D.V.D.; Abou-El-Ardat, K.; Baatout, S.; Sonveaux, P.; Denef, J.-F.; et al. Iodine-Deficiency-Induced Long Lasting Angiogenic Reaction in Thyroid Cancers Occurs Via a Vascular Endothelial Growth Factor–Hypoxia Inducible Factor-1–Dependent, But Not a Reactive Oxygen Species–Dependent, Pathway. *Thyroid* **2012**, *22*, 699–708. [CrossRef] [PubMed]

64. Craps, J.; Joris, V.; De Jongh, B.; Sonveaux, P.; Horman, S.; Lengelé, B.; Bertrand, L.; Many, M.-C.; Colin, I.M.; Gérard, A.-C. Involvement of mTOR and Regulation by AMPK in Early Iodine Deficiency-Induced Thyroid Microvascular Activation. *Endocrinology* **2016**, *157*, 2545–2559. [CrossRef] [PubMed]
65. Ferrara, N. Reprint of Pituitary follicular cells secrete a novel heparin-binding growth factor specific for vascular endothelial cells. *Biochem. Biophys. Res. Commun.* **2012**, *425*, 540–547. [CrossRef]
66. Yang, Z.; Yao, H.; Fei, F.; Li, Y.; Qu, J.; Li, C.; Zhang, S. Generation of erythroid cells from polyploid giant cancer cells: Re-thinking about tumor blood supply. *J. Cancer Res. Clin. Oncol.* **2018**, *144*, 617–627. [CrossRef]
67. Holmes, K.; Roberts, O.L.; Thomas, A.M.; Cross, M.J. Vascular endothelial growth factor receptor-2: Structure, function, intracellular signalling and therapeutic inhibition. *Cell. Signal.* **2007**, *19*, 2003–2012. [CrossRef]
68. Brekken, R.A.; Overholser, J.P.; Stastny, V.; Waltenberger, J.; Minna, J.D.; Thorpe, P.E. Selective inhibition of vascular endothelial growth factor (VEGF) receptor 2 (KDR/Flk-1) activity by a monoclonal anti-VEGF antibody blocks tumor growth in mice. *Cancer Res.* **2000**, *60*, 5117–5124.
69. Cursiefen, C.; Chen, L.; Borges, L.P.; Jackson, D.; Cao, J.; Radziejewski, C.; D'Amore, P.A.; Dana, M.R.; Wiegand, S.J.; Streilein, J.W. VEGF-A stimulates lymphangiogenesis and hemangiogenesis in inflammatory neovascularization via macrophage recruitment. *J. Clin. Investig.* **2004**, *113*, 1040–1050. [CrossRef]
70. Adams, J.; Carder, P.J.; Downey, S.; Forbes, M.A.; MacLennan, K.; Allgar, V.; Kaufman, S.; Hallam, S.; Bicknell, R.; Walker, J.J.; et al. Vascular endothelial growth factor (VEGF) in breast cancer: Comparison of plasma, serum, and tissue VEGF and microvessel density and effects of tamoxifen. *Cancer Res.* **2000**, *60*, 2898–2905. [PubMed]
71. Vacca, A.; Ria, R.; Ribatti, D.; Semeraro, F.; Djonov, V.; Di Raimondo, F.; Dammacco, F. A paracrine loop in the vascular endothelial growth factor pathway triggers tumor angiogenesis and growth in multiple myeloma. *Haematologica* **2003**, *88*, 176–185. [PubMed]
72. Ria, R.; Russo, F.; Cirulli, T.; Massaia, M.; Tosi, P.; Cavo, M.; Guidolin, D.; Ribatti, D.; Dammacco, F.; Vacca, A. A VEGF-dependent autocrine loop mediates proliferation and capillarogenesis in bone marrow endothelial cells of patients with multiple myeloma. *Thromb. Haemost.* **2004**, *92*, 1438–1445. [CrossRef] [PubMed]
73. Yoshinaga, A.; Kajihara, N.; Kukidome, D.; Motoshima, H.; Matsumura, T.; Nishikawa, T.; Araki, E. Hypoglycemia Induces Mitochondrial Reactive Oxygen Species Production Through Increased Fatty Acid Oxidation and Promotes Retinal Vascular Permeability in Diabetic Mice. *Antioxid. Redox Signal.* **2021**, *34*, 1245–1259. [CrossRef]
74. Kumar, S.A.; Hu, X.; Brown, M.; Kuschak, B.; Hernandez, T.A.; Johnston, J.B.; Gibson, S.B. Lysophosphatidic acid receptor expression in chronic lymphocytic leukemia leads to cell survival mediated though vascular endothelial growth factor expression. *Leuk. Lymphoma* **2009**, *50*, 2038–2048. [CrossRef] [PubMed]
75. Sujobert, P.; Bardet, V.; Cornillet-Lefebvre, P.; Hayflick, J.S.; Prie, N.; Verdier, F.; Vanhaesebroeck, B.; Muller, O.; Pesce, F.; Ifrah, N.; et al. Essential role for the p110 isoform in phosphoinositide 3-kinase activation and cell proliferation in acute myeloid leukemia. *Blood* **2005**, *106*, 1063–1066. [CrossRef]
76. Shi, Q.; Le, X.; Abbruzzese, J.L.; Peng, Z.; Qian, C.N.; Tang, H.; Xiong, Q.; Wang, B.; Li, X.C.; Xie, K. Constitutive Sp1 activity is essential for differential constitutive expression of vascular endothelial growth factor in human pancreatic adenocarcinoma. *Cancer Res.* **2001**, *61*, 4143–4154. [PubMed]
77. Hsu, T.-C.; Young, M.R.; Cmarik, J.; Colburn, N.H. Activator protein 1 (AP-1) and nuclear factor κB (NF-κB)–dependent transcriptional events in carcinogenesis. *Free. Radic. Biol. Med.* **2000**, *28*, 1338–1348. [CrossRef]
78. Poulaki, V.; Mitsiades, C.S.; McMullan, C.; Sykoutri, D.; Fanourakis, G.; Kotoula, V.; Tseleni-Balafouta, S.; Koutras, D.A.; Mitsiades, N. Regulation of Vascular Endothelial Growth Factor Expression by Insulin-Like Growth Factor I in Thyroid Carcinomas. *J. Clin. Endocrinol. Metab.* **2003**, *88*, 5392–5398. [CrossRef]
79. Soh, E.Y.; Duh, Q.-Y.; Sobhi, S.A.; Young, D.M.; Epstein, H.D.; Wong, M.G.; Garcia, Y.K.; Min, Y.D.; Grossman, R.F.; Siperstein, A.E.; et al. Vascular Endothelial Growth Factor Expression Is Higher in Differentiated Thyroid Cancer than in Normal or Benign Thyroid 1. *J. Clin. Endocrinol. Metab.* **1997**, *82*, 3741–3747. [CrossRef] [PubMed]
80. Lin, J.-D.; Chao, T.-C. Vascular Endothelial Growth Factor in Thyroid Cancers. *Cancer Biother. Radiopharm.* **2005**, *20*, 648–661. [CrossRef]
81. Lewy-Trenda, I.; Wierzchniewska-Ławska, A. Expression of vascular endothelial growth factor (VEGF) in hu-man thyroid tumors. *Pol. J. Pathol.* **2002**, *53*, 129–132.
82. Presta, M.; Moscatelli, D.; Joseph-Silverstein, J.; Rifkin, D.B. Purification from a human hepatoma cell line of a basic fibroblast growth factor-like molecule that stimulates capillary endothelial cell plasminogen activator production, DNA synthesis, and migration. *Mol. Cell. Biol.* **1986**, *6*, 4060–4066. [CrossRef]
83. Rusnati, M.; Presta, M. Interaction of angiogenic basic fibroblast growth factor with endothelial cell heparan sulfate proteoglycans. *Int. J. Clin. Lab. Res.* **1996**, *26*, 15–23. [CrossRef] [PubMed]
84. Presta, M.; Dell'Era, P.; Mitola, S.; Moroni, E.; Ronca, R.; Rusnati, M. Fibroblast growth factor/fibroblast growth factor receptor system in angiogenesis. *Cytokine Growth Factor Rev.* **2005**, *16*, 159–178. [CrossRef]
85. Eggo, M.C.; Hopkins, J.M.; Franklyn, J.A.; Johnson, G.D.; Sanders, D.S.; Sheppard, M.C. Expression of fibroblast growth factors in thyroid cancer. *J. Clin. Endocrinol. Metab.* **1995**, *80*, 1006–1011. [CrossRef] [PubMed]
86. Shingu, K.; Fujimori, M.; Ito, K.-I.; Hama, Y.; Kasuga, Y.; Kobayashi, S.; Itoh, N.; Amano, J. Expression of Fibroblast Growth Factor-2 and Fibroblast Growth Factor Receptor-1 in Thyroid Diseases: Difference between Neoplasms and Hyperplastic Lesions. *Endocr. J.* **1998**, *45*, 35–43. [CrossRef] [PubMed]

87. Thompson, S.D.; Franklyn, J.A.; Watkinson, J.C.; Verhaeg, J.M.; Sheppard, M.C.; Eggo, M.C. Fibroblast Growth Factors 1 and 2 and Fibroblast Growth Factor Receptor 1 Are Elevated in Thyroid Hyperplasia. *J. Clin. Endocrinol. Metab.* **1998**, *83*, 1336–1341. [CrossRef] [PubMed]
88. Daa, T.; Kodama, M.; Kashima, K.; Yokoyama, S.; Nakayama, I.; Noguchi, S. Identification of basic fibroblast growth factor in papillary carcinoma of the thyroid. *Pathol. Int.* **1993**, *43*, 582–589. [CrossRef] [PubMed]
89. Brew, K.; Nagase, H. The tissue inhibitors of metalloproteinases (TIMPs): An ancient family with structural and functional diversity. *Biochim. Biophys. Acta (BBA)-Bioenerg.* **2010**, *1803*, 55–71. [CrossRef] [PubMed]
90. Quintero-Fabián, S.; Arreola, R.; Becerril-Villanueva, E.; Torres-Romero, J.C.; Arana-Argáez, V.; Lara-Riegos, J.; Ramírez-Camacho, M.A.; Alvarez-Sánchez, M.E. Role of Matrix Metalloproteinases in Angiogenesis and Cancer. *Front. Oncol.* **2019**, *9*, 1370. [CrossRef] [PubMed]
91. Yu, Q.; Stamenkovic, I. Cell surface-localized matrix metalloproteinase-9 proteolytically activates TGF-beta and promotes tumor invasion and angiogenesis. *Genes Dev.* **2000**, *14*, 163–176. [PubMed]
92. Rothhut, B.; Ghoneim, C.; Antonicelli, F.; Soula-Rothhut, M. Epidermal growth factor stimulates matrix metalloproteinase-9 expression and invasion in human follicular thyroid carcinoma cells through Focal adhesion kinase. *Biochimie* **2007**, *89*, 613–624. [CrossRef]
93. Murphy, G. Tissue inhibitors of metalloproteinases. *Genome Biol.* **2011**, *12*, 1–7. [CrossRef]
94. Ria, R.; Prete, F.; Melaccio, A.; Di Meo, G.; Saltarella, I.; Solimando, A.G.; Gurrado, A.; Ferraro, V.; Pasculli, A.; Sgaramella, L.I.; et al. Effect of thyroidectomy on circulating angiogenic cytokines in papillary thyroid carcinoma and benign goiter: Potential for new biomarkers? *Surgery* **2021**, *169*, 27–33. [CrossRef]
95. Saltarella, I.; Morabito, F.; Giuliani, N.; Terragna, C.; Omedè, P.; Palumbo, A.; Bringhen, S.; De Paoli, L.; Martino, E.; LaRocca, A.; et al. Prognostic or predictive value of circulating cytokines and angiogenic factors for initial treatment of multiple myeloma in the GIMEMA MM0305 randomized controlled trial. *J. Hematol. Oncol.* **2019**, *12*, 4. [CrossRef]
96. Jebreel, A.; England, J.; Bedford, K.; Murphy, J.; Karsai, L.; Atkin, S. Vascular endothelial growth factor (VEGF), VEGF receptors expression and microvascular density in benign and malignant thyroid diseases. *Int. J. Exp. Pathol.* **2007**, *88*, 271–277. [CrossRef] [PubMed]
97. Itoh, A.; Iwase, K.; Jimbo, S.; Yamamoto, H.; Yamamoto, N.; Kokubo, M.; Senda, T.; Nakai, A.; Nagagasaka, A.; Nagasaka, T.; et al. Expression of Vascular Endothelial Growth Factor and Presence of Angiovascular Cells in Tissues from Different Thyroid Disorders. *World J. Surg.* **2010**, *34*, 242–248. [CrossRef] [PubMed]
98. Giatromanolaki, A.; Lyberakidis, G.; Lyratzopoulos, N.; Koukourakis, M.I.; Sivridis, E.; Manolas, C. Angiogene-sis and angiogenic factor expression in thyroid cancer. *J BUON* **2010**, *15*, 357–361.
99. Huang, S.-M.; Lee, J.-C.; Wu, T.-J.; Chow, N.-H. Clinical Relevance of Vascular Endothelial Growth Factor for Thyroid Neoplasms. *World J. Surg.* **2001**, *25*, 302–306. [CrossRef] [PubMed]
100. Duick, D.S.; Klopper, J.P.; Diggans, J.C.; Friedman, L.; Kennedy, G.C.; Lanman, R.; McIver, B. The Impact of Benign Gene Expression Classifier Test Results on the Endocrinologist–Patient Decision to Operate on Patients with Thyroid Nodules with Indeterminate Fine-Needle Aspiration Cytopathology. *Thyroid* **2012**, *22*, 996–1001. [CrossRef]
101. Alexander, E.K.; Kennedy, G.C.; Baloch, Z.W.; Cibas, E.S.; Chudova, D.; Diggans, J.; Friedman, L.; Kloos, R.T.; Livolsi, V.A.; Mandel, S.J.; et al. Preoperative Diagnosis of Benign Thyroid Nodules with Indeterminate Cytology. *N. Engl. J. Med.* **2012**, *367*, 705–715. [CrossRef]
102. Alexander, E.K.; Schorr, M.; Klopper, J.; Kim, C.; Sipos, J.; Nabhan, F.; Parker, C.; Steward, D.L.; Mandel, S.J.; Haugen, B.R. Multicenter Clinical Experience with the Afirma Gene Expression Classifier. *J. Clin. Endocrinol. Metab.* **2014**, *99*, 119–125. [CrossRef]
103. Beaudenon-Huibregtse, S.; Alexander, E.K.; Guttler, R.B.; Hershman, J.M.; Babu, V.; Blevins, T.C.; Moore, P.; Andruss, B.; Labourier, E. Centralized Molecular Testing for Oncogenic Gene Mutations Complements the Local Cytopathologic Diagnosis of Thyroid Nodules. *Thyroid* **2014**, *24*, 1479–1487. [CrossRef]
104. González, H.E.; Martínez, J.R.; Vargas-Salas, S.; Solar, A.; Veliz, L.; Cruz, F.; Arias, T.; Loyola, S.; Horvath, E.; Tala, H.; et al. A 10-Gene Classifier for Indeterminate Thyroid Nodules: Development and Multicenter Accuracy Study. *Thyroid* **2017**, *27*, 1058–1067. [CrossRef]
105. Patel, K.N.; Angell, T.E.; Babiarz, J.; Barth, N.M.; Blevins, T.; Duh, Q.-Y.; Ghossein, R.A.; Harrell, R.M.; Huang, J.; Kennedy, G.C.; et al. Performance of a Genomic Sequencing Classifier for the Preoperative Diagnosis of Cytologically Indeterminate Thyroid Nodules. *JAMA Surg.* **2018**, *153*, 817–824. [CrossRef]
106. Pagan, M.; Kloos, R.T.; Lin, C.-F.; Travers, K.J.; Matsuzaki, H.; Tom, E.Y.; Kim, S.Y.; Wong, M.G.; Stewart, A.C.; Huang, J.; et al. The diagnostic application of RNA sequencing in patients with thyroid cancer: An analysis of 851 variants and 133 fusions in 524 genes. *BMC Bioinform.* **2016**, *17* (Suppl. S1), S6. [CrossRef]
107. Cheng, S.; Serra, S.; Mercado, M.; Ezzat, S.; Asa, S. A High-Throughput Proteomic Approach Provides Distinct Signatures for Thyroid Cancer Behavior. *Clin. Cancer Res.* **2011**, *17*, 2385–2394. [CrossRef]
108. Tallini, G.; De Biase, D.; Durante, C.; Acquaviva, G.; Bisceglia, M.; Bruno, R.; Reggiani, M.L.B.; Casadei, G.P.; Costante, G.; Cremonini, N.; et al. BRAF V600E and risk stratification of thyroid microcarcinoma: A multicenter pathological and clinical study. *Mod. Pathol.* **2015**, *28*, 1343–1359. [CrossRef] [PubMed]

109. Xia, F.; Jiang, B.; Chen, Y.; Du, X.; Peng, Y.; Wang, W.; Wang, Z.; Li, X. Prediction of novel target genes and pathways involved in tall cell variant papillary thyroid carcinoma. *Medicine* **2018**, *97*, e13802. [CrossRef]
110. De La Fouchardière, C.; Oussaid, N.; Derbel, O.; Decaussin-Petrucci, M.; Fondrevelle, M.-E.; Wang, Q.; Bringuier, P.-P.; Bournaud-Salinas, C.; Peix, J.-L.; Lifante, J.-C.; et al. Does Molecular Genotype Provide Useful Information in the Management of Radioiodine Refractory Thyroid Cancers? Results of a Retrospective Study. *Target. Oncol.* **2015**, *11*, 71–82. [CrossRef] [PubMed]
111. Han, P.A.; Kim, H.-S.; Cho, S.; Fazeli, R.; Najafian, A.; Khawaja, H.; McAlexander, M.; Dy, B.; Sorensen, M.; Aronova, A.; et al. Association of $BRAF^{V600E}$ Mutation and MicroRNA Expression with Central Lymph Node Metastases in Papillary Thyroid Cancer: A Prospective Study from Four Endocrine Surgery Centers. *Thyroid* **2016**, *26*, 532–542. [CrossRef] [PubMed]
112. Jacques, C.; Guillotin, D.; Fontaine, J.; Franc, B.; Mirebeau-Prunier, D.; Fleury, A.; Malthièry, Y.; Savagner, F. DNA Microarray and miRNA Analyses Reinforce the Classification of Follicular Thyroid Tumors. *J. Clin. Endocrinol. Metab.* **2013**, *98*, E981–E989. [CrossRef] [PubMed]
113. Stokowy, T.; Wojtas, B.; Krajewska, J.; Stobiecka, E.; Dralle, H.; Musholt, T.; Hauptmann, S.; Lange, D.; Hegedüs, L.; Jarząb, B.; et al. A two miRNA classifier differentiates follicular thyroid carcinomas from follicular thyroid adenomas. *Mol. Cell. Endocrinol.* **2015**, *399*, 43–49. [CrossRef] [PubMed]
114. Huang, Y.; Qu, S.; Zhu, G.; Wang, F.; Liu, R.; Shen, X.; Viola, D.; Elisei, R.; Puxeddu, E.; Fugazzola, L.; et al. BRAF V600E Mutation-Assisted Risk Stratification of Solitary Intrathyroidal Papillary Thyroid Cancer for Precision Treatment. *J. Natl. Cancer Inst.* **2018**, *110*, 362–370. [CrossRef]
115. Nucera, C.; Porrello, A.; Antonello, Z.A.; Mekel, M.; Nehs, M.A.; Giordano, T.J.; Gerald, D.; Benjamin, L.E.; Priolo, C.; Puxeddu, E.; et al. B-RafV600E and thrombospondin-1 promote thyroid cancer progression. *Proc. Natl. Acad. Sci. USA* **2010**, *107*, 10649–10654. [CrossRef] [PubMed]
116. Prete, A.; Lo, A.S.; Sadow, P.M.; Bhasin, S.S.; Antonello, Z.A.; Vodopivec, D.M.; Ullas, S.; Sims, J.N.; Clohessy, J.; Dvorak, A.M.; et al. Pericytes Elicit Resistance to Vemurafenib and Sorafenib Therapy in Thyroid Carcinoma via the TSP-1/TGFβ1 Axis. *Clin. Cancer Res.* **2018**, *24*, 6078–6097. [CrossRef]
117. Song, S.; Ewald, A.J.; Stallcup, W.; Werb, Z.; Bergers, G. PDGFRβ+ perivascular progenitor cells in tumours regulate pericyte differentiation and vascular survival. *Nat. Cell Biol.* **2005**, *7*, 870–879. [CrossRef] [PubMed]
118. Klubo-Gwiezdzinska, J.; Junik, R.; Kopczynska, E.; Juraniec, O.; Kardymowicz, H. The comparison of serum vascular endothelial growth factor levels between patients with metastatic and non-metastatic thyroid cancer, and patients with nontoxic multinodular goiter. *Eur. J. Endocrinol.* **2007**, *157*, 521–527. [CrossRef] [PubMed]
119. Nersita, R.; Matrone, A.; Klain, M.; Scavuzzo, F.; Vitolo, G.; Abbondanza, C.; Carlino, M.V.; Giacco, V.; Amato, G.; Carella, C. Decreased serum vascular endothelial growth factor-D levels in metastatic patients with differentiated thyroid carcinoma. *Clin. Endocrinol.* **2011**, *76*, 142–146. [CrossRef] [PubMed]
120. Seybt, T.P.; Ramalingam, P.; Huang, J.; Looney, S.W.; Reid, M.D. Cyclin D1 Expression in Benign and Differentiated Malignant Tumors of the Thyroid Gland: Diagnostic and biologic implications. *Appl. Immunohistochem. Mol. Morphol.* **2012**, *20*, 124–130. [CrossRef]
121. Jeong, S.; Lee, J.; Kim, D.; Seol, M.-Y.; Lee, W.K.; Jeong, J.J.; Nam, K.-H.; Jung, S.G.; Shin, D.Y.; Lee, E.J.; et al. Relationship of Focally Amplified Long Noncoding on Chromosome 1 (FAL1) lncRNA with E2F Transcription Factors in Thyroid Cancer. *Medicine* **2016**, *95*, e2592. [CrossRef] [PubMed]
122. Zhao, D.; Jin, X.; Li, F.; Liang, J.; Lin, Y. Integrin αvβ3 Imaging of Radioactive Iodine-Refractory Thyroid Cancer Using 99mTc-3PRGD2. *J. Nucl. Med.* **2012**, *53*, 1872–1877. [CrossRef]
123. Tuttle, R.M.; Fleisher, M.; Francis, G.L.; Robbins, R.J. Serum Vascular Endothelial Growth Factor Levels Are Elevated in Metastatic Differentiated Thyroid Cancer but Not Increased by Short-Term TSH Stimulation. *J. Clin. Endocrinol. Metab.* **2002**, *87*, 1737–1742. [CrossRef]
124. Sorvillo, F.; Mazziotti, G.; Carbone, A.; Piscopo, M.; Rotondi, M.; Cioffi, M.; Musto, P.; Biondi, B.; Iorio, S.; Amato, G.; et al. Recombinant Human Thyrotropin Reduces Serum Vascular Endothelial Growth Factor Levels in Patients Monitored for Thyroid Carcinoma Even in the Absence of Thyroid Tissue. *J. Clin. Endocrinol. Metab.* **2003**, *88*, 4818–4822. [CrossRef]
125. Wu, F.; Li, F.; Lin, X.; Xu, F.; Cui, R.R.; Zhong, J.Y.; Zhu, T.; Shan, S.K.; Liao, X.B.; Yuan, L.Q.; et al. Exosomes in-creased angiogenesis in papillary thyroid cancer microenvironment. *Endocr. Relat. Cancer* **2019**, *26*, 525–538. [CrossRef]
126. Capp, C.; Wajner, S.M.; Siqueira, D.R.; Brasil, B.A.; Meurer, L.; Maia, A.L. Increased Expression of Vascular Endothelial Growth Factor and Its Receptors, VEGFR-1 and VEGFR-2, in Medullary Thyroid Carcinoma. *Thyroid* **2010**, *20*, 863–871. [CrossRef] [PubMed]
127. Rodríguez-Antona, C.; Pallares, J.; Montero-Conde, C.; Inglada-Pérez, L.; Castelblanco, E.; Landa, I.; Leskelä, S.; Leandro-García, L.J.; López-Jiménez, E.; Letón, R.; et al. Overexpression and activation of EGFR and VEGFR2 in medullary thyroid carcinomas is related to metastasis. *Endocr.-Relat. Cancer* **2010**, *17*, 7–16. [CrossRef] [PubMed]
128. Lodewijk, L.; van Diest, P.; van der Groep, P.; Ter Hoeve, N.; Schepers, A.; Morreau, J.; Bonenkamp, J.; van Engen-van Grunsven, A.; Kruijff, S.; van Hemel, B.; et al. Expression of HIF-1α in medullary thyroid cancer identifies a subgroup with poor prognosis. *Oncotarget* **2017**, *8*, 28650–28659. [CrossRef]
129. Lodewijk, L.; Willems, S.M.; Dreijerink, K.M.A.; de Keizer, B.; van Diest, P.J.; Schepers, A.; Morreau, H.; Bonenkamp, H.J.; Van Engen-van Grunsven, I.A.C.H.; Kruijff, S.; et al. The theranostic target prostate-specific membrane antigen is expressed in medullary thyroid cancer. *Hum. Pathol.* **2018**, *81*, 245–254. [CrossRef] [PubMed]

130. Tokarz, D.; Cisek, R.; Golaraei, A.; Asa, S.; Barzda, V.; Wilson, B.C. Ultrastructural features of collagen in thyroid carcinoma tissue observed by polarization second harmonic generation microscopy. *Biomed. Opt. Express* **2015**, *6*, 3475–3481. [CrossRef] [PubMed]
131. Boufraqech, M.; Nilubol, N.; Zhang, L.; Gara, S.K.; Sadowski, S.M.; Mehta, A.; He, M.; Davis, S.; Dreiling, J.; Copland, J.A.; et al. miR30a Inhibits LOX Expression and Anaplastic Thyroid Cancer Progression. *Cancer Res.* **2015**, *75*, 367–377. [CrossRef]
132. Boufraqech, M.; Patel, D.; Nilubol, N.; Powers, A.S.; King, T.; Shell, J.; Lack, J.; Zhang, L.; Gara, S.K.; Gunda, V.; et al. Lysyl Oxidase Is a Key Player in BRAF/MAPK Pathway-Driven Thyroid Cancer Aggressiveness. *Thyroid* **2019**, *29*, 79–92. [CrossRef]
133. Harburger, D.S.; Calderwood, D. Integrin signalling at a glance. *J. Cell Sci.* **2009**, *122 Pt 2*, 159–163. [CrossRef]
134. Komorowski, J.; Pasieka, Z.; Jankiewicz-Wika, J.; Stepień, H. Matrix Metalloproteinases, Tissue Inhibitors of Matrix Metalloproteinases and Angiogenic Cytokines in Peripheral Blood of Patients with Thyroid Cancer. *Thyroid* **2002**, *12*, 655–662. [CrossRef]
135. Lin, S.Y.; Wang, Y.Y.; Sheu, W.H.-H. Preoperative plasma concentrations of vascular endothelial growth factor and matrix metalloproteinase 9 are associated with stage progression in papillary thyroid cancer. *Clin. Endocrinol.* **2003**, *58*, 513–518. [CrossRef] [PubMed]
136. Cavalheiro, B.G.; Junqueira, C.R.; Brandão, L.G. Ratio of Metalloproteinase 2 to Tissue Inhibitor of Metalloproteinase 2 in Medullary Thyroid Carcinoma. *Arch. Otolaryngol.-Head Neck Surg.* **2009**, *135*, 812. [CrossRef] [PubMed]
137. Cavalheiro, B.G.; Junqueira, C.R.; Brandão, L.G. Expression of Matrix Metalloproteinase 2 (MMP-2) and Tissue Inhibitor of Metalloproteinase 2 (TIMP-2) in Medullary Thyroid Carcinoma: Prognostic Implications. *Thyroid* **2008**, *18*, 865–871. [CrossRef]
138. Marečko, I.; Cvejić, D.; Tatić, S.; Dragutinović, V.; Paunović, I.; Savin, S. Expression of matrix metalloproteinase-2 and its tissue inhibitor-2 in fetal and neoplastic thyroid tissue and their significance as diagnostic and prognostic markers in papillary carcinoma. *Cancer Biomark.* **2012**, *11*, 49–58. [CrossRef]
139. Bumber, B.; Kavanagh, M.M.; Jakovcevic, A.; Sincic, N.; Prstacic, R.; Prgomet, D. Role of matrix metalloproteinases and their inhibitors in the development of cervical metastases in papillary thyroid cancer. *Clin. Otolaryngol.* **2020**, *45*, 55–62. [CrossRef]
140. Luo, D.; Chen, H.; Li, X.; Lu, P.; Long, M.; Peng, X.; Lin, S.; Tan, L.; Zhu, Y.; Ouyang, N.; et al. Activation of the ROCK1/MMP-9 pathway is associated with the invasion and poor prognosis in papillary thyroid carcinoma. *Int. J. Oncol.* **2017**, *51*, 1209–1218. [CrossRef]
141. Meng, X.-Y.; Zhang, Q.; Li, Q.; Lin, S.; Li, J. Immunohistochemical levels of cyclo-oxygenase-2, matrix metalloproteinase-9 and vascular endothelial growth factor in papillary thyroid carcinoma and their clinicopathological correlations. *J. Int. Med. Res.* **2014**, *42*, 619–627. [CrossRef]
142. Wang, N.; Jiang, R.; Yang, J.-Y.; Tang, C.; Yang, L.; Xu, M.; Jiang, Q.-F.; Liu, Z.-M. Expression of TGF-β1, SNAI1 and MMP-9 is associated with lymph node metastasis in papillary thyroid carcinoma. *J. Mol. Histol.* **2013**, *45*, 391–399. [CrossRef] [PubMed]
143. Cabanillas, M.E.; Ryder, M.; Jimenez, C. Targeted Therapy for Advanced Thyroid Cancer: Kinase Inhibitors and Beyond. *Endocr. Rev.* **2019**, *40*, 1573–1604. [CrossRef]
144. Lim, S.M.; Chung, W.Y.; Nam, K.-H.; Kang, S.-W.; Lim, J.Y.; Kim, H.-G.; Shin, S.H.; Sun, J.-M.; Kim, S.-G.; Kim, J.-H.; et al. An open label, multicenter, phase II study of dovitinib in advanced thyroid cancer. *Eur. J. Cancer* **2015**, *51*, 1588–1595. [CrossRef]
145. Eltelety, A.M.; Terris, D.J. Neck Dissection in the Surgical Treatment of Thyroid Cancer. *Endocrinol. Metab. Clin. N. Am.* **2019**, *48*, 143–151. [CrossRef] [PubMed]
146. Sun, Y.; Niu, W.; Du, F.; Du, C.; Li, S.; Wang, J.; Li, L.; Wang, F.; Hao, Y.; Li, C.; et al. Safety, pharmacokinetics, and antitumor properties of anlotinib, an oral multi-target tyrosine kinase inhibitor, in patients with advanced refractory solid tumors. *J. Hematol. Oncol.* **2016**, *9*, 105. [CrossRef]
147. Wells, S.A., Jr.; Robinson, B.G.; Gagel, R.F.; Dralle, H.; Fagin, J.A.; Santoro, M.; Baudin, E.; Elisei, R.; Jarzab, B.; Vasselli, J.R.; et al. Vandetanib in patients with locally advanced or metastatic medullary thyroid cancer: A randomized, double-blind phase III trial. *J. Clin. Oncol.* **2012**, *30*, 134e141. [CrossRef] [PubMed]
148. Leboulleux, S.; Bastholt, L.; Krause, T.; de la Fouchardiere, C.; Tennvall, J.; Awada, A.; Gómez, J.M.; Bonichon, F.; Leenhardt, L.; Soufflet, C.; et al. Vandetanib in locally advanced or metastatic differentiated thyroid cancer: A randomised, double-blind, phase 2 trial. *Lancet Oncol.* **2012**, *13*, 897–905. [CrossRef]
149. Valerio, L.; Pieruzzi, L.; Giani, C.; Agate, L.; Bottici, V.; Lorusso, L.; Cappagli, V.; Puleo, L.; Matrone, A.; Viola, D.; et al. Targeted Therapy in Thyroid Cancer: State of the Art. *Clin. Oncol.* **2017**, *29*, 316–324. [CrossRef]
150. Elisei, R.; Schlumberger, M.J.; Müller, S.P.; Schöffski, P.; Brose, M.S.; Shah, M.H.; Licitra, L.; Jarzab, B.; Medvedev, V.; Kreissl, M.C.; et al. Cabozantinib in Progressive Medullary Thyroid Cancer. *J. Clin. Oncol.* **2013**, *31*, 3639–3646. [CrossRef]
151. Sherman, S.I.; Clary, D.O.; Elisei, R.; Schlumberger, M.J.; Cohen, E.E.W.; Schöffski, P.; Wirth, L.J.; Mangeshkar, M.; Aftab, D.T.; Brose, M.S. Correlative analyses ofRETand RAS mutations in a phase 3 trial of cabozantinib in patients with progressive, metastatic medullary thyroid cancer. *Cancer* **2016**, *122*, 3856–3864. [CrossRef]
152. Capdevila, J.; Iglesias, L.; Halperin, I.; Segura, A.; Martínez-Trufero, J.; Vaz, M.Á.; Corral, J.; Obiols, G.; Grande, E.; Grau, J.J.; et al. Sorafenib in metastatic thyroid cancer. *Endocr.-Relat. Cancer* **2012**, *19*, 209–216. [CrossRef]
153. Brose, M.S.; Nutting, C.M.; Jarzab, B.; Elisei, R.; Siena, S.; Bastholt, L.; de la Fouchardiere, C.; Pacini, F.; Paschke, R.; Shong, Y.K.; et al. Sorafenib in radioactive iodine-refractory, locally advanced or metastatic differentiated thyroid cancer: A randomised, double-blind, phase 3 trial. *Lancet* **2014**, *384*, 319–328. [CrossRef]
154. Sherman, S.I.; Jarzab, B.; Cabanillas, M.E.; Licitra, L.F.; Pacini, F.; Martins, R.; Robinson, B.; Ball, D.; McCaffrey, J.; Shah, M.H.; et al. A phase II trial of the multitargeted kinase inhibitor E7080 in advanced radioiodine (RAI)-refractory differentiated thyroid cancer (DTC). *J. Clin. Oncol.* **2011**, *29*, 5503. [CrossRef]

155. Schlumberger, M.; Tahara, M.; Wirth, L.J.; Robinson, B.; Brose, M.S.; Elisei, R.; Habra, M.A.; Newbold, K.; Shah, M.H.; Hoff, A.O.; et al. Lenvatinib versus Placebo in Radioiodine-Refractory Thyroid Cancer. *N. Engl. J. Med.* **2015**, *372*, 621–630. [CrossRef]
156. Wirth, L.J.; Tahara, M.; Robinson, B.; Francis, S.; Brose, M.S.; Habra, M.A.; Newbold, K.; Kiyota, N.; Dutcus, C.E.; Mathias, E.; et al. Treatment-emergent hypertension and efficacy in the phase 3 Study of (E7080) lenvatinib in differentiated cancer of the thyroid (SELECT). *Cancer* **2018**, *124*, 2365–2372. [CrossRef]
157. National Comprehensive Cancer Network I: NCCN Clinical Practice Guidelines in Oncology—Thyroid Carcinoma v1. 2021. Available online: https://www.nccn.org/professionals/physician_gls/pdf/thyroid_blocks.pdf (accessed on 30 March 2021).
158. Angevin, E.; Lopez-Martin, J.A.; Lin, C.-C.; Gschwend, J.E.; Harzstark, A.; Castellano, D.; Soria, J.-C.; Sen, P.; Chang, J.; Shi, M.; et al. Phase I Study of Dovitinib (TKI258), an Oral FGFR, VEGFR, and PDGFR Inhibitor, in Advanced or Metastatic Renal Cell Carcinoma. *Clin. Cancer Res.* **2013**, *19*, 1257–1268. [CrossRef]
159. Sun, Y.; Du, F.; Gao, M.; Ji, Q.; Li, Z.; Zhang, Y.; Guo, Z.; Wang, J.; Chen, X.; Wang, J.; et al. Anlotinib for the Treatment of Patients with Locally Advanced or Metastatic Medullary Thyroid Cancer. *Thyroid* **2018**, *28*, 1455–1461. [CrossRef]
160. Cohen, E.; Rosen, L.S.; Vokes, E.E.; Kies, M.S.; Forastiere, A.A.; Worden, F.P.; Kane, M.A.; Sherman, E.; Kim, S.; Bycott, P.; et al. Axitinib Is an Active Treatment for All Histologic Subtypes of Advanced Thyroid Cancer: Results From a Phase II Study. *J. Clin. Oncol.* **2008**, *26*, 4708–4713. [CrossRef] [PubMed]
161. Capdevila, J.; Trigo, J.M.; Aller, J.; Manzano, J.L.; Adrián, S.G.; Llopis, C.Z.; Reig, Ò.; Bohn, U.; Cajal, T.R.; Du-ran-Poveda, M.; et al. Axitinib treatment in advanced RAI-resistant differentiated thyroid cancer (DTC) and re-fractory medullary thyroid cancer (MTC). *Eur. J. Endocrinol.* **2017**, *177*, 309–317. [CrossRef] [PubMed]
162. Bible, K.C.; Suman, V.J.; Molina, J.R.; Smallridge, R.C.; Maples, W.J.; Menefee, M.E.; Rubin, J.; Sideras, K.; Morris, J.C.; McIver, B.; et al. Efficacy of pazopanib in progressive, radioiodine-refractory, metastatic differentiated thyroid cancers: Results of a phase 2 consortium study. *Lancet Oncol.* **2010**, *11*, 962–972. [CrossRef]
163. Bible, K.C.; Suman, V.J.; Menefee, M.E.; Smallridge, R.C.; Molina, J.R.; Maples, W.J.; Karlin, N.J.; Traynor, A.M.; Kumar, P.; Goh, B.C.; et al. A multiinstitutional phase 2 trial of pazopanibmonotherapy in advanced anaplastic thyroid cancer. *J. Clin. Endocrinol. Metab.* **2012**, *97*, 3179–3184. [CrossRef] [PubMed]
164. Bible, K.C.; Suman, V.J.; Molina, J.R.; Smallridge, R.C.; Maples, W.J.; Menefee, M.E.; Rubin, J.; Karlin, N.; Sideras, K.; Morris, J.C. III.; et al. A multicenter phase 2 trial of pazopanib in metastatic and progressive medullary thy-roid carcinoma: MC057H. *J. Clin. Endocrinol. Metab.* **2014**, *99*, 1687–1693. [CrossRef] [PubMed]
165. Bible, K.C.; Menefee, M.E.; Lin, C.-C.; Millward, M.J.; Maples, W.J.; Goh, B.C.; Karlin, N.J.; Kane, M.A.; Adkins, D.R.; Molina, J.R.; et al. An International Phase 2 Study of Pazopanib in Progressive and Metastatic Thyroglobulin Antibody Negative Radioactive Iodine Refractory Differentiated Thyroid Cancer. *Thyroid* **2020**, *30*, 1254–1262. [CrossRef] [PubMed]
166. Carr, L.L.; Mankoff, D.A.; Goulart, B.H.; Eaton, K.D.; Capell, P.T.; Kell, E.M.; Bauman, J.E.; Martins, R.G. Phase II Study of Daily Sunitinib in FDG-PET–Positive, Iodine-Refractory Differentiated Thyroid Cancer and Metastatic Medullary Carcinoma of the Thyroid with Functional Imaging Correlation. *Clin. Cancer Res.* **2010**, *16*, 5260–5268. [CrossRef]
167. Bikas, A.; Kundra, P.; Desale, S.; Mete, M.; O'Keefe, K.; Clark, B.G.; Wray, L.; Gandhi, R.; Barett, C.E.; Jelinek, J.S.; et al. Phase 2 clinical trial of sunitinib as adjunctive treatment in patients with advanced differentiated thyroid cancer. *Eur. J. Endocrinol.* **2016**, *174*, 373–380. [CrossRef] [PubMed]
168. Ravaud, A.; de la Fouchardière, C.; Caron, P.; Doussau, A.; Cao, C.D.; Asselineau, J.; Rodien, P.; Pouessel, D.; Nicolli-Sire, P.; Klein, M.; et al. A multicenter phase II study of sunitinib in patients with locally advanced or metastatic differentiated, anaplastic or medullary thyroid carcinomas: Mature data from the THYSU study. *Eur. J. Cancer* **2017**, *76*, 110–117. [CrossRef] [PubMed]
169. Mehnert, J.M.; Varga, A.; Brose, M.S.; Aggarwal, R.R.; Lin, C.-C.; Prawira, A.; De Braud, F.; Tamura, K.; Doi, T.; Piha-Paul, S.A.; et al. Safety and antitumor activity of the anti–PD-1 antibody pembrolizumab in patients with advanced, PD-L1–positive papillary or follicular thyroid cancer. *BMC Cancer* **2019**, *19*, 196. [CrossRef] [PubMed]
170. Antonelli, A.; Ferrari, S.M.; Fallahi, P. Current and future immunotherapies for thyroid cancer. *Expert Rev. Anticancer. Ther.* **2017**, *18*, 149–159. [CrossRef] [PubMed]

cancers

MDPI

Review

Radiomics in Differentiated Thyroid Cancer and Nodules: Explorations, Application, and Limitations

Yuan Cao [1,†], Xiao Zhong [1,†], Wei Diao [1], Jingshi Mu [1], Yue Cheng [2] and Zhiyun Jia [1,*]

[1] Department of Nuclear Medicine, West China Hospital of Sichuan University, Chengdu 610040, China; 2019224020064@stu.scu.edu.cn (Y.C.); 2018324025240@stu.scu.edu.cn (X.Z.); diaowei@stu.scu.edu.cn (W.D.); vivienne0117m@163.com (J.M.)

[2] Department of Radiology, West China Hospital of Sichuan University, Chengdu 610040, China; 2019224025311@stu.scu.edu.cn

* Correspondence: jzygood@scu.edu.cn; Tel.: +86-134-0841-9087

† These authors contributed equally to this work.

Simple Summary: Differentiated thyroid cancer (DTC) is the most common endocrine malignancy with a high incidence rate in females. The COVID-19 epidemic posed an increased risk of treatment delay causing increased DTC morbidity and mortality rate of DTC. Several imaging techniques, including ultrasound (US), magnetic resonance imaging (MRI), and computer tomography (CT), have been applied in the early screening and diagnosis of DTC. However, these traditional methods have limited sensitivity and specificity due to dependence on the experience and skill of the radiologists.

Abstract: Radiomics is an emerging technique that allows the quantitative extraction of high-throughput features from single or multiple medical images, which cannot be observed directly with the naked eye, and then applies to machine learning approaches to construct classification or prediction models. This method makes it possible to evaluate tumor status and to differentiate malignant from benign tumors or nodules in a more objective manner. To date, the classification and prediction value of radiomics in DTC patients have been inconsistent. Herein, we summarize the available literature on the classification and prediction performance of radiomics-based DTC in various imaging techniques. More specifically, we reviewed the recent literature to discuss the capacity of radiomics to predict lymph node (LN) metastasis, distant metastasis, tumor extrathyroidal extension, disease-free survival, and B-Raf proto-oncogene serine/threonine kinase (BRAF) mutation and differentiate malignant from benign nodules. This review discusses the application and limitations of the radiomics process, and explores its ability to improve clinical decision-making with the hope of emphasizing its utility for DTC patients.

Keywords: differentiated thyroid cancer; radiomics; ultrasound; magnetic resonance imaging; computer tomography; prediction; classification

Citation: Cao, Y.; Zhong, X.; Diao, W.; Mu, J.; Cheng, Y.; Jia, Z. Radiomics in Differentiated Thyroid Cancer and Nodules: Explorations, Application, and Limitations. *Cancers* **2021**, *13*, 2436. https://doi.org/10.3390/cancers13102436

Academic Editors: Fabio Medas, Pier Francesco Alesina and Dietmar Georg

Received: 27 April 2021
Accepted: 16 May 2021
Published: 18 May 2021

1. Introduction to Thyroid Cancer

1.1. The Epidemiology and Pathophysiology of Thyroid Cancer

Thyroid cancer is the most common endocrine malignancy and the most commonly diagnosed cancer in people aged 15 to 29 years, and its incidence has continuously increased with 567,233 cases and approximately 41,000 deaths worldwide in 2018 [1,2]. The incidence rate of thyroid cancer is approximately three-fold higher in females than in males but the mortality rate is higher in males than in females [3–5]. In addition, a recent study confirmed that the recurrence rate of well-differentiated thyroid cancer (DTC) is higher in men compared with women. Due to the COVID-19 epidemic, delayed investigations and treatment may further lead to increased morbidity and mortality of thyroid cancer [6]. The various clinical outcomes of thyroid cancer are considered to be related to patient age, sex, tumor type, distant metastases, and invasion of adjacent tissue and lymph nodes [7].

Thyroid tumors are divided into follicular-derived and neuroendocrine C-cell-derived cancers. Greater than 95% of thyroid cancer is DTC, which is follicular-derived thyroid cancer and can be further divided into well-DTC and poorly-DTC (more progressive than well DTC) [8]. Well DTC is a composite of papillary thyroid cancer (PTC), follicular thyroid cancer (FTC), and Hurthle cell thyroid cancer. Of these, papillary thyroid cancer is the most common thyroid cancer with the best prognosis, whereas follicular, Hurthle cell, poorly-differentiated, and C-cell derived thyroid cancers are relatively uncommon but have a high metastatic risk to the lung and bone [7]. Moreover, the increasing diagnostic rate of papillary thyroid cancers is regarded as the leading reason for increasing thyroid cancer incidence, in contrast, the incidence rate of other subtypes has been stable in the past 30 years [9].

Despite the generally stable course, favorable prognosis, and low mortality of thyroid cancer, the rate of local recurrence and distant metastases of DTC approaches 10% to 30%, which depends on the length of follow-up [10,11]. A previous study found that DTC can recur even up to 20 years after the initial diagnosis [12], therefore, a long-term follow-up of patients with DTC is essential [13]. Notably, several studies have investigated the factors related to DTC relapse. However, heterogenicity exists among these studies, and the results indicated the associations between early-onset and recurrence [14]. More specifically, the earlier DTC occurred, the more likely it was to recur. Therefore, timely diagnosis of DTC recurrence is critical.

1.2. Imaging Techniques for DTC Detection

Additionally, the discrimination and identification of thyroid cancer nodules and thyroid benign nodules are important. In most cases, the initial presentation of thyroid cancer is a thyroid nodule [15], however, less than 10% of DTCs appear in the thyroid nodules [16]. Given various factors including age, sex, family history, exposure to radiation, and nodule size that could affect the shift from thyroid nodules to cancer [17], responding to this shift in a timely manner is necessary. Differentiating early malignant tumors from benign tumors and providing definite staging are key challenges for diagnosing and treating thyroid cancer. Moreover, estimating tumor progression or predicting prognosis precisely can significantly aid physicians in making clinical decisions regarding treatment strategies in patients with thyroid cancer. Palpation of the thyroid and cervical lymph nodes remains easiest and least expensive routine detection method, but this method is also the least sensitive [18,19]. In contrast, biopsy and histopathological examination are typically the diagnostic gold standard for thyroid cancer [20]. However, fine-needle aspiration biopsy (FNAB) usually samples a small portion of the lesions; thus, this method could provide limited information regarding tumor heterogeneity and may lead to missed diagnoses. Notably, a proportion of patients are still intractable to invasive examination for screening making it difficult to repeat pathological assessments. Noninvasive imaging examinations including high-resolution ultrasound, magnetic resonance imaging (MRI), computed tomography (CT), single-photon emission computed tomography (SPECT), positron emission tomography (PET), and PET/CT, are also playing an increasingly important role in initial tumor screening, staging, restaging, management, and posttreatment follow-up [21]. Of these, high-resolution ultrasound remains the sole fundamental imaging method in the diagnosis and screening of thyroid nodules and cancer [22]. High-resolution ultrasound is a safe noninvasive imaging technique that could aid in enhancing the early detection of pathologies [23].

Ultrasound is based on the pulse-echo principle that makes it possible to determine the thyroid size, location, number, and morphology of individual nodules, and occult nodules omitted by physical examination [18], and present these findings in a single cross-sectional B-scan image. The suspicious ultrasound features of malignant thyroid nodules exhibit the following characteristics: solid nodule structure, hypoechogenicity, taller-than-wide shape, irregular margin, microcalcification, and invasion of surrounding tissue [18,24]. Nodules that present pure cystic or cystic components that represent greater than 50% of nodule volume tend to be benign [25]. Despite its widespread availability and radiation-free features, the diagnosis significantly relies on the radiologists' experience and subjective judgments, which limits the ability to make an objective diagnosis. Although neck ultrasound is the primary method used to investigate palpable thyroid masses, suspicious neck masses are typically initially screened through CT or MRI examination. Some features may be specific, whereas others may be incidental findings [26]. CT and MRI provide evidence for detecting lymph node metastasis as well as evaluating the invasion of adjacent tissue and organs with the features of cross-sectional imaging and reconstruction function [27]. It has been reported that the CT use rate in the examination of the neck and cervical spine has increased rapidly and is greater than that of ultrasound in the United States [28]. A previous study also verified the value of CT in detecting incidental thyroid nodules and hypothesized that CT imaging may be the current trend rather than ultrasound [29]. Nevertheless, CT also has an obvious limitation given that contrast-enhanced CT with iodinated contrast medium would delay subsequent radioactive iodine therapy [30]. Conversely, based on gadolinium-based contrast agents, MRI can be employed without interfering with radioiodine administration despite the requirement for a longer scan time. In addition, with its higher soft-tissue contrast, MRI combined with diffusion-weighted imaging (DWI) sequences could provide qualitative and quantitative information about tumor lesions at the cell level. DWI has been applied to assess the differentiation of benign and malignant thyroid tumors for several years [31,32]. A recent study verified the potential advantages of DWI in predicting aggressive histological features of thyroid carcinoma [33].

Nuclear medicine examinations have been used in the diagnosis, treatment, and surgical management of thyroid disease. Given the high avidity of radioiodine in functioning thyroid tissues, 131I whole-body scintigraphy (WBS) has a high value in tumor and metastasis detection [34]. WBS is also regarded as a routine diagnostic procedure for DTC patients with thyroidectomy [35]. However, WBS cannot provide a precise anatomic location, which greatly constrains its potential value. Compared with WBS, SPECT/CT not only enables anatomic localization of the tumor but also has higher sensitivity (50%) and specificity (100%) [36]. Besides, PET/CT or PET/MRI is also a relatively high sensitivity imaging technique in the evaluation of recurrent or metastatic tumors. A meta-analysis calculated that the pooled sensitivity was as high as 93.5% for PET/CT in detecting recurrent or metastatic DTC [37]. In addition, PET/CT can detect 21.2% of lymph nodes and soft tissue lesions that were missed by ultrasound [38]. Compared with PET/CT, PET/MRI has low radiation, but the high costs of this method should also be considered. Although some reports have demonstrated the value of the nuclear medicine approach applied in thyroid cancer, underlying issues, such as cost-effectiveness, universality, and radiation, require further discussion. Notwithstanding the above strengths, the current imaging technologies for tumor classification and prediction remain limited. Radiomics is an emerging field that involves segmenting lesions, extracting quantitative radiology features from medical images, and constructing models to classify or predict disease. The current review focuses on the radiomics characteristics of DTC and reviews the classification and prediction ability of radiomics for DTC.

2. Introduction to Radiomics

2.1. The Definition of Radiomics

Radiomics is defined as quantitative mapping that is used to construct a prediction model by extracting and analyzing medical image features related to the prediction target, including clinical endpoints and genomic features [39]. Radiomic features capture tissue and lesion characteristics, such as heterogeneity and shape, and may be used for clinical problem solving alone or in combination with demographic, histologic, genomic, or proteomic data. As an important innovation, medical image analysis automatically extracts a large number of quantitative features of medical images in a high-throughput manner. The use of radiomics in medical image analysis represents a significant improvement [40].

Radiomics research is based on the hypothesis that this type of automatic or semiautomatic software can provide better analysis of medical image data than human doctors due to the increased number of image features revealed by conventional and novel medical imaging that cannot be recognized by human doctors [41]. More specifically, the technology is based on the hypothesis that genomics and proteomics patterns can be expressed in terms of macroscopic image-based features [40].

2.2. Radiomic Features

Compared with the so-called "semantic" qualitative features, which are typically subjectively defined by radiologists, radiologic features can be regarded as quantitative features and are generally divided into shape, first-order statistics, second-order statistics, and higher-order statistics [42]. Familiarity with core principles of radiomic features may facilitate interpretation of results and preselection of features for specific applications.

Shape features represent geometric relations that mainly refer to two-dimensional or three-dimensional image features derived from ROIs, such as tumor volume, surface area, tumor sphericity, and tumor compactness [43].

The first-order statistics features or histogram-based features are derived from the statistical moments of the image intensity histogram and based on the image intensity distribution represented by histograms that characterize the distribution of individual pixel or voxel intensity values within. Features, such as uniformity, asymmetry, kurtosis, and skewness, can also be used to extract other features, such as image energy and entropy [43,44].

Second-order statistical features, which are also known as texture features, quantify intratumoral heterogeneity and explain the spatial interdependence or cooccurrence of information between adjacent voxels [42]. Textural features are not directly computed from the original image but from different descriptive matrices that already encode specific spatial relations between pixels or voxels in the original image. In the original image, there are some matrices of the spatial relationship between the intensity of the encoded image from which a large number of texture features can be calculated. The gray value distribution matrix (GLCM) of cooccurrence voxels in the gray level co-occurrence matrix is one of the most commonly used second-order features in radiomics [45,46]. The neighborhood gray-level different matrix (NGLDM) and the gray-level run-length matrix (GLRLM) are also common. Higher-order statistical features are typically calculated using statistical methods after applying a specific mathematical transformation (filter). For example, repeating patterns, noise suppression, edge enhancement, histogram-oriented gradients, or local binary patterns (LBPs) can be identified. The applied mathematical transformations or filters include Laplacian transformations of Gaussian-filtered images (Laplacian-of-Gaussian), wavelet or Fourier transformations, Minkowski functionals, or fractal analysis [47].

2.3. The Workflow of Radiomics

Radiomics analysis can be achieved by two methods. The first method includes conventional and common typical methods that are used to determine the region of interest (ROI) of the medical image first and then extract the radiomics features from the ROI and analyze the clinical problem [48]. The second method is less applied but pointed out by the previous review, it works based on the radiomics images directly but not the radiomics data derived from conventional images, it is also helpful to recognize ROIs reliably [41].

Radiomics analyses begin with the choice of a disease and image protocol. When targeting disease and image protocols are selected, the classical radiomics process can be divided into the following four steps: selection of the regions of interest, radiomics feature extraction, analysis, and modeling [49]. Figure 1 illustrates the workflow of radiomics for thyroid disease.

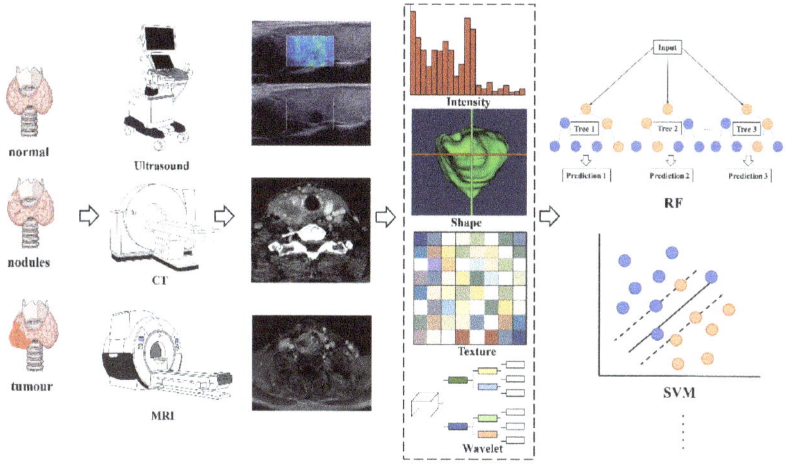

Figure 1. The flowchart shows the workflow of radiomics and its application in thyroid cancer or nodule classification and prediction. Abbreviations: RF—random forest; SVM—support vector machine.

ROIs are commonly delineated by professional radiologists manually or by special software in a semiautomatic or fully automatic manner. In the feature extraction stage, hundreds of candidate radiomic features are typically extracted theoretically to be used as the input of the prediction model, but the number of model parameters will increase exponentially afterward. Moreover, radiation features generally show a high degree of correlation with each other, indicating data redundancy. Thus, some features can be discarded, whereas other features can be grouped and replaced by representative features. Therefore, a large number of candidate features must be removed or transformed via a process called dimensionality reduction [47].

After feature selection, a mathematical model can be established to predict or solve targeted medical problems, such as the existence of specific gene mutations or tumor recurrence. Radiation features can be modeled in many different ways, ranging from statistical models to machine learning methods, depending on the clinical problems to be solved [50]. The most popular algorithms in radiomics are linear regression and logistic regression, decision trees (such as random forests), support vector machines (SVMs), neural networks, and Cox proportional hazards models with censored survival data.

2.4. Clinical Applications of Radiomics

The application and research potential of radiomics are still being explored. However, based on published studies, the clinical application of radiomics can be classified into the following three categories: radiogenomics (linking imaging data to biology), diagnosis of diseases, and clinical outcome prediction, including treatment response, recurrent disease, and survival time [47,51]. However, radiomic studies of thyroid cancer mainly involve the latter two categories.

3. Literature Search Strategy

We conducted a comprehensive literature review from the PubMed, Web of Science and Google Scholar databases for papers published before February 2021, independently. English-language filters were applied in the process of searching. Standard searches were done with the following keywords: 'thyroid cancer', 'differentiated thyroid cancer', 'thyroid nodules', and 'radiomics'. The reference lists were manually checked to identify additional relevant studies. We followed The Preferred Reporting Items for Systematic Reviews and Meta-Analysis (PRISMA) guidelines to select relevant studies [52] (Figure 2).

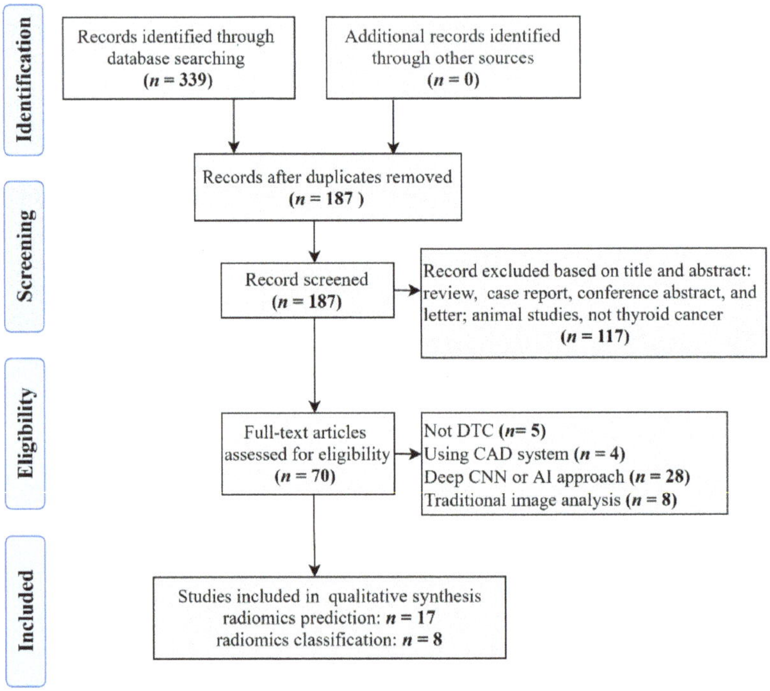

Figure 2. Flow diagram for the identification and exclusion of studies in radiomics application in differentiated thyroid cancer and nodules. Abbreviations: DTC—differentiated thyroid cancer; CAD—computer-aided detection; CNN—convolutional neural networks; AI—artificial intelligence.

4. Radiomics in Thyroid Cancer Prediction

As mentioned above, radiomics aids in cancer detection, diagnosis, prediction of prognosis, evaluation of tumor status, treatment response, and local or distant metastasis [50]. Of these, the predictive value has been determined in various cancers and has been a research hotspot in recent years. Table 1 showed the predictive value of radiomics applied in DTC, Table 1 was organized according to a sequential order of prediction category, imaging method, and published time.

Metastasis is an important indicator of tumor progression [53]. Lymph node (LN) metastasis is closely related to local recurrence, distant metastasis, and thyroid stage, which further indicates the surgical plan [54,55]. Thus, the judgment of LN metastasis is important. Although a small proportion of patients report LN metastasis, those patients with suspicious abnormalities would also be suggested to undergo fine-needle aspiration biopsy (FNA) and prophylactic lymph node dissection (LND). These invasive examinations seem to be unsuitable for those people without LN metastasis. Therefore, it is important to identify a noninvasive approach to pinpoint patients with high-risk LN metastasis in clinical practice. Liu et al. [56] compared the radiomics prediction ability to estimate the LN status among B-mode ultrasound (B-US), strain elastography ultrasound (SE-US) images, and the combination of these two images. As was hypothesized, the combination group showed a better prediction ability than a single image. However, given that only 75 patients were recruited and no validation analysis was performed in this study, the results should be interpreted with caution. Furthermore, the same research team included 450 patients and divided them into training and validation datasets to verify the radiomics evaluation of US thyroid images to predict LN metastasis in PTC patients [57]. This study partly validated their previous conclusion that the features ultimately selected performed equally well regarding the radiomics evaluation. PTC patients with or without LN metastasis showed different radiomics signatures. Jiang et al. [58] extracted radiomics features from both shear-wave elastography (SWE) images and B-mode ultrasound (BMUS) images. They calculated the Rad-score to distinguish patients with high metastasis risk. Then they built and compared the value of radiomics nomogram and clinical nomogram in predicting the LN stage. They concluded that the nomogram based on SEW radiomics signatures performed well in predicting LN status. Li et al. [59] also verified the value of ultrasound radiomics features in predicting LN metastasis. The radiomics features had a larger AUC than the ultrasound features of microcalcifications and an irregular shape.

Although CT and MRI are not exceedingly superior to ultrasound in thyroid cancer diagnosis, CT-based and MRI-based radiomics performed equally as well regarding their predictive value. The ability of CT radiomics signature to predict LN metastasis was initially reported by Lu et al [60]. This group built an SVM model and found that the radiomics signature showed a better predictive value of LN metastasis than any single radiomics signature. They concluded that the radiomics nomogram adds predictive power to LN metastasis. Hu et al. [61] initially applied multimodal MRI radiomics to predict LN metastasis in patients with PTC, and Zhang et al. [62] extracted radiomics features from T2WI and T2WI-fat-suppression (T2WI-FS) images to test and validate the predictive value of LN metastasis. These studies partly demonstrated that MRI-based radiomics can scientifically, quantitatively, and accurately predict LN metastasis in PTC patients, thereby, reducing unnecessary surgery.

LN metastasis is more likely to occur in central regions followed by lateral regions [3]. Lateral LN metastasis exhibits a higher recurrence rate and a poorer prognosis than central LN metastasis [63,64]. A recent study developed an ultrasound-based radiomics nomogram to assess its predictive value for central neck lymph node metastasis in PTC patients [65]. The prediction model showed good accuracy, sensitivity, specificity, and AUC values in both the training dataset and validation dataset. Afterward, the predictive value of ultrasound radiomics for lateral cervical LN metastasis was successively investigated in two studies. Tong et al. [66] retrospectively recruited 840 patients with PTC and extracted radiomics features from their preoperative ultrasound images. These researchers also established a radiomics-based nomogram to predict lateral LN metastasis. This radiomic nomogram presented good discrimination in both training and validation datasets and may therefore have clinical application. More interestingly, one study found a link between ultrasound radiomic features of the primary tumor and the status of lateral LN metastasis [67]. The key and interesting part of this study was that it focused on the radiomics features of thyroid primary tumors in predicting lateral LN metastasis but not the LN itself, which may facilitate the early detection of metastases.

Although the results of the abovementioned studies on the predictive value of ultrasound radiomics were largely positive in nature, the main limitation of the lack of multicenter and external validation could not be overlooked. A recent relatively robust study filled this gap. Yu et al. [3] first focused on the diagnostic value of ultrasound radiomics under a multicenter, cross-machine, multi-operator scenario. Based on B-mode ultrasound images of thyroid lesions, they established and compared four models including clinical statistical model (SM), traditional radiomics model (RM), non-transfer learning model, and transfer learning radiomics (TLR) model to predict the risk of LN metastasis in PTC patients. Of these, the TLR model showed the highest sensitivity and specificity in both the main and external cohorts. Then, a recent study that is in preprint performed an external validation based on CT radiomics indicating the good performance of this method in the prediction of LN metastasis [68]. To some extent, this study adds strength and validity to previous ultrasound-based radiomics studies.

Besides, the predictive value of radiomics was also applied in other aspects, such as the prediction of distant metastasis [69], tumor extrathyroidal extension [70,71], disease-free survival [72], and BRAF mutation [73]. The aggressiveness of tumors is classified based on various features, such as extrathyroidal extension; aggressive pathological subtypes, such as tumors with tall cells, tumors with columnar cells, and the hobnail variant; lymph node involvement; and distant metastasis [74]. A recent study found that multiparametric MRI-based radiomics combined with a machine learning approach can accurately distinguish aggressive PTC patients from nonaggressive patients, which illustrated the role of radiomics in predicting aggressive tumors [75]. Distant metastasis of DTC is uncommon; however, FTC is more likely to have distant metastasis than PTC. It has been reported that the bone metastasis rate in FTC ranges from 7 to 28%, whereas that for PTC is only 1.4–7% [76]. Kwon et al. [69] thus evaluated the capability of ultrasound-based radiomic features to predict distant metastasis of FTC. This study is based on radiomics analysis and a machine learning approach, and multivariate analysis indicated that the radiomic signature and widely invasive histology are related to distant metastasis. Moreover, the AUC of the thyroid ultrasound radiomic signature in predicting distant metastasis was as high as 0.93, demonstrating good predictive performance. The extrathyroidal extension in patients with DTC is also an important factor to consider when determining the surgical modality. Chen et al. [70] selected five CT-based radiomics features that were closely related to the extrathyroidal extension of PTC patients. A CT-based radiomics nomogram was built and showed good predictive value in extrathyroidal extension. This excellent predictive performance for tumor extrathyroidal extension was also verified in an MRI-based radiomics preprint [71]. Regarding "disease-free" cancers, DTC has an overall good disease-free survival after treatment and long-term outcomes [77]. Despite being called a "happy cancer", tumor progression contributes to the 1.4–5.2% mortality rate of thyroid cancer [78,79]. A retrospective study included 768 PTC patients, extracted radiomics features from ultrasound images, and constructed a radiomics signature based on LASSO regression. Finally, a Rad-score was calculated to stratify the patients into high- and low-risk DFS [72]. Furthermore, based on recent progress in molecular genetics, gene-specific information has provided insights into the biology of the tumor, prediction of prognosis, and potential therapeutic targets [80]. The B-Raf proto-oncogene serine/threonine kinase (BRAF) mutation is involved in the pathogenesis of PTC and is related to tumor progression, recurrence, and mortality [73]. In addition, shedding light on the mutational status of thyroid cancer could help clinicians evaluate the tumor response to new drugs, such as tyrosine kinase inhibitors. Thus, if we can predict genes mutated in thyroid cancer through convenient and feasible approaches, this information would contribute to improving tumor diagnosis, judging the prognosis, and personalizing the treatment. To date, two studies have applied radiomics to estimate BRAF mutations in PTC patients [73,81]. These two studies offered a consistent outcome that ultrasound radiomics has a limited value in predicting BRAF nutation. This result indicated that the relationship between ultrasound radiomics and gene mutation may not be as good as expected.

Table 1. Studies used radiomics for the prediction of metastasis, tumor progression, treatment response, and gene mutation.

Reference	Prediction Category	No. Patients	Imaging Method	ROI Segmentation Method	No. Radiomics Features	Model Construction	Validation Method	Sensitivity (%)	Specificity (%)	Accuracy (%)	AUC
Liu et al. (2018) [56]	LNM	75	US and SEUS	manual	US + SWE: 25 US: 36 SWE: 9	SVM	LOOCV	US + SEUS: 77 US: 63 SEUS: 71	US + SEUS: 88 US: 89 SEUS: 75	US + SEUS:85 US: 83 SEUS: 74	US+SEUS: 0.90 US: 0.81 SEUS: 0.80
Liu et al. (2019) [57]	LNM	450	US images	manual	50	SVM	10-fold CV	67.9	72.5	71.1	0.783
Jiang et al. (2019) [58]	LNM	training: 147 EV: 90	SWE images	manual	4	LASSO logistic regression	10-fold CV	training: 80.67 EV: 86.84	training: 82.7 EV: 73.08	training: 78.91 EV: 78.89	training: 0.851 EV: 0.832
Li et al. (2020) [59]	LNM	126	US images	manual	91	hypothesis-testing and bagging	NA	training: 90 test: 72.7	training: 86 test: 80	NA	training: 0.759 test: 0.803
Zhou et al. (2020) [65]	LNM	training: 609 test: 326	US images	manual	23	LASSO logistic regression	NA	training: 82.5 test: 81.6	training: 78.6 test: 81.0	training: 79.8 test: 81.2	training: 0.87 test: 0.858
Tong et al. (2020) [66]	LNM	training: 600 test: 286	US images	manual	21	LASSO logistic regression	NA	training: 74.5 test: 77.4	training: 82.6 test: 83.1	NA	training: 0.877 test:0.862
Park et al. (2020) [67]	LNM	training: 400 test: 368	US images	manual	14	LASSO logistic regression	10-fold CV	NA	NA	NA	training: 0.71 test: 0.621
Yu et al. (2020) [3]	LNM	training: 1013 IT1: 368 IT2: 513	US images	manual	NA	TLR;SM;RM;NTLR	NA	SM: 72 (training); 43 (IT1); 68 (IT2) RM: 71 (training); 36 (IT1); 47 (IT2) NTLR: 75 (training); 71 (IT1); 67 (IT2) TLR: 94 (training); 83 (IT1); 95 (IT2)	SM: 82 (training); 87 (IT1); 67 (IT2) RM: 57 (training); 72 (IT1); 69 (IT2) NTLR: 81 (training); 81 (IT1); 78 (IT2) TLR: 77 (training); 89 (IT1); 75 (IT2)	SM: 77 (training); 61 (IT1); 67 (IT2) RM: 62 (training); 51 (IT1); 60 (IT2) NTLR: 79 (training); 75 (IT1); 73 (IT2) TLR: 84 (training); 86 (IT1); 84 (IT2)	SM: 0.83(training); 0.67(IT1); 0.67(IT2) RM: 0.64(training); 0.55(IT1); 0.57(IT2) NTLR: 0.82(training); 0.81(IT1); 0.79(IT2) TLR: 0.93(training); 0.93(IT1); 0.93(IT2)

Table 1. *Cont.*

Reference	Prediction Category	No. Patients	Imaging Method	ROI Segmentation Method	No. Radiomics Features	Model Construction	Validation Method	Sensitivity (%)	Specificity (%)	Accuracy (%)	AUC
Lu et al. (2019) [60]	LNM	training: 154 test: 67	CT	manual	8 radiomic sub-signatures	SVM	NA	NA	NA	training: 73.4 test: 64.2	training: 0.759 test: 0.706
Hu et al. (2020) [61]	LNM	training: 90 test: 39	MRI	manual	30	LASSO logistic regression	NA	T2WI model: 62.2 DWI model: 86.7 T1C+ model: 68.9 Combined model: 88.9	T2WI model: 87.2 DWI model: 70.2 T1C+ model: 83 Combined model: 72.3	T2WI model: 75.0 DWI model: 78.3 T1C+ model: 76.1 Combined model: 80.4	T2WI model: 0.819 DWI model: 0.826 T1C+ model: 0.808 Combined model: 0.835
Zhang et al. (2020) [62]	LNM	61	MRI	manual	10	RF	LOOCV	T2WI: 83 T2WI-FS: 83	T2WI: 100 T2WI-FS: 90	T2WI: 87 T2WI-FS: 82	T2WI: 0.85 T2WI-FS: 0.80
Kwon et al. (2020) [69]	DM	169	US images	manual	6	SVM	5-fold CV	training: 92 test: 80	training: 87 test: 87	training: 88 test: 85	training: 0.93 test: 0.90
Wang et al. (2019) [75]	Aggressiveness	120	MRI	manual	5	LSSO + GBC LSVM + LRCV LSVM + PAC LSVM + LSVC	10-fold CV	NA	NA	NA	train: 0.874; 0.979;0.971; 0.805; 0.974 test: 0.915; 0.731; 0.731; 0.885; 0.708
Chen et al. (2020) [70]	ETE	training: 437 test: 187	CT	manual	5	LASSO logistic regression	10-fold CV	NA	NA	NA	training: 0.791 test: 0.772
Park et al. (2019) [72]	DFS	768	US images	manual	40	LASSO COX regression	10-fold CV	NA	NA	NA	0.777 (C index)

Table 1. *Cont.*

Reference	Prediction Category	No. Patients	Imaging Method	ROI Segmentation Method	No. Radiomics Features	Model Construction	Validation Method	Sensitivity (%)	Specificity (%)	Accuracy (%)	AUC
Yoon et al. (2020) [73]	BRAF Mutation	training: 387 test: 140	US images	manual	8	LASSO logistic regression	NA	NA	NA	NA	training: 0.718 (C index) test: 0.629 (C index)
Kwon et al. (2020) [81]	BRAF Mutation	96 patients	US images	manual	43	logistic regression SVM RF	5-fold CV	66.8 (mRMR)	61.8 (mRMR)	64.3 (mRMR)	0.65 (mRMR)

Abbreviations: ROI—region of interest; AUC—area under the curve of receiver operating characteristic curve; LMN—lymph node metastasis; US—ultrasound; SEUS—strain elastography ultrasound; SWE—shear-wave elastography; CT—computer tomography; SVM—support vector machine; RF—random forest; LASSO—least absolute shrinkage and selection operator; CV—cross-validation; LOOCV—leave-one-out CV; EV—external validation; TLR—transfer learning radiomics; SM—statistical model; RM—traditional radiomics model; NTLR—non-transfer learning radiomics; IT—independent set; DM—distance metastasis; MRI—magnetic resonance imaging; ETE—extrathyroidal extension; DFS—disease-free survival; LSVM—linear support vector machine; LR—CV-logistic regression classifier with cross-validation; PAC—passive aggressive classifier; LSVC—linear support vector classification; mRMR—minimum redundancy maximum relevance; NA—not applicable.

5. Radiomics in Thyroid Cancer and Nodule Classification

Thyroid cancer nodules are common in thyroid disease. The prevalence of thyroid nodules is approximately 67% in adults [82]. It has been reported that approximately 10% of patients with detected thyroid nodules are diagnosed with malignancy [83]. LN metastasis indicates rapid progression and poor prognosis in thyroid cancer; however, only a small portion of patients will develop metastasis [56]. Therefore, special attention needs to be paid to the differentiation of malignant and benign nodules. Table 2 presents studies focusing on the classification value of radiomics in DTC.

Machine learning or deep learning-based modalities are an important step in the processing of radiomics data. Machine learning approaches typically manually select and delimitate a set of few ROIs on the images; then, machine learning algorithms, such as support vector machine (SVM), random forest, and least absolute shrinkage and selection operator (LASSO), are applied to build a model. Prochazka et al. [84] used histogram analysis and segmentation-based fractal texture analysis algorithms combined with SVM and random forest classifiers to distinguish malignant nodules from benign nodules in ultrasound images. Their results indicated that the histogram feature was the most important parameter in classification, and both SVM (94.64%) and random forests (92.42%) achieved high accuracy. Colakoglu et al. [85] attempted to differentiate benign and malignant thyroid nodules using texture analysis and random forest model construction. After testing the reproducibility of all texture features, they finally screened seven texture features from ultrasound images, including one histogram (HistPerc 99), one HOG (HogO8b2), four GRLMs (GrlmHRLNonUni, GrlmHMGLevNonUni, GrlmNRLNonUni, and GrlmZRLNonUni), and one GLCM (GlcmZ3AngScMom), in a random forest model. The diagnostic sensitivity, specificity, and accuracy were 85.2%, 87.9%, and 86.8%, respectively. Notably, the area under the curve (AUC) of the model was 0.92, indicating good performance. Furthermore, a recent ultrasound-image-based retrospective study recruited 2558 patients (2831 nodules), extracted radiomics features using an in-house texture analysis algorithm, and applied the LASSO method to calculate the radiomics score [86]. They used this radiomics score to determine a cutoff value that can help classify the nodules as benign or malignant. The AUCs of the radiomics score in the training and testing datasets were 0.85 and 0.83, respectively, indicating discriminative power. Furthermore, Yoon et al. [87] also applied texture analysis and the LASSO method in US images to predict malignant thyroid nodules with indeterminate cytology, demonstrating good predictive performance. Zhao et al. [88] compared the diagnostic performance and unnecessary FNAB rate for thyroid nodules of assisted visual-based and radiomic-based machine learning approaches in ultrasound images. In this study, ten machine learning classifiers, including decision tree, naïve Bayes, k nearest neighbors (KNN), logistics regression, SVM, KNN-based bagging, random forest, extremely randomized trees (XGBoost), multilayer perception, and gradient boosting tree classifiers, were verified. The results of the assisted visual-based machine learning approach indicated superior performance in AUC, sensitivity, and specificity in both the training dataset and internal validation dataset. Furthermore, a similar study design was applied to a CT-based radiomics study [89]. This study ultimately included 13 radiomics features after LASSO logistic regression. An SVM model was constructed and compared with seven other machine learning models. The study concluded that the SVM model exhibited good discrimination performance, whereas random forest had the highest stability.

Table 2. Studies used radiomics to differentiate malignant from benign nodules.

Reference	No. Patients/Nodules	Imaging Method	ROI Segmentation	No. Radiomics Features	Model Construction	Validation Method	Sensitivity (%)	Specificity (%)	Accuracy (%)	AUC
Prochazka et al. (2019) [84]	40 nodules in 40 patients	US images	threshold	NA	SVM/RF	LOOCV	NA	NA	NA	RF: 0.9242 SVM: 0.9464
Colakoglu et al. (2019) [85]	235 nodules in 198 patients	US images	manual	7	RF	10-fold CV	85.2	87.9	86.8	0.92
Park et al. (2020) [86]	1624 nodules in 1609 patients training: 1299; test: 325	US images	manual	66	LASSO logistic regression	10-fold CV	70.6	79.8	77.8	0.75
Zhao et al. (2020) [88]	training: 743 nodules in 720 patients test: 106 nodules in 102 patients	US and SWE images	manual	26	SVM	NA	74.4 (US) 70.7 (US + SWE)	72.3 (US) 79.4 (US + SWE)	73.1 (US) 76.2 (US + SWE)	US: 0.798 US + SWE: 0.834
Zhou et al. (2020) [90]	1750 nodules in 1734 patients	US images	semi-automated	NA	Deep learning	NA	training: 90.1 IV: 89.3 EV: 89.5	training: 82.7 IV: 83.5 EV: 84.1	NA	training: 0.96 IV: 0.95 EV: 0.97
Wang et al. (2020) [91]	3120 nodules in 1040 patients	US images	semi-automated /manual	302	SVM	NA	51.19	75.77	66.81	0.6371
Yoon et al. (2020) [87]	155 nodules in 154 patients	US images	manual	15	LASSO logistic regression	10-fold CV	NA	NA	NA	US + Clinical information: 0.839
Yao et al. (2020) [89]	1372 patients	CT images	manual	13	LASSO +RF	10-fold CV	68	82	74	0.82

Abbreviations: ROI—region of interest; AUC—area under the curve of receiver operating characteristic curve; SWE—shear-wave elastography; US—ultrasound; CT—computer tomography; SVM—support vector machine; RF—random forest; LASSO—least absolute shrinkage and selection operator; CV—cross-validation; LOOCV—leave-one-out CV; IV—internal validation; EV—external validation; NA—not applicable.

In addition, the ability to discriminate benign from malignant lesions using a deep learning radiomics approach has also been verified by researchers. Zhou et al. [90] employed the deep learning radiomics method to differentiate benign and malignant thyroid nodules in ultrasound images. This study found that the AUC of deep learning radiomics was greater than that of other deep learning models and traditional naked-eye observations. However, the current limitation of deep learning is its black box issue, making the conclusion difficult to interpret. The abovementioned radiomic-based and deep learning-based classifications are two methods applied in the detection of malignant nodules and metastatic cervical lymph nodes. However, research comparing the diagnostic ability between these two approaches is insufficient but essential. Wang et al. [91] extracted 302-dimensional statistical features from ultrasound images and applied mutual information and linear discriminant analysis to reduce dimensionality. These researchers reported that the accuracy of radiomics for the testing data was 66.81%, which was relatively lower than that of the deep learning approach (74.69%). Although the radiomics approach may not be dominant in this study, the interpretability of deep learning is a long-standing problem that remains elusive.

6. Limitations

Substantial radiomics studies have indicated the predictive value of radiomics in DTC; however, it is undeniable that there are also several limitations in radiomics. First, the 'black box' property of classifiers hampers the causal relationship, and the meaning of radiomics features extracted from grayscale images further hinders data interpretability. Second, radiomics is regarded as a 'population imaging' approach closely relying on different modalities and device parameters, which means variations in imaging protocols among institutions would lead to non-uniform data acquisition and thus influence generalizability. The good classification and prediction performance in a single center might not be generalized to patient cohorts from another center. Therefore, current original studies generally lack external validation. Third, although radiomics partially reflects the information at the molecular biological level, variations in tumor cells and the microenvironment as well as the retrospective nature of the studies represent limit the interpretation of the final results. Notably, based on current studies, the average diagnostic accuracy of radiomics is between 66% and 86%, even worse in the prediction of BRAF mutation, making the economic efficiency is an issue in need of attention and consideration. Furthermore, the reliability of the predictive performance and clinical application may be decreased by discussing the predictive value of radiomics itself without considering the influence of clinical information, such as tumor stages and therapy strategies. More importantly, the ethical issues regarding the use of radiomics in patient stratification and treatment response-based prognosis should also be treated with caution.

7. Conclusions

In summary, radiomics is a hot topic and a rapidly evolving field in medical imaging in general. There are still some technological and ethical limitations of radiomics aforementioned are required to be solved. Nevertheless, increased studies have proved the potential applications of radiomics for both the research and clinical lactation field. For prediction, the radiomics is seemly satisfactory to predict lymph node metastasis, distance metastasis, tumor aggressiveness and extrathyroidal extension, and disease-free survival. While previous original studies consistently negated the value of US radiomics in predicting BRAF mutations in DTC. This result may need to be thoroughly discussed to determine the predictive value of other imaging techniques, such as CT and MRI, and provide a direct or indirect relationship between radiomics and tumor mutations of thyroid cancer in the future study. For diagnosis, the current findings may facilitate breakthroughs in thyroid cancer and nodule classification based on a radiomics approach. These studies demonstrated the usefulness of radiomics in discriminating benign and malignant lesions regardless of the image types (US, CT, or MRI). Further studies should address two important issues: (1) optimize the algorithm and models to improve the accuracy of external validation thereby enhance the diagnostic capacity of radiomics; (2) analyze multi-model or multi-parameters imaging data with a larger sample as well as increase the possibility of clinical transformation.

Author Contributions: Y.C. (Yuan Cao) and X.Z. wrote the first draft of the paper; Y.C. (Yuan Cao), J.M., Y.C. (Yue Cheng) collected and selected the CT, MRI, and U.S. images; Y.C. (Yuan Cao), X.Z., W.D. and Z.J. edited the paper; Z.J. designed the research. All authors have read and agreed to the published version of the manuscript.

Funding: This study was supported by the National Natural Science Foundation of China (Grant Nos. 81771812 and 81971595), the Innovation Spark Project of Sichuan University (Grant No. 2019SCUH0003), and the 1·3·5 Project for Disciplines of Excellence–Clinical Research Incubation Project, West China Hospital, Sichuan University (Grant No. 2020HXFH005).

Institutional Review Board Statement: Not applicable.

Informed Consent Statement: Not applicable.

Data Availability Statement: No new data were created or analyzed in this study. Data sharing is not applicable to this article.

Acknowledgments: The author Yuan Cao thanks her friends Huaqian Zhang and Yun Bai for their guidance on scientific figures drawing.

Conflicts of Interest: The authors declare no conflict of interest.

References

1. Bychkov, A.; Saenko, V.; Nakashima, M.; Mitsutake, N.; Rogounovitch, T.; Nikitski, A.; Orim, F.; Yamashita, S. Patterns of FOXE1 expression in papillary thyroid carcinoma by immunohistochemistry. *Thyroid* **2013**, *23*, 817–828. [CrossRef]
2. Laetitia, G.; Sven, S.; Fabrice, J. Combinatorial Therapies in Thyroid Cancer: An Overview of Preclinical and Clinical Progresses. *Cells* **2020**, *9*, 830. [CrossRef]
3. Yu, J.; Deng, Y.; Liu, T.; Zhou, J.; Jia, X.; Xiao, T.; Zhou, S.; Li, J.; Guo, Y.; Wang, Y.; et al. Lymph node metastasis prediction of papillary thyroid carcinoma based on transfer learning radiomics. *Nat. Commun.* **2020**, *11*, 10. [CrossRef]
4. Sugino, K.; Nagahama, M.; Kitagawa, W.; Ohkuwa, K.; Uruno, T.; Matsuzu, K.; Suzuki, A.; Tomoda, C.; Hames, K.Y.; Akaishi, J.; et al. Distant Metastasis in Pediatric and Adolescent Differentiated Thyroid Cancer: Clinical Outcomes and Risk Factor Analyses. *J. Clin. Endocrinol. Metab.* **2020**, *105*, e3981–e3988. [CrossRef]
5. Piccardo, A.; Siri, G.; Raffa, S.; Castellana, M.; Foppiani, L.; Bottoni, G.; Ugolini, M.; Cistaro, A.; Catrambone, U.; Altrinetti, V.; et al. How to better stratify the risk of differentiated thyroid carcinomas: The key role of radioactive iodine therapy, age, and gender. *Eur. J. Nuclear Med. Mol. Imaging* **2021**, *48*, 822–830. [CrossRef]
6. Liang, W.; Guan, W.; Chen, R.; Wang, W.; Li, J.; Xu, K.; Li, C.; Ai, Q.; Lu, W.; Liang, H.; et al. Cancer patients in SARS-CoV-2 infection: A nationwide analysis in China. *Lancet Oncol.* **2020**, *21*, 335–337. [CrossRef]
7. Cabanillas, M.E.; McFadden, D.G.; Durante, C. Thyroid cancer. *Lancet* **2016**, *388*, 2783–2795. [CrossRef]
8. Howlader, N.; Noone, A.; Krapcho, M.; Miller, D.; Bishop, K.; Altekruse, S. *SEER Cancer Statistics Review, 1975–2013*; National Cancer Institute: Bethesda, MD, USA, 2015.
9. Filetti, S.; Durante, C.; Hartl, D.; Leboulleux, S.; Locati, L.D.; Newbold, K.; Papotti, M.G.; Berruti, A. Thyroid cancer: ESMO Clinical Practice Guidelines for diagnosis, treatment and follow-up†. *Ann. Oncol. Off. J. Eur. Soc. Med. Oncol.* **2019**, *30*, 1856–1883. [CrossRef]
10. Gao, L.; Lin, Y.; Jiang, Y.; Li, H.; Gao, Q.; Xi, X.; Wang, Y.; Yang, X.; Lai, X.; Zhu, S.; et al. Ultrasound characteristics of cervical lesions in patients with radioiodine refractory differentiated thyroid cancer: A strobe-compliant article. *Medicine* **2019**, *98*, e17876. [CrossRef] [PubMed]
11. Mazzaferri, E.L.; Jhiang, S.M. Differentiated thyroid cancer long-term impact of initial therapy. *Trans. Am. Clin. Climatol. Assoc.* **1995**, *106*, 151–168, discussion 168–170. [PubMed]
12. Mazzaferri, E.L.; Kloos, R.T. Clinical review 128: Current approaches to primary therapy for papillary and follicular thyroid cancer. *J. Clin. Endocrinol. Metab.* **2001**, *86*, 1447–1463. [CrossRef]
13. Cooper, D.S.; Doherty, G.M.; Haugen, B.R.; Kloos, R.T.; Lee, S.L.; Mandel, S.J.; Mazzaferri, E.L.; McIver, B.; Sherman, S.I. Tuttle RM: Management guidelines for patients with thyroid nodules and differentiated thyroid cancer. *Thyroid* **2006**, *16*, 109–142. [CrossRef]
14. Naing, S.; Collins, B.J.; Schneider, A.B. Clinical behavior of radiation-induced thyroid cancer: Factors related to recurrence. *Thyroid Off. J. Am. Thyroid. Assoc.* **2009**, *19*, 479–485. [CrossRef]

15. Park, J.Y.; Kim, W.Y.; Hwang, T.S.; Lee, S.S.; Kim, H.; Han, H.S.; Lim, S.D.; Kim, W.S.; Yoo, Y.B.; Park, K.S. BRAF and RAS mutations in follicular variants of papillary thyroid carcinoma. *Endocr. Pathol.* **2013**, *24*, 69–76. [CrossRef]
16. Dean, D.S.; Hay, I.D. Prognostic indicators in differentiated thyroid carcinoma. *Cancer Control. J. Moffitt Cancer Cent.* **2000**, *7*, 229–239. [CrossRef]
17. Hegedüs, L. Clinical practice. The thyroid nodule. *N. Engl. J. Med.* **2004**, *351*, 1764–1771. [CrossRef]
18. Wong, R.; Farrell, S.G.; Grossmann, M. Thyroid nodules: Diagnosis and management. *Med. J. Aust.* **2018**, *209*, 92–98. [CrossRef]
19. Dean, D.S.; Gharib, H. Epidemiology of thyroid nodules. *Best Pract. Res. Clin. Endocrinol. Metab.* **2008**, *22*, 901–911. [CrossRef]
20. Zolotov, S. Genetic Testing in Differentiated Thyroid Carcinoma: Indications and Clinical Implications. *Rambam Maimonides Med. J.* **2016**, *7*, e0009. [CrossRef]
21. Intenzo, C.M.; Dam, H.Q.; Manzone, T.A.; Kim, S.M. Imaging of the thyroid in benign and malignant disease. *Semin. Nuclear Med.* **2012**, *42*, 49–61. [CrossRef]
22. Wang, J.; He, X.; Ma, L.; Li, M.; Sun, L.; Jiang, J.; Zhou, Q. Multimode ultrasonic technique is recommended for the differential diagnosis of thyroid cancer. *PeerJ* **2020**, *8*, e9112. [CrossRef]
23. Sandhu, J.S.; Schmidt, R.A.; La Rivière, P.J. Full-field acoustomammography using an acousto-optic sensor. *Med. Phys.* **2009**, *36*, 2324–2327. [CrossRef]
24. Hoang, J.K.; Lee, W.K.; Lee, M.; Johnson, D.; Farrell, S. US Features of thyroid malignancy: Pearls and pitfalls. *Radiogr. A Rev. Publ. Radiol. Soc. N. Am. Inc.* **2007**, *27*, 847–860, discussion 845–861. [CrossRef]
25. Bonavita, J.A.; Mayo, J.; Babb, J.; Bennett, G.; Oweity, T.; Macari, M.; Yee, J. Pattern recognition of benign nodules at ultrasound of the thyroid: Which nodules can be left alone? *AJR Am. J. Roentgenol.* **2009**, *193*, 207–213. [CrossRef]
26. Hoang, J.K.; Branstetter, B.F.; Gafton, A.R.; Lee, W.K.; Glastonbury, C.M. Imaging of thyroid carcinoma with CT and MRI: Approaches to common scenarios. *Cancer Imaging* **2013**, *13*, 128–139. [CrossRef]
27. Rana, K.A.; Meyer, J.; Ibrahim, S.; Ralls, M.; Kent, P.M. The role of imaging of malignant bone tumors in children and young adults. *Curr. Probl. Cancer* **2013**, *37*, 181–191. [CrossRef]
28. Rao, V.M.; Levin, D.C.; Parker, L.; Frangos, A.J.; Sunshine, J.H. Trends in utilization rates of the various imaging modalities in emergency departments: Nationwide Medicare data from 2000 to 2008. *J. Am. Coll. Radiol.* **2011**, *8*, 706–709. [CrossRef] [PubMed]
29. Hoang, J.K.; Choudhury, K.R.; Eastwood, J.D.; Esclamado, R.M.; Lyman, G.H.; Shattuck, T.M.; Nguyen, X.V. An exponential growth in incidence of thyroid cancer: Trends and impact of CT imaging. *AJNR Am. J. Neuroradiol.* **2014**, *35*, 778–783. [CrossRef]
30. Marcus, C.; Whitworth, P.W.; Surasi, D.S.; Pai, S.I.; Subramaniam, R.M. PET/CT in the management of thyroid cancers. *AJR Am. J. Roentgenol.* **2014**, *202*, 1316–1329. [CrossRef]
31. Erdem, G.; Erdem, T.; Muammer, H.; Mutlu, D.Y.; Firat, A.K.; Sahin, I.; Alkan, A. Diffusion-weighted images differentiate benign from malignant thyroid nodules. *J. Magn. Reson. Imaging JMRI* **2010**, *31*, 94–100. [CrossRef]
32. Schueller-Weidekamm, C.; Kaserer, K.; Schueller, G.; Scheuba, C.; Ringl, H.; Weber, M.; Czerny, C.; Herneth, A. Can Quantitative Diffusion-Weighted MR Imaging Differentiate Benign and Malignant Cold Thyroid Nodules? Initial Results in 25 Patients. *Am. J. Neuroradiol.* **2008**, *30*, 417–422. [CrossRef]
33. Lu, Y.; Moreira, A.L.; Hatzoglou, V.; Stambuk, H.E.; Gonen, M.; Mazaheri, Y.; Deasy, J.O.; Shaha, A.R.; Tuttle, R.M.; Shukla-Dave, A. Using Diffusion-Weighted MRI to Predict Aggressive Histological Features in Papillary Thyroid Carcinoma: A Novel Tool for Pre-Operative Risk Stratification in Thyroid Cancer. *Thyroid* **2015**, *25*, 672–680. [CrossRef]
34. Oh, J.R.; Byun, B.H.; Hong, S.P.; Chong, A.; Kim, J.; Yoo, S.W.; Kang, S.R.; Kim, D.Y.; Song, H.C.; Bom, H.S.; et al. Comparison of ^{131}I whole-body imaging, ^{131}I SPECT/CT, and ^{18}F-FDG PET/CT in the detection of metastatic thyroid cancer. *Eur. J. Nuclear Med. Mol. Imaging* **2011**, *38*, 1459–1468. [CrossRef]
35. Spanu, A.; Nuvoli, S.; Marongiu, A.; Gelo, I.; Mele, L.; Piras, B.; Madeddu, G. Neck lymph node metastasis detection in patients with differentiated thyroid carcinoma (DTC) in long-term follow-up: A (131)I-SPECT/CT study. *BMC Cancer* **2020**, *20*, 239. [CrossRef] [PubMed]
36. Barwick, T.; Murray, I.; Megadmi, H.; Drake, W.M.; Plowman, P.N.; A Akker, S.; Chew, S.L.; Grossman, A.B.; Avril, N. Single photon emission computed tomography (SPECT)/computed tomography using Iodine-123 in patients with differentiated thyroid cancer: Additional value over whole body planar imaging and SPECT. *Eur. J. Endocrinol.* **2010**, *162*, 1131–1139. [CrossRef] [PubMed]
37. Dong, M.-J.; Liu, Z.-F.; Zhao, K.; Ruan, L.-X.; Wang, G.-L.; Yang, S.-Y.; Sun, F.; Luo, X.-G. Value of 18F-FDG-PET/PET-CT in differentiated thyroid carcinoma with radioiodine-negative whole-body scan: A meta-analysis. *Nuclear Med. Commun.* **2009**, *30*, 639–650. [CrossRef]
38. Seo, J.H.; Lee, S.W.; Ahn, B.-C.; Lee, J. Recurrence detection in differentiated thyroid cancer patients with elevated serum level of antithyroglobulin antibody: Special emphasis on using18F-FDG PET/CT. *Clin. Endocrinol.* **2010**, *72*, 558–563. [CrossRef] [PubMed]
39. Lambin, P.; Leijenaar, R.T.; Deist, T.M.; Peerlings, J.; De Jong, E.E.; Van Timmeren, J.; Sanduleanu, S.; LaRue, R.T.; Even, A.J.; Jochems, A.; et al. Radiomics: The bridge between medical imaging and personalized medicine. *Nat. Rev. Clin. Oncol.* **2017**, *14*, 749–762. [CrossRef]
40. Lambin, P.; Rios-Velazquez, E.; Leijenaar, R.; Carvalho, S.; van Stiphout, R.G.; Granton, P.; Zegers, C.M.; Gillies, R.; Boellard, R.; Dekker, A.; et al. Radiomics: Extracting more information from medical images using advanced feature analysis. *Eur. J. Cancer* **2012**, *48*, 441–446. [CrossRef]

41. Conti, A.; Duggento, A.; Indovina, I.; Guerrisi, M.; Toschi, N. Radiomics in breast cancer classification and prediction. In *Seminars in Cancer Biology*; Elsevier: Amsterdam, The Netherlands, 2020.
42. Rizzo, S.; Botta, F.; Raimondi, S.; Origgi, D.; Fanciullo, C.; Morganti, A.G.; Bellomi, M. Radiomics: The facts and the challenges of image analysis. *Eur. Radiol. Exp.* **2018**, *2*, 36. [CrossRef]
43. Van Griethuysen, J.J.M.; Fedorov, A.; Parmar, C.; Hosny, A.; Aucoin, N.; Narayan, V.; Beets-Tan, R.G.H.; Fillion-Robin, J.C.; Pieper, S.; Aerts, H.J.W.L. Computational Radiomics System to Decode the Radiographic Phenotype. *Cancer Res.* **2017**, *77*, e104–e107. [CrossRef] [PubMed]
44. Traverso, A.; Wee, L.; Dekker, A.; Gillies, R. Repeatability and Reproducibility of Radiomic Features: A Systematic Review. *Int. J. Radiat. Oncol. Biol. Phys.* **2018**, *102*, 1143–1158. [CrossRef] [PubMed]
45. Moyaa, L.; Zakeri, H.; Yamazakic, H.; Liuc, W.; Masa, E.; Koshimura, S. 3D gray level co-occurrence matrix and its application to identifying collapsed buildings. *ISPRS J. Photogramm. Remote Sens.* **2019**, *149*, 14–28. [CrossRef]
46. Ergen, B.; Baykara, M. Texture based feature extraction methods for content based medical image retrieval systems. *Bio-Med. Mater. Eng.* **2014**, *24*, 3055–3062. [CrossRef]
47. Mayerhoefer, M.E.; Materka, A.; Langs, G.; Häggström, I.; Szczypiński, P.; Gibbs, P.; Cook, G. Introduction to Radiomics. *J. Nuclear Med. Off. Publ. Soc. Nuclear Med.* **2020**, *61*, 488–495. [CrossRef]
48. Li, R.; Xing, L.; Napel, S.; Rubin, D.L. *Radiomics and Radiogenomics: Technical Basis and Clinical Applications*; CRC Press: Boca Raton, FL, USA, 2019.
49. Kumar, V.; Gu, Y.; Basu, S.; Berglund, A.; Eschrich, S.A.; Schabath, M.B.; Forster, K.; Aerts, H.J.; Dekker, A.; Fenstermacher, D.; et al. Radiomics: The process and the challenges. *Magn. Reson. Imaging* **2012**, *30*, 1234–1248. [CrossRef] [PubMed]
50. Gillies, R.J.; Kinahan, P.E.; Hricak, H. Radiomics: Images Are More than Pictures, They Are Data. *Radiology* **2016**, *278*, 563–577. [CrossRef]
51. Wilson, R.; Devaraj, A. Radiomics of pulmonary nodules and lung cancer. *Transl. Lung Cancer Res.* **2017**, *6*, 86–91. [CrossRef]
52. Moher, D.; Liberati, A.; Tetzlaff, J.; Altman, D.G.; The PRISMA Group. Preferred reporting items for systematic reviews and meta-analyses: The PRISMA statement. *BMJ (Clin. Res. Ed)* **2009**, *339*, b2535. [CrossRef]
53. Wu, Q.; Li, Y.; Wang, Y.; Hu, B. Sonographic features of primary tumor as independent predictive factors for lymph node metastasis in papillary thyroid carcinoma. *Clin. Transl. Oncol. Off. Publ. Fed. Span. Oncol. Soc. Natl. Cancer Inst. Mex.* **2015**, *17*, 830–834. [CrossRef] [PubMed]
54. Hartl, D.M.; Leboulleux, S.; Al Ghuzlan, A.; Baudin, E.; Chami, L.; Schlumberger, M.; Travagli, J.-P. Optimization of staging of the neck with prophylactic central and lateral neck dissection for papillary thyroid carcinoma. *Ann. Surg.* **2012**, *255*, 777–783. [CrossRef] [PubMed]
55. Viola, D.; Materazzi, G.; Valerio, L.; Molinaro, E.; Agate, L.; Faviana, P.; Seccia, V.; Sensi, E.; Romei, C.; Piaggi, P.; et al. Prophylactic central compartment lymph node dissection in papillary thyroid carcinoma: Clinical implications derived from the first prospective randomized controlled single institution study. *J. Clin. Endocrinol. Metab.* **2015**, *100*, 1316–1324. [CrossRef] [PubMed]
56. Liu, T.; Ge, X.; Yu, J.; Guo, Y.; Wang, Y.; Wang, W.; Cui, L. Comparison of the application of B-mode and strain elastography ultrasound in the estimation of lymph node metastasis of papillary thyroid carcinoma based on a radiomics approach. *Int. J. Comput. Assist. Radiol. Surg.* **2018**, *13*, 1617–1627. [CrossRef] [PubMed]
57. Liu, T.; Zhou, S.; Yu, J.; Guo, Y.; Wang, Y.; Zhou, J.; Chang, C. Prediction of Lymph Node Metastasis in Patients With Papillary Thyroid Carcinoma: A Radiomics Method Based on Preoperative Ultrasound Images. *Technol. Cancer Res. Treat.* **2019**, *18*, 1533033819831713. [CrossRef] [PubMed]
58. Jiang, M.; Li, C.; Tang, S.; Lv, W.; Yi, A.; Wang, B.; Yu, S.; Cui, X.; Dietrich, C.F. Nomogram Based on Shear-Wave Elastography Radiomics Can Improve Preoperative Cervical Lymph Node Staging for Papillary Thyroid Carcinoma. *Thyroid* **2020**, *30*, 885–897. [CrossRef] [PubMed]
59. Li, F.; Pan, D.; He, Y.; Wu, Y.; Peng, J.; Li, J.; Wang, Y.; Yang, H.; Chen, J. Using ultrasound features and radiomics analysis to predict lymph node metastasis in patients with thyroid cancer. *BMC Surg.* **2020**, *20*, 315. [CrossRef]
60. Lu, W.; Zhong, L.Z.; Dong, D.; Fang, M.J.; Dai, Q.; Leng, S.Y.; Zhang, L.W.; Sun, W.; Tian, J.; Zheng, J.J.; et al. Radiomic analysis for preoperative prediction of cervical lymph node metastasis in patients with papillary thyroid carcinoma. *Eur. J. Radiol.* **2019**, *118*, 231–238. [CrossRef]
61. Hu, W.; Wang, H.; Wei, R.; Wang, L.; Dai, Z.; Duan, S.; Ge, Y.; Wu, P.-Y.; Song, B. MRI-based radiomics analysis to predict preoperative lymph node metastasis in papillary thyroid carcinoma. *Gland. Surg.* **2020**, *9*, 1214–1226. [CrossRef]
62. Zhang, H.; Hu, S.; Wang, X.; He, J.; Liu, W.; Yu, C.; Sun, Z.; Ge, Y.; Duan, S. Prediction of Cervical Lymph Node Metastasis Using MRI Radiomics Approach in Papillary Thyroid Carcinoma: A Feasibility Study. *Technol. Cancer Res. Treat.* **2020**, *19*, 1533033820969451. [CrossRef]
63. Randolph, G.W.; Duh, Q.Y.; Heller, K.S.; LiVolsi, V.A.; Mandel, S.J.; Steward, D.L.; Tufano, R.P.; Tuttle, R.M. The prognostic significance of nodal metastases from papillary thyroid carcinoma can be stratified based on the size and number of metastatic lymph nodes, as well as the presence of extranodal extension. *Thyroid* **2012**, *22*, 1144–1152. [CrossRef]
64. Ito, Y.; Tomoda, C.; Uruno, T.; Takamura, Y.; Miya, A.; Kobayashi, K.; Matsuzuka, F.; Kuma, K.; Miyauchi, A. Ultrasonographically and anatomopathologically detectable node metastases in the lateral compartment as indicators of worse relapse-free survival in patients with papillary thyroid carcinoma. *World J. Surg.* **2005**, *29*, 917–920. [CrossRef] [PubMed]

65. Zhou, S.C.; Liu, T.T.; Zhou, J.; Huang, Y.X.; Guo, Y.; Yu, J.H.; Wang, Y.Y.; Chang, C. An Ultrasound Radiomics Nomogram for Preoperative Prediction of Central Neck Lymph Node Metastasis in Papillary Thyroid Carcinoma. *Front. Oncol.* **2020**, *10*, 1591. [CrossRef] [PubMed]
66. Tong, Y.; Li, J.; Huang, Y.; Zhou, J.; Liu, T.; Guo, Y.; Yu, J.; Zhou, S.; Wang, Y.; Chang, C. Ultrasound-Based Radiomic Nomogram for Predicting Lateral Cervical Lymph Node Metastasis in Papillary Thyroid Carcinoma. *Acad. Radiol.* **2020**. [CrossRef] [PubMed]
67. Park, V.Y.; Han, K.; Kim, H.J.; Lee, E.; Youk, J.H.; Kim, E.-K.; Moon, H.J.; Yoon, J.H.; Kwak, J.Y. Radiomics signature for prediction of lateral lymph node metastasis in conventional papillary thyroid carcinoma. *PLoS ONE* **2020**, *15*, e0227315. [CrossRef] [PubMed]
68. Han, Z.-J.; Wei, P.; Ding, Z.; Luo, D.; Qian, L.; Zhou, J.; Wang, H.; Cai, W.; Zhang, M. Computed Tomography Radiomics for the Preoperative Prediction of Cervical Lymph Node Metastasis in Papillary Thyroid Carcinoma: Development and External Validation. *Res. Sq.* **2020**. Available online: https://www.researchsquare.com/article/rs-26914/v1 (accessed on 18 November 2020).
69. Kwon, M.R.; Shin, J.H.; Park, H.; Cho, H.; Kim, E.; Hahn, S.Y. Radiomics Based on Thyroid Ultrasound Can Predict Distant Metastasis of Follicular Thyroid Carcinoma. *J. Clin. Med.* **2020**, *9*, 2156. [CrossRef] [PubMed]
70. Chen, B.; Zhong, L.Z.; Dong, D.; Zheng, J.J.; Fang, M.J.; Yu, C.Y.; Dai, Q.; Zhang, L.W.; Tian, J.; Lu, W.; et al. Computed Tomography Radiomic Nomogram for Preoperative Prediction of Extrathyroidal Extension in Papillary Thyroid Carcinoma. *Front. Oncol.* **2019**, *9*, 9. [CrossRef] [PubMed]
71. Wei, R.; Wang, H.; Wang, L.; Hu, W.; Sun, X.; Dai, Z.; Zhu, J.; Li, H.; Ge, Y.; Song, B. Radiomics Based on Multiparametric MRI for Extrathyroidal Extension Feature Prediction in Papillary Thyroid Cancer. *BMC Med. Imaging* **2020**, *21*, 1–8.
72. Park, V.; Han, K.; Lee, E.; Kim, E.-K.; Moon, H.J.; Yoon, J.H.; Kwak, J.Y. Association between radiomics signature and disease-free survival in conventional papillary thyroid carcinoma. *Sci. Rep.* **2019**, *9*, 1–7. [CrossRef]
73. Yoon, J.H.; Han, K.; Lee, E.; Lee, J.; Kim, E.-K.; Moon, H.J.; Park, V.; Nam, K.H.; Kwak, J.Y. Radiomics in predicting mutation status for thyroid cancer: A preliminary study using radiomics features for predicting BRAFV600E mutations in papillary thyroid carcinoma. *PLoS ONE* **2020**, *15*, e0228968. [CrossRef]
74. Song, E.; Jeon, M.J.; Oh, H.-S.; Han, M.; Lee, Y.-M.; Kim, T.Y.; Chung, K.-W.; Kim, W.B.; Shong, Y.K.; Song, D.E.; et al. Do aggressive variants of papillary thyroid carcinoma have worse clinical outcome than classic papillary thyroid carcinoma? *Eur. J. Endocrinol.* **2018**, *179*, 135–142. [CrossRef]
75. Wang, H.; Song, B.; Ye, N.R.; Ren, J.L.; Sun, X.L.; Dai, Z.D.; Zhang, Y.; Chen, B.H.T. Machine learning-based multiparametric MRI radiomics for predicting the aggressiveness of papillary thyroid carcinoma. *Eur. J. Radiol.* **2020**, *122*, 7. [CrossRef] [PubMed]
76. Schadow, S.; Simons, V.S.; Lochnit, G.; Kordelle, J.; Gazova, Z.; Siebert, H.C.; Steinmeyer, J. Metabolic Response of Human Osteoarthritic Cartilage to Biochemically Characterized Collagen Hydrolysates. *Int. J. Mol. Sci.* **2017**, *18*, 207. [CrossRef] [PubMed]
77. Wang, X.; Zhang, C.; Srivastava, A.; Yu, W.; Liu, C.; Wei, D.; Li, Y.; Yang, J. Risk Factors That Influence Surgical Decision-Making for Patients with Low-Risk Differentiated Thyroid Cancer with Tumor Diameters of 1–4 cm. *Cancer Manag. Res.* **2020**, *12*, 12423–12428. [CrossRef]
78. Cho, B.Y.; Choi, H.S.; Park, Y.J.; Lim, J.A.; Ahn, H.Y.; Lee, E.K.; Kim, K.W.; Yi, K.H.; Chung, J.K.; Youn, Y.K.; et al. Changes in the clinicopathological characteristics and outcomes of thyroid cancer in Korea over the past four decades. *Thyroid* **2013**, *23*, 797–804. [CrossRef]
79. Londero, S.C.; Krogdahl, A.; Bastholt, L.; Overgaard, J.; Pedersen, H.B.; Hahn, C.H.; Bentzen, J.; Schytte, S.; Christiansen, P.; Gerke, O.; et al. Papillary thyroid carcinoma in Denmark, 1996–2008: Outcome and evaluation of established prognostic scoring systems in a prospective national cohort. *Thyroid* **2015**, *25*, 78–84. [CrossRef]
80. Xing, M.; Alzahrani, A.S.; Carson, K.A.; Viola, D.; Elisei, R.; Bendlova, B.; Yip, L.; Mian, C.; Vianello, F.; Tuttle, R.M.; et al. Association between BRAF V600E mutation and mortality in patients with papillary thyroid cancer. *Jama* **2013**, *309*, 1493–1501. [CrossRef]
81. Kwon, M.R.; Shin, J.H.; Park, H.; Cho, H.; Hahn, S.Y.; Park, K.W. Radiomics Study of Thyroid Ultrasound for Predicting BRAF Mutation in Papillary Thyroid Carcinoma: Preliminary Results. *AJNR Am. J. Neuroradiol.* **2020**, *41*, 700–705. [CrossRef]
82. Guth, S.; Theune, U.; Aberle, J.; Galach, A.; Bamberger, C.M. Very high prevalence of thyroid nodules detected by high frequency (13 MHz) ultrasound examination. *Eur. J. Clin. Investig.* **2009**, *39*, 699–706. [CrossRef] [PubMed]
83. Brito, J.P.; Morris, J.C.; Montori, V.M. Thyroid cancer: Zealous imaging has increased detection and treatment of low risk tumours. *BMJ (Clin. Res. Ed)* **2013**, *347*, f4706. [CrossRef]
84. Prochazka, A.; Gulati, S.; Holinka, S.; Smutek, D. Classification of Thyroid Nodules in Ultrasound Images Using Direction-Independent Features Extracted by Two-Threshold Binary Decomposition. *Technol. Cancer Res. Treat.* **2019**, *18*, 1533033819830748. [CrossRef]
85. Colakoglu, B.; Alis, D.; Yergin, M. Diagnostic Value of Machine Learning-Based Quantitative Texture Analysis in Differentiating Benign and Malignant Thyroid Nodules. *J. Oncol.* **2019**, *2019*, 7. [CrossRef] [PubMed]
86. Park, V.Y.; Lee, E.; Lee, H.S.; Kim, H.J.; Yoon, J.; Son, J.; Song, K.; Moon, H.J.; Yoon, J.H.; Kim, G.R.; et al. Combining radiomics with ultrasound-based risk stratification systems for thyroid nodules: An approach for improving performance. *Eur. Radiol.* **2021**, *31*, 2405–2413. [CrossRef]
87. Yoon, J.; Lee, E.; Kang, S.-W.; Han, K.; Park, V.Y.; Kwak, J.Y. Implications of US radiomics signature for predicting malignancy in thyroid nodules with indeterminate cytology. *Eur. Radiol.* **2021**, *2021*, 1–9.

88. Zhao, C.-K.; Ren, T.-T.; Yin, Y.-F.; Shi, H.; Wang, H.-X.; Zhou, B.-Y.; Wang, X.-R.; Li, X.; Zhang, Y.-F.; Liu, C.; et al. A Comparative Analysis of Two Machine Learning-Based Diagnostic Patterns with Thyroid Imaging Reporting and Data System for Thyroid Nodules: Diagnostic Performance and Unnecessary Biopsy Rate. *Thyroid* **2021**, *31*, 470–481. [CrossRef]
89. Yao, X.; Ge, Y.; Wu, Q.; Zhu, H.; Zhai, J. Construction and Validation of Two-Level CT-Based Radiomics Models Used for Thyroid Cancer Screening in the Population. 2020. Available online: https://ssrn.com/abstract=3703901 (accessed on 18 November 2020).
90. Zhou, H.; Jin, Y.; Dai, L.; Zhang, M.; Qiu, Y.; Wang, K.; Tian, J.; Zheng, J. Differential diagnosis of benign and malignant thyroid nodules using deep learning radiomics of thyroid ultrasound images. *Eur. J. Radiol.* **2020**, *127*, 108992. [CrossRef]
91. Wang, Y.F.; Yue, W.W.; Li, X.L.; Liu, S.Y.; Guo, L.H.; Xu, H.X.; Zhang, H.Y.; Yang, G. Comparison Study of Radiomics and Deep Learning-Based Methods for Thyroid Nodules Classification Using Ultrasound Images. *IEEE Access* **2020**, *8*, 52010–52017. [CrossRef]

cancers MDPI

Review

Differentiated Thyroid Cancer: A Health Economic Review

Klaas Van Den Heede [1,2,*], Neil S. Tolley [1,3], Aimee N. Di Marco [1,3] and Fausto F. Palazzo [1,3]

1 Department of Endocrine & Thyroid Surgery, Hammersmith Hospital, London W12 0HS, UK; n.tolley@imperial.ac.uk (N.S.T.); a.di-marco@imperial.ac.uk (A.N.D.M.); f.palazzo@imperial.ac.uk (F.F.P.)
2 Department of General and Endocrine Surgery, OLV Hospital, 9300 Aalst, Belgium
3 Department of Surgery and Cancer, Imperial College, London SW7 2AZ, UK
* Correspondence: klaas.vandenheede@nhs.net

Simple Summary: This review reflects on health economic considerations associated with the increasing diagnosis and treatment of differentiated thyroid cancer. Analysis of different relevant health economic topics, such as overdiagnosis, overtreatment, surgical costs, and costs of follow-up are being addressed. Several unanswered research questions such as optimising molecular markers for diagnosis, active surveillance of primary tumours, and improved risk stratification and survivorship care all influence future healthcare expenditures.

Abstract: The incidence of differentiated thyroid cancer (DTC) is rising, mainly because of an increased detection of asymptomatic thyroid nodularity revealed by the liberal use of thyroid ultrasound. This review aims to reflect on the health economic considerations associated with the increasing diagnosis and treatment of DTC. Overdiagnosis and the resulting overtreatment have led to more surgical procedures, increasing health care and patients' costs, and a large pool of community-dwelling thyroid cancer follow-up patients. Additionally, the cost of thyroid surgery seems to increase year on year even when inflation is taken into account. The increased healthcare costs and spending have placed significant pressure to identify potential factors associated with these increased costs. Some truly ground-breaking work in health economics has been undertaken, but more cost-effectiveness studies and micro-cost analyses are required to evaluate expenses and guide future solutions.

Keywords: cost-benefit analysis; economics; medical; thyroid neoplasms

Citation: Van Den Heede, K.; Tolley, N.S.; Di Marco, A.N.; Palazzo, F.F. Differentiated Thyroid Cancer: A Health Economic Review. *Cancers* **2021**, *13*, 2253. https://doi.org/10.3390/cancers13092253

Academic Editor: Fabio Medas

Received: 18 April 2021
Accepted: 5 May 2021
Published: 7 May 2021

Publisher's Note: MDPI stays neutral with regard to jurisdictional claims in published maps and institutional affiliations.

1. Introduction

Thyroid nodules are common and increase with age, especially in iodine-deficient areas [1]. One-third of screened adult cohorts in Europe have a thyroid abnormality on ultrasound [2]. Detected thyroid nodules are investigated to establish a benign or malignant diagnosis and the treatment plan for each of these outcomes is informed by national and international guidelines [3,4]. However, the guidelines rarely include economic considerations.

Differentiated thyroid cancer (DTC), an umbrella term for papillary thyroid cancer (PTC), follicular thyroid cancer (FTC), and Hürthle cell thyroid cancer (HTC) represents approximately 95% of all thyroid cancers [5]. The incidence of DTC has been increasing for the last three decades, but the disease-specific mortality remains stable. Most patients have an excellent prognosis, so the increasing diagnoses have created a vast pool of thyroid cancer survivors that require follow-up. This paper aims to reflect on the health economic considerations associated with the increasing diagnosis and treatment of DTC.

2. Epidemiology of DTC

The incidence of DTC is rising worldwide [6]. In 2020, 448,915 new cases of thyroid cancer were estimated, with an age-standardised rate of 10.1/100,000 and 3.1/100,000 in women and men, respectively (Global Cancer Observatory, IARC). In the United Kingdom (UK), where thyroid cancer incidence is lower than most other European countries, it has increased by 68% over the last decade with 3700 new thyroid cancers diagnosed a year. The expectation is a further rise to 11 cases per 100,000 by 2035 (Cancer Research UK). In 2019, 52,070 new cases were estimated in the United States (US) [7]. If the rising trend in incidence is maintained, thyroid cancer should become the fourth most common cancer in the United States by 2030 [8]. Despite the progressive increase in incidence, the disease-specific mortality in the US has increased marginally from 0.40 to 0.46 per 100,000 and can be accounted for by the advanced and dedifferentiated cancers that occur most commonly in an ageing population [9]. In 2020, 43,646 patients died from thyroid cancer (27,740 women and 15,906 men) (Global Cancer Observatory, IARC), almost no change from the 40,000 estimated global deaths in 2012 [6]. These trends of incidence and mortality are seen across the developed world, with pockets of extreme increase in incidence in countries where thyroid screening has been adopted, such as in South Korea [5,10,11]. The rate of incidental DTC however has remained stable in autopsy studies since 1970 [12].

The rising incidence of DTC applies primarily in high-income countries where incidence rates are more than two-fold higher than low and middle-income countries [6]. International comparisons can be difficult due to differences in the reporting and treatment of the disease. However, even within the same country different rates of DTC diagnosis exist, usually coinciding with a different medical ethos, healthcare structure, and/or funding strategy as noted in regions of Belgium and Brazil [13–15]. In the US, social-economic group and race are also influential with a higher incidence of thyroid cancer found in white patients with a higher income and health insurance levels [16].

The increasing incidence of thyroid cancer is driven by early-stage DTC without any increase of note in mortality or any increase in the known risk factors [5]. Despite an increase in exposure from medical conditions and their treatments, the overall environmental radiation burden has declined [17–20].

Iodine deficiency [21] predisposes to goitre and thyroid nodularity which are also risk factors for thyroid cancer diagnosis [5]. A meta-analysis reported a PTC/FTC ratio of 3.4–6.5:1 compared to a ratio of 0.19–1.7:1 in iodine-deficient areas [22]. Chronic iodine deficiency may also be a risk factor for anaplastic thyroid cancer [5,23] but overall, there is no epidemiological overlap between the surge in DTC and iodine deficient areas.

In light of the above considerations, whilst the hypothesis of increased population exposure to known or some unrecognised carcinogens is a potential explanation for the thyroid cancer epidemic, this remains somewhat unlikely.

3. Overdiagnosis and Overtreatment

It is probable that the single most important cause of the rising DTC incidence over the last few decades has been the increased detection of asymptomatic thyroid nodularity revealed by the liberal use of thyroid ultrasound. This has unveiled a huge reservoir of mainly benign but sometimes malignant disease. The junction at which diagnosis becomes overdiagnosis is the point at which the identification of disease does not lead to overall population benefit. Overtreatment is an almost inevitable product of overdiagnosis and is observed when a disease is diagnosed and optimally treated but the net result is an unfavourable balance between patient benefit and the overall adverse effects of care. This risk was recognised almost 30 years ago [24] as increasing access to ever-improving imaging techniques replaced medical examination.

The widespread use of neck ultrasound has led to either a preoperative increased detection of early-stage tumours and/or indirectly to thyroid surgery where incidental thyroid cancers, mainly papillary thyroid carcinomas under 10 mm (papillary thyroid microcarcinomas (PTMC)), are found. From 1975 to 2009, the proportion of incidental PTMC has increased from 25% to 39% [25]. In some European countries and the US, 45 to 70% of thyroid malignancies are considered "over diagnosed", based on studies comparing the expected and observed prevalence of thyroid cancer [26]. This conclusion is also inferred by the rise of early-stage thyroid cancer and the incongruity of there being more cancer with no change in mortality over decades [27]. The alternative explanation, that early diagnosis coupled with excellent treatment has compensated for a real thyroid cancer epidemic, appears less substantiated.

Overdiagnosis and overtreatment are clear generic population-based concepts but are more difficult to define at an individual level since it has not been possible to reliably predict the natural history of an individual PTMC in a specific patient. The early diagnosis of a PTMC will have saved some patients from a late diagnosis and despite the excellent overall prognosis some PTMC may become larger and metastasise or manifest an aggressive clinical behaviour even without enlargement. However, it remains the case that at autopsy after deaths unrelated to thyroid cancer 6.7–16.1% of thyroids present one or more foci of PTMC [12] so that the vast majority of newly diagnosed PTMC is implicitly of no clinical significance. The diagnosis and treatment of PTMC offers no benefit to the patient in the vast majority of cases. Apart from some difficult to identify patients who will benefit, most are exposed to potential morbidity without gain. In addition to the personal risk of surgery, one must consider the psychological effects of a cancer diagnosis that is cancer in name but infrequently in behaviour. A frequently overlooked additional consequence of the surge in DTC diagnoses is the drain on healthcare resources.

The overdetection and treatment of PTMC comes with an economic cost irrespective of whether it is treated surgically or subjected to a surveillance programme. These costs must be balanced against the consequences of a delayed diagnosis in the minority of patients that may come to harm if a timely cancer diagnosis is not made. This argument effectively overlaps with the health economic debate that applies to cancer screening in general. Does thyroid cancer screening fit the cancer screening principle that a presumptive diagnosis of subclinical disease and an early diagnosis improves outcome? [28]. For screening to be effective, the time interval between a disease becoming detectable by the screening tool and the presentation of clinically detectable disease must be shown to be detrimental to the patient [29]. For a screening program to be considered the disease must be common, have an identifiable risk group and the screening tool must be both sensitive and specific. There is no evidence that this applies to thyroid cancer. A Polish group reviewed 4701 patients surgically treated for thyroid cancer [27] with patients divided according to whether the diagnosis was made with a clinical presentation or without symptoms or risk factors. The asymptomatic group predictably presented a lower TNM stage, a lower rate of multifocality, and no characteristics of aggressive clinical behaviour. The use of screening results in the diagnosis of indolent cases and may lead to overdiagnosis and overtreatment. Very few countries have implemented a thyroid ultrasound screening program for thyroid cancer and several governments have now acknowledged the possible detrimental effects of unwarranted neck ultrasound use in asymptomatic patients.

In an attempt to reduce unstructured neck ultrasound screening in the UK, only a thyroid specialist should request a thyroid ultrasound [30]. The American Preventive Service Task Force (USPSTF) recently released its guidelines, in which it strongly recommends against using neck ultrasound for thyroid cancer screening in asymptomatic patients [31]. The impact of changing guidelines was seen in South Korea where screening with neck ultrasound for thyroid cancer became part of a National Cancer Control Program in 1999 [32], creating an epidemic of low-risk PTC. After recognising the morbidity of unnecessary thyroid surgery due to the thyroid screening this practice was discouraged from 2014 with a corresponding decrease in the incidence of thyroid cancer and the number of thyroid operations decreased significantly [33]. However, if patients do not undergo surgery for PTMC, the management dilemmas and costs associated with an active surveillance (AS) programme with repeated clinical review and ultrasounds is also problematic since a reliable predictor of progression is still not available [34,35].

4. The Indeterminate Thyroid Nodule

The detection of a thyroid nodule begins a cascade of investigations with neck ultrasound and fine-needle aspiration (FNA) at the heart of the algorithm. Benign cytology should allow patient discharge in most cases. Since it is not always possible to unequivocally exclude malignancy at FNA cytology, surgery may be recommended for these 'indeterminate' lesions. However, the cancer rate at final histology after surgery is less than 30% [36]. The problem of indeterminate cytology and 70% of unnecessary thyroid operations may be addressed in some cases with the identification of mutations in molecular panels that are promising [37,38]. Molecular testing, however, adds further expense to the diagnostic workup (£2160–£2880) [39] and usually reduces the risk of rather than guaranteeing the absence of cancer. A recent review of available molecular panels concluded that the more accurate molecular-based test methods are still expensive and restricted to a few, highly specialised and centralised laboratories [40]. Molecular testing is therefore not currently provided by taxpayer-funded healthcare systems since value (benefit/cost) remains unproven.

The cost of mutation panels however needs to be put in the context of the potential saving of unnecessary surgery and the benefit of patient discharge, assuming that this actually occurs. Several cost-effectiveness studies have been performed, comparing lobectomy to genetic testing [37], molecular panel testing [41], or lobectomy and frozen section to total thyroidectomy for thyroid nodules suspicious of cancer [42]. Most studies suggest that a diagnostic lobectomy remains overall preferable to genetic testing as a strategy for ruling out the malignancy of indeterminate thyroid nodules. The conclusions are determined principally by the consequence of "closure" after a hemithyroidectomy versus living under surveillance after using molecular panels which appears to remain the recommendation. A systematic review concluded that the test specificity had to be >68% and the amount of surgery decreased by over 50% for molecular testing to be cost-effective [39]. This health economics model confirmed that molecular evaluation of thyroid nodules with indeterminate cytology could generate positive health outcomes by reducing the rate of unnecessary surgery on benign nodules and may find traction as the costs of the tests decrease.

5. Surgery as the Solution?

Thyroid surgery is becoming increasingly expensive. A large population-based study demonstrated increasing patient charges for both inpatient and outpatient elective thyroid surgery, with increasing costs of £644 or 4.31% every year between 2006 and 2014, after controlling for multiple clinical and demographic variables and adjusting for inflation [43]. There is ample evidence that a thyroid lobectomy presents no survival difference compared to a total thyroidectomy in low-risk PTC less than four centimetres in diameter [44]. Hemithyroidectomy has the advantage of retaining natural thyroid function in 80% or more of patients and avoids permanent hypoparathyroidism and its sequelae. The disadvantages of a hemithyroidectomy are the reduction of efficacy of thyroglobulin as a tumour marker, the preclusion of radioiodine as adjuvant treatment, and a higher risk of requiring a second operation for local recurrence. Overall, the 2015 American Thyroid Association guidelines conclude that a lobectomy is an acceptable treatment primarily to avoid the morbidity of total thyroidectomy documented in lower volume practices [3] rather than because it is a better option from an oncological point of view.

Most thyroid surgery in the US and many parts of the world is performed by low-volume general, ENT, and, to a lesser extent, maxillofacial surgeons [45]. Whilst a hemithyroidectomy in low-risk thyroid cancer may offer lower morbidity with unchanged cancer efficacy [46] the cost considerations appear to have taken a back seat. The Quality Adjusted Life Year (QALY) can be used in the assessment of the value of medical interventions [47]. If the Incremental Cost-Effectiveness Ratio (ICER) is applied to the treatment of a solitary thyroid nodule with an FNA biopsy that is 'suspicious for cancer' a hemithyroidectomy alone does not appear to be the most cost-effective and appears to be inferior in cost-effectiveness compared to a total thyroidectomy. This calculation is based on a model that includes the accuracy of a frozen section and the rate of injury to the recurrent laryngeal nerve (RLN). Unfortunately, the study failed to factor in the varying rate of malignancy for an FNA biopsy and calculated just 12 months of the life-long hormonal replacement, long-term permanent nerve palsy, and permanent hypocalcaemia. Equally a thorough costing of ultrasound surveillance of the neck was also insufficiently assessed but is likely to add additional cost to the hemithyroidectomy group [42]. As the study was published before the 2015 ATA guidelines, the higher rate of completion thyroidectomy might have altered the cost-effectiveness analysis.

A more recent cost-effectiveness analysis compared total thyroidectomy versus lobectomy for small (2 cm) nodules suspicious for PTC (defined as Bethesda V) [48]. The authors conclude that a total thyroidectomy protocol produced an incremental cost of £1929 and incremental effectiveness of minus 0.24 QALY as compared to the lobectomy protocol. The consecutive sensitivity analysis demonstrated that total thyroidectomy apparently only becomes a cost-effective strategy if the risk of stages III and IV PTC is 82.4% among patients with Bethesda V cytology on preoperative FNA. These counterintuitive findings may be related to the quantification of the risk of morbidity (hypothyroidism, hypoparathyroidism, or unilateral RLN injury) after lobectomy was estimated at up to 50% which is high compared to national registry data [49]. Whether the true cost of follow-up and additional imaging rather than a cheaper nurse led thyroglobulin follow-up have been contemplated was not clearly stated. One feature that is not quantified adequately is the cost of lifelong physician follow-up and frequent office ultrasound in the lobectomy group that is likely to make the surveillance of anything less than a total thyroidectomy more expensive.

6. Surgical Technology: A Cost-Effective Addition?

As stated above, the cost of thyroid surgery seems to increase year on year even when inflation is taken into account. In part this may be caused by the increasing use of technology aimed to improve outcomes. The morbidity after thyroid surgery is low when performed by high-volume surgeons [50,51] and the real-world results suggest a gross underreporting of surgical morbidity [52]. Hypoparathyroidism, recurrent laryngeal nerve palsy, and post-operative haemorrhage reduce QoL and add cost to the overall treatment of thyroid cancer [52]. Costs can be reduced with appropriate postoperative hypocalcaemia protocols [53] and the cost of care is consistently lower in high-volume hospitals in the USA mainly due to reduced length of stay but other variations remain unexplained [54]. One possible variable relates to the use of technological adjuncts.

To reduce the morbidity of thyroid surgery, many technical aids have been developed and advocated. These include nerve monitoring devices, vessel sealing devices, autofluorescence technology, and new surgical approaches, such as robotic thyroid approaches and more recently transoral surgery. Naturally, these devices may have advantages to offer in some cases, possibly reducing morbidity or the time of surgery, but always at a cost. The technology adds to the total costs associated with thyroid surgery, as was demonstrated using the Nationwide Inpatient Sample (NIS) database [55] and Premier Healthcare Database [43]. However, often the enthusiasm for new technology has meant that a rigorous cost-effectiveness/value analysis is not performed until the devices have become ingrained in surgical practice. It is clear that some technology may be expensive but more cost-effective than cheaper solutions [56]. For example, energy-based devices for sealing, cutting, and/or secondary haemostasis are now widely used and preferred to the clamp-and-tie approach for this reason [57]. The various technologies (ultrasonic, bipolar, and advanced bipolar) have proven efficacy and safety [57–61] and a pooled cost-effectiveness meta-analysis showed an 8.7% reduction in procedure costs, derived primarily from a reduction in operating time costs, across surgical procedures ($p = 0.029$) [62].

The efficacy data on intraoperative neuromonitoring (IONM) of the RLN and EBSLN in thyroidectomy are now extensive, but it remains controversial whether the use of IONM can reduce the rate of permanent RLN injury in thyroid surgery. Most device users are reluctant to return to thyroid surgery without the device [63] but there has been an attempt to address the value of IONM [64–66]. The most recent one evaluated the cost-effectiveness of IONM using a Markov chain model, in the setting of a bilateral thyroidectomy [64]. The ICER between the use and non-use of IONM was £33,401 per QALY with the conclusion that this is an acceptable cost in avoiding bilateral RLN palsy and tracheostomy. However, the cost-utility analysis did not confirm these results completely, reporting visual identification of the RLN led to a cost saving of £129 and £496 per patient, and an improvement of 0.001 and 0.004 QALY, over selective IONM and universal IONM, respectively. It was concluded that if the RLN injury were decreased by 50.4% or more with IONM compared to visual identification, the selective use of IONM in high-risk cases would be the most cost-effective solution [65]. Another analysis failed to demonstrate cost-effectivity in a realistic clinical setting [66]. The use of IONM has however become the standard of care irrespective of the value considerations in most developed countries and has a key role in training to which a price cannot be attached as cannot the value of avoidance of bilateral nerve palsy provided by IONM [67].

Autofluorescence of the parathyroid glands and the use of indocyanine green (ICG) to evaluate their vascularisation is another new surgical technique that recently has been developed [68–70]. Time will tell whether this adds value in the event that hypoparathyroidism can be prevented with the associated costs of life-long supplements and end-organ damage including renal impairment.

The costs of novel surgical approaches such as robotic transaxillary thyroidectomy and transoral endoscopic thyroidectomy vestibular approach (TOETVA), which have as the main feature avoiding a neck scar [71], are yet to be evaluated from a health economics point of view. The widespread use of robotic thyroid surgery in Korea has been ascribed to extensive government support, economic interests, and the higher surgical fees associated with the technique [72]. One analysis has compared transoral endoscopic thyroidectomy vestibular approach and transcervical approach thyroidectomy but omitted conventional surgery as a control. Differences in mean variable direct cost for lobectomy and total thyroidectomy were £918 and £745, respectively, due to the longer operating time and different energy-based devices (open versus keyhole) used [73].

7. Follow-Up: The Gift That Keeps on Giving?

Current European, British, and American guidelines recommend regular follow-up of DTC after surgery in order to detect early recurrence, supervise TSH suppression, and manage any surgical complications. It is recommended that it be undertaken by a member of the multidisciplinary team according to the established local protocols [3,30,74]. Surgical morbidity after total thyroidectomy adds significantly to the expenses of surgical treatment. Only a few studies have evaluated the cost-effectiveness of different management strategies for vocal fold paralysis and (temporary) hypoparathyroidism [75–77].

Lifelong surveillance with hormone replacement or TSH suppression has a cost, and this is increasing cumulatively as the number of thyroid cancers treated with surgery increases coupled with the progressive improvement in generic life expectancy. The low yield of cancer recurrence in all but the most aggressive forms of thyroid cancer has called into question the value of thyroid cancer follow-up, especially three-monthly follow-ups advocated by some in the first year and the Thyrogen®-stimulated (Sanofi Belgium, Machelen, Flemish Brabant, Belgium) risk stratification [78].

More than 750,000 thyroid cancer survivors are living in the United States today [25,79,80]. Eighty percent of new thyroid cancer patients are under 65 years of age and the 20-year disease-specific survival is over 90%. The cost of the follow-up of 750,000 patients has to be contextualised with thyroid mortality of just 0.4% of all cancer deaths in the United States [81]. The increasing detection of thyroid cancer and the ageing general population suggest that the thyroid cancer follow-up numbers will continue to rise significantly [82]. The current and projected healthcare-related costs attributable to well-differentiated thyroid cancer care have been studied by Lubitz and colleagues [83]. The total estimated costs associated with WDTC care in 2013 exceeded £1.15 billion in the US alone. The initial treatment including diagnostics, surgery, and adjuvant radioactive iodine (RAI) accounts for £473 million (or 41% of the total annual costs), and an alarming, £428 million (37% of total costs) is taken by the management of the follow-up. There are also hidden costs related to medical practitioner activity and the cost to society as workdays are lost to attend for investigations and doctor visits are not calculated in this budget calculation.

8. Active Surveillance of PTMC

Having established that PTMC can be treated conservatively does not mean that the individuals diagnosed with a usually indolent benign behaving thyroid lesion stop being patients. Indeed, avoiding surgery in PTMC may actually be more expensive than surgery as it is replaced by "active surveillance (AS)".

Japanese data have explored AS for the management of incidentally identified uncomplicated PTMC. Long-term longitudinal follow-up studies in Japan have demonstrated that PTMC can safely be treated conservatively with no significant morbidity and no increase in disease-specific mortality [84–86]. Following 1235 patients for up to 227 months with biopsy-confirmed thyroid malignancy showed 0% distant metastatic rates and the small percentage of patients with tumour progression or new lymph node metastases showed excellent outcomes with rescue surgery [35,46]. Given the absence of reliable predictors of which PTMC will remain dormant and which will develop into clinically significant disease, the active surveillance patients are monitored radiologically at variable intervals indefinitely. The cost implication of identifying an indolent thyroid cancer whether followed by surgery or AS is rarely considered, nor indeed the psychological impact of a "cancer" diagnosis that stays with the patient indefinitely.

It has been shown that in an American and Canadian context nonoperative management of PTMC is associated with a modest decrement in QoL. Indeed, a thyroid lobectomy appeared cost-effective and is associated with an ICER of £3192/QALY, well below the study's willingness-to-pay threshold [87]. Deterministic sensitivity analysis revealed that the cost-effectiveness was highly dependent on the relative disutility of AS, meaning the patient-specific QoL decrement due to AS, as well as on the remaining life expectancy after diagnosis. It remains clear that the diagnosis of PTMC is undesirable both for the patient and the healthcare system except for the minority that develops a true PTC. A recent meta-analysis demonstrated tumour growth in 4.4% of 4156 patients with AS for low-risk PTMC, with only 1.0% developing cervical lymph node metastasis, and 0.04% developing metastatic disease over a pooled mean period of 44 months [88].

9. Healthcare Structure and the Growing Cost of Care

Healthcare is funded differently around the world. A broadly speaking socialised healthcare model where treatment is free at the point of access dominates in most of Northern Europe and hybrid schemes with co-payment exist through most of the European Union. Private insurance-based models or self-funded healthcare exists elsewhere. In other words, providing a health episode in some contexts is a societal burden and others an item of service that is associated with a fee and therefore potential profit. The epidemic in thyroid cancer may therefore be seen as a health economic crisis or a wealth opportunity depending on the context in which medicine is practiced.

Studies to explore the economics of the increase in thyroid cancer diagnosis and the associated increase in thyroidectomy rates depending on the health model can be difficult to interpret. In general, cost-effectiveness analyses are hypothetical and present inherent limitations with reproducibility, mainly because of changes in values (probability and cost) over time and the varying model designs [48].

Existing studies on thyroid cancer cost rarely provide a holistic view of the different factors associated with the excess expenditures. Calculations are not contextualised with other cancers and offer an annual estimate of expenditure, without considering the effect of concurrent medical conditions, mental health, and functional status on healthcare expenditures that are paramount to develop future solutions [89,90].

A recent SEER-database study projects the estimated lifetime cost for a hypothetical cohort of individuals with thyroid cancer to be £24,981 per patient, ranging from £24,074 to £42,201 for those with local or metastatic disease respectively. The total cost for an incident cohort of thyroid cancer diagnosed in 2010 was approximately £1 billion and projected to increase to more than £1.7 billion for the 2019 cohort. The total medical cost including diagnosis, treatment, and management for the cohorts diagnosed between 2010 and 2019 is approximately £13.4 billion [91]. Based on the SEER/Medicare data, Boltz et al. estimated the first-year cost for non-metastatic DTC of £12,744 per patient [92]. Berger et al. analysed 183 metastatic thyroid cancers (2003–2005) using a US health insurance claim database estimating the first-year costs to be £43,416 per patient [93]. Another recent study used different US data sources including Medical Expenditure Panel Survey (MEPS) data to estimate the annual direct spending for thyroid cancer to be £3.9 billion in the United States [94]. Lubitz et al, again using the SEER data, conducted a stacked cohort cost analysis from 1985–2013 to estimate current and future healthcare expenditures attributable to well-differentiated thyroid cancer. The current societal costs were estimated to be £1.1 billion in 2013 and predicted to be £2.5 billion in 2030 based on present thyroid cancer incidence trends. The problem is not confined to the US healthcare model.

In Brazil, thyroid cancer increased in incidence from 1.51/100,000 to 4.57/100,000 between 2008 and 2018 with an almost unchanged mortality rate (0.30 to 0.36) [14]. A significant increase in the number of thyroid investigation tools (US, FNA) and treatment/follow-up procedures (surgery, low dose RAI, US) was noted in all geographic regions during the same period. However, procedures related to more aggressive thyroid cancers (neck dissection, high dose RAI) decreased. Costs of thyroid US increased by 91%, FNA costs by 128%, treatment-related costs by 120%. This resulted in immediate costs to the Brazilian public health system of £29.5 million over 8 years. A similar picture has been highlighted in Australia where the estimated economic burden of "excess" thyroidectomies in New South Wales has been demonstrated as significant [95]. The incidence of DTC and total thyroidectomy both doubled between 2003 and 2012, while the mortality rate remained unchanged. The projected increase of 2196 thyroidectomy procedures translated into an additional cost of over £10 million in surgery-related healthcare expenditure alone over a decade. A similar picture has been found in Hong Kong where numbers of thyroidectomies for cancer increased even excluding incidental PTMC [96] with the associated cost implications of £8334 per patient in the first year.

There are of course large differences in healthcare costs in different countries and comparing different healthcare and reimbursement systems is challenging [97]. One study performed a cost-analysis of thyroid cancer care between the United States and France identifying that the US healthcare system spends nearly £7200 more per patient for initial 1-year management of PTC than in France. The main components contributing to this cost disparity were hospital facility (70%) and nuclear medicine (19%) reimbursements, despite a lesser duration of stay and lower use of RAI in the United States. Most studies, unfortunately, fail to consider the costs of lifelong thyroid substitution and monitoring of long-term follow-up. It is indeed probable that the annual follow-up cost matches the original larger outlay of surgery as previously suggested. In a publicly funded healthcare system, this substantial cost impacts the funds available for the care of other pathologies [83].

An American study calculated the excess healthcare expenditures of the community-dwelling thyroid cancer patients compared to non-cancer controls in a propensity score-matched analysis [98]. The yearly average total healthcare expenditures among adults with thyroid cancer were significantly higher compared to propensity score-matched controls (£6896 vs £4194, p = <0.001). Similar observations were found in terms of inpatient and outpatient expenditures.

10. Do Guidelines Help Control Costs?

Cancer guidelines focus almost exclusively on best care. Cost of care tends to not be considered at all or to be an afterthought years after the implementation. A recent study used a microsimulation model to compare the cost-effectiveness of the revised 2015 ATA guidelines to the 2009 guidelines [99]. One of the aims of these revised guidelines was to reduce the number of total thyroidectomies and surgical complications and, therefore, potentially cost. The study illustrates that the ATA 2015 guideline patient generated greater average QALYs (13.09 vs 12.43) at a lower average cost per patient (£10,612 vs £14,386) [99].

Reducing the cost of care is not only relevant to socialised medicine since it can also have an impact on personal wellbeing and cause insecurities regarding personal wealth with the associated QoL considerations. Financial difficulties are reported by 43% of thyroid cancer survivors and are associated with worse anxiety and depression [81]. A South Korean retrospective cohort study calculated an average personal medical cost of £2547 per patient after diagnosis of thyroid cancer at 2 years [100]. Fighting cancer can be a costly battle and understanding the relationship between patient-reported financial toxicity (FT) and health outcomes can help to support post-treatment cancer survivors. Incorporation of FT assessment into survivorship care planning could enhance clinical assessment of thyroid cancer patients, help address the dynamic and persistent challenges of survivorship, and help identify those most in need of intervention across the cancer care continuum [101].

11. Future Considerations

Impalpable thyroid cancers detected by ultrasound have almost always an excellent prognosis. The precursor lesions of DTC are not well-established and recognised pathology lesions, but there is no clear demarcation that differentiates precancerous from cancerous lesions. If these were to be reclassified as an indolent lesion of epithelial origin (IDLE), the need for aggressive therapy and screening would be mitigated [102]. Therefore, the re-definition of these lesions as "papillary lesions in situ" as precursors of malignant tumours might be beneficial in reducing the overdiagnosis and overtreatment of patients with thyroid nodules [103]. Being able to select which patients would develop more aggressive disease will have huge impact on healthcare costs for DTC.

Surgical complications from an often-unnecessary operation, the emotional distress linked to the diagnosis of 'cancer', and the stress of follow-up, as well as the financial burden to the individual and society, should not be ignored. The problem affects wealthy countries where the steep rise in thyroid ultrasound and FNA has been driven by access to diagnostic imaging. The reversal or slowing down of this trend requires an understanding of the pathology at all medical levels but is not easy to solve [104]. Education whilst helpful clashes with the realities of defensive medicine where the fear of litigation can intimidate doctors towards more investigations, more interventions, and endless follow-up that transforms every person into a lifelong patient. Future research should be directed towards micro-cost analyses to identify potential factors associated with the increased costs. Cost-effectiveness studies with QALY and ICER calculations should be implemented in future guidelines on treatment, surgical, and follow-up strategy.

Some ground-breaking work in health economics has been undertaken, but more needs to be done on to stem the tide and avert medical bankruptcy. Some changes that have been shown to help are the centralisation of cancer care for an economy of scale and quality assurance that comes from group practice and a multidisciplinary environment.

However, a broader, international approach is required to address the problem of overdiagnosis and overtreatment of thyroid cancer, facilitated by data collection, health economic assessment, subspecialisation, and international health policy that together may find a balance between expenses and clinical benefit for the patient. International societies will have to incorporate health economic considerations into their guidelines. The revised 2015 ATA guidelines stated several research questions that remain unanswered to date: optimising molecular markers for diagnosis, AS of DTC primary tumours, and improved risk stratification and survivorship care. Potential answers could all influence future healthcare expenditures.

12. Conclusions

The current thyroid cancer 'pandemic' is caused primarily by small PTCs that may have caused no harm in most patients, if left undiagnosed. Regardless of the followed guidelines, healthcare, and insurance system, substantial resources are being used for the diagnosis, treatment, and follow-up of this potentially indolent condition. Increased healthcare costs and spending have placed significant pressure to identify potential factors associated with these increased costs and find solutions. The next decade will determine whether as clinicians we can reverse current trends in the ever-increasing cost of thyroid cancer care.

13. Take Home Messages

- The main cause of the rising incidence of DTC incidence over the last decades has been the increased detection of asymptomatic thyroid nodularity revealed by the liberal use of thyroid ultrasound.
- After controlling for multiple clinical and demographic variables, and adjusting for inflation, the cost of thyroid surgery is still increasing.
- The cost of long-term follow-up, active surveillance, and excess healthcare expenditures of the community-dwelling thyroid cancer 'survivors' has to be evaluated in light of the different healthcare models.
- Future research should be directed towards micro-cost analyses to identify potential factors associated with the increased costs.
- Cost-effectiveness studies with QALY and ICER calculations should be implemented in future guidelines on treatment, surgical, and follow-up strategy.

14. Notes

1. For international comparison between studies and data, all monetary values have been expressed in pound sterling (£) at the time of writing: 1 GBP = 1.39 $US = 1.17 EUR = AUD 1.80.
2. A brief summary contextualising health economic terms and concepts used in this manuscript can be found as Supplementary Material [105–109].

Supplementary Materials: The following are available online at https://www.mdpi.com/article/10.3390/cancers13092253/s1, Supplementary Material: Summary of Health Economic Terms and Concepts.

Author Contributions: K.V.D.H., was involved in the study design, literature search, analysis and interpretation of data, and drafting of the manuscript—N.S.T., was involved in the study design, and critical revision of the manuscript—A.N.D.M., was involved in the study design, and critical revision of the manuscript—F.F.P., was involved in the study design, analysis and interpretation of data, and critical revision of the manuscript. All authors have contributed substantially to the work reported. All authors have read and agreed to the published version of the manuscript.

Funding: This research received no external funding.

Conflicts of Interest: The authors declare no conflict of interest.

References

1. Vanderpump, M.P. The Epidemiology of Thyroid Disease. *Br. Med. Bull.* **2011**, *99*, 39–51. [CrossRef] [PubMed]
2. Reiners, C.; Wegscheider, K.; Schicha, H.; Theissen, P.; Vaupel, R.; Wrbitzky, R.; Schumm-Draeger, P.M. Prevalence of Thyroid Disorders in the Working Population of Germany: Ultrasonography Screening in 96,278 Unselected Employees. *Thyroid* **2004**, *14*, 926–932. [CrossRef] [PubMed]
3. Haugen, B.R.; Alexander, E.K.; Bible, K.C.; Doherty, G.M.; Mandel, S.J.; Nikiforov, Y.E.; Pacini, F.; Randolph, G.W.; Sawka, A.M.; Schlumberger, M.; et al. 2015 American Thyroid Association Management Guidelines for Adult Patients with Thyroid Nodules and Differentiated Thyroid Cancer: The American Thyroid Association Guidelines Task Force on Thyroid Nodules and Differentiated Thyroid Cancer. *Thyroid* **2016**, *26*, 1–133. [CrossRef]
4. Filetti, S.; Durante, C.; Hartl, D.; Leboulleux, S.; Locati, L.D.; Newbold, K.; Papotti, M.G.; Berruti, A.; ESMO Guidelines Committee. Thyroid Cancer: ESMO Clinical Practice Guidelines for Diagnosis, Treatment and Follow-Up. *Ann. Oncol.* **2019**, *30*, 1856–1883. [CrossRef]

5. Pellegriti, G.; Frasca, F.; Regalbuto, C.; Squatrito, S.; Vigneri, R. Worldwide Increasing Incidence of Thyroid Cancer: Update on Epidemiology and Risk Factors. *J. Cancer Epidemiol.* **2013**, *2013*, 965212. [CrossRef] [PubMed]
6. La Vecchia, C.; Malvezzi, M.; Bosetti, C.; Garavello, W.; Bertuccio, P.; Levi, F.; Negri, E. Thyroid Cancer Mortality and Incidence: A Global Overview. *Int. J. Cancer* **2015**, *136*, 2187–2195. [CrossRef]
7. Siegel, R.L.; Miller, K.D.; Jemal, A. Cancer Statistics, 2019. *CA Cancer J. Clin.* **2019**, *69*, 7–34. [CrossRef]
8. Rahib, L.; Smith, B.D.; Aizenberg, R.; Rosenzweig, A.B.; Fleshman, J.M.; Matrisian, L.M. Projecting Cancer Incidence and Deaths to 2030: The Unexpected Burden of Thyroid, Liver, and Pancreas Cancers in the United States. *Cancer Res.* **2014**, *74*, 2913–2921. [CrossRef]
9. Chen, A.Y.; Jemal, A.; Ward, E.M. Increasing Incidence of Differentiated Thyroid Cancer in the United States, 1988–2005. *Cancer* **2009**, *115*, 3801–3807. [CrossRef]
10. Ahn, H.S.; Kim, H.J.; Welch, H.G. Korea's Thyroid-Cancer "Epidemic"—Screening and Overdiagnosis. *N. Engl. J. Med.* **2014**, *371*, 1765–1767. [CrossRef] [PubMed]
11. Smittenaar, C.R.; Petersen, K.A.; Stewart, K.; Moitt, N. Cancer Incidence and Mortality Projections in the UK until 2035. *Br. J. Cancer* **2016**, *115*, 1147–1155. [CrossRef] [PubMed]
12. Furuya-Kanamori, L.; Bell, K.J.L.; Clark, J.; Glasziou, P.; Doi, S.A.R. Prevalence of Differentiated Thyroid Cancer in Autopsy Studies over Six Decades: A Meta-Analysis. *J. Clin. Oncol.* **2016**, *34*, 3672–3679. [CrossRef]
13. Decallonne, B.; van den Bruel, A.; Macq, G.; Elaut, N.; de Schutter, H. The Impact of Regional Variation in Clinical Practice on Thyroid Cancer Diagnosis: A National Population-Based Study. *Eur. Thyroid J.* **2020**, *9*, 32–39. [CrossRef] [PubMed]
14. Janovsky, C.; Bittencourt, M.S.; Novais, M.A.P.; Maciel, R.M.B.; Biscolla, R.P.M.; Zucchi, P. Thyroid Cancer Burden and Economic Impact on the Brazilian Public Health System. *Arch. Endocrinol. Metab.* **2018**, *62*, 537–544. [CrossRef] [PubMed]
15. Van den Bruel, A.; Francart, J.; Dubois, C.; Adam, M.; Vlayen, J.; de Schutter, H.; Stordeur, S.; Decallonne, B. Regional Variation in Thyroid Cancer Incidence in Belgium Is Associated with Variation in Thyroid Imaging and Thyroid Disease Management. *J. Clin. Endocrinol. Metab.* **2013**, *98*, 4063–4071. [CrossRef]
16. Golden, S.H.; Brown, A.; Cauley, J.A.; Chin, M.H.; Gary-Webb, T.L.; Kim, C.; Sosa, J.A.; Sumner, A.E.; Anton, B. Health Disparities in Endocrine Disorders: Biological, Clinical, and Nonclinical Factors—An Endocrine Society Scientific Statement. *J. Clin. Endocrinol. Metab.* **2012**, *97*, E1579–E1639. [CrossRef]
17. Jegerlehner, S.; Bulliard, J.L.; Aujesky, D.; Rodondi, N.; Germann, S.; Konzelmann, I.; Chiolero, A.; Group, N.W. Overdiagnosis and Overtreatment of Thyroid Cancer: A Population-Based Temporal Trend Study. *PLoS ONE* **2017**, *12*, e0179387. [CrossRef] [PubMed]
18. Demoury, C.; de Schutter, H.; Faes, C.; Carbonnelle, S.; Fierens, S.; Molenberghs, G.; van Damme, N.; van Bladel, L.; van Nieuwenhuyse, A.; Vleminckx, C. Thyroid Cancer Incidence Near Nuclear Sites in Belgium: An Ecological Study at Small Geographical Level. *Int. J. Cancer* **2020**, *146*, 3034–3043. [CrossRef]
19. Schlumberger, M.; le Guen, B. Nuclear-Power-Plant Accidents: Thyroid Cancer Incidence and Radiation-Related Health Effects from the Chernobyl Accident. *Med. Sci.* **2012**, *28*, 746–756. [CrossRef]
20. Morris, L.G.T. Thyroid Cancer Screening after Nuclear Accidents. *JAMA Otolaryngol. Head Neck Surg.* **2019**, *145*, 79. [CrossRef]
21. Zimmermann, M.B.; Boelaert, K. Iodine Deficiency and Thyroid Disorders. *Lancet Diabetes Endocrinol.* **2015**, *3*, 286–295. [CrossRef]
22. Lind, P.; Langsteger, W.; Molnar, M.; Gallowitsch, H.J.; Mikosch, P.; Gomez, I. Epidemiology of Thyroid Diseases in Iodine Sufficiency. *Thyroid* **1998**, *8*, 1179–1183. [CrossRef] [PubMed]
23. Besic, N.; Hocevar, M.; Zgajnar, J. Lower Incidence of Anaplastic Carcinoma after Higher Iodination of Salt in Slovenia. *Thyroid* **2010**, *20*, 623–626. [CrossRef] [PubMed]
24. Black, W.C.; Welch, H.G. Advances in Diagnostic Imaging and Overestimations of Disease Prevalence and the Benefits of Therapy. *N. Engl. J. Med.* **1993**, *328*, 1237–1243. [CrossRef]
25. Davies, L.; Welch, H.G. Increasing Incidence of Thyroid Cancer in the United States, 1973–2002. *JAMA* **2006**, *295*, 2164–2167. [CrossRef]
26. Fagin, J.A.; Wells, S.A., Jr. Biologic and Clinical Perspectives on Thyroid Cancer. *N. Engl. J. Med.* **2016**, *375*, 1054–1067. [CrossRef]
27. Kaliszewski, K.; Diakowska, D.; Wojtczak, B.; Rudnicki, J. Cancer Screening Activity Results in Overdiagnosis and Overtreatment of Papillary Thyroid Cancer: A 10-Year Experience at a Single Institution. *PLoS ONE* **2020**, *15*, e0236257. [CrossRef]
28. Obuchowski, N.A.; Graham, R.J.; Baker, M.E.; Powell, K.A. Ten Criteria for Effective Screening: Their Application to Multislice CT Screening for Pulmonary and Colorectal Cancers. *AJR Am. J. Roentgenol.* **2001**, *176*, 1357–1362. [CrossRef] [PubMed]
29. Black, W.C.; Welch, H.G. Screening for Disease. *AJR Am. J. Roentgenol.* **1997**, *168*, 3–11. [CrossRef]
30. Mitchell, A.L.; Gandhi, A.; Scott-Coombes, D.; Perros, P. Management of Thyroid Cancer: United Kingdom National Multidisciplinary Guidelines. *J. Laryngol. Otol.* **2016**, *130*, S150–S160. [CrossRef] [PubMed]
31. Jin, J. JAMA PATIENT PAGE. The US Preventive Services Task Force. *JAMA* **2016**, *315*, 1804. [CrossRef] [PubMed]
32. Ahn, H.S.; Kim, H.J.; Kim, K.H.; Lee, Y.S.; Han, S.J.; Kim, Y.; Ko, M.J.; Brito, J.P. Thyroid Cancer Screening in South Korea Increases Detection of Papillary Cancers with No Impact on Other Subtypes or Thyroid Cancer Mortality. *Thyroid* **2016**, *26*, 1535–1540. [CrossRef] [PubMed]
33. Ahn, H.S.; Welch, H.G. South Korea's Thyroid-Cancer "Epidemic"—Turning the Tide. *N. Engl. J. Med.* **2015**, *373*, 2389–2390. [CrossRef]

34. Leboulleux, S.; Tuttle, R.M.; Pacini, F.; Schlumberger, M. Papillary Thyroid Microcarcinoma: Time to Shift from Surgery to Active Surveillance? *Lancet Diabetes Endocrinol.* **2016**, *4*, 933–942. [CrossRef]
35. Ito, Y.; Oda, H.; Miyauchi, A. Insights and Clinical Questions About the Active Surveillance of low-Risk Papillary Thyroid Microcarcinomas [Review]. *Endocr. J.* **2016**, *63*, 323–328. [CrossRef] [PubMed]
36. Inabnet, W.B., 3rd; Palazzo, F.; Sosa, J.A.; Kriger, J.; Aspinall, S.; Barczynski, M.; Doherty, G.; Iacobone, M.; Nordenstrom, E.; Scott-Coombes, D.; et al. Correlating the Bethesda System for Reporting Thyroid Cytopathology with Histology and Extent of Surgery: A Review of 21,746 Patients from Four Endocrine Surgery Registries across Two Continents. *World J. Surg.* **2020**, *44*, 426–435. [CrossRef] [PubMed]
37. Balentine, C.J.; Vanness, D.J.; Schneider, D.F. Cost-Effectiveness of Lobectomy versus Genetic Testing (Afirma(R)) for Indeterminate Thyroid Nodules: Considering the Costs of Surveillance. *Surgery* **2018**, *163*, 88–96. [CrossRef]
38. Nikiforova, M.N.; Mercurio, S.; Wald, A.I.; Barbi de Moura, M.; Callenberg, K.; Santana-Santos, L.; Gooding, W.E.; Yip, L.; Ferris, R.L.; Nikiforov, Y.E. Analytical Performance of the ThyroSeq v3 Genomic Classifier for Cancer Diagnosis in Thyroid Nodules. *Cancer* **2018**, *124*, 1682–1690. [CrossRef]
39. Labourier, E. Utility and Cost-Effectiveness of Molecular Testing in Thyroid Nodules with Indeterminate Cytology. *Clin. Endocrinol. (Oxf)* **2016**, *85*, 624–631. [CrossRef]
40. Sciacchitano, S.; Lavra, L.; Ulivieri, A.; Magi, F.; de Francesco, G.P.; Bellotti, C.; Salehi, L.B.; Trovato, M.; Drago, C.; Bartolazzi, A. Comparative Analysis of Diagnostic Performance, Feasibility and Cost of Different Test-Methods for Thyroid Nodules with Indeterminate Cytology. *Oncotarget* **2017**, *8*, 49421–49442. [CrossRef]
41. Labourier, E.; Shifrin, A.; Busseniers, A.E.; Lupo, M.A.; Manganelli, M.L.; Andruss, B.; Wylie, D.; Beaudenon-Huibregtse, S. Molecular Testing for miRNA, mRNA, and DNA on Fine-Needle Aspiration Improves the Preoperative Diagnosis of Thyroid Nodules with Indeterminate Cytology. *J. Clin. Endocrinol. Metab.* **2015**, *100*, 2743–2750. [CrossRef]
42. Leiker, A.J.; Yen, T.W.; Cheung, K.; Evans, D.B.; Wang, T.S. Cost Analysis of Thyroid Lobectomy and Intraoperative Frozen Section versus Total Thyroidectomy in Patients with a Cytologic Diagnosis of "Suspicious for Papillary Thyroid Cancer". *Surgery* **2013**, *154*, 1307–1313. [CrossRef] [PubMed]
43. Sahli, Z.T.; Zhou, S.; Sharma, A.K.; Segev, D.L.; Massie, A.; Zeiger, M.A.; Mathur, A. Rising Cost of Thyroid Surgery in Adult Patients. *J. Surg. Res.* **2021**, *260*, 28–37. [CrossRef]
44. Adam, M.A.; Pura, J.; Gu, L.; Dinan, M.A.; Tyler, D.S.; Reed, S.D.; Scheri, R.; Roman, S.A.; Sosa, J.A. Extent of Surgery for Papillary Thyroid Cancer Is Not Associated with Survival: An Analysis of 61,775 Patients. *Ann. Surg.* **2014**, *260*, 601–605, discussion 605–607. [CrossRef]
45. Gourin, C.G.; Tufano, R.P.; Forastiere, A.A.; Koch, W.M.; Pawlik, T.M.; Bristow, R.E. Volume-Based Trends in Thyroid Surgery. *Arch. Otolaryngol. Head Neck Surg.* **2010**, *136*, 1191–1198. [CrossRef] [PubMed]
46. Lee, J.; Park, J.H.; Lee, C.R.; Chung, W.Y.; Park, C.S. Long-Term Outcomes of Total Thyroidectomy versus Thyroid Lobectomy for Papillary Thyroid Microcarcinoma: Comparative Analysis after Propensity Score Matching. *Thyroid* **2013**, *23*, 1408–1415. [CrossRef] [PubMed]
47. Bravo Vergel, Y.; Sculpher, M. Quality-Adjusted Life Years. *Pract. Neurol.* **2008**, *8*, 175–182. [CrossRef]
48. Al-Qurayshi, Z.; Farag, M.; Shama, M.A.; Ibraheem, K.; Randolph, G.W.; Kandil, E. Total Thyroidectomy versus Lobectomy in Small Nodules Suspicious for Papillary Thyroid Cancer: Cost-Effectiveness Analysis. *Laryngoscope* **2020**, *130*, 2922–2926. [CrossRef] [PubMed]
49. Aspinall, S.; Oweis, D.; Chadwick, D. Effect of Surgeons' Annual Operative Volume on the Risk of Permanent Hypoparathyroidism, Recurrent Laryngeal Nerve Palsy and Haematoma Following Thyroidectomy: Analysis of United Kingdom Registry of Endocrine and Thyroid Surgery (UKRETS). *Langenbecks Arch. Surg.* **2019**, *404*, 421–430. [CrossRef]
50. Nouraei, S.A.; Virk, J.S.; Middleton, S.E.; Aylin, P.; Mace, A.; Vaz, F.; Kaddour, H.; Darzi, A.; Tolley, N.S. A National Analysis of Trends, Outcomes and Volume-Outcome Relationships in Thyroid Surgery. *Clin. Otolaryngol.* **2017**, *42*, 354–365. [CrossRef]
51. Lorenz, K.; Raffaeli, M.; Barczynski, M.; Lorente-Poch, L.; Sancho, J. Volume, Outcomes, and Quality Standards in Thyroid Surgery: An Evidence-Based Analysis-European Society of Endocrine Surgeons (ESES) Positional Statement. *Langenbecks Arch. Surg.* **2020**, *405*, 401–425. [CrossRef]
52. Patel, N.; Scott-Coombes, D. Impact of Surgical Volume and Surgical Outcome Assessing Registers on the Quality of Thyroid Surgery. *Best Pract. Res. Clin. Endocrinol. Metab.* **2019**, *33*, 101317. [CrossRef] [PubMed]
53. Mercante, G.; Anelli, A.; Giannarelli, D.; Giordano, D.; Sinopoli, I.; Ferreli, F.; Digiesi, G.; Appetecchia, M.L.; Barnabei, A.; Cristalli, G.; et al. Cost-Effectiveness in Transient Hypocalcemia Post-Thyroidectomy. *Head Neck* **2019**, *41*, 3940–3947. [CrossRef] [PubMed]
54. Wu, S.Y.; Terrell, J.; Park, A.; Perrier, N. Understanding Thyroidectomy Cost Variations among National Cancer Institute-Designated Cancer Centers. *World J. Surg.* **2020**, *44*, 385–392. [CrossRef]
55. Biron, V.L.; Bang, H.; Farwell, D.G.; Bewley, A.F. National Trends and Factors Associated with Hospital Costs Following Thyroid Surgery. *Thyroid* **2015**, *25*, 823–829. [CrossRef]
56. Russell, L.B.; Gold, M.R.; Siegel, J.E.; Daniels, N.; Weinstein, M.C. The Role of Cost-Effectiveness Analysis in Health and Medicine. Panel on Cost-Effectiveness in Health and Medicine. *JAMA* **1996**, *276*, 1172–1177. [CrossRef] [PubMed]
57. Garas, G.; Okabayashi, K.; Ashrafian, H.; Shetty, K.; Palazzo, F.; Tolley, N.; Darzi, A.; Athanasiou, T.; Zacharakis, E. Which Hemostatic Device in Thyroid Surgery? A Network Meta-Analysis of Surgical Technologies. *Thyroid* **2013**, *23*, 1138–1150. [CrossRef]

58. Van Slycke, S.; Gillardin, J.P.; van den Heede, K.; Minguet, J.; Vermeersch, H.; Brusselaers, N. Comparison of the Harmonic Focus and the Thunderbeat for Open Thyroidectomy. *Langenbecks Arch. Surg.* **2016**, *401*, 851–859. [CrossRef] [PubMed]
59. Konturek, A.; Szpyra, B.; Stopa-Barczynska, M.; Barczynski, M. Energy-Based Devices for Hemostasis in Thyroid Surgery. *Gland Surg.* **2020**, *9*, S153–S158. [CrossRef]
60. Contin, P.; Goossen, K.; Grummich, K.; Jensen, K.; Schmitz-Winnenthal, H.; Buchler, M.W.; Diener, M.K. ENERgized Vessel Sealing Systems versus CONventional Hemostasis Techniques in Thyroid Surgery—The ENERCON Systematic Review and Network Meta-Analysis. *Langenbecks Arch. Surg.* **2013**, *398*, 1039–1056. [CrossRef]
61. Hua, N.; Quimby, A.E.; Johnson-Obaseki, S. Comparing Hematoma Incidence between Hemostatic Devices in Total Thyroidectomy: A Systematic Review and Meta-Analysis. *Otolaryngol. Head Neck Surg.* **2019**, *161*, 770–778. [CrossRef]
62. Cheng, H.; Soleas, I.M.; Ferko, N.C.; Cameron, C.G.; Clymer, J.W.; Amaral, J.F. Hospital Costs Associated with Thyroidectomy Performed with a Harmonic Device Compared to Conventional Techniques: A Systematic Review and Meta-Analysis. *J. Med. Econ.* **2016**, *19*, 750–758. [CrossRef]
63. Tae, K. Cost-Effectiveness of Intraoperative Neural Monitoring in Thyroid Surgery: Comment on "Analyzing Cost-Effectiveness of Neural-Monitoring in Recurrent Laryngeal Nerve Recovery Course in Thyroid Surgery". *Gland Surg.* **2019**, *8*, 304–306. [CrossRef] [PubMed]
64. Al-Qurayshi, Z.; Kandil, E.; Randolph, G.W. Cost-Effectiveness of Intraoperative Nerve Monitoring in Avoidance of Bilateral Recurrent Laryngeal Nerve Injury in Patients Undergoing Total Thyroidectomy. *Br. J. Surg.* **2017**, *104*, 1523–1531. [CrossRef]
65. Rocke, D.J.; Goldstein, D.P.; de Almeida, J.R. A Cost-Utility Analysis of Recurrent Laryngeal Nerve Monitoring in the Setting of Total Thyroidectomy. *JAMA Otolaryngol. Head Neck Surg.* **2016**, *142*, 1199–1205. [CrossRef] [PubMed]
66. Wang, T.; Kim, H.Y.; Wu, C.W.; Rausei, S.; Sun, H.; Pergolizzi, F.P.; Dionigi, G. Analyzing Cost-Effectiveness of Neural-Monitoring in Recurrent Laryngeal Nerve Recovery Course in Thyroid Surgery. *Int. J. Surg.* **2017**, *48*, 180–188. [CrossRef] [PubMed]
67. Schneider, R.; Randolph, G.W.; Dionigi, G.; Wu, C.W.; Barczynski, M.; Chiang, F.Y.; Al-Quaryshi, Z.; Angelos, P.; Brauckhoff, K.; Cernea, C.R.; et al. International Neural Monitoring Study Group Guideline 2018 Part I: Staging Bilateral Thyroid Surgery with Monitoring Loss of Signal. *Laryngoscope* **2018**, *128* (Suppl. 3), S1–S17. [CrossRef]
68. Vlasses, P.H.; Besarab, A.; Lottes, S.R.; Conner, D.P.; Green, P.J.; Gault, M.H. False-Positive Digoxin Measurements Due to Conjugated Metabolite Accumulation in Combined Renal and Hepatic Dysfunction. *Am. J. Nephrol.* **1987**, *7*, 355–359. [CrossRef]
69. Van Slycke, S.; van den Heede, K.; Brusselaers, N.; Vermeersch, H. Feasibility of Autofluorescence for Parathyroid Glands During Thyroid Surgery and the Risk of Hypocalcemia: First Results in Belgium and Review of the Literature. *Surg. Innov.* **2020**, 1553350620980263. [CrossRef]
70. Di Marco, A.N.; Palazzo, F.F. Near-Infrared Autofluorescence in Thyroid and Parathyroid Surgery. *Gland Surg.* **2020**, *9*, S136–S146. [CrossRef]
71. Aidan, P.; Arora, A.; Lorincz, B.; Tolley, N.; Garas, G. Robotic Thyroid Surgery: Current Perspectives and Future Considerations. *ORL J. Otorhinolaryngol. Relat. Spec.* **2018**, *80*, 186–194. [CrossRef]
72. Lee, S.R.; Lee, E.S.; Eum, H.L.; Lee, Y.J.; Lee, S.W.; Park, J.Y.; Suh, D.S.; Kim, D.Y.; Kim, S.H.; Kim, Y.M.; et al. New Surgical Technique for Robotic Myomectomy: Continuous Locking Suture on Myoma (LSOM) Technique. *J. Clin. Med.* **2021**, *10*, 654. [CrossRef]
73. Razavi, C.R.; Tanavde, V.A.; Kim, A.S.; Shaear, M.; Tufano, R.P.; Russell, J.O. The Variable Direct Cost and Cost Drivers of Transoral Endoscopic Thyroidectomy Vestibular *Approach. Gland Surg.* **2021**, *10*, 521–528. [CrossRef] [PubMed]
74. Luster, M.; Aktolun, C.; Amendoeira, I.; Barczynski, M.; Bible, K.C.; Duntas, L.H.; Elisei, R.; Handkiewicz-Junak, D.; Hoffmann, M.; Jarzab, B.; et al. European Perspective on 2015 American Thyroid Association Management Guidelines for Adult Patients with Thyroid Nodules and Differentiated Thyroid Cancer: Proceedings of an Interactive International Symposium. *Thyroid* **2019**, *29*, 7–26. [CrossRef] [PubMed]
75. Nicholson, K.J.; Smith, K.J.; McCoy, K.L.; Carty, S.E.; Yip, L. A Comparative Cost-Utility Analysis of Postoperative Calcium Supplementation Strategies Used in the Current Management of Hypocalcemia. *Surgery* **2020**, *167*, 137–143. [CrossRef]
76. Gardner, G.M.; Smith, M.M.; Yaremchuk, K.L.; Peterson, E.L. The Cost of Vocal Fold Paralysis after Thyroidectomy. *Laryngoscope* **2013**, *123*, 1455–1463. [CrossRef] [PubMed]
77. Naunheim, M.R.; Song, P.C.; Franco, R.A.; Alkire, B.C.; Shrime, M.G. Surgical Management of Bilateral Vocal Fold Paralysis: A Cost-Effectiveness Comparison of Two Treatments. *Laryngoscope* **2017**, *127*, 691–697. [CrossRef]
78. Orlov, S.; Salari, F.; Kashat, L.; Freeman, J.L.; Vescan, A.; Witterick, I.J.; Walfish, P.G. Post-Operative Stimulated Thyroglobulin and Neck Ultrasound as Personalized Criteria for Risk Stratification and Radioactive Iodine Selection in Low- and Intermediate-Risk Papillary Thyroid Cancer. *Endocrine* **2015**, *50*, 130–137. [CrossRef]
79. Cheng, S.Y.; Ringel, M.D. Frontiers in Thyroid Cancer: December 2009. *Thyroid* **2009**, *19*, 1297–1298. [CrossRef]
80. Lubitz, C.C.; Sosa, J.A. The Changing Landscape of Papillary Thyroid Cancer: Epidemiology, Management, and the Implications for Patients. *Cancer* **2016**, *122*, 3754–3759. [CrossRef]
81. Mongelli, M.N.; Giri, S.; Peipert, B.J.; Helenowski, I.B.; Yount, S.E.; Sturgeon, C. Financial Burden and Quality of Life among Thyroid Cancer Survivors. *Surgery* **2020**, *167*, 631–637. [CrossRef]
82. Enewold, L.; Zhu, K.; Ron, E.; Marrogi, A.J.; Stojadinovic, A.; Peoples, G.E.; Devesa, S.S. Rising Thyroid Cancer Incidence in the United States by Demographic and Tumor Characteristics, 1980–2005. *Cancer Epidemiol. Biomarkers Prev.* **2009**, *18*, 784–791. [CrossRef]

83. Lubitz, C.C.; Kong, C.Y.; McMahon, P.M.; Daniels, G.H.; Chen, Y.; Economopoulos, K.P.; Gazelle, G.S.; Weinstein, M.C. Annual Financial Impact of Well-Differentiated Thyroid Cancer Care in the United States. *Cancer* **2014**, *120*, 1345–1352. [CrossRef]
84. Ito, Y.; Uruno, T.; Nakano, K.; Takamura, Y.; Miya, A.; Kobayashi, K.; Yokozawa, T.; Matsuzuka, F.; Kuma, S.; Kuma, K.; et al. An Observation Trial without Surgical Treatment in Patients with Papillary Microcarcinoma of the Thyroid. *Thyroid* **2003**, *13*, 381–387. [CrossRef]
85. Ito, Y.; Miyauchi, A. Nonoperative Management of Low-Risk Differentiated Thyroid Carcinoma. *Curr. Opin. Oncol.* **2015**, *27*, 15–20. [CrossRef] [PubMed]
86. Miyauchi, A. Clinical Trials of Active Surveillance of Papillary Microcarcinoma of the Thyroid. *World J. Surg.* **2016**, *40*, 516–522. [CrossRef]
87. Venkatesh, S.; Pasternak, J.D.; Beninato, T.; Drake, F.T.; Kluijfhout, W.P.; Liu, C.; Gosnell, J.E.; Shen, W.T.; Clark, O.H.; Duh, Q.Y.; et al. Cost-Effectiveness of Active Surveillance versus Hemithyroidectomy for Micropapillary Thyroid Cancer. *Surgery* **2017**, *161*, 116–126. [CrossRef]
88. Saravana-Bawan, B.; Bajwa, A.; Paterson, J.; McMullen, T. Active Surveillance of Low-Risk Papillary Thyroid Cancer: A Meta-Analysis. *Surgery* **2020**, *167*, 46–55. [CrossRef] [PubMed]
89. Reeve, B.B.; Potosky, A.L.; Smith, A.W.; Han, P.K.; Hays, R.D.; Davis, W.W.; Arora, N.K.; Haffer, S.C.; Clauser, S.B. Impact of Cancer on Health-Related Quality of Life of Older Americans. *J. Natl. Cancer Inst.* **2009**, *101*, 860–868. [CrossRef]
90. Meraya, A.M.; Raval, A.D.; Sambamoorthi, U. Chronic Condition Combinations and Health Care Expenditures and Out-of-Pocket Spending Burden among Adults, Medical Expenditure Panel Survey, 2009 and 2011. *Prev. Chronic Dis.* **2015**, *12*, E12. [CrossRef] [PubMed]
91. Aschebrook-Kilfoy, B.; Schechter, R.B.; Shih, Y.C.; Kaplan, E.L.; Chiu, B.C.; Angelos, P.; Grogan, R.H. The Clinical and Economic Burden of a Sustained Increase in Thyroid Cancer Incidence. *Cancer Epidemiol. Biomarkers Prev.* **2013**, *22*, 1252–1259. [CrossRef]
92. Boltz, M.M.; Hollenbeak, C.S.; Schaefer, E.; Goldenberg, D.; Saunders, B.D. Attributable Costs of Differentiated Thyroid Cancer in the Elderly Medicare Population. *Surgery* **2013**, *154*, 1363–1369, discussion 1369–1370. [CrossRef]
93. Berger, A.; Edelsberg, J.; Chung, K.; Nguyen, A.; Stepan, D.; Oster, G. Healthcare (HC) Utilization and Costs in Patients (pts) with Newly Diagnosed Metastatic Thyroid Cancer (mTC). *J. Clin. Oncol.* **2007**, *25*, 170–182. [CrossRef]
94. Iadeluca, L.; Mardekian, J.; Chander, P.; Hopps, M.; Makinson, G.T. The Burden of Selected Cancers in the US: Health Behaviors and Health Care Resource Utilization. *Cancer Manag. Res.* **2017**, *9*, 721–730. [CrossRef]
95. Furuya-Kanamori, L.; Sedrakyan, A.; Onitilo, A.A.; Bagheri, N.; Glasziou, P.; Doi, S.A.R. Differentiated Thyroid Cancer: Millions Spent with No Tangible Gain? *Endocr. Relat. Cancer* **2018**, *25*, 51–57. [CrossRef]
96. Lang, B.H.; Wong, C.K.; Chan, C.T. Initial Attributable Cost and Economic Burden of Clinically-Relevant Differentiated Thyroid Cancer: A Health Care Service Provider Perspective. *Eur. J. Surg. Oncol.* **2015**, *41*, 758–765. [CrossRef] [PubMed]
97. Finnerty, B.M.; Brunaud, L.; Mirallie, E.; McIntyre, C.; Aronova, A.; Fahey, T.J., 3rd; Zarnegar, R. Cost Disparity between Health Care Systems—It's Not the Surgeons: A Cost Analysis of Thyroid Cancer Care between the United States and France. *Surgery* **2016**, *159*, 132–140. [CrossRef] [PubMed]
98. Bhattacharjee, S.; Khobrani, M.; Alrabiah, Z.; Bilal, J.; Riaz, I.B. Healthcare Expenditures among Community-Dwelling Adults with Thyroid Cancer in the United States: A Propensity Score Matched Analysis. *Heliyon* **2019**, *5*, e01995. [CrossRef]
99. White, C.; Weinstein, M.C.; Fingeret, A.L.; Randolph, G.W.; Miyauchi, A.; Ito, Y.; Zhan, T.; Ali, A.; Gazelle, G.S.; Lubitz, C.C. Is Less More? A Microsimulation Model Comparing Cost-Effectiveness of the Revised American Thyroid Association's 2015 to 2009 Guidelines for the Management of Patients with Thyroid Nodules and Differentiated Thyroid Cancer. *Ann. Surg.* **2020**, *271*, 765–773. [CrossRef]
100. Hyun, M.K.; Kim, J.H.; Kwon, J.W. Incidence of Thyroid Cancer and Medical Cost among Patients with Newly Diagnosed Thyroid Nodules in Korea: A Retrospective Cohort Study Using Nationwide Data. *J. Cancer Res. Ther.* **2019**, *15*, 676–680. [CrossRef] [PubMed]
101. Ver Hoeve, E.S.; Ali-Akbarian, L.; Price, S.N.; Lothfi, N.M.; Hamann, H.A. Patient-Reported Financial Toxicity, Quality of Life, and Health Behaviors in Insured US Cancer Survivors. *Support Care Cancer* **2021**, *29*, 349–358. [CrossRef] [PubMed]
102. Esserman, L.J.; Thompson, I.M.; Reid, B.; Nelson, P.; Ransohoff, D.F.; Welch, H.G.; Hwang, S.; Berry, D.A.; Kinzler, K.W.; Black, W.C.; et al. Addressing Overdiagnosis and Overtreatment in Cancer: A Prescription for Change. *Lancet Oncol.* **2014**, *15*, e234–e242. [CrossRef]
103. Canberk, S. Precursor and Borderline Lesions of the Thyroid (Indolent Lesions of Epithelial Origin): From Theory to Practice. *Gland Surg.* **2020**, *9*, 1724–1734. [CrossRef] [PubMed]
104. Schnadig, V.J. Overdiagnosis of Thyroid Cancer: Is This Not an Ethical Issue for Pathologists as Well as Radiologists and Clinicians? *Arch. Pathol. Lab. Med.* **2018**, *142*, 1018–1020. [CrossRef]
105. Culyer, A.J.; Newhouse, J.P. *Handbook of Health Economics*; Elsevier North Holland: Amsterdam, The Netherlands, 2000.
106. Neumann, P.J.; Sanders, G.D. Cost-Effectiveness Analysis 2.0. *N. Engl. J. Med.* **2017**, *376*, 203–205. [CrossRef] [PubMed]
107. Xu, X.; Grossetta Nardini, H.K.; Ruger, J.P. Micro-costing studies in the health and medical literature: Protocol for a systematic review. *Syst. Rev.* **2014**, *3*, 47. [CrossRef] [PubMed]
108. Rutter, C.M.; Zaslavsky, A.M.; Feuer, E.J. Dynamic microsimulation models for health outcomes: A review. *Med. Decis. Making.* **2011**, *31*, 10–18. [CrossRef] [PubMed]
109. Latouche, G.; Ramaswami, V. *Introduction to Matrix Analytic Methods in Stochastic Modeling*; SIAM: Philadelphia, PA, USA, 1999.

cancers

MDPI

Article

^{18}F-FDG-PET/CT in Patients with Advanced, Radioiodine Refractory Thyroid Cancer Treated with Lenvatinib

Freba Ahmaddy [1], Caroline Burgard [1], Leonie Beyer [1], Viktoria Florentine Koehler [2], Peter Bartenstein [1,3,4], Matthias P. Fabritius [5], Thomas Geyer [5], Vera Wenter [1], Harun Ilhan [1,3,4], Christine Spitzweg [2,3,4] and Andrei Todica [1,3,4,*]

1 Department of Nuclear Medicine, University Hospital, LMU Munich, 81377 Munich, Germany; Freba.Ahmaddy@med.uni-muenchen.de (F.A.); Caroline.Burgard@med.uni-muenchen.de (C.B.); Leonie.Beyer@med.uni-muenchen.de (L.B.); Peter.Bartenstein@med.uni-muenchen.de (P.B.); Vera.Wenter@med.uni-muenchen.de (V.W.); Harun.Ilhan@med.uni-muenchen.de (H.I.)
2 Department of Internal Medicine IV, University Hospital, LMU Munich, 81377 Munich, Germany; Viktoria.Koehler@med.uni-muenchen.de (V.F.K.); Christine.Spitzweg@med.uni-muenchen.de (C.S.)
3 Comprehensive Cancer Center (CCC LMU), University Hospital, LMU Munich, 81377 Munich, Germany
4 Interdisciplinary Center for Thyroid Carcinoma (ISKUM), University Hospital, LMU Munich, 81377 Munich, Germany
5 Department of Radiology, University Hospital, LMU Munich, 81377 Munich, Germany; Matthias.Fabritius@med.uni-muenchen.de (M.P.F.); Thomas.Geyer@med.uni-muenchen.de (T.G.)
* Correspondence: Andrei.Todica@med.uni-muenchen.de; Tel.: +49-89-4400-74653

Simple Summary: In patients with advanced radioiodine refractory differentiated thyroid carcinoma (DTC), therapeutic options are limited. In the "Study of (E7080) Lenvatinib in Differentiated Cancer of the Thyroid (SELECT)", Lenvatinib significantly prolonged the progression-free survival, resulting in a more frequent use in clinical practice for this patient group. Due to considerable side effects, an accurate assessment of response to treatment is crucial in these patients. Therefore, we aimed to improve treatment individualization and reduce unnecessary therapies by selecting patients who will most likely benefit from Lenvatinib treatment using 2-deoxy-2-[^{18}F] fluoro-D-glucose positron-emission-tomography/computed-tomography.

Abstract: Background: The tyrosine kinase inhibitor (TKI) Lenvatinib represents one of the most effective therapeutic options in patients with advanced radioiodine refractory differentiated thyroid carcinoma (DTC). We aimed to assess the role of 2-deoxy-2-[^{18}F] fluoro-D-glucose positron-emission-tomography/computed-tomography (^{18}F-FDG-PET/CT) in the monitoring of functional tumor response compared to morphological response. Methods: In 22 patients, a modified Positron Emission Tomography Response Criteria In Solid Tumors (mPERCIST) evaluation before treatment with Lenvatinib and at 3 and 6 month follow up was performed. Further PET-parameters and morphologic tumor response using Response Evaluation Criteria in Solid Tumors (RECIST) 1.1 were assessed and their prediction of progression-free survival (PFS) and disease-specific survival (DSS) was evaluated. Results: Most patients were rated stable in morphological evaluation and progressive using a metabolic response. All patients who responded to therapy through RECIST showed a decline in nearly all Positron Emission Tomography (PET)-parameters. For both time-points, non-responders according to mPERCIST showed significantly lower median PFS and DSS, whereas according to RECIST, only DSS was significantly lower. Conclusion: Tumor response assessment by ^{18}F-FDG-PET outperforms morphological response assessment by CT in patients with advanced radioiodine refractory DTC treated with Lenvatinib, which seems to be correlated with clinical outcomes.

Keywords: differentiated thyroid cancer; radioiodine refractory; Lenvatinib; ^{18}F-FDG-PET/CT

Citation: Ahmaddy, F.; Burgard, C.; Beyer, L.; Koehler, V.F.; Bartenstein, P.; Fabritius, M.P.; Geyer, T.; Wenter, V.; Ilhan, H.; Spitzweg, C.; et al. ^{18}F-FDG-PET/CT in Patients with Advanced, Radioiodine Refractory Thyroid Cancer Treated with Lenvatinib. *Cancers* **2021**, *13*, 317. https://doi.org/10.3390/cancers13020317

Received: 14 December 2020
Accepted: 14 January 2021
Published: 16 January 2021

Publisher's Note: MDPI stays neutral with regard to jurisdictional claims in published maps and institutional affiliations.

1. Introduction

Differentiated thyroid cancer (DTC) is the most frequent endocrine malignancy comprising the papillary (PTC), follicular (FTC) and poorly differentiated (PDTC) histological subtypes [1]. Although most patients with DTC can be cured by total thyroidectomy and radioiodine treatment (RAI; 10-year survival rate >90%) [2], approximately 5–10% of patients with DTC develop an aggressive disease with distant metastases and loss of 131-iodine avidity [3,4]. Inoperable metastatic and/or radioiodine refractory DTC is associated with a less favorable prognosis, with 10-year survival rates between 25% and 40%. Distant metastases most frequently occur in the lungs (50%), bones (25%) or both (20%) and less frequently at other sites (5%) [1,3,5,6]. In these patients, therapeutic options are limited.

Tyrosine kinase inhibitors (TKIs), which inhibit VEGF (vascular endothelial growth factor) receptor signaling and tumor angiogenesis, improve progression-free survival (PFS) in patients with structurally progressive, radioiodine refractory DTC [7–10]. Lenvatinib is an oral, multitargeted TKI targeting VEGFRs 1–3, FGFRs (fibroblast growth factor receptors) 1–4, PDGFR (platelet-derived growth factor receptor) α, RET (rearranged during transfection receptor tyrosine kinase) and c-KIT (receptor for stem cell factor) signaling networks [11,12]. In the placebo-controlled phase 3 "Study of (E7080) Lenvatinib in Differentiated Cancer of the Thyroid (SELECT)", Lenvatinib significantly prolonged progression-free survival (PFS), resulting in approval by the US Food and Drug Administration and European Medicines Agency in 2015 [13].

Accurate assessment of treatment response is crucial to discriminate between responders and non-responders thereby avoiding inefficient therapy and its potential adverse effects. The current standard for monitoring tumor response is measurement of change in tumor size based on anatomical imaging techniques such as computed tomography (CT); this technique has been most frequently assessed by the Response Evaluation Criteria in Solid Tumors (RECIST) [14], which were updated (RECIST 1.1 criteria) in 2009 [15]. As newer cancer treatments are cytostatic rather than cytotoxic, functional changes are expected to precede the morphologic changes and therefore 2-deoxy-2-[^{18}F] fluoro-D-glucose positron emission tomography/computed tomography (^{18}F-FDG-PET/CT) has the potential to improve diagnostic accuracy and prediction of the course of tumor development [16,17]. Wahl et al. described the Positron Emission Tomography Response Criteria In Solid Tumors (PERCIST) in 2009 to provide a structured guidance for response assessment using ^{18}F-FDG-PET [18]. However, data on potential ^{18}F-FDG-PET/CT applications in staging and restaging of advanced radioiodine refractory DTC is limited.

The aim of this study was to assess the role of ^{18}F-FDG-PET in the monitoring of functional tumor response (modified PERCIST 1.0 and quantitative PET-parameters) in comparison to morphological response (RECIST 1.1) in combined ^{18}F-FDG-PET/CT and thereby predicting both PFS and disease-specific survival (DSS) in patients with advanced radioiodine refractory DTC receiving Lenvatinib treatment.

2. Results

2.1. Patient Characteristics

Twenty-two patients (11 female) with advanced radioiodine refractory DTC fulfilled the inclusion criteria. The mean age at primary presentation was 53.1 ± 13.1 years and 60.8 ± 13.7 years at Lenvatinib treatment start. For most of the patients (n = 12), the histological subtype was FTC, followed by 7 PDTC and 3 PTC patients. Ten patients initially presented with stage IV, 9 patients with stage III and 3 patients with stage II DTC according to the seventh edition of the American Joint Committee on Cancer (AJCC) tumor-node-metastasis (TNM) staging system. A total of 4 out of 12 patients with FTC showed vascular invasion. Histopathological data of study patients are presented in Tables S1 and S3 in the supplements. Seven patients already showed distant metastases at primary presentation (5/7 patients with pulmonary metastases). At Lenvatinib treatment start, the majority of the patients (n = 20) showed advanced metastatic disease and in 14 patients, more than one site was affected. Metastatic sites were most frequently the lung (n = 19), followed by lymph nodes (n = 12), bone (n = 5), pleura (n = 2), liver (n = 2), subcutaneous metastases (n = 1), brain (n = 1) and kidney (n = 1). Local recurrence occurred in 6/22 patients (2/6 without distant metastases). Mean Thyroglobulin (Tg)-level at treatment start was 3950 ± 7062 ng/mL.

Prior to start of Lenvatinib treatment, all patients had total thyroidectomy with or without lymphadenectomy. Surgery had been followed by RIT for remnant ablation. Additionally, 15/22 patients received more than two courses of RIT (range 2–11), 12/22 patients had undergone further surgery/metastasectomy, 13/22 had received external beam radiotherapy, 9/22 patients had been treated with TKIs other than Lenvatinib (Sorafenib n = 7, Pazopanib n = 3, Cabozantinib n = 2), 2/22 had received chemotherapy and one patient had undergone redifferentiation therapy with Dabrafenib. Single-patient characteristics are presented in Table S1 in the supplemental information.

In 14/22 patients, treatment was initiated at full dose (daily dose of 24 mg per day) and 8/22 patients received reduced dosage (20 mg per day n = 1, 18 mg per day n = 3, 14 mg per day n = 3, 10 mg per day n = 1). The mean Lenvatinib dose during treatment was 17.7 ± 4.2 mg/die. Dose interruptions and incremental reductions in the dose because of toxic effects were seen in 16/22 patients. The most frequent adverse effects were hypertension (n = 14), fatigue (n = 12), decreased appetite (n = 12), diarrhea (n = 11) and nausea (n = 6).

2.2. *Evaluation of Treatment Response*

The median duration of treatment with Lenvatinib was 11.0 months (interquartile range, IQR 25% 5.2–IQR 75% 26.3). The median follow-up time was 17.0 months (IQR 25% 9.8–IQR 75% 27.0). By the time the follow-up period ended, 11/22 patients were still on Lenvatinib treatment. The mean time from baseline ^{18}F-FDG-PET/CT to treatment initiation was 1.2 months (range 0–4.0), the first follow-up ^{18}F-FDG-PET/CT was performed after a mean of 3.7 months (range 2.0–6.0) and the second follow-up occurred after a mean of 5.6 months (range 3.0–8.0).

2.2.1. Treatment Response According to mPERCIST and RECIST

After 3.7 ± 1.0 months, data of 19 patients were available for response evaluation. Of those 19 patients, 12/19 patients showed disease control (DC) according to mPERCIST and 14/19 showed DC according to RECIST, whereas 7/19 patients showed progressive disease (PD) according to mPERCIST and 5/19 patients according to RECIST. None of the enrolled patients showed complete response (CR) in morphological evaluation (RECIST), though 3 patients showed CR in a metabolic assessment (see Figure 1a).

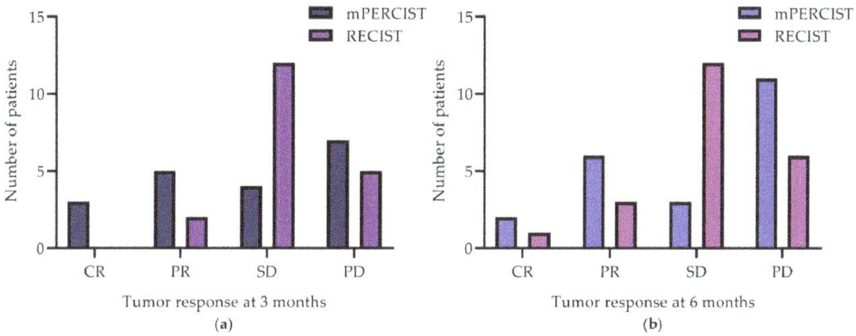

Figure 1. Tumor response evaluation by mPERCIST and RECIST criteria at 3 month (**a**) and 6 month (**b**) follow-up imaging. mPERCIST, modified Positron Emission Tomography Response Criteria In Solid Tumors; RECIST, Response Evaluation Criteria in Solid Tumors; CR, complete response; PR, partial response; SD, stable disease; PD, progressive disease.

After 5.7 ± 1.4 months, 22 patients were evaluated. Compared to baseline, more patients showed PD (mPERCIST/RECIST: 11/6), but 2 patients indicated CR according to mPERCIST and one patient according to RECIST (see Figure 1b).

For both evaluation time-points, the majority of patients were rated SD in morphological evaluation (3 months: $n = 12$, 6 months: $n = 12$), while there was more heterogeneity in metabolic treatment response, with most patients presenting with PD. Details of treatment response at 3 and 6 months are presented in Figure 1 and single-patient course of disease are summarized in Table S2 in the supplemental file.

2.2.2. Additional Single PET-Parameters

When evaluating single PET-parameters (mean/maximum standardized uptake value ($SUV_{mean/max}$), Metabolic Tumor Volume (MTV) and Total Lesion Glycolysis (TLG)) additionally to mPERCIST classification according to peak standardized uptake value (SUV_{peak}) measurements, all responders (RECIST) showed a decline in all PET-parameters from baseline to the 3 month follow-up and from baseline to the 6 month follow-up, except SUV_{mean} from baseline to the 6 month follow-up.

The mean changes of all PET-parameters over 6 months follow-up divided into DC/PD (RECIST) and significant differences between groups are shown in Table 1 and Figure 2. For both time-points, DC patients showed significantly lower SUV_{peak} (3 months: $p = 0.004$, 6 months: $p = 0.023$), SUV_{max} (3 months: $p = 0.003$, 6 months: $p = 0.008$), MTV (3 months: $p = 0.010$, 6 months: $p = 0.006$) and TLG values (3 months: $p = 0.019$, 6 months: $p = 0.011$). One patient was excluded due to not measurable uptake in baseline ^{18}F-FDG-PET/CT. The percentage change of Tg-levels from baseline to the 3 month follow up and baseline to the 6 month follow-up ^{18}F-FDG-PET/CT showed no significant difference between DC and PD patients (baseline to 3 months: −41% ± 72%, $p = 0.853$; baseline to 6 months: −45% ± 73%, $p = 0.436$).

Table 1. Mean changes and SD (%) of PET-parameters in patients with DC and PD according to RECIST from baseline to 3 and 6 month follow-up imaging.

Mean Change ±SD (%)	SUV_{peak}	SUV_{mean}	SUV_{max}	MTV	TLG
		Baseline to 3 Month Follow-Up			
DC (n = 13/18)	−43% ± 45%	−12% ± 28%	−33% ± 35%	−56% ± 38%	−56% ± 42%
PD (n = 5/19)	49% ± 84%	12% ± 51%	66% ± 62%	439% ± 718%	797% ± 1489%
p-value	0.004 **	0.336	0.003 **	0.010 *	0.019 *
		Baseline to 6 Month Follow-Up			
DC (n = 15/21)	−42% ± 57%	−2% ± 21%	−24% ± 35%	−23% ± 152%	−10% ± 189%
PD (n = 6/22)	36% ± 81%	9% ± 46%	49% ± 68%	394% ± 652%	687% ± 1358%
p-value	0.023 *	0.677	0.008 **	0.006 **	0.011 *

DC, disease control; PD, progressive disease; SD, standard deviation; SUV, standard uptake value; MTV, metabolic tumor volume; TLG, total lesion glycolysis; * *p*-value < 0.05; ** *p*-value < 0.01.

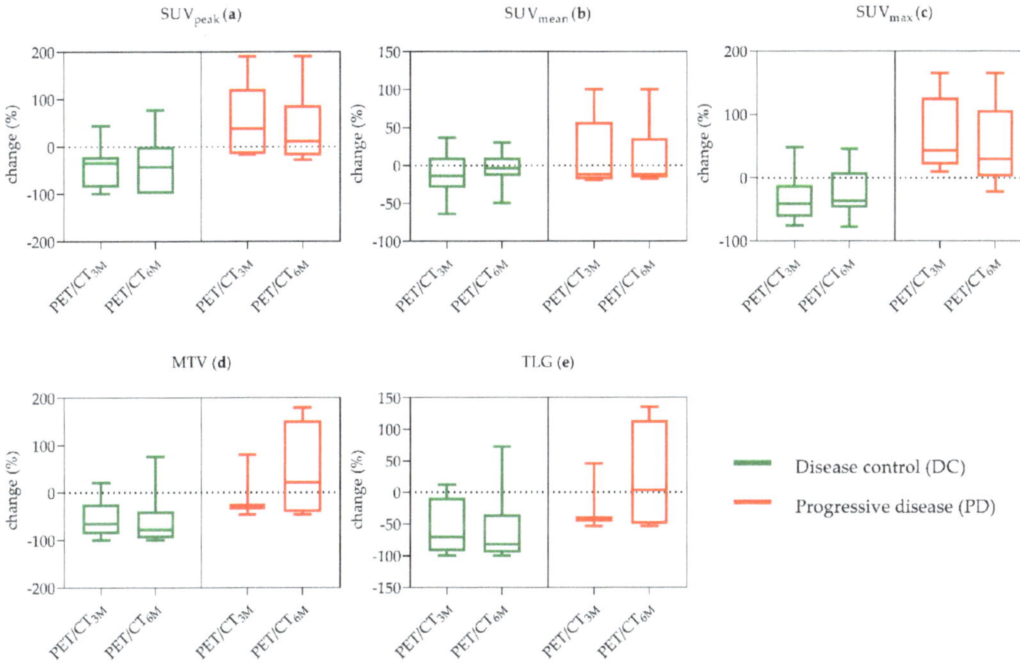

Figure 2. Mean changes of PET-parameters (**a**) SUV_{peak}, (**b**) SUV_{mean}, (**c**) SUV_{max}, (**d**) MTV and (**e**) TLG in patients with DC and PD according to RECIST from baseline to 3 and 6 month follow-up imaging. 3M, 3 months; 6M, 6 months; DC, disease control; PD, progressive disease; SUV, standard uptake value; MTV, metabolic tumor volume; TLG, total lesion glycolysis.

2.3. Outcome Analysis

During the follow-up period, 13/22 patients progressed (according to RECIST). The mean PFS was 12.5 ± 9.2 months. At the end of the study, 12/22 patients had died of thyroid cancer. The mean DSS was 14.2 ± 9.1 months. For detailed PFS and DSS of all patients, see Table S2 in the supplemental information.

PD according to mPERCIST was correlated with worse outcomes and significantly lower PFS and DSS for both time-points. Patients with PD at 3 month follow-up showed a significant lower median PFS (4.0 vs. 24 months, p = 0.008) and DSS (20.0 months vs. median not reached for responders, p = 0.015) compared to DC (see Figure 3a,c). At the 6 month follow-up, mPERCIST also showed significant differences for both PFS and DSS (PFS 4.0 vs. 15.0 months, p = 0.003; DSS 9.0 months vs. the median not reached for responders, p = 0.001) between DC and PD (see Figure 3b,d).

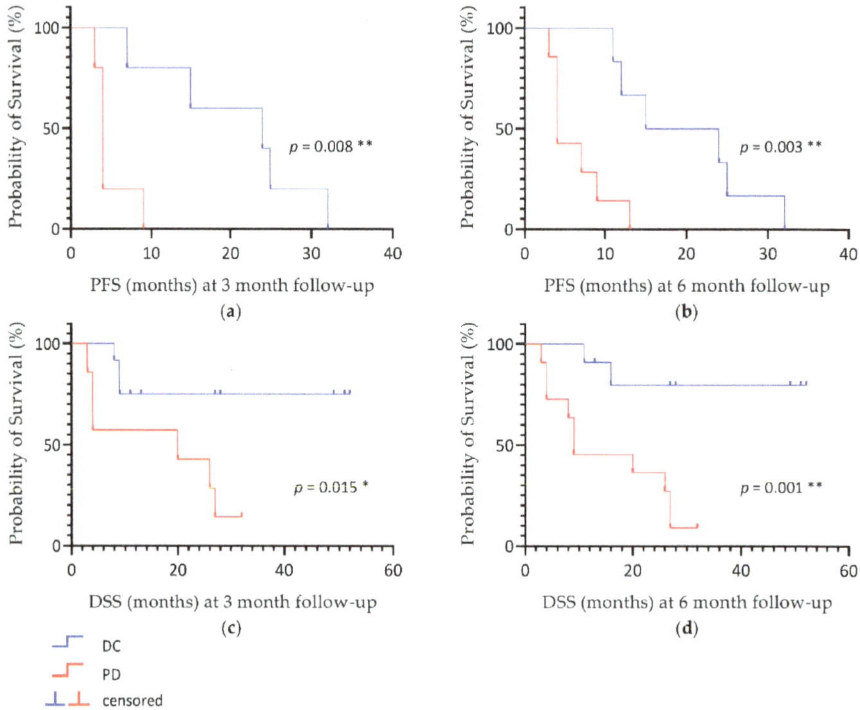

Figure 3. Kaplan-Meier estimate of PFS (**a**,**b**) and DSS (**c**,**d**) according to mPERCIST criteria for 3 and 6 month follow-up imaging. PFS, progression-free survival; DSS, disease-specific survival; DC, disease control; PD, progressive disease; * p-value < 0.05; ** p-value < 0.01.

According to the RECIST criteria, PFS did not differ between PD and DC patients at 3 months (15.0 versus 4.0 months, $p = 0.196$) and 6 months (13.0 versus 4.0 months, $p = 0.114$). Patients with PD by RECIST showed a significantly lower median DSS at 3 months (4.0 months versus median not reached, $p = 0.046$) and 6 months (6.5 months versus median not reached, $p = 0.039$; see Table 2).

Table 2. Association of PD and DC according to mPERCIST and RECIST to PFS and DSS at the 3 month and 6 month follow-ups.

p-Value	mPERCIST		RECIST	
	3 Months	6 Months	3 Months	6 Months
PFS	0.008 **	0.003 **	0.196	0.114
DSS	0.015 *	0.001 **	0.046 *	0.039 *

mPERCIST, modified Positron Emission Tomography Response Criteria In Solid Tumors; RECIST, Response Evaluation Criteria in Solid Tumors; DC, disease control; PD, progressive disease; * p-value < 0.05; ** p-value < 0.01.

All other PET-parameters showed no significant association to PFS and DSS for both time-points.

3. Discussion

In the present study, we investigated the role of ^{18}F-FDG-PET/CT for monitoring functional tumor response in comparison to morphological imaging and its ability to predict PFS and DSS in patients with advanced, radioiodine refractory DTC undergoing

Lenvatinib treatment. Our results demonstrate that functional imaging is able to evaluate tumor response in a more differentiated manner than morphological imaging only. In our series, all patients who responded to therapy showed a decline in all PET-parameters except SUV_{mean}, whereas a lack of functional tumor response was associated with a worse outcome (PFS and DSS). PET-parameters SUV_{peak}, SUV_{max}, MTV and TLG at 3 and 6 month follow-ups were significantly higher in patients with disease progression and could serve as additional markers for monitoring early tumor response and outcome.

The current standard for monitoring treatment response and progression in clinical trials is the change in tumor size assessed by RECIST. To date, the current guidelines do not give specific recommendations for response monitoring in patients with DTC outside clinical trials and response assessment by PERCIST is not mentioned [19]. Since clinical patient management and treatment planning depend on response monitoring through imaging, clinical decisions may vary based on different imaging modalities.

^{18}F-FDG-PET/CT combines functional and morphological imaging. Measurement of glucose metabolism varies less than tumor size measurements and can better distinguish between active tumor and post-therapeutic changes [20,21]. Tumor response evaluation using ^{18}F-FDG-PET/CT showed promising results for several cancer entities, such as breast, lung and pancreatic cancer [17,21–23]. In addition, many previous studies have shown the important role of ^{18}F-FDG-PET/CT in staging and follow-up of patients with advanced, metastatic DTC [24–26] and its valuable role in patients with metastatic DTC under treatment with TKIs [27,28]. However, to date the number of studies in patients with DTC undergoing Lenvatinib treatment is limited and no standardized treatment assessment has been proposed so far.

Tumor FDG-uptake can be measured in various ways. Firstly, we used the single-lesion method according to Wahl et al. [29], which was shown to be superior to the five-lesion method [22,30]. Secondly, in accordance to Fendler et al., we used peak standardized uptake value corrected for body weight (SUV_{peak}) instead of lean body mass corrected SUV (SUL_{peak}) as proposed by PERCIST 1.0, because the main objective is the percentage change of SUV from baseline to follow-up imaging and should therefore not be a significant confounder [31]. Riedl et al. could also show that response classification was unchanged when SUV_{max} was used instead of SUL_{peak} in patients with metastatic breast cancer [22]. Thus, we measured the SUV_{peak} of the most active lesion, which may differ in consecutive scans. Furthermore, we assessed the PET-parameters SUV_{mean}, SUV_{max}, MTV and TLG to identify possible other measures since technical methods for quantitative measurement are under continuous improvement [32].

Novel cancer therapies, such as TKI treatment, are cytostatic rather than cytotoxic and therefore may not result in a significant decrease of tumor size [33,34]. Additionally, certain metastasis localizations such as bone metastasis do not frequently show morphological changes after therapy [22]. Thus, differentiation of tumor response categorization in CR, PR, SD and PD in these patients by morphological imaging is limited. However, FDG-uptake in tumor cells is known to correlate with disease prognosis [35] and, as precision therapy is evolving, the current monitoring of treatment response does not seem to have been adjusted accordingly.

Whereas the majority of patients in our study were categorized as SD by RECIST 1.1 on CT at both follow-up times, our data show that patients were categorized in a more differentiated manner by mPERCIST using ^{18}F-FDG-PET. This finding is in line with the study of Riedl et al., who reported that patients with metastatic breast cancer with SD and PD by RECIST were frequently classified worse by PERCIST [22].

Based on these differences in categorization of patients, Kaplan-Meier analysis demonstrated significant distinction between DC and PD. Tumor response by mPERCIST was significantly correlated with PFS and DSS, whereas tumor response by morphological imaging showed no significant correlation. In our study, responses determined by using the RECIST 1.1 criteria at 3 and 6 months was found to be statistically significant for DSS, but the association was lower compared to the mPERCIST response, indicating that mPERCIST detects progression more precisely than RECIST. All other PET-parameters ($SUV_{mean/max}$, MTV and TLG) showed no significant association with PFS and DSS. These findings are consistent with the results reported by Riedl et al. [22] and could subsequently lead to earlier change of therapy in patients considered SD by RECIST but do not show therapy response by mPERCIST. The association of metabolic response with survival benefit has already been shown in several other solid tumors such as breast cancer [36].

In this study, a decline of nearly all PET-parameters was found in patients with DC. Studies on the role of the PET-parameter SUV_{max} in DTC patients are limited. In line with our data, Carr et al. showed that patients with metastatic DTC or medullary thyroid carcinoma treated with Sunitinib showing DC had a significant decline in average and mean percentage change SUV_{max} compared to patients with progressive disease [27]. A significant decline in SUV_{max} could also be shown in patients with radioiodine refractory DTC treated with Apatinib, whereas in DTC patients treated with Vandetanib, no correlation between SUV_{max} and DC could be found [37]. To date, SUV_{max} is the most commonly used semiquantitative PET-parameter due to its simple application but there are more and more studies suggesting the use of SUV_{peak} alternatively [38]. Since SUV_{peak} is measured in a larger VOI than the single-pixel SUV_{max}, it appears to be more robust to image noise.

The volume-related PET-parameters MTV and TLG could also show promising results in metastatic DTC patients. The study by Manohar et al. showed that these parameters can be used for dynamic risk stratification regarding PFS [39]. TLG appeared promising in some cancers such as colorectal cancer and brain tumors, but not in others such as sarcomas [40–43]. Data from Lee et al. showed that in patients with pancreatic cancer, TLG was an independent prognostic factor for predicting recurrence-free and overall survival, whereas Benz et al. reported that TLG was less accurate in predicting tumor response in sarcomas compared to SUV_{mean} and SUV_{max} [23,40]. The same was shown for MTV, which was found to be useful for treatment response assessment in non-small cell lung cancer (NSCLC) and pancreatic cancer [23,44]. Furthermore, it was demonstrated to be an independent prognostic factor for DSS in patients with cervical cancer treated by radical surgery and could independently predict survival in patients with locally advanced squamous cell cervical carcinoma [45,46]. Indeed, in our analysis, volume related PET-parameters (MTV and TLG) were found to be useful tools to distinguish DC from PD but failed to provide prognostic value in terms of PFS and DSS. SUV_{mean} showed the weakest correlation with tumor response in our study. In contrast, Werner et al. identified a SUV_{mean} of less than 4.0 before treatment in medullary thyroid carcinoma as a predictor of longer PFS [20]. Consequently, all PET-parameters except for SUV_{mean} seem to be a useful tool and may be evaluated alongside SUV_{peak} as suggested in PERCIST 1.1 criteria [29].

The percentage change of Tg-levels from baseline to 3 month- and baseline to 6 month follow-up ^{18}F-FDG-PET/CT showed no significant difference between DC and PD patients. One possible explanation for the missing correlation between Tg and ^{18}F-FDG-PET/CT might be the different de-differentiation level of the thyroid cancer patients treated with Lenvatinib.

To our knowledge, this is the first study attempting to address the impact of using different imaging modalities and therefore different evaluation criteria for treatment response in patients with advanced, radioiodine refractory DTC undergoing Lenvatinib treatment. However, the role of ^{18}F-FDG-PET/CT and the selection of the optimal PET-parameters for monitoring of functional tumor response in patients with advanced, radioiodine refractory DTC undergoing Lenvatinib treatment will have to be verified in prospective trials in larger patient cohorts.

Our study has several limitations. Due to the retrospective design of the study, the span between baseline imaging and initiation of treatment and the intervals of follow-up imaging varied between patients and follow-up imaging at 3 months was not available in all patients. Furthermore, due to the small cohort, the rarity of the disease and heterogeneity in patient cohort (histology, stage of disease), statistical power of the analysis is limited.

4. Materials and Methods

4.1. Study Population

For this retrospective study, we selected patients with advanced, radioiodine-refractory PTC, FTC and PDTC undergoing Lenvatinib treatment at the department of endocrinology (University Hospital, LMU Munich, Munich, Germany) between May 2015 and August 2019. Patients were eligible for inclusion in this study when the time span between baseline ^{18}F-FDG-PET/CT and initiation of treatment was less than 4 months and follow-up imaging was performed after 3 $\pm$ 3 months and/or 6 $\pm$ 3 months at the Department of Nuclear Medicine (University Hospital, LMU Munich, Munich, Germany).

All patients had extended disease, were radioiodine-refractory and had at least one FDG-positive lesion, except for one patient at baseline PET scan. Lenvatinib treatment was initiated based on a multidisciplinary tumor board decision.

4.2. Ethics Statement

The study was approved by the local ethics committee (Ethics committee of the Medical Faculty,

University Hospital, LMU Munich, Munich, Germany, IRB #20-736, 21.09.2020) and has been conducted in accordance with the ethical standards of the Declaration of Helsinki and national and international guidelines. The requirement to obtain informed consent was waived due to the retrospective design of this study.

4.3. Imaging Techniques

Patients fasted at least 6 h (demanded glucose level <160 mg/dL). Prior to the injection of approximately 250 MBq ^{18}F-FDG whole-body, ^{18}F-FDG-PET/CT images were acquired using a Biograph 64 TruePoint w/TrueV and Biograph mCT Flow 20-4R PET/CT scanner (Siemens, Healthcare GmbH, Erlangen, Germany) and were initiated approximately 60 min after intravenous tracer administration. After intravenous injection of a contrast agent (Ultravist 300, Bayer Vital GmbH, Leverkusen, Germany or Imeron 350, 2.5 mL/s, Bracco Imaging Deutschland GmbH, Konstanz, Germany) diagnostic CT scans of the neck, thorax, abdomen and pelvis (100–190 mAs; 120 kV) were acquired.

To depict the venous phase, initiation of CT acquisition was delayed 90 s after injection of the contrast agent.

4.4. Response Evaluation

Complete response (CR), partial response (PR) and stable disease (SD) were considered as disease control (DC), remaining patients were categorized as progressive disease (PD) using both RECIST 1.1 in CT and modified PERCIST criteria (mPERCIST) in ^{18}F-FDG-PET of combined ^{18}F-FDG-PET/CT.

4.4.1. RECIST 1.1

The implementation of the evaluation criteria RECIST 1.1 is based on the original publication of Eisenhauer et al. [15]. RECIST 1.1 was performed by an experienced radiologist using mint Lesion version 3.7 software (Mint Medical GmbH, Heidelberg, Germany) without knowledge of the results of the PET studies. A maximum of 3 to 5 target lesions were measured (max. 2 target lesions per organ) and at least 2 non-target lesions at baseline, 3 month and 6 month follow-up CT-scans. Time-point responses were then evaluated automatically. A relative increase of 20% and an absolute increase of at least 5 mm in target sum were considered as PD, while a decrease of 30% in target sum was considered PR.

4.4.2. mPERCIST and Other PET-Parameters

Semi-automated measurements of PET-parameters in ^{18}F-FDG-PET of the entire tumor burden in all patients were performed by an experienced nuclear medicine physician using image fusion software (Hybrid Viewer 2.6, Hermes Medical Solutions, Stockholm, Sweden) [29]. First the background was measured in the healthy liver to ensure the technical comparability of PET studies and to determine if the target tumor lesion shows sufficiently high glucose uptake with a minimum threshold for measurability defined as 1.5 × (mean value of normal liver) + 2 × (standard deviation of liver) or greater at baseline. For measurements of the background activity a fixed 3-cm diameter spherical volume of interest (VOI) was placed in the right side of the liver. Furthermore, a new lesion or unequivocal progression in the follow-up PET scan was rated as progressive disease changes, even if the target lesion at baseline did not show the minimum glucose uptake.

To assess treatment response by mPERCIST change in peak standardized uptake value (SUV_{peak}) was measured in the tumor region with the highest radiotracer uptake, which describes the average SUV computed in a fixed 1-mL sphere recommended by PERCIST instead of the widely used single-pixel maximum standardized uptake value (SUV_{max}) to avoid noise errors [18,29]. In a slight modification to the PERCIST 1.0 criteria, the quantitative PET-parameter was adjusted to body weight (SUV_{peak} in g/mL) rather than the body surface area (SUL_{peak}), as previously described by Fendler et al. for the single most active lesion in the patient at baseline, 3 month and 6 month follow-up [31]. A 1 mL spherical VOI was placed at the focus of the single active lesion and the highest SUV_{peak} value was computed automatically. The single most active lesion presents the target lesion, from which it is assumed to correspond to the worst behaving portion of the tumor. The percentage changes in SUV_{peak} from the reference baseline scan to 3 month and 6 month follow-up scans were assessed in all patients. In mPERCIST, decrease greater than or equal to 30% in SUV_{peak} was considered as PR and increase greater than 30% as PD (see Table 3).

Table 3. mPERCIST criteria from Wahl [29], modified by Fendler et al. [31].

Response Criteria	
Complete response (CR)	Normalization of all lesions to SUVpeak less than mean liver SUV and indistinguishable from surrounding background
Partial response (PR)	>30% decrease in SUVpeak; minimum 0.8 unit decrease in SUVpeak
Stable disease (SD)	Does not meet other criteria
Progressive disease (PD)	>30% increase in SUVpeak; minimum 0.8 unit increase in SUVpeak>75% increase in TLG

Outcome determination is measured on the single most active lesion on each scan (not necessarily the same lesion). Standardized uptake value (SUV).

All further PET-parameters were derived through segmentation of all tumor lesions: mean/maximum standardized uptake value ($SUV_{mean/max}$), Metabolic Tumor Volume (MTV) and Total Lesion Glycolysis (TLG). MTV was defined by volume delineation and TLG was calculated as (MTV x SUV_{mean}) [23]. All areas with physiological, non-tumoral ^{18}F-FDG-uptake were excluded. Response was determined separately in all PET-parameters using the same criteria for percentage change except for TLG, which had to show an increase of greater than 75% according to Wahl et al. to be assessed as PD (see Table 3) [29].

4.5. Outcome Analysis

PFS was defined as the time between treatment start and disease progression according to RECIST 1.1. Disease-specific survival (DSS) was calculated from the time of baseline ^{18}F-FDG-PET/CT until time of death. The observation period ended on 26th of May 2020.

4.6. Statistical Analysis

Ordinal and continuous variables are presented as median (interquartile range, IQR) or mean ± standard deviation (SD). Change in % was calculated using the following formula: ((value of follow-up PET)/(value of baseline PET) − 1) × 100. The Mann-Whitney u test was used to compare mean percentage changes between DC and PD patients. Survival analysis using Kaplan-Meier analysis was performed for PFS and DSS according to the mPERCIST and RECIST 1.1 criteria for 3 month and 6 month follow-ups. Quantitative survival data are given as median in months. Log rank test was used to compare survival rates between subgroups. *p*-values ≤ 0.05 were considered to indicate statistical significance. All analyses were performed using SPSS computer software (SPSS Statistics 25, IBM).

5. Conclusions

In conclusion, our study suggests that in patients with advanced radioiodine refractory DTC undergoing Lenvatinib treatment, tumor response evaluation by ^{18}F-FDG-PET/CT outperforms morphological response evaluation using CT and furthermore appears to be stronger correlated with outcome analysis. Monitoring tumor response with ^{18}F-FDG-PET/CT in these patients has the potential to improve treatment individualization and avoid ineffective therapies by selecting patients who will most likely benefit from Lenvatinib treatment. Therefore, tumor response assessed by ^{18}F-FDG-PET/CT is a highly promising modality in order to increase diagnostic accuracy in these patients and should be further investigated.

Supplementary Materials: The following are available online at https://www.mdpi.com/2072-6694/13/2/317/s1, Table S1: Patient Characteristics, Table S2: Single-Patient Course of Disease.

Author Contributions: Conceptualization, F.A., L.B. and A.T.; methodology, F.A., L.B., C.B. and A.T.; software, F.A. and C.B.; validation, F.A., L.B. and A.T.; formal analysis, T.G.; investigation, F.A. and V.F.K.; data curation, F.A., C.B. and V.F.K.; writing—original draft preparation, F.A., L.B. and A.T.; writing—review and editing, F.A., L.B., V.W., H.I., M.P.F., C.S. and A.T.; supervision, P.B., C.S. and A.T. All authors have read and agreed to the published version of the manuscript.

Funding: Vera Wenter was financially supported by the Kuhbier-Langewiesche foundation and the Bavarian Equal Opportunities Sponsorship (BGF). The foundation had no role in study design, data collection and analysis, decision to publish, or preparation of the manuscript. No other potential conflicts of interest relevant to this article exist.

Institutional Review Board Statement: The study was conducted according to the guidelines of the Declaration of Helsinki, and approved by the Ethics Committee of the Medical Faculty, University Hospital, LMU Munich, Munich, Germany (IRB #20-736, 21.09.2020).

Informed Consent Statement: Informed consent was obtained from all subjects involved in the study.

Data Availability Statement: The data presented in this study are available upon reasonable request from the corresponding author.

Acknowledgments: This study is part of the doctoral thesis of Freba Ahmaddy. Vera Wenter was financially supported by the Bavarian Equal Opportunities Sponsorship (BGF) to promote equal opportunities for women in research and teaching. The sponsorship did not influence the study design, data collection and analysis, decision to publish, or preparation of the manuscript.

Conflicts of Interest: The authors declare no conflict of interest.

References

1. Schlumberger, M.; Sherman, S.I. Approach to the patient with advanced differentiated thyroid cancer. *Eur. J. Endocrinol.* **2012**, *166*, 5–11. [CrossRef] [PubMed]
2. Links, T.P.; van Tol, K.M.; Jager, P.L.; Plukker, J.T.; Piers, D.A.; Boezen, H.M.; Dullaart, R.P.; de Vries, E.G.; Sluiter, W.J. Life expectancy in differentiated thyroid cancer: A novel approach to survival analysis. *Endocr. Relat. Cancer* **2005**, *12*, 273–280. [CrossRef] [PubMed]
3. Durante, C.; Haddy, N.; Baudin, E.; Leboulleux, S.; Hartl, D.; Travagli, J.P.; Caillou, B.; Ricard, M.; Lumbroso, J.D.; De Vathaire, F.; et al. Long-term outcome of 444 patients with distant metastases from papillary and follicular thyroid carcinoma: Benefits and limits of radioiodine therapy. *J. Clin. Endocrinol. Metab.* **2006**, *91*, 2892–2899. [CrossRef] [PubMed]
4. Eustatia-Rutten, C.F.; Corssmit, E.P.; Biermasz, N.R.; Pereira, A.M.; Romijn, J.A.; Smit, J.W. Survival and death causes in differentiated thyroid carcinoma. *J. Clin. Endocrinol. Metab.* **2006**, *91*, 313–319. [CrossRef] [PubMed]
5. Schlumberger, M. Management of refractory thyroid cancers. *Ann. D'endocrinol.* **2011**, *72*, 149–157. [CrossRef]
6. Schlumberger, M.J. Diagnostic follow-up of well-differentiated thyroid carcinoma: Historical perspective and current status. *J. Endocrinol. Investig.* **1999**, *22*, 3–7.

7. Brose, M.S.; Nutting, C.M.; Jarzab, B.; Elisei, R.; Siena, S.; Bastholt, L.; de la Fouchardiere, C.; Pacini, F.; Paschke, R.; Shong, Y.K.; et al. Sorafenib in radioactive iodine-refractory, locally advanced or metastatic differentiated thyroid cancer: A randomised, double-blind, phase 3 trial. *Lancet* **2014**, *384*, 319–328. [CrossRef]
8. Nair, A.; Lemery, S.J.; Yang, J.; Marathe, A.; Zhao, L.; Zhao, H.; Jiang, X.; He, K.; Ladouceur, G.; Mitra, A.K.; et al. FDA Approval Summary: Lenvatinib for Progressive, Radio-iodine-Refractory Differentiated Thyroid Cancer. *Clin. Cancer Res.* **2015**, *21*, 5205–5208. [CrossRef]
9. Schneider, T.C.; Abdulrahman, R.M.; Corssmit, E.P.; Morreau, H.; Smit, J.W.; Kapiteijn, E. Long-term analysis of the efficacy and tolerability of sorafenib in advanced radio-iodine refractory differentiated thyroid carcinoma: Final results of a phase II trial. *Eur. J. Endocrinol.* **2012**, *167*, 643–650. [CrossRef]
10. Cabanillas, M.E.; Habra, M.A. Lenvatinib: Role in thyroid cancer and other solid tumors. *Cancer Treat. Rev.* **2016**, *42*, 47–55. [CrossRef]
11. Matsui, J.; Funahashi, Y.; Uenaka, T.; Watanabe, T.; Tsuruoka, A.; Asada, M. Multi-kinase inhibitor E7080 suppresses lymph node and lung metastases of human mammary breast tumor MDA-MB-231 via inhibition of vascular endothelial growth factor-receptor (VEGF-R) 2 and VEGF-R3 kinase. *Clin. Cancer Res.* **2008**, *14*, 5459–5465. [CrossRef] [PubMed]
12. Matsui, J.; Yamamoto, Y.; Funahashi, Y.; Tsuruoka, A.; Watanabe, T.; Wakabayashi, T.; Uenaka, T.; Asada, M. E7080, a novel inhibitor that targets multiple kinases, has potent antitumor activities against stem cell factor producing human small cell lung cancer H146, based on angiogenesis inhibition. *Int. J. Cancer* **2008**, *122*, 664–671. [CrossRef] [PubMed]
13. Schlumberger, M.; Tahara, M.; Wirth, L.J.; Robinson, B.; Brose, M.S.; Elisei, R.; Habra, M.A.; Newbold, K.; Shah, M.H.; Hoff, A.O.; et al. Lenvatinib versus placebo in radioiodine-refractory thyroid cancer. *N. Engl. J. Med.* **2015**, *372*, 621–630. [CrossRef] [PubMed]
14. Therasse, P.; Arbuck, S.G.; Eisenhauer, E.A.; Wanders, J.; Kaplan, R.S.; Rubinstein, L.; Verweij, J.; Van Glabbeke, M.; van Oosterom, A.T.; Christian, M.C.; et al. New guidelines to evaluate the response to treatment in solid tumors. European Organization for Research and Treatment of Cancer, National Cancer Institute of the United States, National Cancer Institute of Canada. *J. Natl. Cancer Inst.* **2000**, *92*, 205–216. [CrossRef] [PubMed]
15. Eisenhauer, E.A.; Therasse, P.; Bogaerts, J.; Schwartz, L.H.; Sargent, D.; Ford, R.; Dancey, J.; Arbuck, S.; Gwyther, S.; Mooney, M.; et al. New response evaluation criteria in solid tumours: Revised RECIST guideline (version 1.1). *Eur. J. Cancer* **2009**, *45*, 228–247. [CrossRef] [PubMed]
16. Ziai, D.; Wagner, T.; El Badaoui, A.; Hitzel, A.; Woillard, J.B.; Melloni, B.; Monteil, J. Therapy response evaluation with FDG-PET/CT in small cell lung cancer: A prognostic and comparison study of the PERCIST and EORTC criteria. *Cancer Imaging* **2013**, *13*, 73–80. [CrossRef]
17. Yamamoto, Y.; Kameyama, R.; Murota, M.; Bandoh, S.; Ishii, T.; Nishiyama, Y. Early assessment of therapeutic response using FDG PET in small cell lung cancer. *Mol. Imaging Biol.* **2009**, *11*, 467–472. [CrossRef]
18. Joo Hyun, O.; Lodge, M.A.; Wahl, R.L. Practical PERCIST: A Simplified Guide to PET Response Criteria in Solid Tumors 1.0. *Radiology* **2016**, *280*, 576–584. [CrossRef]
19. Haugen, B.R.; Alexander, E.K.; Bible, K.C.; Doherty, G.M.; Mandel, S.J.; Nikiforov, Y.E.; Pacini, F.; Randolph, G.W.; Sawka, A.M.; Schlumberger, M.; et al. 2015 American Thyroid Association Management Guidelines for Adult Patients with Thyroid Nodules and Differentiated Thyroid Cancer: The American Thyroid Association Guidelines Task Force on Thyroid Nodules and Differentiated Thyroid Cancer. *Thyroid* **2016**, *26*, 1–133. [CrossRef]
20. Jacene, H.A.; Leboulleux, S.; Baba, S.; Chatzifotiadis, D.; Goudarzi, B.; Teytelbaum, O.; Horton, K.M.; Kamel, I.; Macura, K.J.; Tsai, H.L.; et al. Assessment of interobserver reproducibility in quantitative 18F-FDG PET and CT measurements of tumor response to therapy. *J. Nucl. Med.* **2009**, *50*, 1760–1769. [CrossRef]
21. Hildebrandt, M.G.; Gerke, O.; Baun, C.; Falch, K.; Hansen, J.A.; Farahani, Z.A.; Petersen, H.; Larsen, L.B.; Duvnjak, S.; Buskevica, I.; et al. [18F]Fluorodeoxyglucose (FDG)-Positron Emission Tomography (PET)/Computed Tomography (CT) in Suspected Recurrent Breast Cancer: A Prospective Comparative Study of Dual-Time-Point FDG-PET/CT, Contrast-Enhanced CT, and Bone Scintigraphy. *J. Clin. Oncol.* **2016**, *34*, 1889–1897. [CrossRef] [PubMed]
22. Riedl, C.C.; Pinker, K.; Ulaner, G.A.; Ong, L.T.; Baltzer, P.; Jochelson, M.S.; McArthur, H.L.; Gonen, M.; Dickler, M.; Weber, W.A. Comparison of FDG-PET/CT and contrast-enhanced CT for monitoring therapy response in patients with metastatic breast cancer. *Eur. J. Nucl. Med. Mol. Imaging* **2017**, *44*, 1428–1437. [CrossRef]
23. Lee, J.W.; Kang, C.M.; Choi, H.J.; Lee, W.J.; Song, S.Y.; Lee, J.H.; Lee, J.D. Prognostic Value of Metabolic Tumor Volume and Total Lesion Glycolysis on Preoperative ^{18}F-FDG PET/CT in Patients with Pancreatic Cancer. *J. Nucl. Med.* **2014**, *55*, 898–904. [CrossRef]
24. Zoller, M.; Kohlfuerst, S.; Igerc, I.; Kresnik, E.; Gallowitsch, H.J.; Gomez, I.; Lind, P. Combined PET/CT in the follow-up of differentiated thyroid carcinoma: What is the impact of each modality? *Eur. J. Nucl. Med. Mol. Imaging* **2007**, *34*, 487–495. [CrossRef] [PubMed]
25. Vural, G.U.; Akkas, B.E.; Ercakmak, N.; Basu, S.; Alavi, A. Prognostic significance of FDG PET/CT on the follow-up of patients of differentiated thyroid carcinoma with negative 131I whole-body scan and elevated thyroglobulin levels: Correlation with clinical and histopathologic characteristics and long-term follow-up data. *Clin. Nucl. Med.* **2012**, *37*, 953–959. [CrossRef]

26. Dong, M.J.; Liu, Z.F.; Zhao, K.; Ruan, L.X.; Wang, G.L.; Yang, S.Y.; Sun, F.; Luo, X.G. Value of 18F-FDG-PET/PET-CT in differentiated thyroid carcinoma with radioiodine-negative whole-body scan: A meta-analysis. *Nucl. Med. Commun.* **2009**, *30*, 639–650. [CrossRef] [PubMed]
27. Carr, L.L.; Mankoff, D.A.; Goulart, B.H.; Eaton, K.D.; Capell, P.T.; Kell, E.M.; Bauman, J.E.; Martins, R.G. Phase II study of daily sunitinib in FDG-PET-positive, iodine-refractory differentiated thyroid cancer and metastatic medullary carcinoma of the thyroid with functional imaging correlation. *Clin. Cancer Res.* **2010**, *16*, 5260–5268. [CrossRef]
28. Marotta, V.; Ramundo, V.; Camera, L.; Del Prete, M.; Fonti, R.; Esposito, R.; Palmieri, G.; Salvatore, M.; Vitale, M.; Colao, A.; et al. Sorafenib in advanced iodine-refractory differentiated thyroid cancer: Efficacy, safety and exploratory analysis of role of serum thyroglobulin and FDG-PET. *Clin. Endocrinol.* **2013**, *78*, 760–767. [CrossRef]
29. Wahl, R.L.; Jacene, H.; Kasamon, Y.; Lodge, M.A. From RECIST to PERCIST: Evolving Considerations for PET response criteria in solid tumors. *J. Nucl. Med.* **2009**, *50* (Suppl 1), 122s–150s. [CrossRef]
30. Pinker, K.; Riedl, C.C.; Ong, L.; Jochelson, M.; Ulaner, G.A.; McArthur, H.; Dickler, M.; Gönen, M.; Weber, W.A. The Impact That Number of Analyzed Metastatic Breast Cancer Lesions Has on Response Assessment by 18F-FDG PET/CT Using PERCIST. *J. Nucl. Med.* **2016**, *57*, 1102–1104. [CrossRef]
31. Michl, M.; Lehner, S.; Paprottka, P.M.; Ilhan, H.; Bartenstein, P.; Heinemann, V.; Boeck, S.; Albert, N.L.; Fendler, W.P. Use of PERCIST for Prediction of Progression-Free and Overall Survival After Radioembolization for Liver Metastases from Pancreatic Cancer. *J. Nucl. Med.* **2016**, *57*, 355–360. [CrossRef] [PubMed]
32. Devriese, J.; Beels, L.; Maes, A.; Van de Wiele, C.; Pottel, H. Impact of PET reconstruction protocols on quantification of lesions that fulfil the PERCIST lesion inclusion criteria. *EJNMMI Phys.* **2018**, *5*, 35. [CrossRef] [PubMed]
33. Choi, H. Response evaluation of gastrointestinal stromal tumors. *Oncologist* **2008**, *13* (Suppl 2), 4–7. [CrossRef] [PubMed]
34. Costelloe, C.M.; Chuang, H.H.; Madewell, J.E.; Ueno, N.T. Cancer Response Criteria and Bone Metastases: RECIST 1.1, MDA and PERCIST. *J. Cancer* **2010**, *1*, 80–92. [CrossRef] [PubMed]
35. Bénard, F.; Sterman, D.; Smith, R.J.; Kaiser, L.R.; Albelda, S.M.; Alavi, A. Prognostic value of FDG PET imaging in malignant pleural mesothelioma. *J. Nucl. Med.* **1999**, *40*, 1241–1245.
36. Bruzzi, P.; Del Mastro, L.; Sormani, M.P.; Bastholt, L.; Danova, M.; Focan, C.; Fountzilas, G.; Paul, J.; Rosso, R.; Venturini, M. Objective response to chemotherapy as a potential surrogate end point of survival in metastatic breast cancer patients. *J. Clin. Oncol.* **2005**, *23*, 5117–5125. [CrossRef]
37. Leboulleux, S.; Bastholt, L.; Krause, T.; de la Fouchardiere, C.; Tennvall, J.; Awada, A.; Gómez, J.M.; Bonichon, F.; Leenhardt, L.; Soufflet, C.; et al. Vandetanib in locally advanced or metastatic differentiated thyroid cancer: A randomised, double-blind, phase 2 trial. *Lancet Oncol.* **2012**, *13*, 897–905. [CrossRef]
38. Sher, A.; Lacoeuille, F.; Fosse, P.; Vervueren, L.; Cahouet-Vannier, A.; Dabli, D.; Bouchet, F.; Couturier, O. For avid glucose tumors, the SUV peak is the most reliable parameter for [(18)F]FDG-PET/CT quantification, regardless of acquisition time. *EJNMMI Res.* **2016**, *6*, 21. [CrossRef]
39. Manohar, P.M.; Beesley, L.J.; Bellile, E.L.; Worden, F.P.; Avram, A.M. Prognostic Value of FDG-PET/CT Metabolic Parameters in Metastatic Radioiodine-Refractory Differentiated Thyroid Cancer. *Clin. Nucl. Med.* **2018**, *43*, 641–647. [CrossRef]
40. Benz, M.R.; Allen-Auerbach, M.S.; Eilber, F.C.; Chen, H.J.; Dry, S.; Phelps, M.E.; Czernin, J.; Weber, W.A. Combined assessment of metabolic and volumetric changes for assessment of tumor response in patients with soft-tissue sarcomas. *J. Nucl. Med.* **2008**, *49*, 1579–1584. [CrossRef]
41. Robbins, R.J.; Wan, Q.; Grewal, R.K.; Reibke, R.; Gonen, M.; Strauss, H.W.; Tuttle, R.M.; Drucker, W.; Larson, S.M. Real-time prognosis for metastatic thyroid carcinoma based on 2-[18F]fluoro-2-deoxy-D-glucose-positron emission tomography scanning. *J. Clin. Endocrinol. Metab.* **2006**, *91*, 498–505. [CrossRef] [PubMed]
42. Guillem, J.G.; Moore, H.G.; Akhurst, T.; Klimstra, D.S.; Ruo, L.; Mazumdar, M.; Minsky, B.D.; Saltz, L.; Wong, W.D.; Larson, S. Sequential preoperative fluorodeoxyglucose-positron emission tomography assessment of response to preoperative chemoradiation: A means for determining longterm outcomes of rectal cancer. *J. Am. Coll. Surg.* **2004**, *199*, 1–7. [CrossRef] [PubMed]
43. Erdi, Y.E.; Macapinlac, H.; Rosenzweig, K.E.; Humm, J.L.; Larson, S.M.; Erdi, A.K.; Yorke, E.D. Use of PET to monitor the response of lung cancer to radiation treatment. *Eur. J. Nucl. Med.* **2000**, *27*, 861–866. [CrossRef] [PubMed]
44. Sharma, A.; Mohan, A.; Bhalla, A.S.; Sharma, M.C.; Vishnubhatla, S.; Das, C.J.; Pandey, A.K.; Sekhar Bal, C.; Patel, C.D.; Sharma, P.; et al. Role of Various Metabolic Parameters Derived From Baseline 18F-FDG PET/CT as Prognostic Markers in Non-Small Cell Lung Cancer Patients Undergoing Platinum-Based Chemotherapy. *Clin. Nucl. Med.* **2018**, *43*, e8–e17. [CrossRef] [PubMed]
45. Marti, J.L.; Morris, L.G.T.; Ho, A.S. Selective use of radioactive iodine (RAI) in thyroid cancer: No longer "one size fits all". *Eur. journal Surg. Oncol.* **2018**, *44*, 348–356. [CrossRef]
46. Liang, Y.; Li, X.; Wan, H.; Fang, Y.; Zheng, R.; Zhang, W.; Liu, Y.; Chen, C.; Wu, N. Prognostic Value of Volume-Based Metabolic Parameters Obtained by 18F-FDG-PET/CT in Patients With Locally Advanced Squamous Cell Cervical Carcinoma. *J. Comput. Assist. Tomogr.* **2018**, *42*, 429–434. [CrossRef]

cancers 2020, 12, 3637

Article

Evaluation of Clinicopathological and Molecular Parameters on Disease Recurrence of Papillary Thyroid Cancer Patient: A Retrospective Observational Study

Salvatore Sorrenti [1,†], Giovanni Carbotta [1,†], Filippo Maria Di Matteo [1], Antonio Catania [1], Daniele Pironi [1], Francesco Tartaglia [1], Danilo Tarroni [1], Federica Gagliardi [1], Domenico Tripodi [1], Mikiko Watanabe [2], Stefania Mariani [2], Eleonora D'Armiento [3], Poupak Fallahi [4], Alessandro Sindoni [5], Corrado De Vito [5], Alessandro Antonelli [4], Salvatore Ulisse [1,*] and Enke Baldini [1]

1 Department of Surgical Sciences, "Sapienza" University of Rome, 00161 Rome, Italy; salvatore.sorrenti@uniroma1.it (S.S.); giovanni.carbotta@uniroma1.it (G.C.); filippomaria.dimatteo@uniroma1.it (F.M.D.M.); Antonio.Catania@uniroma1.it (A.C.); daniele.pironi@uniroma1.it (D.P.); francesco.tartaglia@uniroma1.it (F.T.); danilo.tarroni@uniroma1.it (D.T.); federica.gagliardi@uniroma1.it (F.G.); domenico.tripodi@uniroma1.it (D.T.); enke.baldini@uniroma1.it (E.B.)

2 Department of Experimental Medicine, "Sapienza" University of Rome, 00161 Rome, Italy; mikiko.watanabe@uniroma1.it (M.W.); s.mariani@uniroma1.it (S.M.)

3 Department of Internal Medicine and Medical Specialties, "Sapienza" University of Rome, 00161 Rome, Italy; eleonora.darmiento@uniroma1.it

4 Department of Clinical and Experimental Medicine, University of Pisa, 56126 Pisa, Italy; poupak.fallahi@unipi.it (P.F.); alessandro.antonelli@med.unipi.it (A.A.)

5 Department of Public Health and Infectious Diseases, "Sapienza" University of Rome, 00161 Rome, Italy; alessandro.sindoni@uniroma1.it (A.S.); corrado.devito@uniroma1.it (C.D.V.)

* Correspondence: salvatore.ulisse@uniroma1.it

† These authors contributed equally to this work.

Received: 14 October 2020; Accepted: 2 December 2020; Published: 4 December 2020

Simple Summary: Papillary thyroid cancer (PTC) patients are staged according to the Tumor-Node-Metastasis staging system (TNM). This work was aimed at comparing the usefulness of the 8th edition of TNM (TNM-8), currently used, and that of the previous one (TNM-7) for predicting disease-free interval (DFI) in a cohort of 1148 patients. Moreover, clinicopathological and molecular factors were statistically evaluated in order to determine which of these was/were the best predictor(s) of DFI. Results obtained from the multivariate analysis indicated that advanced tumor stages were independent risk factors for a lower DFI regardless of TNM, but the statistical model created with the TNM-7 was most accurate. When stage-determining factors were included individually in the multivariate analysis, LN metastases, tall cell variant, and age emerged as independent risk factors for a shorter DFI, with lateral LN metastases being the most relevant. No molecular parameters could improve the prediction of DFI provided by LN metastases.

Abstract: The American Joint Committee on Cancer has revised the Tumor-Node-Metastasis (TNM) staging system for papillary thyroid cancer (PTC) patients. We examined the impact of this new classification (TNM-8) on patient stratification and estimated the prognostic value of clinicopathological features for the disease-free interval (DFI) in a cohort of 1148 PTC patients. Kaplan–Meier analyses showed that all clinicopathological parameters analyzed, except age and multifocality, were associated significantly with DFI. Cox regression identified tall cell PTC variant and stage as independent risk factors for DFI. When the stage was replaced with age, tumor size, and lymph node (LN) metastases in the set of covariates, the lateral LN metastases stood out as the strongest independent predictor of DFI, followed by tall cell variant and age. A noteworthy result emerging from these analyzes is that regression models had lower Akaike and Bayesian information criterions if variables were categorized based on the TNM-7. In addition, we examined data from a different PTC patient cohort, acquired from The Cancer Genome Atlas database, to verify whether the DFI prediction could be enhanced by further clinicopathological and molecular parameters. However, none of these was found to be a significant predictor of DFI in the Cox model.

Keywords: papillary thyroid cancer; prognosis; TNM; histology; multifocality; lymph node metastasis; vascular invasion; autoimmune thyroid diseases

---

1. Introduction

Accurate staging of patients affected by differentiated thyroid cancer (DTC) is of crucial importance to ensure the appropriate therapeutic strategy and follow-up, and to ensure the patients' quality of life [1]. To date, several staging systems aimed at estimating the risk of disease-related death or disease relapse/persistence are available. The most employed one is the Tumor-Node-Metastasis (TNM) classification, developed by the American Joint Committee on Cancer (AJCC) [2,3]. The latest version of the TNM system (8th edition/TNM-8) was significantly amended in 2016 with respect to the previous version (7th edition/TNM-7) released in 2009 [3,4]. The 8th edition, while maintaining the classical anatomic extension of the disease as its groundwork, incorporates biological and molecular markers to create a more personalized prognostic stratification [4]. Based on TNM-8, many DTC patients are now included in lower stages and considered to have a reduced risk of dying from thyroid cancer [3,5]. However, in DTC patients the risk of disease recurrence is considerably higher than the risk of disease-related mortality, which makes the TNM staging system, designed to foresee patient survival, uninformative for the prediction of disease recurrence [1,6]. In 2009 the American Thyroid Association (ATA) endorsed a validated risk-stratification system for DTC recurrence in which TNM parameters were implemented by clinicopathological features (i.e., tumor histology, vascular invasion, radioactive iodine uptake, post-operative thyroglobulin serum level, etc.) to divide patients in three risk categories (low, intermediate, and high) [6–8]. Although this model was recognized as a valuable tool in clinical practice, in 2015 the ATA substituted the three-risk-categories-model with a continuum risk model varying from very low risk to high risk of recurrence [1,5]. In the latter, besides TNM and clinicopathological parameters, mutations of BRAF and TERT genes were included [1,6]. In the TNM-8 it has been recommended to take note, in individual patient records, of a number of molecular and clinicopathological parameters that, even if not included in the actual staging system, could be evaluated for inclusion in the next TNM edition [3,4]. They comprise the microscopic extrathyroidal extension, location and number of metastatic lymph nodes, number of lymph nodes sampled and size of the largest metastatic one, extranodal extension, histological subtypes, vascular invasion, postoperative thyroglobulin (Tg) serum level, extension of surgical resection, and molecular characterization [3,9]. In the present work, we retrospectively investigated a case study comprising 1148 patients affected by papillary thyroid cancer (PTC) to evaluate: (i) the effect of the new TNM-8 staging system on patients' risk stratification compared to the previous TNM-7; (ii) the prognostic value of a number of clinicopathological and molecular parameters determined by proportional hazards regression (Cox regression).

2. Results

We first evaluated the impact of the new TNM-8 on patients' risk stratification compared to the previous TNM-7. In this regard, 1113 patients for whom all clinical data required were available, were staged according to both TNM systems. Since in the TNM-8 the patients' age cutoff has been shifted from 45 to 55 years, the percentage of younger patients (age $<$ 55 years) in our case study increased from 46.4% (516/1113) in TNM-7 to 68.6% (764/1113) in TNM-8. Due to the lack of distant metastases, all these patients were classified as stage I regardless of TNM edition. As expected, among older patients (age > 55 years) we observed a considerable reduction in the relative frequencies of individuals at stage III and IV, with a concomitant increase in those at stage I and II, moving from TNM-7 to TNM-8 (Figure 1). As noted in Figure 1, classification of PTC according to TNM-8 led to a considerable downstaging of patients.

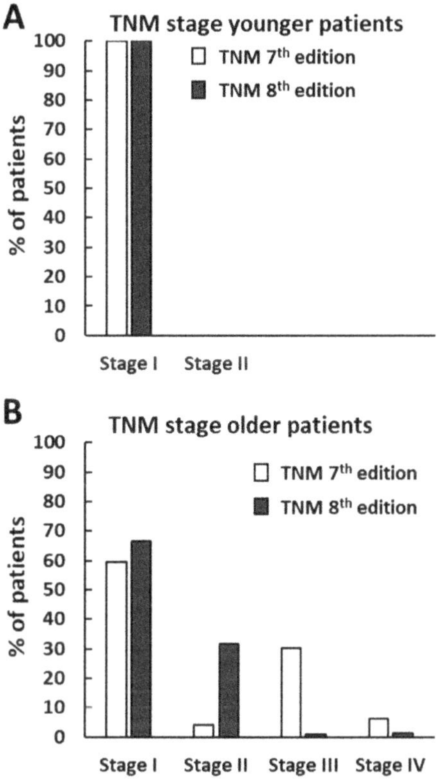

Figure 1. Distribution of 1113 papillary thyroid cancer (PTC) patients according to the 7th or the 8th Tumor-Node-Metastasis (TNM) staging system. (**A**) displays the staging of patients younger than 45 years (516 out of 1113 patients) according to the TNM-7 or younger than 55 years (764 out of 1113 patients) according to the TNM-8. (**B**) displays the distribution of stages for older patients as defined in the 7th or the 8th TNM edition.

Univariate analysis was performed to evaluate the association of several clinicopathological parameters, including age at diagnosis, gender, autoimmune thyroid disease (AITD), tumor histology, size (T), lymph node metastases (N), stage, multifocality, capsular, muscle, and vascular invasion, with PTC recurrences. Since some categories were poorly represented, especially among tumor sizes and stages, they were combined with other categories to avoid the inclusion of too small groups in the statistics (see Section 4). As shown in Table 1, all the parameters analyzed with the exclusion of age and multifocality were significantly associated with PTC recurrences. In particular, the PTC sclerosing and tall cell variants and lymph node metastases had a very strong correlation with recurrences (Cramer's V index > 0.25).

Table 1. Univariate analysis of the association between clinicopathological parameters and PTC recurrences. AITD, Autoimmune Thyroid Disease. *p*-values < 0.05 are evidenced in bold.

Clinicopathological Parameters	No Recurrences	Recurrences	Cramer's V Index	*p*-Value
Median age (range)	47 year (12–80 year)	48 (23–85 year)	-	0.906
	Age			
≥55 year	621	32	-	0.118
<55 year	288	23		
≥45 year	419	25	-	0.926
<45 year	490	30		
	Gender			
Male	192	24	0.125	**<0.001**
Female	717	31		
	AITD			
Yes	238	5	0.091	**0.005**
No	671	50		
	PTC variants			
classical	545	16	0.291	**<0.001**
follicular	232	8		
sclerosing	84	23		
tall cell	21	7		
	T (7th edition)			
T1–T2	716	12	-	**0.028**
T3–T4	193	9		
	T (8th edition)			
T1a–T3a	732	15	0.094	**0.004**
T3b–T4	177	11		
	N			
N0	663	7	0.647	**<0.001**
N1a	71	3		
N1b	33	42		
	Stage (7th edition)			
Stages I–II	787	15	-	**0.001**
Stages III–IV	120	10		
	Stage (8th edition)			
Stage I	844	18	-	**<0.001**
Stages II–IV	65	8		
	Multifocality			
Yes	208	8	-	0.412
No	701	19		
	Capsular invasion			
Yes	197	11	0.077	**0.019**
No	712	16		
	Muscle invasion			
Yes	76	7	-	**0.015**
No	833	24		
	Vascular invasion			
Yes	46	5	-	**0.013**
No	863	22		

These observations were confirmed by the Kaplan–Meier analysis, reported in Figure 2. All clinicopathological parameters, with the exception of age and multifocality, were found to impact significantly on disease-free interval (DFI). Patients classified as T1a and T1b had the same DFI.

We finally created Cox regression models to predict the probability of DFI as a function of different sets of independent variables. Clinical parameters were categorized as in the univariate analysis (see Table 1). The first series of covariates included gender, histological variants (classical, follicular, sclerosing, and tall cell), AITD, multifocality, stage, capsular, muscle, and vascular invasion. Tall cell variant and stage turned out to be significant predictors of DFI (see Table 2), and the stage was significant either if calculated with the 7th or with the 8th edition. Of note is that using TNM-7 instead of TNM-8, the Akaike information criterion (AIC) decreased by about 12 units, indicating a significant improvement of the model.

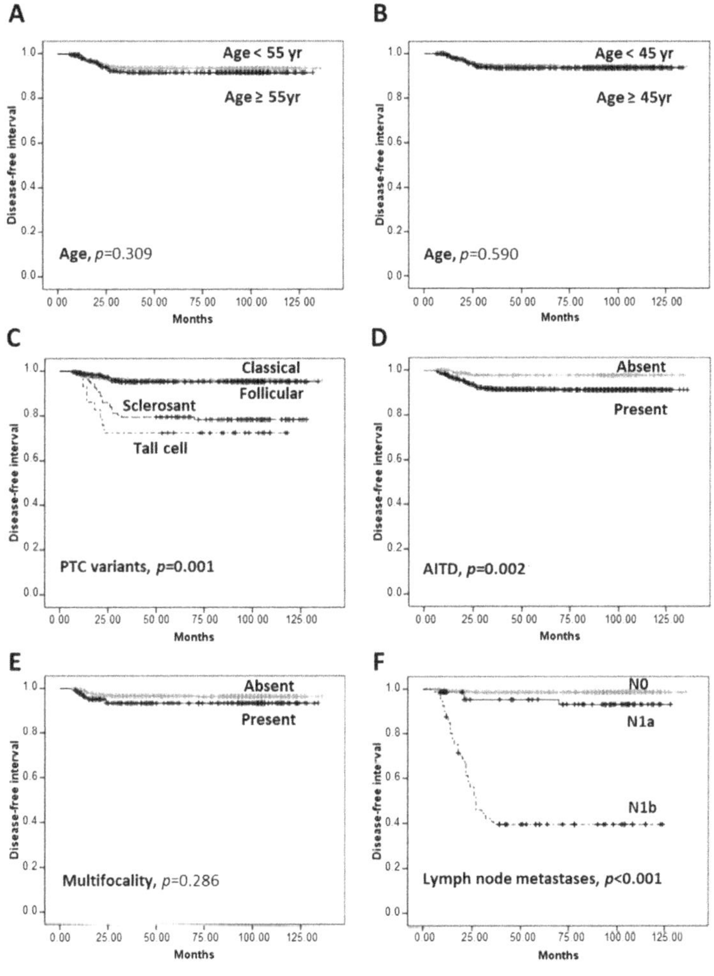

Figure 2. *Cont.*

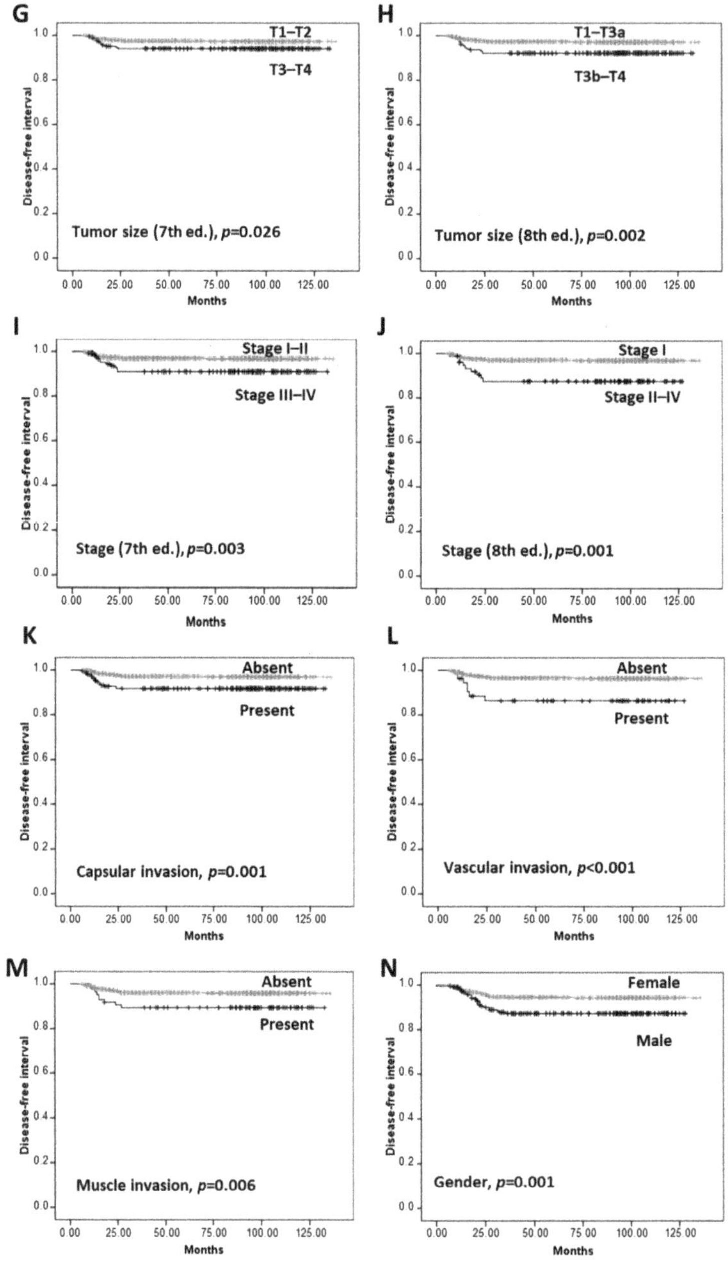

Figure 2. Kaplan–Meier analysis. Kaplan–Meier curves with Mantel–Cox log-rank statistical text were made to estimate the impact on disease-free interval (DFI) at age <55 years or ≥55 year (**A**), age <45 years or ≥45 years (**B**), PTC histological variants (**C**), AITD (**D**), multifocality (**E**), lymph node metastases (**F**), tumor size (7th edition) (**G**), tumor size (8th edition) (**H**), stage (7th edition) (**I**), stage (8th edition) (**J**), capsular invasion (**K**), vascular invasion (**L**), muscle invasion (**M**), or gender (**N**). *p* values < 0.05 are evidenced in bold.

Table 2. Cox regression for the prediction of DFI was performed with stage and other clinicopathological parameters. The table shows predictors retained in the model after backward selection. The variables entered in the analysis were: gender, histological variants, AITD, multifocality, stage (8th or 7th edition), capsular, muscle, and vascular invasion. HR: hazard ratio. CI: confidence interval. AIC: Akaike information criterion. BIC: Bayesian information criterion. *p*-values < 0.05 are evidenced in bold.

Cox Regression with TMN-8					
Clinicopathological Parameters	**HR**	**95% CI**	***p*-Value**	**AIC**	**BIC**
Sex	2.207	0.96–5.06	0.062		
Histological variant					
Classic	1	—	—		
Follicular	0.57	0.16–2.03	0.387	308.74	343.1
Sclerosing	2.22	0.81–6.08	0.122		
Tall-cell	4.08	1.12–15.10	**0.035**		
Stage	4.28	1.76–10.43	**0.001**		
Cox Regression with TMN-7					
Clinicopathological Parameters	**HR**	**95% CI**	***p*-Value**	**AIC**	**BIC**
Histological variant					
Classic	1	—	—		
Follicular	0.66	0.18–2.37	0.524	296.403	315.89
Sclerosing	2.43	0.88–6.69	0.085		
Tall-cell	4.31	1.17–15.83	**0.028**		
Stage	1.95	1.27–2.98	**0.002**		

We then replaced stage with stage-related parameters, so that the new set of covariates comprised lymph node metastases, tumor size, dichotomized age at diagnosis, gender, histological variants, AITD, multifocality, muscle and vascular invasion (see Table 3). Capsular invasion was excluded due to its collinearity with tumor size (variance inflation factor > 5). In this setting, the presence of lymph node metastases beyond the central compartment (N1b) was the independent variable most strongly associated with DFI (Hazard Ratio = 37.55, $p < 0.001$). Although in the univariate analysis dichotomous age was not significantly associated with recurrences or DFI, in Cox regression it became a significant predictor both applying the 55-year and 45-year threshold. When the hazard function was generated with T and age categorized according to the TNM-7 edition, the sclerosing and tall cell variants also displayed significant hazard ratios. Moreover, this model had lower AIC and BIC than that resulting from categories based on TNM-8, similarly to what was observed for the Cox regression including stage.

After that, we sought to verify if the DFI prediction could be strengthened by combining lymph node metastases and age with further histological and molecular parameters that were not available for our patients. These data were acquired from a previous study by the Cancer Genome Atlas Research Network for Cancer Genomics [10–12]. Specifically, we considered lymph node metastases, age, number of total non-silent mutations, number of CpGT mutations, BRAF-RAF score, ERK score, miRNA cluster, RPPA cluster, ploidy, differentiation score, and follicular component. Univariate analysis showed that BRAF-RAF score ($p = 0.014$), differentiation score ($p = 0.045$), and lymph node metastases ($p = 0.005$) associated significantly with recurrences. Nonetheless, adding all the above variables with $p < 0.25$ in the univariate analysis to lymph node metastases and age in the Cox regression did not improve significantly the prediction of DFI. Considering a subgroup of patients ($n = 310$) for which lymph node metastases were categorized as N0, N1a, and N1b in the database, N1b displayed the highest hazard ratio and significance, similar to what emerged from the analysis of our patient cohort (Table 3). In particular, N1a showed a HR of 6.53 (95% CI 1.14–37.37, $p < 0.05$) and N1b had a HR of 14.46 (95% CI 2.29–91.07, $p < 0.01$).

Table 3. Cox regression for the prediction of DFI performed with stage-determining factors and other clinicopathological parameters. The table shows predictors retained in the model after backward selection. The variables entered in the model were: gender, histological variants, AITD, multifocality, dichotomized age, T, N, muscle and vascular invasion. HR: hazard ratio. CI: confidence interval. AIC: Akaike information criterion. BIC: Bayesian information criterion. p-values < 0.05 are evidenced in bold.

Cox Regression with TMN-8					
Clinicopathological Parameters	**HR**	**95% CI**	***p*-Value**	**AIC**	**BIC**
Age (<55 year and ≥55 year)	2.907	1.24–6.81	**0.014**	238.59	253.2
Lymph node metastasis					
N0	1	—	—		
N1a	3.75	0.77–18.24	0.101		
N1b	37.55	14.79–95.34	**<0.001**		
Cox Regression with TMN-7					
Clinicopathological Parameters	**HR**	**95% CI**	***p*-Value**	**AIC**	**BIC**
Age (<45 year and ≥45 year)	3.5	1.16–10.55	**0.026**	202.97	241.94
Histological variant					
lassic	1	—	—		
Follicular	1.53	0.37–6.29	0.556		
Sclerosing	3.42	1.04–6.69	**0.042**		
Tall-cell	7.22	1.69–30.80	**0.008**		
T (T1–T2 and T3–T4)	0.607	0.343–1.075	0.087		
Lymph node metastasis					
N0	1	—	—		
N1a	4.22	0.84–21.27	0.081		
N1b	34.72	10.43–115.601	**<0.001**		

3. Discussion

Follicular thyroid cell-derived tumors are the most common endocrine malignancy and the fifth most common cancer in women [13–15]. Its annual incidence, about 3% of all cancer, has been shown to more than double over the last decades as a result of the improved ability to diagnose malignant transformation in small thyroid nodules [14,15]. The differentiated papillary (PTC) and follicular (FTC) carcinomas represent most of the epithelial thyroid cancers, which may progressively dedifferentiate giving rise to the more aggressive poorly DTC (PDTC), and to the incurable anaplastic thyroid carcinomas (ATC) [16]. Although the prognosis of DTC patients is favorable, with a 5-years-survival rate of nearly 98%, about 20% of them face the morbidity of disease recurrence [1,2,14,15]. The TNM staging system elaborated by the AJCC based on clinicopathological parameters is the most widely used approach to predict thyroid cancer survival, but it is much less reliable in discriminating patients with a higher risk of developing relapses over time [1–3]. The TNM has been significantly revised in 2016 (TNM-8), with respect to its previous version (TNM-7) [3,4,9]. Various reports have documented the ability of the TNM-8 to better predict the disease-specific survival (DSS) in DTC patients, but we could not verify this point because none of the patients examined died due to PTC [17–28]. It has to be mentioned, however, that in one of these studies it was shown that the new TNM improved the prediction of DSS for PTC, but not for FTC patients [23]. In addition, reasonable concerns have been raised for patients in the 45–54 age range, classified in stages III or IV by the TNM-7 but currently considered in stages I or II by the TNM-8, for whom the severity of the disease could be underestimated [24].

In the present study, as expected, the comparison of the two TNM systems in 1113 PTC patients evidenced a considerable patient downstaging by TNM-8, in agreement with a number of earlier reports [5,17–28]. Even though TNM staging was conceived to predict DSS, some studies showed that both TNM-7 and TNM-8 were significantly associated with disease-free survival and that TNM-8 allowed better discrimination of the recurrence risk over time [25,27,29]. In our case study we found analogous results, but the differences between curves created with TNM-7 and TNM-8 stages and T were much less evident in our Kaplan–Meier analysis due to the need for combining some categories to fulfill statistical requirements. However, when the Cox regression analysis was performed with parameters classified according to TNM-7 instead of TNM-8, lower Akaike Information Criterion (AIC) and Bayesian Information Criterion (BIC) values were obtained, indicating that the model based on TNM-7 should be preferred. This statement would seem to be in contrast with the conclusions of other authors about the superior predictive performance of TNM-8 over TNM-7 for DFI. However, it has to be mentioned that these authors focused attention on HRs of individual predictors, while we evaluated the virtue of model fit. Our findings are in line with a previous work showing that in patients above 55 years, pT7 was superior to pT8 in predicting DFI [28].

In the framework of The Cancer Genome Atlas (TCGA) project, a comprehensive multiplatform analysis was carried out to determine the genomic landscape of 496 PTC cases, and a reclassification of PTC into molecular subtypes was proposed to improve clinicopathological grading and management of patients [12]. In this study, the lowest thyroid differentiation score (TDS) was assigned to a tall cell-like tumor cluster, which was associated with more advanced stage and higher risk, while the classical PTC (CPTC) had an intermediate TDS, and the follicular variant (FVPTC) maintained a high TDS [12]. These results were corroborated by a subsequent multicenter retrospective study including 6282 cases of PTC [29]. Differential risk patterns of disease recurrence and patient mortality were determined for the three major PTC variants, with increasing aggressiveness from the FVPTC to the CPTC, up to the tall cell PTC (TCPTC) [30]. The results of our study do not confirm a higher recurrence-free probability for FVPTC compared to CPTC, whereas the DFI probability was significantly reduced for the tall cell and sclerosing PTC variants. The partial discrepancy of our findings with the previous ones is probably because, due to the numerical scarcity of relapses in FVPTC, we could not distinguish between encapsulated/well-demarcated noninvasive forms and infiltrative FVPTC.

When in our regression analysis the TNM stage was replaced by stage-related parameters analyzed as independent variables, lymph node metastasis and age dichotomized in <55 years and ≥55 years emerged as the only significant predictors of DFI. Taking advantage of a PTC cohort of patients derived from the TCGA, we sought to verify whether, besides lymph node metastasis and age, the DFI prediction could be improved by additional histological and molecular parameters not available for our case study. The results obtained demonstrated that only a couple of them (BRAF-RAF score and differentiation score) were significantly associated with recurrences, and none of the parameters selected for the Cox regression impacted significantly on the model. Additionally, in this PTC cohort, lateral lymph node involvement represented the best predictor of DFI, with the N1b category (spreading beyond the central compartment) having the highest HR.

4. Materials and Methods

4.1. Patients

In this study, we retrospectively analyzed 1148 patients affected by PTC enrolled in the period 1995–2018 at the Umberto I hospital, Department of Surgical Sciences of the Sapienza University of Rome. The case study included 883 females and 265 males with a median age of 47 years (range 12–88 years). All subjects gave their informed consent for inclusion before they participated in the study. The study was conducted in accordance with the Declaration of Helsinki, and the protocol was approved by the Ethics Committee of the Umberto I hospital (Protocol No. 2615). Of the 1148 patients, 1127 patients had a total thyroidectomy, while 21 patients had a lobectomy. Post-surgical RAI was performed on 565 patients, but not on 583 patients including 486 pT1a cases and 97 pT1b cases. Thyroid hormone replacement was applied following international guidelines recommendations [1–3,31,32]. For each patient, data regarding age at diagnosis, gender, absence or presence of autoimmune thyroid disease (AITD), tumor size, occurrence of lymph nodal or distant metastases, histology, multifocality, capsular invasion, vascular invasion, and muscle infiltration were collected. All patients were staged according to either the TNM-7 or the TNM-8. Histopathological diagnoses were made based on the WHO classification [11]. In particular, the main PTC variants observed included: 683 classical, 279 follicular, 121 diffuse sclerosing, and 32 tall cell variants. Of the 1148 patients, 283 were affected by AITD, 276 by chronic lymphocytic thyroiditis, and 7 by Graves' disease. The follow-up was available for 964 patients with a mean duration of 69.51 months (range 12–136 months, Table 1). Of these, 13 patients died for causes not related to PTC. In patients not affected by AITD, recurrences were diagnosed by neck ultrasonography, measurement of serum Tg levels, either in basal conditions or following recombinant human TSH stimulation (rhTSH), fine needle aspiration cytology (FNAC), and/or Tg determination in the FNA wash-out from lymph nodes [33], ^{131}I whole-body scan, or histological analysis following surgical resection of the lesion. The same was applied to AITD patients with positive Tg auto-antibodies with the exclusion of Tg measurements. During the follow-up, we observed 11 persistence (diagnosed before 12 months from the initial therapy) and 55 recurrences, including 54 lymph node metastases and 1 lung metastasis. In addition, we used data previously obtained from a study that described the genomic landscape of 496 PTC, with 396 of which follow-up was available [11–14].

4.2. Statistical Analysis

To avoid bias in the univariate and multivariate analyses, variable categories containing a small number of events, whose statistical results were unreliable, were merged with larger categories. Thus, in accordance with TNM-7, we divided tumor sizes (T) in T1 + T2 and T3 + T4, and tumor stages (S) in S1 + S2 and S3 + S4. The tumor sizes as defined by the TNM-8 were classified in T1 + T2 + T3a and T3b + T4, and the tumor stages in S1 and S2 + S3 + S4. Univariate analyses were executed for each clinical parameter in relation to the presence/absence of recurrence. Statistical comparison between recurrent and non-recurrent patients was carried out with the Chi-square test or the Fisher exact test for categorical variables, and with the Mann–Whitney test for continuous variables (not normally distributed). Where a significance was found in the Chi-square test, the Cramer's V was used as a post-test to determine the strength of association between variables. Kaplan–Meier curves were created to estimate the DFI in patient groups, and differences were statistically evaluated by the log-rank test. Finally, Cox regression was performed to quantify the hazard ratios of several explanatory variables, both continuous and categorical. The selection of covariates was made by including all parameters with a p-value < 0.25 in the univariate analysis, together with those of known clinical significance. Proportional hazards assumption and absence of multi-collinearity were preliminarily assessed for these covariates. The backward stepwise approach was used for the model selection. Data analyses were done by using the SPSS software for Windows (SPSS, Inc., Chicago, IL, USA), considering the probability value <0.05 as the threshold limit for statistical significance.

5. Conclusions

In conclusion, our study evidenced that lymph node metastases display a predictive value for DFI of PTC patients far higher than other clinical, histological, and molecular parameters currently available. Hence, it would be desirable to try to further improve the prediction of the DFI by employing more in-depth analysis of lymph node characteristics, through both instrumental and molecular investigations.

Author Contributions: S.S., G.C., F.M.D.M., A.C., D.P. and F.T. collected all the clinical data; E.B., M.W., S.M., F.G., D.T. (Danilo Tarroni), D.T. (Domenico Tripodi) and E.D. created the database; P.F., A.S., C.D.V., E.B., M.W. and S.M. ran the statistical analysis; S.S., A.A., S.U. and E.B. wrote the manuscript. All authors have read and agreed to the published version of the manuscript.

Funding: This research received no external funding.

Conflicts of Interest: The authors declare no conflict of interest.

References

1. Haugen, B.R.; Alexander, E.K.; Bible, K.C.; Doherty, G.M.; Mandel, S.J.; Nikiforov, Y.E.; Pacini, F.; Randolph, G.W.; Sawka, A.M.; Schlumberger, M.; et al. 2015 American Thyroid Association management guidelines for adult patients with thyroid nodules and differentiated thyroid cancer: The American Thyroid Association guidelines task force on thyroid nodules and differentiated thyroid cancer. *Thyroid* **2016**, *26*, 1–133. [CrossRef] [PubMed]
2. Filetti, S.; Durante, C.; Hartl, D.; Leboulleux, S.; Locati, L.D.; Newbold, K.; Papotti, M.G.; Berruti, A.; ESMO Guidelines Committee. Thyroid cancer: ESMO clinical practice guidelines for diagnosis, treatment and follow-up. *Ann. Oncol.* **2019**, *30*, 1856–1883. [CrossRef] [PubMed]
3. Tuttle, R.M.; Haugen, B.; Perrier, N.D. Updated American Joint Committee on Cancer/Tumor-Node-Metastasis Staging System for Differentiated and Anaplastic Thyroid Cancer (Eighth Edition): What Changed and Why? *Thyroid* **2017**, *27*, 751–756. [CrossRef] [PubMed]
4. Amin, M.B.; Greene, F.L.; Edge, S.B.; Compton, C.C.; Gershenwald, J.E.; Brookland, R.K.; Meyer, L.; Gress, D.M.; Byrd, D.R.; Winchester, D.P. The eighth edition AJCC cancer staging manual: Continuing to build a bridge from a population-based to a more "personalized" approach to cancer staging. *Cancer J. Clin.* **2017**, *67*, 93–99. [CrossRef]
5. Lamartina, L.; Grani, G.; Arvat, E.; Nervo, A.; Zatelli, M.C.; Rossi, R.; Puxeddu, E.; Morelli, S.; Torlontano, M.; Massa, M.; et al. 8th edition of the AJCC/TNM staging system of thyroid cancer: What to expect (ITCO#2). *Endocr. Relat. Cancer* **2018**, *25*, L7–L11. [CrossRef]
6. Tuttle, R.M.; Alzahrani, A.S. Risk stratification in differentiated thyroid cancer: From detection to final follow-up. *J. Clin. Endocrinol. Metab.* **2019**, *104*, 4087–4100. [CrossRef]
7. Tuttle, R.M.; Tala, H.; Shah, J.; Leboeuf, R.; Ghossein, R.; Gonen, M.; Brokhin, M.; Omry, G.; Fagin, J.A.; Shaha, A. Estimating risk of recurrence in differentiated thyroid cancer after total thyroidectomy and radioactive iodine remnant ablation: Using response to therapy variables to modify the initial risk estimates predicted by the new American Thyroid Association staging system. *Thyroid* **2010**, *20*, 1341–1349. [CrossRef]
8. Castagna, M.G.; Maino, F.; Cipri, C.; Belardini, V.; Theodoropoulou, A.; Cevenini, G.; Pacini, F. Delayed risk stratification, to include the response to initial treatment (surgery and radioiodine ablation), has better outcome predictivity in differentiated thyroid cancer patients. *Eur. J. Endocrinol.* **2011**, *165*, 441–446. [CrossRef]
9. Tuttle, M.; Morris, L.F.; Haugen, B.; Shah, J.; Sosa, J.A.; Rohren, E.; Subramaniam, R.M.; Hunt, J.L.; Perrier, N.D. Thyroid differentiated and anaplastic carcinoma. In *AJCC Cancer Staging Manual*, 8th ed.; Amin, M.B., Edge, S.B., Greene, F., Byrd, D., Brookland, R.K., Washington, M.K., Gershenwald, J.E., Compton, C.C., Hess, K.R., Sullivan, D.C., et al., Eds.; Springer International Publishing: New York, NY, USA, 2017; pp. 425–434.
10. Cerami, E.; Gao, J.; Dogrusoz, U.; Gross, B.E.; Sumer, S.O.; Aksoy, B.A.; Jacobsen, A.; Byrne, C.I.; Heuer, M.L.; Larsson, E.; et al. The cBio cancer genomics portal: An open platform for exploring multidimensional cancer genomics data. *Cancer Discov.* **2012**, *2*, 401–404. [CrossRef]
11. Gao, J.; Aksoy, B.A.; Dogrusoz, U.; Dresdner, G.; Gross, B.; Sumer, S.O.; Sun, Y.; Jacobsen, A.; Sinha, R.; Larsson, E.; et al. Integrative analysis of complex cancer genomics and clinical profiles using the cBioPortal. *Sci. Signal.* **2013**, *6*, pl1. [CrossRef]
12. Cancer Genome Atlas Research Network. Integrated genomic characterization of papillary thyroid carcinoma. *Cell* **2014**, *159*, 676–690. [CrossRef] [PubMed]
13. National Cancer Institute. 2019 SEER Cancer Statistics Review, 1975–2016. Available online: https://seer.cancer.gov/archive/csr/1975_2016/ (accessed on 16 June 2020).
14. Siegel, R.L.; Miller, K.D.; Jemal, A. Cancer statistics. *CA Cancer J. Clin.* **2019**, *69*, 7–34. [CrossRef] [PubMed]
15. Bray, F.; Ferlay, J.; Soerjomataram, I.; Siegel, R.L.; Torre, L.A.; Jemal, A. Global cancer statistics 2018: GLOBOCAN estimates of incidence and mortality worldwide for 36 cancers in 185 countries. *Cancer J. Clin.* **2018**, *68*, 394–424. [CrossRef] [PubMed]
16. Nikiforv, Y.E.; Biddinger, P.W.; Thompson, L.D.R. *Diagnostic Pathology and Molecular Genetics of the Thyroid*; Lippincott Williams & Wilkins: Philadelphia, PA, USA, 2009.
17. Zhi, J.; Wu, Y.; Hu, L.; Zhao, J.; Liu, H.; Ruan, X.; Hou, X.; Zhang, J.; Zheng, X.; Gao, M. Assessment of the prognostic value and N1b changes of the eighth TNM/AJCC staging system for differentiated thyroid carcinoma. *Int. J. Clin. Oncol.* **2020**, *25*, 59–66. [CrossRef]

18. Pontius, L.N.; Oyekunle, T.O.; Thomas, S.M.; Stang, M.T.; Scheri, R.P.; Roman, S.A.; Sosa, J.A. Projecting survival in papillary thyroid cancer: A comparison of the seventh and eighth editions of the American Joint Commission on Cancer/Union for International Cancer Control staging systems in two contemporary national patient cohorts. *Thyroid* **2017**, *27*, 1408–1416. [CrossRef]
19. Van Velsen, E.F.S.; Stegenga, M.T.; van Kemenade, F.J.; Kam, B.L.R.; van Ginhoven, T.M.; Visser, W.E.; Peeters, R.P. Comparing the Prognostic Value of the Eighth Edition of the American Joint Committee on Cancer/Tumor Node Metastasis Staging System Between Papillary and Follicular Thyroid Cancer. *Thyroid* **2018**, *28*, 976–981. [CrossRef]
20. Ghaznavi, S.A.; Ganly, I.; Shaha, A.R.; English, C.; Wills, J.; Tuttle, R.M. Using the American Thyroid Association Risk-Stratification System to Refine and Individualize the American Joint Committee on Cancer Eighth Edition Disease-Specific Survival Estimates in Differentiated Thyroid Cancer. *Thyroid* **2018**, *28*, 1293–1300. [CrossRef]
21. Tam, S.; Boonsripitayanon, M.; Amit, M.; Fellman, B.M.; Li, Y.; Busaidy, N.L.; Cabanillas, M.E.; Dadu, R.; Sherman, S.; Waguespack, S.G.; et al. Survival in Differentiated Thyroid Cancer: Comparing the AJCC Cancer Staging Seventh and Eighth Editions. *Thyroid* **2018**, *28*, 1301–1310. [CrossRef]
22. Kim, M.; Kim, W.G.; Oh, H.S.; Park, S.; Kwon, H.; Song, D.E.; Kim, T.Y.; Shong, Y.K.; Kim, W.B.; Sung, T.Y.; et al. Comparison of the Seventh and Eighth Editions of the American Joint Committee on Cancer/Union for International Cancer Control Tumor-Node-Metastasis Staging System for Differentiated Thyroid Cancer. *Thyroid* **2017**, *27*, 1149–1155. [CrossRef]
23. Kim, M.; Kim, H.I.; Jeon, M.J.; Kim, H.K.; Kim, E.H.; Yi, H.S.; Kim, E.S.; Kim, H.; Kim, B.H.; Kim, T.Y.; et al. Eighth edition of tumor-node-metastasis staging system improve survival predictability for papillary, but not follicular thyroid carcinoma: A multicenter cohort study. *Oral Oncol.* **2018**, *87*, 97–103. [CrossRef]
24. Shteinshnaider, M.; Muallem Kalmovich, L.; Koren, S.; Or, K.; Cantrell, D.; Benbassat, C. Reassessment of Differentiated Thyroid Cancer Patients Using the Eighth TNM/AJCC Classification System: A Comparative Study. *Thyroid* **2018**, *28*, 201–209. [CrossRef] [PubMed]
25. Shaha, A.R.; Migliacci, J.C.; Nixon, I.J.; Wang, L.Y.; Wong, R.J.; Morris, L.G.T.; Patel, S.G.; Shah, J.P.; Tuttle, R.M.; Ganly, I. Stage migration with the new American Joint Committee on Cancer (AJCC) staging system (8th edition) for differentiated thyroid cancer. *Surgery* **2019**, *165*, 6–11. [CrossRef] [PubMed]
26. Chereau, N.; Oyekunle, O.T.; Zambeli-Ljepović, A.; Kazaure, H.S.; Roman, S.A.; Menegaux, F.; Sosa, J.A. Predicting recurrence of papillary thyroid cancer using the eighth edition of the AJCC/UICC staging system. *Br. J. Surg.* **2019**, *106*, 889–897. [CrossRef] [PubMed]
27. Nam, S.H.; Bae, M.R.; Roh, J.L.; Gong, G.; Cho, K.J.; Choi, S.H.; Nam, S.Y.; Kim, S.Y. A comparison of the 7th and 8th editions of the AJCC staging system in terms of predicting recurrence and survival in patients with papillary thyroid carcinoma. *Oral Oncol.* **2018**, *87*, 158–164. [CrossRef] [PubMed]
28. Tran, B.; Roshan, D.; Abraham, E.; Wang, L.; Garibotto, N.; Wykes, J.; Campbell, P.; Ebrahimi, A. An Analysis of the American Joint Committee on Cancer 8th Edition T Staging System for Papillary Thyroid Carcinoma. *J. Clin. Endocrinol. Metab.* **2018**, *103*, 2199–2206. [CrossRef] [PubMed]
29. Kim, K.; Kim, J.K.; Lee, C.R.; Kang, S.W.; Lee, J.; Jeong, J.J.; Nam, K.H.; Chung, W.Y. Comparison of long-term prognosis for differentiated thyroid cancer according to the 7th and 8th editions of the AJCC/UICC TNM staging system. *Ther. Adv. Endocrinol. Metab.* **2020**, *11*, 2042018820921019. [CrossRef]
30. Shi, X.; Liu, R.; Basolo, F.; Giannini, R.; Shen, X.; Teng, D.; Guan, H.; Shan, Z.; Teng, W.; Musholt, T.J.; et al. Differential Clinicopathological Risk and Prognosis of Major Papillary Thyroid Cancer Variants. *J. Clin. Endocrinol. Metab.* **2016**, *101*, 264–274. [CrossRef]
31. Singer, P.A.; Cooper, D.S.; Daniels, G.H.; Ladenson, P.W.; Greenspan, F.S.; Levy, E.G.; Braverman, L.E.; Clark, O.H.; McDougall, I.R.; Ain, K.V.; et al. Treatment guidelines for patients with thyroid nodules and well-differentiated thyroid cancer. American Thyroid Association. *Arch. Intern. Med.* **1996**, *156*, 2165–2172. [CrossRef]

32. Cooper, D.S.; Doherty, G.M.; Haugen, B.R.; Kloos, R.T.; Lee, S.L.; Mandel, S.J.; Mazzaferri, E.L.; McIver, B.; Sherman, S.I.; Tuttle, R.M.; et al. Management guidelines for patients with thyroid nodules and differentiated thyroid cancer. *Thyroid* **2006**, *16*, 109–142. [CrossRef]
33. Baldini, E.; Sorrenti, S.; Di Gioia, C.; De Vito, C.; Antonelli, A.; Gnessi, L.; Carbotta, G.; D'Armiento, E.; Miccoli, P.; De Antoni, E.; et al. Cervical lymph node metastases from thyroid cancer: Does thyroglobulin and calcitonin measurement in fine needle aspirates improve the diagnostic value of cytology? *BMC Clin. Pathol.* **2013**, *13*, e7. [CrossRef]

cancers

MDPI

Article

Effects of the Minimal Extrathyroidal Extension on Early Response Rates after (Adjuvant) Initial Radioactive Iodine Therapy in PTC Patients

Freba Ahmaddy [1,†], Vera Wenter [1,†], Harun Ilhan [1], Daniel Wacker [1], Marcus Unterrainer [1], Thomas Knösel [2], Peter Bartenstein [1], Christine Spitzweg [3], Sebastian Lehner [1,4] and Andrei Todica [1,*]

1 Department of Nuclear Medicine, University Hospital, LMU Munich, 81377 Munich, Germany; Freba.Ahmaddy@med.uni-muenchen.de (F.A.); Vera.Wenter@med.uni-muenchen.de (V.W.); Harun.Ilhan@med.uni-muenchen.de (H.I.); Daniel_Wacker@web.de (D.W.); Marcus.Unterrainer@med.uni-muenchen.de (M.U.); Peter.Bartenstein@med.uni-muenchen.de (P.B.); Sebastian.Lehner@med.uni-muenchen.de (S.L.)

2 Institute of Pathology, Ludwig-Maximilians-University of Munich, 81377 Munich, Germany; Thomas.Knoesel@med.uni-muenchen.de

3 Department of Internal Medicine IV, University Hospital, LMU Munich, 81377 Munich, Germany; Christine.Spitzweg@med.uni-muenchen.de

4 Ambulatory Healthcare Center Dr. Neumaier & Colleagues, Radiology, Nuclear Medicine, Radiation Therapy, 93053 Regensburg, Germany

* Correspondence: andrei.todica@med.uni-muenchen.de; Tel.: +49-89-4400-74653

† These two authors contributed equally to this work.

Received: 11 September 2020; Accepted: 11 November 2020; Published: 13 November 2020

Simple Summary: The aim of our retrospective study was to evaluate the impact of minimal extrathyroidal extension on early response rate after (adjuvant) initial radioactive iodine therapy in patients with papillary thyroid cancer (PTC). We found that response rates after radioactive iodine (RAI) therapy in PTC patients were achieved irrespective of minimal extrathyroidal extension (mETE). Nonetheless, the risk of lymph node metastases involvement was significantly higher in the mETE patient group.

Abstract: Background: Extrathyroidal extension of differentiated thyroid cancer is a poor outcome factor but seems to be less significant in minimal extrathyroidal extension (mETE). However, the impact of mETE on response rate after (adjuvant) initial radioactive iodine (RAI) therapy remains unclear. We therefore compared response rates of patients with classical and follicular variants of papillary thyroid cancer (PTC) according to the updated eighth tumor-node-metastasis (TNM) classification to a control group. Methods: 455 patients with T3 (primary tumor > 4 cm) PTC according to the seventh classification who underwent total thyroidectomy followed by RAI therapy were screened. Patients formerly classified as T3 PTC solely due to mETE were reclassified into patients with T1 (primary tumor ≤ 2 cm) or T2 (primary tumor > 2 cm but ≤ 4 cm) +mETE and compared to a control group of T1/T2 −mETE PTC patients. Results: 138/455 patients were reclassified as T1/2 +mETE and compared to 317/455 T1/T2 −mETE control patients. At initial presentation, +mETE patients showed significantly higher rates of cervical lymph node metastases (p-value 0.001). Response rates were comparable in both groups (p-value n.s.). N1a/N1b-stage (Hazard ratio, HR 0.716; 95% CI 0.536–0.956, p-value 0.024) was identified as an independent prognostic factor for lower response rates. Conclusion: Response rates after RAI therapy were comparable in PTC patients irrespective of mETE but with higher rates of lymph node metastases.

Keywords: differentiated thyroid cancer; papillary thyroid cancer; minimal extrathyroidal extension; radioactive iodine therapy

1. Introduction

The extent of cancer at time of diagnosis is a key factor to assess the chance of successful treatment outcome [1]. In papillary thyroid cancer (PTC), there is general consensus that gross extrathyroidal extension (ETE) affects prognosis [2–4]. However, there has been considerable debate over the years regarding the most appropriate treatment for patients with minimal ETE (mETE), defined as extension to perithyroidal soft tissue or sternothyroid muscle [5–9]. Since January 2018, the new eighth edition of the TNM staging system (published in October 2016) has been used to classify patients with differentiated thyroid cancer (DTC) and predict disease mortality. Several substantial modifications were made to the seventh Union for International Cancer Control/American Joint Committee on Cancer (UICC/AJCC) tumor-node-metastasis (TNM) staging system to improve prognostic power, guide best treatment, and change towards the current trend of "personalized medicine" and risk adapted therapy concepts [10,11].

As a key change, mETE detected only on histological examination is no longer a determinant of the T-stage within the TNM classification [12]. The former T3 category included any tumor with >4 cm limited to the thyroid gland or tumors of any size with minimal ETE. In the updated eighth AJCC/TNM staging system, DTC with tumor size of ≤4 cm limited to thyroid gland is staged T1/2-disease regardless of the presence of mETE. Considering the initial risk stratification proposed by the 2015 American Thyroid Association (ATA), the presence of mETE alone upstages low-risk patients to the intermediate-risk group [11]. Therefore, the presence of mETE has a direct impact on clinical patient management.

The impact of mETE on the clinical outcome is still a matter of debate. Some studies suggest that mETE has no impact on the disease-free survival [6,8,13,14], whereas others could not confirm this data [15–17] and report a worse outcome in these patients. These studies focused on long-term outcomes. Undoubtedly, long-term outcomes remain the most crucial endpoint, but on a day to day basis, initial presentation of patients influences clinical decisions, and early response to therapy determines the clinical follow-up examinations (e.g., dynamic risk stratification according to the latest ATA guidelines).

Therefore, the aim of the present study was to investigate the initial clinical presentation and the effect on early response rates in PTC patients treated at our institute, which were reclassified as PTC T1/2 with mETE (+mETE) according to the updated eighth TNM staging system and compared to a control group consisting of PTC T1/2 without mETE (−mETE).

2. Results

2.1. Group Analysis

2.1.1. Patient Characteristics

Patient characteristics are summarized in Table 1. At initial presentation, +mETE patients showed significantly higher rates of cervical lymph node (N1a/N1b-stage) metastases (46% in +mETE patients (63/138) versus 29% in −mETE patients (91/317), *p*-value 0.001). Furthermore, higher initial radioactive iodine (RAI) activity was administered in +mETE patients as compared to the control group (4.6 ± 2.1 GBq in +mETE patients versus 3.3 ± 1.0 GBq in −mETE patients, *p*-value 0.001). Regarding histology, +mETE patients had significantly more often classical PTC than the follicular variant of PTC (75% in +mETE patients (103/138) versus 62% in −mETE (197/317), $p = 0.010$).

2.1.2. Outcome Analysis

Six to nine months after RAI therapy, the number of patients presenting without detectable Tg (stimulated Tg < 0.5 ng/mL) was comparable in both groups (77% in +mETE patients (106/138) and

81% in −mETE patients (258/317), *p*-value 0.262). Likewise, 97% of +mETE patients (134/138) and 99% of −mETE patients (313/317), *p*-value 0.241) did not present with relevant residual, cervical, or distant pathological uptake (*p*-value 0.387). Therefore, responder rates (combination of stimulated Tg < 0.5 ng/mL, no relevant uptake in the I-131 whole body scan, unremarkable neck ultrasonography) were similar in both groups (76% in +mETE patients (100/138) and 72% in −mETE patients (242/317), *p*-value 0.379). Furthermore, patients showed comparable responder rates irrespective of the histological subtype (*p*-value = 0.908). The outcome of the whole group is shown in Table 1.

Table 1. Patient characteristics and outcome analysis of the entire group.

n = 455 (100%)	T1/2 +mETE *n* = 138 (30%)	T1/2 −mETE *n* = 317 (70%)	*p* Value
	Patient characteristics		
Age (years)	57 ± 16	55 ± 14	0.054 †
Female sex–no. (%)	95 (69%)	234 (74%)	0.276 ‡
Tumor size (mm)	14.9 ± 8.4	14.4 ± 8.7	0.551 †
Classical PTC	103 (75%)	197 (62%)	0.010 ‡
N1a/N1b-stage–no. (%)	63 (46%)	91 (29%)	0.001 ‡
Mean initial RAI activity (GBq)	4.6 ± 2.1	3.3 ± 1.0	0.001 †
	Outcome analysis		
Tg-level < 0.5 ng/mL after TSH-stimulation	106 (77%)	258 (81%)	0.262 ‡
No pathological uptake in WBS–no. (%)	128 (93%)	291 (92%)	0.729 ‡
Unremarkable neck ultrasonography	134 (97%)	313 (99%)	0.241 ‡
Responder rates–no. (%)	100 (76%)	242 (72%)	0.379 ‡

‡ $\chi 2$
† *t*-test

mETE, minimal extrathyroidal extension; PTC, papillary thyroid carcinoma; T, tumor; N, nodus; RAI, radioactive iodine; GBq, gigabecquerel; Tg, thyroglobulin; TSH, Thyroid-stimulating hormone; WBS, whole body scan; responder rates: combination of stimulated Tg < 0.5 ng/mL, no relevant uptake in the I-131 whole body scan, unremarkable neck ultrasonography.

Both groups showed no significant differences in terms of age (57 ± 16 years in +mETE patients and 55 ± 14 in −mETE patients, *p*-value 0.504), sex (69% female in +mETE patients (95/138) and 74% in −mETE patients (234/317), *p*-value 0.276) and tumor size (14.9 ± 8.4 mm in +mETE patients and 14.4 ± 8.7 mm in −mETE patients, *p*-value 0.551).

2.2. Subgroup Analysis

2.2.1. N0/Nx-Subgroup Outcome Analysis

In the N0/Nx-subgroup analysis, 301 patients (75 +mETE patients, 226 −mETE patients) were evaluated. In total, 189/301 (62.7%) patients presented with N0-stage and 112/301 (37.3%) patients with Nx-stage. No significant differences were found between the two groups in terms of Tg responder rates after stimulation (89% in +mETE patients (67/75) and 88% in −mETE patients (199/226), *p*-value 0.764) as well as non-pathological cervical or distant iodine uptake (93% in +mETE patients (70/75) and 94% in −mETE patients (212/226), *p*-value 0.884). Responder rates were identical in both groups (84% in +mETE patients (63/75) and 84% in −mETE patients (190/226), *p*-value 0.988). Findings are presented in Table 2.

Table 2. Outcome analysis of the subgroups: N0/Nx and N1a/N1b.

Outcome Parameters	N0/Nx $n = 301$		p Value	N1a/1b $n = 154$		p Value
	+mETE $n = 75$ (25%)	−mETE $n = 226$ (75%)		+mETE $n = 63$ (41%)	−mETE $n = 91$ (59%)	
Outcome analysis						
Tg-level < 0.5 ng/mL after TSH-stimulation	67 (89%)	199 (88%)	0.764 ‡	39 (62%)	59 (65%)	0.710 ‡
No pathological uptake in WBS–no. (%)	70 (93%)	212 (94%)	0.884 ‡	58 (92%)	79 (87%)	0.307 ‡
Responder rates–no. (%)	63 (84%)	190 (84%)	0.0.988 ‡	37 (59%)	52 (57%)	0.845 ‡

‡ χ2
† t-test

Responder rates: combination of stimulated Tg < 0.5 ng/mL, no relevant uptake in the I-131 whole body scan, unremarkable neck ultrasonography.

2.2.2. N1a/N1b-Subgroup Outcome Analysis

In the N1a/N1b-subgroup analysis, 154 patients were included (63 +mETE patients, 91 −mETE patients). In total, 113/154 (73.4%) patients presented with N1a-stage and 41/154 (26.6%) patients with N1b-stage. In patients with N1a-stage, a mean of 19 ± 13 lymph nodes was removed, and in patients with N1b, 30 ± 20 lymph nodes were removed ($p = 0.001$). There was no significant difference between the two groups in terms of Tg responder rates after stimulation (62% in +mETE patients (39/63) and 65% in −mETE patients (59/91), $p = 0.710$) and relevant iodine uptake in the whole body scan (92% in +mETE patients (58/63) and 87% in −mETE patients (79/91), p-value 0.307). Overall, responder rates in this subgroup also were comparable irrespective of mETE (59% in +mETE patients (37/63) and 57% in −mETE patients (52/91), p-value 0.845). All data regarding treatment success after follow-up are summarized in Table 2. Irrespective of mETE, in the N1a/N1b-subgroup, subgroup responder rates were significantly lower than in the N0/Nx-subgroup (59% versus 84% in +mETE and 57% versus 84% in −mETE patients, p-value 0.001, respectively). In Figure 1, responder rates for the entire group and N0/Nx- and N1a/N1b-subgroups are presented. No differences in responder rates of the entire group as well as among subgroups could be found, irrespective of the presence of mETE.

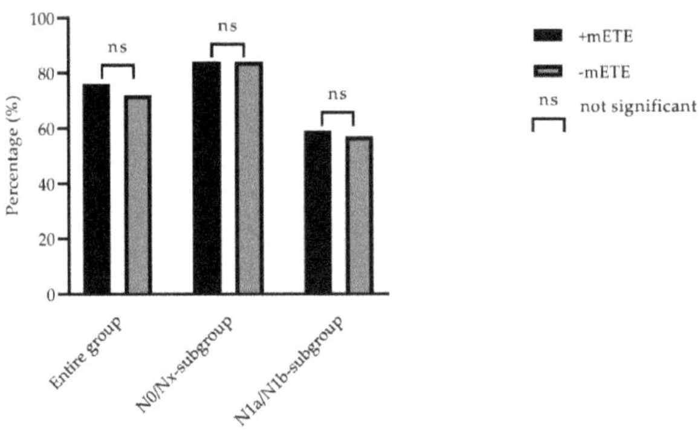

Figure 1. Responder rates (in %) of the entire group and the N-subgroup. No significant differences were found regarding responder rates in the entire group and among N0/Nx- and N1a/N1b-subgroups.

Of note, patients with N1a/N1b-status and +mETE received a significantly higher initial radioiodine activity as compared to patients from the −mETE group (6.3 ± 1.7 GBq versus 3.8 ± 1.1 GBq, *p*-value 0.001). In patients with higher administered RAI activity (≥7400 MBq), significantly more patients showed +mETE compared to patients with lower (≤3700 MBq) administered RAI activity (49/57 (86%) patients with high RAI activity versus 89/398 (22%) patients with low RAI activity, *p*-value 0.001). Furthermore, significantly more patients with higher administered RAI activity showed N1-stage (52/57 (91%) patients with high RAI activity versus 102/398 (26%) patients with low RAI activity, *p*-value 0.001). Significantly more patients with higher administered RAI activity showed poorer response rates compared to patients with lower administered RAI activity (25/57 (49%) patients with high RAI activity versus 88/398 (22%) patients with low RAI activity, *p*-value 0.001).

2.2.3. Uni- and Multivariate Analysis

To analyze possible risk factors for poorer outcomes, we performed a univariate and a multivariate analysis. Of the factors regarding primary presentation of patients, age ≥ 55 years at initial presentation was significantly associated with poorer outcome (Hazard ratio, HR = 7.605, p = 0.006), whereas gender (HR = 10.675, p = 0.104), histological subtype (HR = 8.123, p = 0.746), and the presence of mETE (HR = 9.556, p = 0.256) were not associated with poorer outcome. Regarding TNM-staging, N1a/N1b-stage (HR = 7.239, p = 0.001) was the only unfavorable prognostic factor for poorer outcome, whereas T-stage > T1 (HR = 8.837, p = 0.251) was not associated with lower responder rates. Furthermore, a mean initial I-131-dose of ≥7400 MBq (HR = 14.028, p = 0.026) was associated with significantly poorer outcome in the univariate analysis. In the multivariate analysis, N1a/N1b-stage was the only independent unfavorable prognostic factor for treatment success (HR = 0.716, p = 0.024). Age ≥ 55 years at initial presentation (HR = 1.003, p = 0.405) and mean initial I-131-dose of ≥7400 MBq (HR = 0.915, p = 0.672) were not significantly associated with poorer outcome in the multivariate analysis. All risk factors are summarized in Table 3.

Table 3. Prognostic risk factors for poorer responder rates (uni-/multivariate analysis).

Covariate	Level	Response Rate (Univariate Analysis)		Response Rate (Multivariate Analysis)	
		HR (95% CI)	***p* Value**	**HR (95% CI)**	***p* Value**
Gender	Female Male	Ref 10.675 (6.752–14.577)	0.104		
Age (years)	<55 ≥55	Ref 7.605 (7.220–7.989)	0.006	Ref 1.003 (0.995–1.012)	0.405
Histology	Classical PTC Follicular variant PTC	Ref 8.123 (7.451–8.796)	0.746		
T-stage	T 1>T1	Ref 8.837 (7.081–10.592)	0.251		
N-stage	N0, Nx N1a, N1b	Ref 10.737 (6.917–14.557)	< 0.001	Ref 0.716 (0.536–0.956)	0.024
mETE	−mETE +mETE	Ref 9.556 (6.757–12.355)	0.256		
Mean initial RAI dose (GBq)	≤3.7 ≥7.4	Ref 14.028 (5.044–23.012)	0.026	Ref 0.915 (0.605–1.383)	0.672

T, tumor; N, nodus; mETE, minimal extrathyroidal extension; GBq, gigabecquerel; HR, hazard ratio; CI, confidence interval; RAI, radioactive iodine.

3. Discussion

Extrathyroidal extension of thyroid cancer has been recognized as a factor of poor outcome [2,3]. More recent analyses have suggested that mETE is less significant for patient outcome than gross extension [5–7,18,19]. The updated eighth edition of the AJCC/TNM staging system removed the subclassification of mETE, resulting in a downstaging of T3 tumors ≤ 4 cm. However, the impact of mETE on treatment success after initial RAI therapy still remains a matter of debate. Although TNM-staging is mainly associated with the disease specific mortality risk, it still influences the clinical patient management. We therefore evaluated the primary presentation and the early treatment response in our patient cohort with or without mETE.

Firstly, we compared +mETE patients to a control group with matched histology, age, sex, and tumor size. Secondly, we subdivided patients in subgroups with N0/Nx- and N1a/N1b- stages to analyze the study group in more detail. These more homogenous subgroups were supposed to improve data quality, as confounding factors could be better analyzed.

Overall, our data suggested that mETE does not affect treatment success. Indeed, analyzing biochemical (Tg-levels) and structural (uptake in WBS and ultrasound) characteristics, comparable responder rates were found in both groups (+mETE vs. −mETE). These findings mirror data by Arora et al. and Kim et al., where the presence of mETE was not an independent predictive factor of recurrence [9,20]. Furthermore, the study by Ito et al. showed that mETE was not associated with recurrence in contrast to gross ETE. Thus, they suggested not using mETE as an indicator for poor prognosis [6].

Nevertheless, our data indicate that +mETE patients have a significantly higher risk of presenting with lymph node metastases at initial presentation as compared to −mETE patients. This is in line with the study of Kim et al. who reported that patients with gross or mETE were more likely to have nodal metastases in the central or the lateral neck compartments [20]. Shin et al. showed that there was no significant difference in recurrence between +mETE and −mETE patients; although lymph node metastases were an independent factor for the increased risk of mETE, it did not affect recurrence-free survival [7]. On the contrary, data in a recent meta-analysis from Diker-Cohen et al. indicated that, in patients with N1a/N1b disease, the presence of mETE did further increase the risk of recurrence, yet still within the low risk category [21]. Overall, our analysis identified N1a/N1b-stage as the only risk factor for lower responder rates in the multivariate analysis. Overall, our data indicate that patients with mETE have a higher risk of systemic disease. Therefore, since a prophylactic lymph node neck dissection is not suggested in patients with T1/T2 disease, precise perioperative diagnostic examinations (ultrasound, post-treatment WBS) are crucial in this cohort to exclude lymph node metastases [11].

In our study, response rates were similar in the N0/Nx- and the N1a/N1b-stage subgroup analysis. Nonetheless, it needs to be emphasized that, in this N-stage subgroup, +mETE patients received a significantly higher activity as compared to patients without mETE. Seo et al. compared the outcome after (adjuvant) initial RAI therapy in patients with lymph node metastases and mETE treated with standard activity (3.0 GBq) or a low-dose activity (1.1 GBq) and found no significant differences between both regiments regarding the initial response rate as well as during the follow-up within the first years (mean follow-up time of 45 months) [22]. Therefore, it is very unlikely that the significantly higher treatment activity in our +mETE group might have led to a significant bias in this study.

Patients with higher administered RAI activity had a worse treatment response compared to patients treated with lower RAI activity. This finding was to be expected, since significantly more patients with lymph node metastases were treated with higher doses. It is well known that patients with lymph node metastases show poorer treatment response [23].

It needs to be highlighted that patients included in this retrospective study come from a historical collective. Therefore, patients received relatively high doses of RAI, which was in line with the German and institutional guidelines at the time of treatment. However, current guidelines trend towards decreasing radioiodine doses, which was supported by the two prospective studies "Ablation with low-dose radioiodine and thyrotropin alfa in thyroid cancer" (HiLo) and "Strategies of radioiodine ablation in patients with low-risk thyroid cancer" (ESTIMABL) [24,25]. Compared to current guidelines, especially +mETE patients with lymph node metastases were most likely overtreated with RAI.

As the majority of PTC cases comprise classical and follicular variants of PTC, only these histological subgroups were included in our study [26]. Patients with classical PTC had mETE significantly more often as compared to patients with the follicular variant of PTC. This finding is in line with the study of Yu et al., who also reported significantly higher rates of ETE in classical PTC patients. Response rates in our patient cohort were comparable in both groups. Yu et al. also showed that no differences in outcome could be found between classical and follicular variants of PTC patients [27].

Our study has several limitations. First, there may have been a selection bias because of the retrospective design. Secondly, in our study, patients with mETE were treated with significantly higher radioiodine doses. Higher doses were administered because mETE was considered as a risk factor at the time of inclusion. Furthermore +mETE patients presented more often with lymph node metastases.

Thyroglobulin antibodies are only present in a minority of the patients and therefore could not be included in the analysis in a convincing way. This is indeed a limitation of the study, which cannot be overcome. However, although the recovery is less sensitive than the direct measurement of the antibodies, we are convinced that an undisturbed recovery adds confidence for the validity of the measured thyroglobulin.

Furthermore, primary surgical procedures were performed in different hospitals. Therefore, histological tissue or slides were not available, and only the original pathology reports were reviewed. However, we only included patients with detailed reports indicative for reclassification.

4. Materials and Methods

4.1. Study Population

We retrospectively reviewed consecutive patients with pT1-T3 PTC from our institutional data base who underwent total thyroidectomy followed by RAI therapy at the Department of Nuclear Medicine (University Hospital, LMU Munich) between January 2010 and June 2015. Epidemiological and clinical features of these patients were assessed (age at diagnosis, gender, TNM stage, tumor size, presence of ETE, resection margins). Patients initially classified as PTC T3 solely due to mETE (according to the seventh UICC/AJCC TNM staging system) were reclassified according to the updated eighth UICC/AJCC TNM staging system into the subgroup of T1/2 +mETE. These patients were compared to a control group consisting of PTC patients classified as T1/2 −mETE according to former and updated TNM classifications. Pathological reports from the referring hospitals were reviewed and reclassified according to the updated TNM staging system. Since the majority of PTC cases comprise classical and follicular variants of PTC, we only investigated these histological subgroups in our study. Patients with aggressive histological subtypes of PTC, distant metastases diagnosed from clinical examination or imaging (cM1-stage), or unresectable carcinomas or positive resection margins (R1/R2-stage) were excluded.

For our study, a total of 1140 patients were screened, and 638 patients with PTC were evaluated. A total of 164 patients were retrospectively reclassified as T1/2 with mETE (T1/2 +mETE); 346 T1/2 patients without mETE (T1/2 −mETE) served as a control group. A total of 46 patients remained T3 according to former and updated TNM staging systems and were consequently excluded, and 24 patients were excluded due to aggressive histological subtypes of PTC. A total of 455 patients fulfilled the inclusion criteria. The majority of patients (300/455, 65.9%) showed classical variant of PTC. For subgroup analysis of N0/Nx patients, we defined N0- and Nx-status according to Robinson et al. Patients with T1-stage were staged as N0 after examination of ≥6 lymph nodes and patients with T2 after ≥9 lymph nodes [28]. All other patients were staged Nx.

4.2. Ethics Statement

The study was approved by the local ethics committee (Ethics committee of the Medical Faculty, University Hospital, LMU Munich, Munich, Germany, IRB #20-210) and was conducted in accordance with the ethical standards according to the Declaration of Helsinki and according to national and international guidelines. The requirement to obtain informed consent was waived due to the retrospective design of this study.

4.3. Treatment

All patients underwent total thyroidectomy with or without lymphadenectomy. Surgery was followed by (adjuvant) initial radioactive iodine therapy [29]. Prior to RAI therapy, patients were stimulated with recombinant human TSH (rhTSH, Thyrogen®, Sanofi Genzyme, Cambridge, MA, United States) i. m. on two consecutive days or underwent hormone withdrawal prior to RAI therapy to achieve TSH levels ≥ 30μU/mL according to current guideline recommendations [11]. The administered radioiodine activity depended on the tumor stage as well as on the time of inclusion and ranged from 2.0 to 7.4 GBq I-131 (54–200 mCi).

4.4. Follow-Up and Outcome

Outcome of RAI therapy was assessed six to nine months after initial therapy. The follow up was based on physical examination, neck ultrasound, determination of the level of stimulated thyroglobulin (Tg)-level by two assays (Roche Elecsys® Tg II, Roche Diagnostics GmbH, Mannheim, Germany) with a measuring range of the Roche assay as 0.04–500 ng/mL with a theoretical lower limit of detection of 0.04 ng/mL and a theoretical lower limit of quantitation of 0.1 ng/mL with an error of < 30% or Siemens Immulite with an analytical sensitivity of 0.2 ng/mL and a functional sensitivity of 0.5 ng/mL), and Tg-recovery (Roche Elecsys® Tg II Confirmatory Test) as well as a diagnostic I-131 whole body scintigraphy (WBS), which was performed approximately 72 h after application of 370 MBq I-131 (10 mCi) in hypothyroidism or after administration of rhTSH i.m. on two consecutive days. In case of any pathological finding in the WBS, an additional single-photon-emission computed-tomography (SPECT)/low dose computer-tomography (CT) of the relevant region was performed (most often neck and thorax). Three days after stimulation, Tg and Tg recovery were determined.

Patients were classified as responders to adjuvant radioiodine therapy if stimulated Tg-levels were lower than 0.5 ng/ml, the thyroid bed was empty or showed a hyperechoic region, and no suspicious lymph nodes were found in the neck ultrasound and if the uptake in the thyroid bed was rated as non-relevant and no pathological uptake was seen outside the thyroid bed according to the WBS. In addition, if a second radioiodine treatment was needed for any given reason, the adjuvant radioiodine therapy was considered as inadequate.

4.5. Subgroup Analysis

At initial presentation, +mETE patients presented significantly more often with lymph node metastases (N1-stage 46% in +mETE patients vs. 29% in −mETE patients) as presented in Table 1. Therefore, we performed a subgroup analysis. We compared patients without local lymph node metastases (N0-stage) or with unknown lymph node status (Nx-stage) to patients with local lymph node metastases in the central (N1a-stage) or the latero-cervical compartment (N1b-stage) to identify possible influence of N-stage regarding response rate.

4.6. Statistical Analysis

All continuous variables (age, tumor size, I-131-dose) were expressed as mean ± standard deviation (SD). Unpaired Student´s t-test was used to compare metric variables (age, tumor size, I-131-dose). Chi-squared test was used to compare categorial variables (gender, N-Stage, uptake in whole body scan, Tg-level after TSH stimulation, TSH stimulation by rhTSH, re-therapy courses). Parameters that showed significant influence on success rate in the univariate analysis were included in the multivariate analysis. Vice versa parameters with p values ≥ 0.5 were not included in the multivariate analysis. The multivariate regression model was applied to analyze prognostic factors associated with treatment success. A p-value ≤ 0.05 was considered statistically significant. All analyses were performed using SPSS computer software (SPSS Statistics 25, IBM).

5. Conclusions

In conclusion, early treatment response in patients with classical or follicular variants of T1/T2 PTC is not significantly affected by the presence of mETE. Despite a higher incidence of lymph node metastases in patients with mETE, prophylactic lymphadenectomy is not suggested in patients in the T1/T2-stage. Therefore, accurate perioperative patient workup, including cervical neck ultrasound and post-treatment WBS, remains crucial.

Author Contributions: Authors contributed equally to this work; F.A., V.W.; conceptualization, A.T., F.A., D.W.; writing—original draft preparation, F.A., V.W.; supervision, A.T., H.I., C.S., S.L., P.B., M.U., T.K.; writing—review and editing, A.T., P.B., H.I.; visualization, F.A., M.U.; project administration, P.B., A.T., F.A.; data curation, F.A., D.W.; resources, F.A., D.W. All authors have read and agreed to the published version of the manuscript.

Funding: This work was financially supported by the Kuhbier-Langewiesche foundation and the Bavarian Equal Opportunities Sponsorship (BGF). The foundation had no role in study design, data collection and analysis, decision to publish, or preparation of the manuscript. No other potential conflicts of interest relevant to this article exist.

Acknowledgments: A significant part of this work originated from the doctoral thesis of Daniel Wacker. Vera Wenter was financially supported by the Bavarian Equal Opportunities Sponsorship (BGF) to promote equal opportunities for women in research and teaching. The sponsorship did not influence study design, data collection and analysis, decision to publish, or preparation of the manuscript.

Conflicts of Interest: The authors declare that they have no conflict of interest.

References

1. Edge, S.B.; Compton, C.C. The American Joint Committee on Cancer: The 7th edition of the AJCC cancer staging manual and the future of TNM. *Ann. Surg. Oncol.* **2010**, *17*, 1471–1474. [CrossRef]
2. Ito, Y.; Kudo, T.; Kobayashi, K.; Miya, A.; Ichihara, K.; Miyauchi, A. Prognostic factors for recurrence of papillary thyroid carcinoma in the lymph nodes, lung, and bone: Analysis of 5,768 patients with average 10-year follow-up. *World J. Surg.* **2012**, *36*, 1274–1278. [CrossRef] [PubMed]
3. Verburg, F.A.; Mäder, U.; Tanase, K.; Thies, E.-D.; Diessl, S.; Buck, A.K.; Luster, M.; Reiners, C. Life expectancy is reduced in differentiated thyroid cancer patients >/= 45 years old with extensive local tumor invasion, lateral lymph node, or distant metastases at diagnosis and normal in all other DTC patients. *J. Clin. Endocrinol. Metab.* **2013**, *98*, 172–180. [CrossRef] [PubMed]
4. Andersen, P.E.; Kinsella, J.; Loree, T.R.; Shaha, A.R.; Shah, J.P. Differentiated carcinoma of the thyroid with extrathyroidal extension. *Am. J. Surg.* **1995**, *170*, 467–470. [CrossRef]
5. Yin, D.-T.; Yu, K.; Lu, R.-Q.; Li, X.; Xu, J.; Lei, M. Prognostic impact of minimal extrathyroidal extension in papillary thyroid carcinoma. *Medicine (Baltimore)* **2016**, *95*, e5794. [CrossRef]
6. Ito, Y.; Tomoda, C.; Uruno, T.; Takamura, Y.; Miya, A.; Kobayashi, K.; Matsuzuka, F.; Kuma, K.; Miyauchi, A. Prognostic significance of extrathyroid extension of papillary thyroid carcinoma: Massive but not minimal extension affects the relapse-free survival. *World J. Surg.* **2006**, *30*, 780–786. [CrossRef]
7. Shin, J.H.; Haa, T.K.; Parka, H.K.; Ahna, M.S.; Kima, K.H.; Baea, K.B.; Kima, T.H.; Choia, C.S.; Kimb, T.K.; Baec, S.K.; et al. Implication of minimal extrathyroidal extension as a prognostic factor in papillary thyroid carcinoma. *Int. J. Surg.* **2013**, *11*, 944–947. [CrossRef]
8. Al-Qurayshi, Z.; Shama, M.A.; Randolph, G.W.; Kandil, E. Minimal extrathyroidal extension does not affect survival of well-differentiated thyroid cancer. *Endocr. Relat. Cancer* **2017**, *24*, 221–226. [CrossRef]
9. Arora, N.; Turbendian, H.K.; Scognamiglio, T.; Wagner, P.L.; Goldsmith, S.J.; Zarnegar, R.; Fahey, T.J. Extrathyroidal extension is not all equal: Implications of macroscopic versus microscopic extent in papillary thyroid carcinoma. *Surgery* **2008**, *144*, 942–947. [CrossRef]

10. Amin, M.B.; Greene, F.L.; Edge, S.B.; Compton, C.C.; Gershenwald, J.E.; Brookland, R.K.; Meyer, L.; Gress, D.M.; Byrd, D.R.; Winchester, D.P. The Eighth Edition AJCC Cancer Staging Manual: Continuing to build a bridge from a population-based to a more "personalized" approach to cancer staging. *CA Cancer J. Clin.* **2017**, *67*, 93–99. [CrossRef]
11. Haugen, B.R.; Alexander, E.K.; Bible, K.C.; Doherty, G.M.; Mandel, S.J.; Nikiforov, Y.E.; Pacini, F.; Randolph, G.W.; Sawka, A.M.; Schlumberger, M.; et al. 2015 American Thyroid Association Management Guidelines for Adult Patients with Thyroid Nodules and Differentiated Thyroid Cancer: The American Thyroid Association Guidelines Task Force on Thyroid Nodules and Differentiated Thyroid Cancer. *Thyroid* **2016**, *26*, 1–133. [CrossRef] [PubMed]
12. Perrier, N.D.; Brierley, J.D.; Tuttle, R.M. Differentiated and anaplastic thyroid carcinoma: Major changes in the American Joint Committee on Cancer eighth edition cancer staging manual. *CA Cancer J. Clin.* **2018**, *68*, 55–63. [CrossRef] [PubMed]
13. Kluijfhout, W.P.; Pasternak, J.D.; Kwon, J.S.; Lim, J.; Shen, W.T.; Gosnell, J.E.; Khanafshar, E.; Duh, Q.-Y.; Suh, I. Microscopic Positive Tumor Margin Does Not Increase the Risk of Recurrence in Patients with T1-T2 Well-Differentiated Thyroid Cancer. *Ann. Surg. Oncol.* **2016**, *23*, 1446–1451. [CrossRef] [PubMed]
14. Woo, C.G.; Sung, C.O.; Choi, Y.M.; Kim, W.G.; Kim, T.Y.; Shong, Y.K.; Kim, W.B.; Hong, S.J.; Song, D.E. Clinicopathological Significance of Minimal Extrathyroid Extension in Solitary Papillary Thyroid Carcinomas. *Ann. Surg. Oncol.* **2015**, *22* (Suppl. 3), S728–S733. [CrossRef]
15. Radowsky, J.S.; Howard, R.S.; Burch, H.B.; Stojadinovic, A. Impact of degree of extrathyroidal extension of disease on papillary thyroid cancer outcome. *Thyroid* **2014**, *24*, 241–244. [CrossRef]
16. Santos, M.J.; Bugalho, M.J. Papillary thyroid carcinoma: Different clinical behavior among pT3 tumors. *Endocrine* **2016**, *53*, 754–760. [CrossRef]
17. Youngwirth, L.M.; Adam, M.A.; Scheri, R.P.; Roman, S.A.; Sosa, J.A. Extrathyroidal Extension Is Associated with Compromised Survival in Patients with Thyroid Cancer. *Thyroid* **2017**, *27*, 626–631. [CrossRef]
18. Nixon, I.J.; Ganly, I.; Patel, S.; Palmer, F.L.; Whitcher, M.M.; Tuttle, R.M.; Shaha, A.R.; Shah, J.P. The impact of microscopic extrathyroid extension on outcome in patients with clinical T1 and T2 well-differentiated thyroid cancer. *Surgery* **2011**, *150*, 1242–1249. [CrossRef]
19. Hay, I.D.; Johnson, T.R.; Thompson, G.B.; Sebo, T.J.; Reinalda, M.S. Minimal extrathyroid extension in papillary thyroid carcinoma does not result in increased rates of either cause-specific mortality or postoperative tumor recurrence. *Surgery* **2016**, *159*, 11–19. [CrossRef]
20. Kim, J.W.; Roh, J.-L.; Gong, G.; Cho, K.-J.; Choi, S.-H.; Nam, S.Y.; Kim, S.Y. Extent of Extrathyroidal Extension as a Significant Predictor of Nodal Metastasis and Extranodal Extension in Patients with Papillary Thyroid Carcinoma. *Ann. Surg. Oncol.* **2017**, *24*, 460–468. [CrossRef]
21. Diker-Cohen, T.; Hirsch, D.; Shimon, I.; Bachar, G.; Akirov, A.; Duskin-Bitan, H.; Robenshtok, E. Impact of Minimal Extra-Thyroid Extension in Differentiated Thyroid Cancer: Systematic Review and Meta-analysis. *J. Clin. Endocrinol. Metab.* **2018**. [CrossRef] [PubMed]
22. Seo, M.; Kim, Y.S.; Lee, J.C.; Han, M.W.; Kim, E.S.; Kim, K.B.; Park, S.H. Low-Dose Radioactive Iodine Ablation Is Sufficient in Patients With Small Papillary Thyroid Cancer Having Minor Extrathyroidal Extension and Central Lymph Node Metastasis (T3 N1a). *Clin. Nucl. Med.* **2017**, *42*, 842–846. [CrossRef] [PubMed]
23. Hughes, C.J.; Shaha, A.R.; Shah, J.P.; Loree, T.R. Impact of lymph node metastasis in differentiated carcinoma of the thyroid: A matched-pair analysis. *Head Neck.* **1996**, *18*, 127–132. [CrossRef]
24. Mallick, U.; Harmer, C.; Yap, B.; Wadsley, J.; Clarke, S.; Moss, L.; Nicol, A.; Clark, P.M.; Farnell, K.; McCready, R.; et al. Ablation with low-dose radioiodine and thyrotropin alfa in thyroid cancer. *N. Engl. J. Med.* **2012**, *366*, 1674–1685. [CrossRef]
25. Schlumberger, M.; Catargi, B.; Borget, I.; Pharm, D.; Deandreis, D.; Zerdoud, S.; Bridji, B.; Bardet, S.; Leenhardt, L.; Bastie, D.; et al. Strategies of radioiodine ablation in patients with low-risk thyroid cancer. *N. Engl. J. Med.* **2012**, *366*, 1663–1673. [CrossRef]
26. Henke, L.E.; Pfeifer, J.D.; Baranski, T.J.; DeWees, T.; Grigsby, P.W. Long-term outcomes of follicular variant vs. classic papillary thyroid carcinoma. *Endocr. Connect.* **2018**, *7*, 1226–1235. [CrossRef]
27. Yu, X.-M.; Schneider, D.F.; Leverson, G.; Chen, H.; Rebecca, S. Follicular variant of papillary thyroid carcinoma is a unique clinical entity: A population-based study of 10,740 cases. *Thyroid* **2013**, *23*, 1263–1268. [CrossRef]

28. Robinson, T.J.; Thomas, S.; Dinan, M.A.; Roman, S.; Sosa, J.A.; Hyslop, T. How Many Lymph Nodes Are Enough? Assessing the Adequacy of Lymph Node Yield for Papillary Thyroid Cancer. *J. Clin. Oncol.* **2016**, *34*, 3434–3439. [CrossRef]
29. Ruel, E.; Thomas, S.; Dinan, M.; Perkins, J.M.; Roman, S.A.; Sosa, J.A. Adjuvant radioactive iodine therapy is associated with improved survival for patients with intermediate-risk papillary thyroid cancer. *J. Clin. Endocrinol. Metab.* **2015**, *100*, 1529–1536. [CrossRef]

Cancers 2020, 12, 3268

MDPI

Article

Results and Clinical Interpretation of Germline *RET* Analysis in a Series of Patients with Medullary Thyroid Carcinoma: The Challenge of the Variants of Uncertain Significance

Giovanni Innella [1,2], Cesare Rossi [1], Maria Romagnoli [1], Andrea Repaci [3], Davide Bianchi [4], Maria Elena Cantarini [5], Davide Martorana [6], Lea Godino [1], Andrea Pession [2,5], Antonio Percesepe [6], Uberto Pagotto [2,3] and Daniela Turchetti [1,2,*]

1 Division of Medical Genetics, Azienda Ospedaliero-Universitaria di Bologna, 40138 Bologna, Italy; giovanni.innella@studio.unibo.it (G.I.); cesare.rossi@unibo.it (C.R.); maria.romagnoli@uslcentro.toscana.it (M.R.); lea.godino@aosp.bo.it (L.G.)

2 Department of Medical and Surgical Sciences, University of Bologna, 40138 Bologna, Italy; andrea.pession@unibo.it (A.P.); uberto.pagotto@unibo.it (U.P.)

3 Endocrinology and Diabetes Prevention and Care Unit, Department of Medical and Surgical Sciences, University of Bologna, 40138 Bologna, Italy; rep.rep@libero.it

4 Division of Endocrinology, Ospedale di Bentivoglio, 40010 Bentivoglio (BO), Italy; davide.bianchi@ausl.bo.it

5 Division of Pediatric Oncology, Azienda Ospedaliero-Universitaria di Bologna, 40138 Bologna, Italy; mariaelena.cantarini@aosp.bo.it

6 Division of Medical Genetics, Azienda Ospedaliero-Universitaria di Parma, 43126 Parma, Italy; dmartorana@ao.pr.it (D.M.); antonio.percesepe@unipr.it (A.P.)

* Correspondence: daniela.turchetti@unibo.it; Tel.: +39-051-208-0904

Received: 2 October 2020; Accepted: 3 November 2020; Published: 5 November 2020

Simple Summary: About 25% of Thyroid Carcinomas of Medullary type occur in carriers of hereditary alterations in the *RET* gene. Different alterations are associated with different risks (highest, high, and moderate) and management depends on risk category. We explored prevalence, clinical presentation and management of inherited *RET* variants in patients tested at our center. We found inherited *RET* variants in 31.9% of tested individuals: the vast majority of patients with Medullary Thyroid Carcinoma who had a family history positive for the disease was found to carry a *RET* change, but also 14.3% of those with no family history tested positive, supporting the recommendation to perform genetic testing in all cases of Medullary Thyroid Carcinoma. For known variants, findings in our patients were consistent with available risk classification. Besides, we obtained evidence supporting the classification of two rare variants of uncertain clinical significance (p.Ser904Phe and p.Asp631_Leu633delinsGlu), which may help future management of carriers.

Abstract: Germline *RET* variants are responsible for approximately 25% of medullary thyroid carcinoma (MTC) cases. Identification of *RET* variant carriers allows for the adoption of preventative measures which are dependent on the risk associated with the specific alteration. From 2002 to 2020, at our cancer genetics clinic, *RET* genetic testing was performed in 163 subjects (102 complete gene analyses and 61 targeted analyses), 72 of whom presented with MTC. A germline *RET* variant was identified in 31.9% of patients affected by MTC (93.8% of those having positive family history and 14.3% of clinically sporadic cases). Subsequent target testing in relatives allowed us to identify 22 asymptomatic carriers, who could undertake appropriate screening. Overall, patients with germline *RET* variants differed significantly from those who tested negative by family history ($p < 0.001$) and mean age at MTC diagnosis (44.45 vs. 56.42 years; $p = 0.010$), but the difference was not significant when only carriers of moderate risk variants were considered (51.78 vs. 56.42 years; $p = 0.281$). Out of

12 different variants detected in 49 patients, five (41.7%) were of uncertain significance (VUS). For two of these, p.Ser904Phe and p.Asp631_Leu633delinsGlu, co-segregation and genotype/phenotype analysis, matched with data from the literature, provided evidence supporting their classification in the moderate and the highest/high risk class (with a MEN2B phenotype), respectively.

Keywords: *RET*; medullary thyroid carcinoma; clinical management; variants of uncertain significance

---

1. Introduction

Medullary thyroid carcinoma (MTC) accounts for 4–10% of all thyroid cancer cases [1,2] and originates from the parafollicular cells of the thyroid or C-cells, physiologically responsible for the secretion of calcitonin; C-cell hyperplasia (CCH) is considered as the first stage of histological progression that evolves into MTC [3,4]. Among MTC cases, around 25% present in the context of an inherited syndrome, whereas the remaining 75% are sporadic [5–7]. Inherited MTC syndromes include multiple endocrine neoplasia type 2 (MEN2A and MEN2B) and familial MTC (FMTC) [8,9]. MTC is associated with pheocromocytoma (PCC) and parathyroid hyperplasia/primary hyperparathyroidism (PHPT) in MEN2A, [10,11], and with PCC, marfanoid habitus and ganglioneuromatosis of the gut and oral mucosa in MEN2B [12]; conversely, FMTC is characterized by multiple cases of MTC in the family, with no other clinical manifestations [13].

Both MEN2 and FMTC are caused by germline, activating variants in the *RET* proto-oncogene following an autosomal dominant pattern of transmission [14,15]. Nevertheless, different *RET* mutations confer different cancer risks [16–19], which has led to recommendations for management of the carriers based on the level of risk associated with the specific mutation [20]. In this regard, the American Thyroid Association (ATA) stratified *RET* mutations into distinct risk levels, in order to define the most appropriate management for each known mutation. Former classification provided for a stratification into four risk levels (from D to A from the highest to the lowest level of risk) [21], while the 2015 guideline revision combined levels A and B for a total of three risk levels: highest (HST), high (H) and moderate (MOD) [22].

The ATA's recommended management consists of prophylactic thyroidectomy to be performed as soon as possible in carriers of HST and H risk level variants (within the first year of life and within 5 years, respectively), while for carriers of MOD risk level variants, it is suggested to perform annual serum calcitonin screening, and prophylactic thyroidectomy should be performed when values become elevated. Screening for PCC (annual dosing of plasma and urinary catecholamines and metabolites) should start at 11 years for carriers of H/HST variants and at 16 years for carriers of MOD variants. For carriers of H and MOD variants, biochemical screening for PHPT is also recommended (annual dosing of serum calcium and parathyroid hormone), starting at 8 and 20 years, respectively [21–23].

Of course, a stratification by risk is possible only for known, recurrent mutations, for which genotype–phenotype correlations have been clearly established. Conversely, the detection of a novel or rare mutation in a family poses serious counselling and management issues, as the associated risk is mostly unknown. In these cases, until genotype–phenotype correlations are clarified, risk and subsequent management of healthy carrier cannot be based on standard guidelines and need to be evaluated case-by-case, possibly on the basis of clinical and family history of the carriers, which however, may be informative only for large families with many well characterized members [24].

The aim of the study was to analyze the experience of our center with *RET* genetic testing in order to (a) explore prevalence, clinical significance and genotype–phenotype correlations of germline *RET* mutations, (b) collect information which could potentially contribute to defining the clinical role of the variants of uncertain significance (VUS) encountered at our center, and (c) discuss the approach to management of carriers of novel and rare *RET* mutations.

2. Results

2.1. Clinical Characteristics and Genetic Test Results

Among subjects submitted to *RET* analysis in our laboratory, 117/163 (71.8%) had personal and/or family history of MTC (114) or CCH (3), while the remaining had personal and/or family history of other pathologies possibly related to *RET* alterations (PCC, PHPT, intestinal ganglioneuromatosis). The list of cases included in the study is reported in Table S1.

A germline *RET* variant was identified in 49/163 (30.1%) subjects: 15/102 (14.7%) index cases, who underwent a complete gene analysis, and 34/61 (55.7%) relatives of a *RET* carrier, who underwent a targeted search for a known variant. Considering only the 72 patients affected by MTC/CCH, a germline *RET* variant was identified in 23 (31.9%), with 15/16 (93.8%) of these having positive family history and 8/56 (14.3%) of sporadic cases. Finally, considering only patients with CCH, 1/3 (33.3%) carried a variant of *RET*.

Mean age at MTC diagnosis was 44.45 years in patients with germline *RET* variants (pathogenetic or considered likely pathogenetic) and 56.42 years in patients with no variants detected ($p = 0.010$). Among patients with known cancer staging, 42.9% of those with *RET* variants and 36.4% of those with negative analysis had locally advanced disease (T > 1). All four MTC patients who also displayed other manifestations of MEN2 were found to carry a pathogenic germline *RET* variant.

2.2. RET Test Results and Clinical Correlations

Twelve different *RET* variants were identified in our sample: seven previously classified in a specific risk class (one of HST risk level, two of H risk level, four of MOD risk level) (Table 1) and five unclassified. The HST risk level variant p.Met918Thr was identified in a sporadic case of MEN2B, as well as in an external patient for whom phenotype was not detailed. H risk level variants were identified in two cases of familial MEN2A. MOD risk level variants were found in 34 subjects of 13 families; all belonged to A risk class (the lowest risk level) in the previous classification.

Table 1. *RET* classified variants detected in the population under study.

Nucleotide Variant	Aminoacidic Change	ATA Risk Level	N. Families	N. Carriers	MTC/tot Carriers [a] (%)	PCC/Tot Carriers [a] (%)	PHPT/Tot Carriers [a] (%)	MEN2B Manifestations [b]/Tot Carriers [a] (%)
c.2671T > C	p.Ser891Ala	MOD	1	1	0/1 (0.0)	0/1 (0.0)	0/1 (0.0)	0/1 (0.0)
c.2410G > A	p.Val804Met	MOD	5	14	6/12 (50.0)	0/12 (0.0)	0/12 (0.0)	0/12 (0.0)
c.2370G > T	p.Leu790Phe	MOD	1	9	7/9 (77.8)	1/9 (11.1)	0/9 (0.0)	0/9 (0.0)
c. 2304G > C	p.Glu768Asp	MOD	2	10	3/10 (30.0)	0/10 (0.0)	0/10 (0.0)	0/10 (0.0)
c.1901G > T	p.Cys634Phe	H	1	1	1/1 (100.0)	1/1 (100.0)	0/1 (0.0)	0/1 (0.0)
c.1901G > A	p.Cys634Tyr	H	0	1	1/1 (100.0)	1/1 (100.0)	0/1 (0.0)	0/1 (0.0)
c.2753T > C	p.Met918Thr	HST	2	2	2/2 (100.0)	0/1 (0.0)	0/1 (0.0)	1/1 (100.0)

[a] Only carriers with known clinical information were included; [b] Including marfanoid habitus, ganglioneuromatosis of the gut and oral mucosa, mild dysmorphic features. Abbreviations: ATA = American Thyroid Association; MTC = medullary thyroid carcinoma; PCC = pheocromocytoma; PHPT = primary hyperparathyroidism; MOD = moderate; H = high; HST = highest.

Overall, patients with germline *RET* variants significantly differed from those testing negative by the presence of family history (68.2% vs. 2.1%; $p < 0.001$) and by mean age at MTC diagnosis (44.45 vs. 56.42; $p = 0.010$). When comparing carriers of MOD risk variants with wild-type *RET* patients, the presence of family history was still significantly more frequent in the former group (72.2% vs. 2.1%; $p < 0.001$), while mean age at MTC diagnosis did not differ significantly (51.78 vs. 56.42; $p = 0.281$). Indeed, mean age at MTC diagnosis was 51.78 years among carriers of MOD risk variants, compared to 11.5 years in carriers of HST/H risk level variants ($p < 0.001$). The comparison of clinical features of patients with MTC according to test results is shown in Table 2.

Table 2. Clinical characteristics of MTC patients according to test result.

Feature	*RET* VARIANT DETECTED				*p* Value		
	NONE	ALL	MOD	HST/H	(NONE vs. ALL)	(NONE vs. MOD)	(MOD vs. HST/H)
Age at diagnosis of MTC (mean)	56.42	44.45	51.78	11.50	0.010	0.281	<0.001
Sex, n. Female/tot (%)	32/48 (66.7)	13/22 (59.1)	10/18 (55.6)	3/4 (75.0)	0.597	0.408	0.616
Presence of other tumors, n./tot (%)	14/48 (29.2)	6/22 (27.3)	4/18 (22.2)	2/4 (50.0)	1.000	0.759	0.292
Positive family history, n./tot (%)	1/48 (2.1)	15/22 (68.2)	13/18 (72.2)	2/4 (50.0)	<0.001	<0.001	0.565
Stage, n. T > 1/tot[a] (%)	8/22 (36.4)	3/7 (42.9)	2/6 (33.3)	1/1 (100.0)	1.000	1.000	0.429

[a] Information on stage was available for 29 patients.

2.3. Families with Unclassified Variants

Twelve individuals were carriers of variants for which the associated risk has not been clearly established. Overall, five VUS were found: one in multiple individuals from a single family, while the others were identified in individual subjects. Details on the variants are shown in Table 3.

Table 3. Frequency and predictions of unclassified variants identified.

Nucleotide Variant	Aminoacidic Change	Allele Frequency [a]	Mean Conservation Score [b]	Clinvar Class	Varsome Class (Computational Verdicts)	N. Carriers (n. Affected by MTC)
c.2711C > T	p.Ser904Phe	NP	5.5799	LP	LP (10 D vs. 1 B)	8 (5)
c.2372A > T	p.Tyr791Phe	0.00209	5.34	CI	LB (8 D vs. 3 B)	1 (1)
c.2129A > G	p.Lys710Arg	0.00000816	3.72	US	US (8 D vs. 3 B)	1 (0)
c.1946C > T	p.Ser649Leu	0.0003164	4.34	CI	LP (11 D vs. 0 B)	1 (1)
c.1893_1898del CGAGCT	p.Asp631_Leu 633delinsGlu	NP	1.2967	NP	LP (1 D vs. 0 B)	1 (1)

[a] From gnomAD exomes; [b] From GERP (Genomic Evolutionary Rate Profiling http://mendel.stanford.edu/SidowLab/downloads/gerp/). Abbreviations: P = pathogenic; LP = likely pathogenic; NP = not present; D = deleterious; B = benign; LB = likely benign; CI = conflicting interpretations; US = uncertain significance.

The p.Ser904Phe variant was found in a family with several members affected by MTC (Figure 1): eight individuals were tested and found to carry the variant, while two other relatives were obligate carriers. Out of 10 carriers, seven developed slowly progressing MTC at an average age of 46.3 years and none manifested other *RET*-related problems. p.Ser904Phe is a rare variant previously reported in one family with father and son affected by adult-onset MTC [25]; therefore, the associated risk is still unclear. Cosci et al. [26], through in silico and in vitro analyses, showed that the variant has relatively high transforming activity but low aggressiveness and suggested to assign the variant to the lowest ATA risk level A. Consistently, the segregation of the variant in our family and the clinical history of carriers showed that, although highly penetrant, this variant causes late-onset, slowly progressing MTC, leading us to hypothesize that the screening recommended for carriers of lowest-risk mutations may be appropriate for healthy carriers of the p.Ser904Phe variant.

The p.Tyr791Phe variant was found in a patient with MTC diagnosed at 22 years of age and a negative family history for endocrine diseases. The variant, first reported in patients with Hirschsprung disease [27], MTC [28,29] and PCC [30], involves a highly conserved amino acid and used to be regarded as pathogenic based on in silico predictions. More recently, the evidence that the variant has similar frequencies in affected and unaffected subjects [31,32] is more common in the population than expected for a disease-causing variant [33,34], fails to co-segregate with the disease in some families [35,36] and co-occurred with a pathogenic variant in some patients [37,38] led researchers to reconsider it as likely benign. In our patient, however, the young age at MTC diagnosis raises the suspicion that this variant may have, to some extent, favored the development of MTC, possibly interacting with other factors in a multifactorial context, or that she carries a pathogenic variant undetected by the multigene test performed.

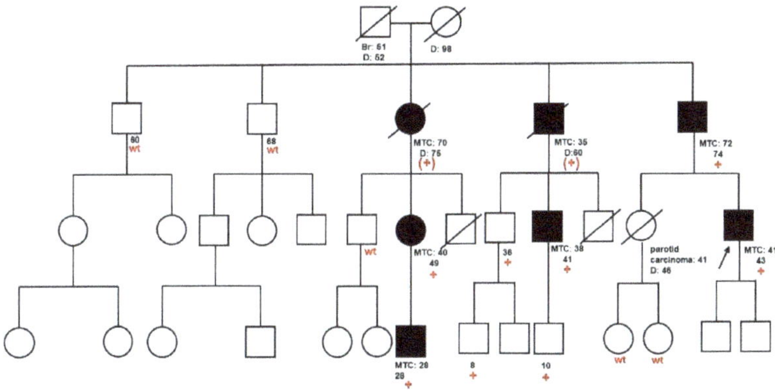

Figure 1. Family tree of family 91-O-03. We report the age at diagnosis of MTC and the age at death or at the last follow-up of patients evaluated at our clinic and/or who developed MTC; in red, we indicate the result of *RET* analysis ("+" = carrier of p.Ser904Phe variant; "(+)" = obligate carrier of the variant; "wt" = testing negative).

The p.Lys710Arg variant was found in a single 76-year-old patient who had PHPT and elevated serum calcitonin, who underwent a multigene analysis for hyperparathyroidism. This variant, very rare in population databases, has never been reported in patients affected by conditions known to be *RET*-related. The lysine residue substituted by arginine at codon 710 of the protein is highly conserved, but there is a small physicochemical difference between the two amino acids; consequently, computational predictors give conflicting results on the potential impact of this missense change, which is currently classified as of uncertain significance. As the clinical picture of our patient is not strongly suggestive of a *RET*-related condition, it is likely that this variant did not play a significant role in his disorder.

The p.Ser649Leu variant was found in a patient with MTC diagnosed at 59 years of age and a negative family history for endocrine diseases who also carried the common p.Val804Met variant, belonging to the MOD risk level. Her unaffected daughter was found to carry only the p.Val804Met variant, demonstrating that the two variants are "in trans" in the proband. The variant is rare in population databases and multiple lines of computational evidence reported by Varsome support its deleterious effect on the gene or gene product, but conflicting interpretations regarding its pathogenicity are present in the literature [36,39]. The evidence that, in our patient, the p.Ser649Leu variant is present "in trans" with a known pathogenic variant is against its pathogenicity, although an additive effect in combination with p.Val804Met cannot be excluded.

The p.Asp631_Leu633delinsGlu (c.1893_1898delCGAGCT) variant causes an in-frame deletion of two amino acids; the nomenclature reflects the fact that the deletion starts at the third base of the Asp631 codon and extends through Glu632 up to the second base of Leu633, resulting in deletion of Glu632 and Leu633 and a change of the Asp631 codon into glutamic acid. The deletion was identified in a female child with neonatal onset of abdominal distension, constipation and vomiting, with subsequent growth retardation, who was diagnosed with abdominal-pelvic plexiform ganglioneuroma when she was 2 years old. This patient also displayed lesions consistent with neurofibromas at the buttocks, mild dysmorphic features and nodules at the upper lip and was diagnosed with MTC and parathyroid adenoma when she was 7 years old. This clinical picture, resembling the MEN2B phenotype, led us to perform *RET* testing. The p.Asp631_Leu633delinsGlu variant is not reported in population databases, or in the medical literature; therefore, its clinical impact was completely unknown. Segregation analysis undertaken in the family demonstrated that it occurred "de novo", supporting its pathogenicity. Generally, *RET* defects associated with MEN2 and FMTC are typically gain of function, while deletions of part of the gene are mostly expected to cause loss of function; however, cases of *RET* deletions associated with MEN2 have been reported [40]. Moreover, Borganzone et al. studied a similar somatic alteration of *RET*, p.Glu632_Leu633del (c.1894_1899delGAGCTG), and demonstrated that this in-frame deletion reduces the spacing between two Cysteine residues, causing ligand-independent constitutive dimerization and activation of RET. Remarkably, RET activation was even greater in this case compared to activation induced by the frequent mutation p.Cys634Arg [41,42]. Although in our variant the deletion is shifted by 1 bp compared to the somatic mutation described by Borganzone et al., it results in the deletion of two amino acids in the same location; thus, the final effect—that is, the constitutive activation of RET signaling—is likely to be the same. Collectively taken, the "de novo" origin in our patient, her clinical phenotype and the functional data support the hypothesis that the p.Asp631_Leu633delinsGlu variant is causative of MEN2B and should be assigned to the HST/H risk class.

3. Discussion

Since the important role of *RET* alterations in the pathogenesis of MTC has been ascertained, it is considered appropriate to perform the analysis of this gene in all individuals diagnosed with primary CCH, MTC or MEN2, either sporadic or familial [3]. The identification of positive subjects is in fact important for the management of patients and especially of their healthy relatives, who could benefit from specific surveillance programs and/or prophylactic treatments [43,44]. The aim of this study was to critically analyze our experience with *RET* testing.

Among the 72 individuals affected by MTC or CCH who underwent *RET* analysis at our laboratory between 2002 and 2020, 23 (31.9%) were found to carry a germline *RET* variant. As expected, a positive family history increased the chance of finding a variant: out of 16 subjects who had positive family history, 15 had a detectable *RET* variant. In the only familial case where the analysis was negative (subject 51), the patient had been treated at 32 years of age for primary CCH and her father had died at 43 years of age for MTC; given the strong suspicion of an underlying genetic cause, a second-level analysis was performed using the NGS multi-gene panel for endocrine tumors, but no variants were found. Despite the negative test results, the early age of onset and the family history are suspicious for an undetected MTC-predisposing gene defect.

Germline *RET* variants were identified in eight of 56 subjects with apparently sporadic MTC (14.3%, slightly higher than the 4–10% reported in the literature [26,45–47]), confirming the importance of screening *RET* in all cases of MTC, even when the family history is negative [48]. Indeed, testing allowed us to reclassify as hereditary a fraction of apparently sporadic cases and led us to extend genetic testing to 18 relatives, eight of whom (44.4%), belonging to three distinct families, were found to carry the variant (p.Val804Met in all cases) and were therefore able to benefit from specific surveillance.

Among patients with CCH, 1/3 (33.3%) carried a *RET* variant (of MOD risk level); actually, she was an asymptomatic patient who was found to have inherited the familial variant and subsequently undertook the surveillance program that led to the diagnosis of CCH. On one hand, this may have represented a successful instance of early diagnosis, provided that CCH is a precursor condition for MTC; on the other hand, we cannot be sure that this benign finding would eventually evolve into a malignant condition and this may have been, conversely, a case of overdiagnosis and overtreatment.

Taking into account clinical features and genetic test results shows that wild-type *RET* patients and carriers of MOD risk level variants only differ by family history ($p < 0.001$), but not by clinical characteristics such as mean age at diagnosis of MTC and cancer stage. This is also supported by the fact that among 40 individuals found to carry variants assigned to MOD risk level or the p.Ser904Phe variant (excluding those for whom we have no clinical information), 22 had not developed primary CCH or MTC at the time of the last follow-up (55.0%): 4/9 of those over 60 years of age (44.4%), 8/18 of those between 40 and 60 years of age (44.4%), 8/11 of those between 20 and 40 years of age (72.7%) and 2/2 of those under 20 years of age (100.0%). Several lines of evidence have suggested that the aggressiveness of MTC does not depend on the presence, absence or type of *RET* variant (which mainly affects the age at onset of the disease) but on the stage and the age at diagnosis of the disease [20], which are the strongest predictors of survival for patients with MTC; therefore, our data further support the appropriateness of the non-invasive screening recommended by current guidelines for healthy carriers of MOD risk level variants.

For carriers of variants with unclear associated risk, however, until the genotype–phenotype correlations are clarified, the attempt to assess the risk and respective proper management of healthy carriers only relies on the clinical history of carriers—which, however, can provide meaningful information only when large families with many characterized members are available—or on any significant biomolecular evidence.

Thus, in the 91-O-03 family, the availability of several genetically and clinically characterized members allowed us to provide evidence that the p.Ser904Phe variant is highly penetrant (7/10 of carriers developed MTC, 70%) but leads to the development of slowly-progressing MTC at relatively advanced age (average age at diagnosis: 46.3 years), suggesting that recommended screening for carriers of lower risk mutations is appropriate for healthy carriers of this variant.

Moreover, in the case of the p.Asp631_Leu633delinsGlu variant, the clinical picture of the patient and the "de novo" origin, associated with the functional studies on a very similar variant [41,42], provide convincing evidence in favor of the pathogenicity of p.Asp631_Leu633delinsGlu and of its assignment to the HST/H risk level category. Of note, clinical manifestations in this patient were consistent with MEN2B, a phenotype that has been reported to be associated in 95% of cases with the p.Met918Thr variant and in 2–3% of cases with the p.Ala883Phe variant [49]. Both these variants affect residues located in the substrate specificity pocket of the central catalytic core of the tyrosine kinase domain and likely cause RET activation by altering its substrate specificity [50]. Conversely, p.Asp631_Leu633delinsGlu affects residues located at a great distance in a different domain (the cysteine-rich extracellular domain). Mutations in this domain are expected to cause RET activation by inducing its disulfide-linked dimerization and are generally associated with a MEN2A/FMTC phenotype, which gives a new perspective in the view of elucidating molecular mechanisms leading to the more severe MEN2B phenotype. Rarely, a MEN2B-like phenotype has been described in patients carrying two *RET* variants (bi-allelic or *in-cis* on the same allele) [51,52]. It can be hypothesized that, although different, all these defects result in a particularly intense RET activation and that the higher the activation level, the more severe is the phenotype.

Among the families with MOD risk level variants, the case of the 228-O-18 family, carrying the p.Leu790Phe variant, is worthy of consideration. In this family, the p.Leu790Phe variant was found in nine individuals, four of whom developed MTC; intriguingly, three of these individuals were also affected by neurofibromatosis 1 (NF1), caused by a mutation of the *NF1* gene inherited from the other parental branch, and one developed a PCC. The p.Leu790Phe variant is classified at the lowest risk level and is generally associated exclusively with MTC [53]; it is therefore possible that, in this individual, the risk of developing a PCC was greater than that of the ordinary carriers of this variant, due to the co-presence of the mutation of *NF1*, another gene whose alterations are associated with an increased risk of developing PCC.

One limitation of this study is that most patients underwent the analysis of selected *RET* exons through Sanger sequencing, which is expected to be less sensitive if compared to whole-gene NGS-based analysis. However, since all the variants identified were found using the Sanger method, and the percentage of individuals is in line with data previously reported in the literature (even slightly higher for sporadic cases), we can conclude that this testing approach demonstrated satisfactory accuracy in finding *RET* variants, supporting the evidence that most clinically relevant variants reside in known mutational hotspots [54].

4. Materials and Methods

4.1. Patients

From 2002 to 2020, in our laboratory, *RET* molecular analysis was performed in a total of 163 subjects, 102 of which underwent a complete gene analysis, while in the other 61, the targeted search for a family mutation was performed. In total, 120 of these subjects had participated in genetic counseling at our Cancer Genetics Clinic in Bologna based on personal history of a possible *RET*-related condition or identification of a *RET* mutation in the family; after verifying the presence of criteria for *RET* testing, informed consent was collected and a venous blood sample was drawn. For the other 43 subjects, blood sample was sent to our laboratory by external centers with the request for *RET* analysis, after informed consent had been collected by the requesting physician.

4.2. Clinical Data

The phenotype leading to the suspicion of a *RET* variant in the family, and therefore the reason for *RET* analysis, was known for 140 of the 163 analyzed subjects. Of these, main clinical information regarding families with MTC, including disease status, age at diagnosis and family history, was available for all the patients who came to our clinic for genetic counseling and for the other 15 subjects sent from external physicians. This and any other information, such as stage of MTC, survival status and presence of any further pathologies, was collected during genetic counseling and/or derived from medical records and pathology reports.

4.3. RET Analysis

Genomic DNA was isolated from peripheral blood-EDTA using the QIAmp DNA Blood Mini Kit according the manufacturer's protocol (Qiagen, Valencia, CA, USA).

From 2002 to June 2019, sequencing of exons 5, 8, 10, 11, 13, 14, 15 and 16 of *RET* (RefSeq.NM_020975.5) was performed through bidirectional Sanger sequencing: briefly, PCR amplifications of target exons were carried out with FastStartTaq DNA polymerase (Roche, Basel, Switzerland), followed by standard dideoxy sequencing, and run on a ABI3730 DNA analyzer (Applied Biosystems, Foster City, CA, USA). PCR and sequencing conditions, as well as the primer sequences, are available upon request. Chromatograms were analyzed for variants using the software Sequencer (Gene Code Corporation, Ann Arbor, MI, USA). According to the ARUP database as of January 2020 (https://arup.utah.edu/database/MEN2/MEN2_display.php) exons 5, 8, 10, 11, 13, 14, 15 and 16 cover all but one (Exon 7: c.1513_1518delGAGGGG: p.E505_G506del) of the *RET* mutations described in the literature.

Since July 2019, the entire RET cds (20 exons) has been included in an NGS panel (IAD177392-ThermoFisher Scientific) comprising 27 genes related to MEN2, pheochromocytoma and renal carcinoma and run on an Ion S5 next-generation sequencing system followed by analysis with the Ion Reporter Software (ThermoFisher Scientific, Waltham, MA, USA). The mean amplicon coverage and the target base coverage at > 100x for multiple experiments were > 800x and > 97%, respectively: these parameters guarantee a sensitivity of > 99% for the test. All the variants of interest were confirmed through Sanger sequencing.

Overall, 157 patients underwent Sanger sequencing analysis and 6 the NGS panel analysis.

4.4. Interpretation of Unclassified Variants

Rare/novel variants whose associated risk was unknown were evaluated through a review of the information available in the following public databases: gnomAD, ClinVar, varsome. In particular, for each variant, the classification in the mutational databases, the frequency in the population databases, the conservation of the substituted amino acids, the results of in silico predictions about the effect of the variant on the protein and the results of any functional assay were evaluated. All databases were last consulted on 15 September 2020. Moreover, reports about these variants possibly present in the literature were researched and evaluated. Finally, when possible, segregation of the variant in the family was assessed, in particular for variants classified as probably pathogenic and if/when other cases of MTC were present in the family.

4.5. Statistical Analysis

All available data were entered anonymously into a dedicated database and were analyzed by using the statistical package IBM-SPSS Statistics (Ver. 25 for Windows, IBM Co., Armonk, NY, USA). Means, standard deviation (SD), ranges and frequencies were used as descriptive statistics. The Fisher's exact test was used for dichotomous variables and the independent t-test to analyze differences between two group means. Two-tailed p values lower than 0.05 were considered statistically significant. For the analysis, carriers of the p.Ser904Phe variant were included in the MOD category and the carrier of p.Asp631_Leu633delinsGlu variant in the HST/H category. Carriers of the other VUS were excluded from the analysis.

5. Conclusions

The results of our study provide support to the recommendation that *RET* genetic screening should be performed in all MTC cases, regardless of the family history of patients and their clinical presentation, and according to the appropriateness of ATA's guidelines for clinical management of carriers of MOD risk level mutations. It is also highlighted that *RET* molecular analysis leads to the detection of a substantial proportion of variants associated with unknown risks, which poses serious challenges to the counselling and management of the patients and the family. However, co-segregation analysis in the family, genotype/phenotype analysis and a careful revision of the databases and literature proves helpful, at least in some of the cases, in order to tentatively assign the case to one of the known risk classes and inform management accordingly. This approach led us to provide evidence supporting the classification of p.Ser904Phe as the lowest risk level variant and of p.Asp631_Leu633delinsGlu as a novel variant responsible for MEN2B of HST/H risk level.

Supplementary Materials: The following are available online at http://www.mdpi.com/2072-6694/12/11/3268/s1, Table S1: Case series under study.

Author Contributions: Conceptualization: D.T. and G.I.; methodology: D.T., G.I., C.R., L.G.; patient identification and clinical characterization: A.R., D.B., D.M., M.E.C., U.P., A.P. (Antonio Percesepe), A.P. (Andrea Pession); data curation: M.R.; writing—original draft preparation: G.I., D.T.; writing—review and editing: C.R. All authors have read and agreed to the published version of the manuscript.

Funding: This research received no external funding.

Conflicts of Interest: The authors declare no conflict of interest.

References

1. Omur:, O.; Baran, Y. An update on molecular biology of thyroid cancers. *Crit. Rev. Oncol. Hematol.* **2014**, *90*, 233–252. [CrossRef] [PubMed]
2. Kondo, T.; Ezzat, S.; Asa, S.L. Pathogenetic mechanisms in thyroid follicular-cell neoplasia. *Nat. Rev. Cancer* **2006**, 6292–6306. [CrossRef] [PubMed]
3. Salehian, B.; Samoa, R. RET gene abnormalities and thyroid disease: Who should be screened and when. *J. Clin. Res. Pediatr. Endocrinol.* **2013**, *5* (Suppl. 1), 70–78. [CrossRef] [PubMed]
4. Yadav, M.; Agrawal, V.; Pani, K.C.; Verma, R.; Jaiswal, S.; Mishra, A.; Pandey, R. C-cell hyperplasia in sporadic and familial medullary thyroid carcinoma. *Indian J. Pathol. Microbiol.* **2018**, *61*, 485–488. [CrossRef] [PubMed]
5. Roman, S.; Lin, R.; Sosa, J.A. Prognosis of MTC: Demographic, clinical, and pathologic predictors of survival in 1252 cases. *Cancer* **2006**, *107*, 2134–2142. [CrossRef] [PubMed]
6. Figlioli, G.; Landi, S.; Romei, C.; Elisei, R.; Gemignani, F. MTC (MTC) and RET proto-oncogene: Mutation spectrum in the familial cases and a meta-analysis of studies on the sporadic form. *Mutat Res.* **2013**, *752*, 36–44. [CrossRef]

7. Raue, F.; Frank-Raue, K. Das medulläre Schilddrüsenkarzinom und die multiple endokrine Neoplasie Typ 2 [MTC and multiple endocrine neoplasia type 2]. *Dtsch Med. Wochenschr.* **2020**, *10*. [CrossRef]
8. Wohllk, N.; Schweizer, H.; Erlic, Z.; Schmid, K.W.; Walz, M.K.; Raue, F.; Neumann, H.P. Multiple endocrine neoplasia type 2. *Best Pr. Res. Clin. Endocrinol. Metab.* **2010**, *24*, 371–387. [CrossRef]
9. Moline, J.; Eng, C. Multiple endocrine neoplasia type 2: An overview. *Genet. Med.* **2011**, *13*, 755–764. [CrossRef]
10. Howe, J.R.; Norton, J.A.; Wells, S.A., Jr. Prevalence of pheochromocytoma and hyperparathyroidism in multiple endocrine neoplasia type 2A: Results of long-term follow-up. *Surgery* **1993**, *114*, 1070–1077.
11. Larsen, L.V.; Mirebeau-Prunier, D.; Imai, T.; Alvarez-Escola, C.; Hasse-Lazar, K.; Censi, S.; Castroneves, L.A.; Sakurai, A.; Kihara, M.; Horiuchi, K.; et al. Primary hyperparathyroidism as first manifestation in multiple endocrine neoplasia type 2A: An international multicenter study. *Endocr. Connect.* **2020**, *9*, 489–497. [CrossRef]
12. Brauckhoff, M.; Machens, A.; Hess, S.; Lorenz, K.; Gimm, O.; Brauckhoff, K.; Sekulla, C.; Dralle, H. Premonitory symptoms preceding metastatic medullary thyroid cancer in MEN 2B: An exploratory analysis. *Surgery* **2008**, *144*, 1044–1053. [CrossRef]
13. Donis-Keller, H.; Dou, S.; Chi, D.; Carlson, K.M.; Toshima, K.; Lairmore, T.C.; Howe, J.R.; Moley, J.F.; Goodfellow, P.; Wells, S.A., Jr. Mutations in the RET proto-oncogene are associated with MEN 2A and FMTC. *Hum. Mol. Genet.* **1993**, *2*, 851–856. [CrossRef] [PubMed]
14. Mulligan, L.M.; Kwok, J.B.; Healey, C.S.; Elsdon, M.J.; Eng, C.; Gardner, E.; Love, D.R.; Mole, S.E.; Moore, J.K.; Papi, L.; et al. Germ-line mutations of the RET proto-oncogene in multiple endocrine neoplasia type 2A. *Nature* **1993**, *363*, 458–460. [CrossRef] [PubMed]
15. Mulligan, L.M. RET revisited: Expanding the oncogenic portfolio. *Nat. Rev. Cancer* **2014**, *14*, 173–186. [CrossRef]
16. Eng, C.; Clayton, D.; Schuffenecker, I.; Lenoir, G.; Cote, G.; Gagel, R.F.; van Amstel, H.K.; Lips, C.J.; Nishisho, I.; Takai, S.I.; et al. The relationship between specific RET proto-oncogene mutations and disease phenotype in multiple endocrine neoplasia type 2. International RET mutation consortium analysis. *JAMA* **1996**, *276*, 1575–1579. [CrossRef]
17. Yip, L.; Cote, G.J.; Shapiro, S.E.; Ayers, G.D.; Herzog, C.E.; Sellin, R.V.; Sherman, S.I.; Gagel, R.F.; Lee, J.E.; Evans, D.B. Multiple endocrine neoplasia type 2: Evaluation of the genotype-phenotype relationship. *Arch. Surg.* **2003**, *138*, 409–416. [CrossRef]
18. Hedayati, M.; Zarif Yeganeh, M.; Sheikholeslami, S.; Afsari, F. Diversity of mutations in the RET proto-oncogene and its oncogenic mechanism in medullary thyroid cancer. *Crit. Rev. Clin. Lab. Sci.* **2016**, *53*, 217–227. [CrossRef]
19. Raue, F.; Frank-Raue, K. Update on Multiple Endocrine Neoplasia Type 2: Focus on MTC. *J. Endocr. Soc.* **2018**, *2*, 933–943. [CrossRef]
20. Voss, R.K.; Feng, L.; Lee, J.E.; Perrier, N.D.; Graham, P.H.; Hyde, S.M.; Nieves-Munoz, F.; Cabanillas, M.E.; Waguespack, S.G.; Cote, G.J.; et al. MTC in MEN2A: ATA Moderate- or High-Risk RET Mutations Do Not Predict Disease Aggressiveness. *J. Clin. Endocrinol. Metab.* **2017**, *102*, 2807–2813. [CrossRef]
21. Kloos, R.T.; Eng, C.; Evans, D.B.; Francis, G.L.; Gagel, R.F.; Gharib, H.; Moley, J.F.; Pacini, F.; Ringel, M.D.; Schlumberger, M.; et al. Medullary thyroid cancer: Management guidelines of the American Thyroid Association. *Thyroid* **2009**, *19*, 565–612. [CrossRef] [PubMed]
22. Wells, S.A., Jr.; Asa, S.L.; Dralle, H.; Elisei, R.; Evans, D.B.; Gagel, R.F.; Lee, N.; Machens, A.; Moley, J.F.; Pacini, F.; et al. Revised American Thyroid Association guidelines for the management of MTC. *Thyroid* **2015**, *25*, 567–610. [CrossRef] [PubMed]
23. Haugen, B.R.; Alexander, E.K.; Bible, K.C.; Doherty, G.M.; Mandel, S.J.; Nikiforov, Y.E.; Pacini, F.; Randolph, G.W.; Sawka, A.M.; Schlumberger, M.; et al. 2015 American Thyroid Association Management Guidelines for Adult Patients with Thyroid Nodules and Differentiated Thyroid Cancer: The American Thyroid Association Guidelines Task Force on Thyroid Nodules and Differentiated Thyroid Cancer. *Thyroid* **2016**, *26*, 1–133. [CrossRef] [PubMed]
24. Machens, A.; Lorenz, K.; Weber, F.; Dralle, H. Genotype-specific progression of hereditary medullary thyroid cancer. *Hum. Mutat.* **2018**, *39*, 860–869. [CrossRef]

25. Elisei, R.; Tacito, A.; Ramone, T.; Ciampi, R.; Bottici, V.; Cappagli, V.; Viola, D.; Matrone, A.; Lorusso, L.; Valerio, L.; et al. Twenty-Five Years Experience on RET Genetic Screening on Hereditary MTC: An Update on The Prevalence of Germline RET Mutations. *Genes* **2019**, *10*, 698. [CrossRef]
26. Cosci, B.; Vivaldi, A.; Romei, C.; Gemignani, F.; Landi, S.; Ciampi, R.; Tacito, A.; Molinaro, E.; Agate, L.; Bottici, V.; et al. In silico and in vitro analysis of rare germline allelic variants of RET oncogene associated with medullary thyroid cancer. *Endocr. Relat. Cancer* **2011**, *18*, 603–612. [CrossRef]
27. Seri, M.; Yin, L.; Barone, V.; Bolino, A.; Celli, I.; Bocciardi, R.; Pasini, B.; Ceccherini, I.; Lerone, M.; Kristoffersson, U.; et al. Frequency of RET mutations in long- and short-segment Hirschsprung disease. *Hum. Mutat.* **1997**, *9*, 243–249. [CrossRef]
28. Berndt, I.; Reuter, M.; Saller, B.; Frank-Raue, K.; Growth, P.; Grussendorf, M.; Raue, F.; Ritter, M.M.; Höppner, W. A new hot spot for mutations in the ret protooncogene causing familial MTC and multiple endocrine neoplasia type 2A. *J. Clin. Endocrinol. Metab.* **1998**, *83*, 770–774. [CrossRef]
29. Tamanaha, R.; Camacho, C.P.; Ikejiri, E.S.; Maciel, R.M.; Cerutti, J.M. Y791F RET mutation and early onset of MTC in a Brazilian kindred: Evaluation of phenotype-modifying effect of germline variants. *Clin. Endocrinol.* **2007**, *67*, 806–808. [CrossRef]
30. Neumann, H.P.; Bausch, B.; McWhinney, S.R.; Bender, B.U.; Gimm, O.; Franke, G.; Schipper, J.; Klisch, J.; Altehoefer, C.; Zerres, K.; et al. Germ-line mutations in nonsyndromic pheochromocytoma. *N. Engl. J. Med.* **2002**, *346*, 1459–1466. [CrossRef]
31. Vierhapper, H.; Bieglmayer, C.; Heinze, G.; Baumgartner-Parzer, S. Frequency of RET proto-oncogene mutations in patients with normal and with moderately elevated pentagastrin-stimulated serum concentrations of calcitonin. *Thyroid* **2004**, *14*, 580–583. [CrossRef]
32. Toledo, R.A.; Loureço, D.M., Jr.; Camacho, C.; Lindsey, S.; Cerutti, J.; Maciel, R.M.; Toledo, S.P. RET Y791F: Alone or accompanied? *Arch. Endocrinol. Metab.* **2015**, *59*, 476–477. [CrossRef] [PubMed]
33. Amendola, L.M.; Dorschner, M.O.; Robertson, P.D.; Salama, J.S.; Hart, R.; Shirts, B.H.; Murray, M.L.; Tokita, M.J.; Gallego, C.J.; Kim, D.S.; et al. Actionable exomic incidental findings in 6503 participants: Challenges of variant classification. *Genome Res.* **2015**, *25*, 305–315. [CrossRef]
34. Toledo, R.A.; Hatakana, R.; Lourenço, D.M., Jr.; Lindsey, S.C.; Camacho, C.P.; Almeida, M.; Lima, J.V., Jr.; Sekiya, T.; Garralda, E.; Naslavsky, M.S.; et al. Comprehensive assessment of the disputed RET Y791F variant shows no association with MTC susceptibility. *Endocr. Relat. Cancer* **2015**, *22*, 65–76. [CrossRef]
35. Vestergaard, P.; Vestergaard, E.M.; Brockstedt, H.; Christiansen, P. Codon Y791F mutations in a large kindred: Is prophylactic thyroidectomy always indicated? *World J. Surg.* **2007**, *31*, 996–1004. [CrossRef]
36. Erlic, Z.; Hoffmann, M.M.; Sullivan, M.; Franke, G.; Peczkowska, M.; Harsch, I.; Schott, M.; Gabbert, H.E.; Valimäki, M.; Preuss, S.F.; et al. Pathogenicity of DNA variants and double mutations in multiple endocrine neoplasia type 2 and von Hippel-Lindau syndrome. *J. Clin. Endocrinol. Metab.* **2010**, *95*, 308–313. [CrossRef]
37. Toledo, R.A.; Wagner, S.M.; Coutinho, F.L.; Lourenço, D.M., Jr.; Azevedo, J.A.; Longuini, V.C.; Reis, M.T.; Siqueira, S.A.; Lucon, A.M.; Tavares, M.R.; et al. High penetrance of pheochromocytoma associated with the novel C634Y/Y791F double germline mutation in the RET protooncogene. *J. Clin. Endocrinol. Metab.* **2010**, *95*, 1318–1327. [CrossRef]
38. Pęczkowska, M.; Kowalska, A.; Sygut, J.; Waligórski, D.; Malinoc, A.; Janaszek-Sitkowska, H.; Prejbisz, A.; Januszewicz, A.; Neumann, H.P. Testing new susceptibility genes in the cohort of apparently sporadic phaeochromocytoma/paraganglioma patients with clinical characteristics of hereditary syndromes. *Clin. Endocrinol.* **2013**, *79*, 817–823. [CrossRef] [PubMed]
39. Colombo-Benkmann, M.; Li, Z.; Riemann, B.; Hengst, K.; Herbst, H.; Keuser, R.; Gross, U.; Rondot, S.; Raue, F.; Senninger, N.; et al. Characterization of the RET protooncogene transmembrane domain mutation S649L associated with nonaggressive medullary thyroid carcinoma. *Eur. J. Endocrinol.* **2008**, *158*, 811–816. [CrossRef]
40. Latteyer, S.; Klein-Hitpass, L.; Khandanpour, C.; Zwanziger, D.; Poeppel, T.D.; Schmid, K.W.; Führer, D.; Moeller, L.C. A 6-Base Pair in Frame Germline Deletion in Exon 7 of RET Leads to Increased RET Phosphorylation, ERK Activation, and MEN2A. *J. Clin. Endocrinol. Metab.* **2016**, *101*, 1016–1022. [CrossRef] [PubMed]
41. Bongarzone, I.; Vigano, E.; Alberti, L., Mondellini, P.; Uggeri, M.; Pasini, B.; Borrello, M.G.; Pierotti, M.A. The Glu632-Leu633 deletion in cysteine rich domain of Ret induces constitutive dimerization and alters the processing of the receptor protein. *Oncogene* **1999**, *18*, 4833–4838. [CrossRef]

42. Ceccherini, I.; Pasini, B.; Pacini, F.; Gullo, M.; Bongarzone, I.; Romei, C.; Santamaria, G.; Matera, I.; Mondellini, P.; Scopsi, L.; et al. Somatic in frame deletions not involving juxtamembranous cysteine residues strongly activate the RET proto-oncogene. *Oncogene* **1997**, *14*, 2609–2612. [CrossRef]
43. Mulligan, L.M. 65 YEARS OF THE DOUBLE HELIX: Exploiting insights on the RET receptor for personalized cancer medicine. *Endocr. Relat. Cancer* **2018**, *25*, T189–T200. [CrossRef] [PubMed]
44. Krampitz, G.W.; Norton, J.A. RET gene mutations (genotype and phenotype) of multiple endocrine neoplasia type 2 and familial MTC. *Cancer* **2014**, *120*, 1920–1931. [CrossRef]
45. Elisei, R.; Romei, C.; Cosci, B.; Agate, L.; Bottici, V.; Molinaro, E.; Sculli, M.; Miccoli, P.; Basolo, F.; Grasso, L.; et al. RET genetic screening in patients with medullary thyroid cancer and their relatives: Experience with 807 individuals at one center. *J. Clin. Endocrinol. Metab.* **2007**, *92*, 4725–4729. [CrossRef]
46. Bugalho, M.J.; Domingues, R.; Santos, J.R.; Catarino, A.L.; Sobrinho, L. Mutation analysis of the RET proto-oncogene and early thyroidectomy: Results of a Portuguese cancer centre. *Surgery* **2007**, *141*, 90–95. [CrossRef]
47. Wiench, M.; Wygoda, Z.; Gubala, E.; Wloch, J.; Lisowska, K.; Krassowski, J.; Scieglinska, D.; Fiszer-Kierzkowska, A.; Lange, D.; Kula, D.; et al. Estimation of risk of inherited medullary thyroid carcinoma in apparent sporadic patients. *J. Clin. Oncol.* **2001**, *19*, 1374–1380. [CrossRef]
48. Romei, C.; Cosci, B.; Renzini, G.; Bottici, V.; Molinaro, E.; Agate, L.; Passannanti, P.; Viola, D.; Biagini, A.; Basolo, F.; et al. RET genetic screening of sporadic medullary thyroid cancer (MTC) allows the preclinical diagnosis of unsuspected gene carriers and the identification of a relevant percentage of hidden familial MTC (FMTC). *Clin. Endocrinol.* **2011**, *74*, 241–247. [CrossRef]
49. Mulligan, L.M.; Marsh, D.J.; Robinson, B.G.; Schuffenecker, I.; Zedenius, J.; Lips, C.J.; Gagel, R.F.; Takai, S.I.; Noll, W.W.; Fink, M.; et al. Genotype-phenotype correlation in multiple endocrine neoplasia type 2: Report of the International RET Mutation Consortium. *J. Intern. Med.* **1995**, *238*, 343–346. [CrossRef] [PubMed]
50. Gimm, O.; Marsh, D.J.; Andrew, S.D.; Frilling, A.; Dahia, P.L.; Mulligan, L.M.; Zajac, J.D.; Robinson, B.G.; Eng, C. Germline dinucleotide mutation in codon 883 of the RET proto-oncogene in multiple endocrine neoplasia type 2B without codon 918 mutation. *J. Clin. Endocrinol. Metab.* **1997**, *82*, 3902–3904. [CrossRef]
51. Iwashita, T.; Murakami, H.; Kurokawa, K.; Kawai, K.; Miyauchi, A.; Futami, H.; Qiao, S.; Ichihara, M.; Takahashi, M. A two-hit model for development of multiple endocrine neoplasia type 2B by RET mutations. *Biochem. Biophys. Res. Commun.* **2000**, *268*, 804–808. [CrossRef]
52. Miyauchi, A.; Futami, H.; Hai, N.; Yokozawa, T.; Kuma, K.; Aoki, N.; Kosugi, S.; Sugano, K.; Yamaguchi, K. Two germline missense mutations at codons 804 and 806 of the RET proto-oncogene in the same allele in a patient with multiple endocrine neoplasia type 2B without codon 918 mutation. *Jpn. J. Cancer Res.* **1999**, *90*, 1–5. [CrossRef] [PubMed]
53. Bihan, H.; Murat, A.; Fysekidis, M.; Al-Salameh, A.; Schwartz, C.; Baudin, E.; Thieblot, P.; Borson-Chazot, F.; Guillausseau, P.J.; Cardot-Bauters, C.; et al. The clinical spectrum of RET proto-oncogene mutations in codon 790. *Eur. J. Endocrinol.* **2013**, *169*, 271–276. [CrossRef]
54. Margraf, R.L.; Crockett, D.K.; Krautscheid, P.M.; Seamons, R.; Calderon, F.R.; Wittwer, C.T.; Mao, R. Multiple endocrine neoplasia type 2 RET protooncogene database: Repository of MEN2-associated RET sequence variation and reference for genotype/phenotype correlations. *Hum. Mutat.* **2009**, *30*, 548–556. [CrossRef]

MDPI
St. Alban-Anlage 66
4052 Basel
Switzerland
Tel. +41 61 683 77 34
Fax +41 61 302 89 18
www.mdpi.com

Cancers Editorial Office
E-mail: cancers@mdpi.com
www.mdpi.com/journal/cancers

www.ingramcontent.com/pod-product-compliance
Ingram Content Group UK Ltd.
Pitfield, Milton Keynes, MK11 3LW, UK
UKHW060123010826
14089UKWH00006B/120

9 783036 553344